Theoretical Basis FOR NURSING

5TH EDITION

Theoretical Basis FOR NURSING

5TH EDITION

Melanie McEwen, PhD, RN, CNE, ANEF

Professor
University of Texas Health Science Center at Houston
School of Nursing
Houston, Texas

Evelyn M. Wills, PhD, RN

Professor (Retired)
Department of Nursing
College of Nursing & Allied Health Professions
University of Louisiana at Lafayette
Lafayette, Louisiana

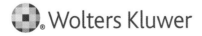 Wolters Kluwer

Philadelphia • Baltimore • New York • London
Buenos Aires • Hong Kong • Sydney • Tokyo

Acquisitions Editor: Christina Burns
Development Editor: Michael Kerns
Editorial Coordinator: Tim Rinehart
Editorial Assistant: Kaitlin Campbell
Production Project Manager: Kim Cox
Design Coordinator: Elaine Kasmer
Illustration Coordinator: Jennifer Clements
Manufacturing Coordinator: Karin Duffield
Prepress Vendor: Absolute Service, Inc.

Fifth Edition

Library of Congress Cataloging-in-Publication Data

Names: McEwen, Melanie, author. | Wills, Evelyn M., author.
Title: Theoretical basis for nursing / Melanie McEwen, Evelyn M. Wills.
Description: Fifth edition. | Philadelphia : Wolters Kluwer, [2018] |
   Includes bibliographical references and index.
Identifiers: LCCN 2017049174 | ISBN 9781496351203
Subjects: | MESH: Nursing Theory
Classification: LCC RT84.5 | NLM WY 86 | DDC 610.73—dc23 LC record available at
https://lccn.loc.gov/2017049174

RRS1712

To Kaitlin and Grant—You have helped me broaden my thoughts and consider all kinds of possibilities; I hope I've done the same for you.

Also for Helen and Keith—Our children chose well. Besides, you have given us Madelyn, Logan, Brenna, Liam, Lucy, Andrew, Michael, and Jacob; they are gifts beyond words.

Melanie McEwen

To Tom, Paul, and Vicki, who light up my life, and to Marian, who left us for a better place. You were always my best listener. To Teddy, Gwen, Merlyn, and Madelyn, who have been so patient and loving during this process.

My deepest gratitude to Leslie, who has supported me through this writing process.

Evelyn M. Wills

CONTRIBUTORS

Sattaria Smith Dilks, DNP, APRN-BC, FNP, PMHNP/CNS
Professor and Co-Coordinator Graduate Program
College of Nursing
McNeese State University
Lake Charles, Louisiana
Chapter 14: Theories From the Behavioral Sciences

Joan C. Engebretson, DrPH, AHN-BC, RN, FAAN
Judy Fred Professor in Nursing
University of Texas Health Science Center at Houston
School of Nursing, Department of Family Nursing
Houston, Texas
Chapter 13: Theories From the Sociologic Sciences

Melinda Granger Oberleitner, DNS, RN
Associate Dean, College of Nursing & Allied Health Professions
Professor, Department of Nursing
SLEMCO/BORSF Endowed Professor of Nursing
University of Louisiana at Lafayette
Lafayette, Louisiana
Chapter 17: Theories, Models, and Frameworks From Leadership and Management
Chapter 21: Application of Theory in Nursing Administration and Management

Cathy L. Rozmus, PhD, RN
PARTNERS Endowed Professorship in Nursing
Vice Dean
Department of Family Health
The University of Texas Health Science Center at Houston
School of Nursing
Houston, Texas
Chapter 16: Ethical Theories and Principles

Jeffrey P. Spike, PhD
Professor of Family and Community Medicine
The University of Texas Health Science Center at Houston
School of Medicine
Professor, Department of Management, Policy, and Community Health
University of Texas Health Science Center School of Public Health
Houston, Texas
Chapter 16: Ethical Theories and Principles

REVIEWERS

Cynthia Dakin, PhD, RN
Director of Graduate Studies
Associate Professor
Department of Nursing
Elms College
Chicopee, Massachusetts

Janet DuPont, RNC-OB, MSN, MEd, PhD
Master of Science in Nursing Instructor/Developer
Nursing Program
Norwich University
Northfield, Vermont

Ruth Neese, PhD, RN, CEN
Assistant Professor
Department of Nursing
Indian River State College
Fort Pierce, Florida

Brandon N. Respress, PhD, RN, MPH, MSN
Assistant Professor
College of Nursing and Health Innovation
University of Texas at Arlington
Arlington, Texas

Jacqueline Saleeby, PhD, RN, CS
Associate Professor
Department of Nursing
Maryville University
St. Louis, Missouri

Stephen J. Stapleton, PhD, MS, RN, CEN, FAEN
Associate Professor
Mennonite College of Nursing
Illinois State University
Normal, Illinois

Kathleen Williamson, MSN, PhD, RN
Associate Professor and Chair
Wilson School of Nursing
Midwestern State University
Wichita Falls, Texas

Cindy Zellefrow, DNP, MSEd, RN, LSN, APHN-BC
Assistant Professor of Clinical Practice
Assistant Director, Center for Transdisciplinary and
Evidence-based Practice
College of Nursing
The Ohio State University
Columbus, Ohio

PREFACE

Rare is the student who enrolls in a nursing program and is excited about the requirement of taking a course on theory. Indeed, many fail to see theory's relevance to the real world of nursing practice and often have difficulty applying the information in later courses and in their research. This book is the result of the frustration felt by a group of nursing instructors who met a number of years ago to adopt a textbook for a theory course. Indeed, because of student complaints and faculty dissatisfaction, we were changing textbooks yet again. A fairly lengthy discussion arose in which we concluded that the available books did not meet the needs of our students or course faculty. We were determined to write a book that was a general overview of theory per se, stressing how it is—and should be—used by nurses to improve practice, research, education, and management/leadership.

As in past editions, an ongoing review of trends in nursing theory and nursing science has shown an increasing emphasis on middle range theory, evidence-based practice (EBP), and situation-specific theories. To remain current and timely, in this fifth edition, we have added a new chapter entitled "Ethical Theories and Principles," presenting information on these topics and describing how they relate to theory in nursing. We have also included new middle range and situation-specific nursing theories as well as new "shared" theories from non-nursing disciplines. One notable addition is a significant section discussing Complexity Science and Complex Adaptive Systems in Chapter 13 (Theories From the Sociologic Sciences) helping to explain their importance to nursing. Updates and application examples have been added throughout the discussions on the various theories.

Organization of the Text

Theoretical Basis for Nursing is designed to be a basic nursing theory textbook that includes the essential information students need to understand and apply theory in practice, research, education, and administration/management.

The book is divided into four units. **Unit I, Introduction to Theory**, provides the background needed to understand what theory is and how it is used in nursing. It outlines tools and techniques used to develop, analyze, and evaluate theory so that it can be used in nursing practice, research, administration and management, and education. In this unit, we have provided a balanced view of "hot" topics (e.g., philosophical world views and utilization of shared or borrowed theory). Also, rather than espousing one strategy for activities such as concept development and theory evaluation, we have included a variety of strategies.

Unit II, Nursing Theories, focuses largely on the grand nursing theories and begins with a chapter describing their historical development. This unit divides the grand nursing theories into three groups based on their focus (human needs, interactive process, and unitary process). The works of many of the grand theorists are briefly summarized in Chapters 7, 8, and 9. Because this volume is intended to serve as a broad foundation, these analyses provide the reader with enough information to understand the basis of the work and to whet the reader's appetite to select one or more for further study rather than delving into significant detail.

Chapters 10 and 11 cover the significant topic of middle range nursing theory. Chapter 10 presents a detailed overview of the origins and growth of middle range theory in nursing and gives numerous examples of how middle range theories have been developed by nurses. Chapter 11 provides an overview of some of the growing number of middle range nursing theories. The theories presented include some of the most commonly used middle range nursing theories (e.g., Pender's Health Promotion Model and Leininger's Culture Care Diversity and Universality Theory) as well as some that are less well known but have a growing body of research support (e.g., Meleis's Transitions Theory, the Theory of Unpleasant Symptoms, and the Uncertainty in Illness Theory). The intent is to provide a broad range of middle range theories to familiarize the reader with examples and to encourage them to search for others appropriate to their practice or research. Ultimately, it is hoped that readers will be challenged to develop new theories that can be used by nurses.

Chapter 12, which discusses EBP, explains and defines the idea/process of EBP and describes how it relates to nursing theory and application of theory in nursing practice and research. The chapter concludes with a short presentation and review of five different EBP models that have been widely used by nurses and are well supported in the literature.

Unit III, Shared Theories Used by Nurses, is rather unique in nursing literature. Our book acknowledges that "shared" or "borrowed" theories are essential to nursing and negates the idea that the use of shared theory in practice or research is detrimental. In this unit, we have identified some of the most significant theories that have been developed outside of the discipline of nursing but are continually used in nursing. We have organized these theories based on broad disciplines: theories from the sociologic sciences, behavioral sciences, biomedical sciences, and philosophy as well as from administration, management, and learning. Each of these chapters was written by a nurse with both educational and practical experience in his or her respective area. These theories are presented with sufficient information to allow the reader to understand the theories and to recognize those that might be appropriate for his or her own work. These chapters also provide original references and give examples of how the concepts, theories, and models described have been used by other nurses.

Chapter 16, new to the fifth edition, describes ethical theories and principles that apply to nursing practice. This addition was suggested by nursing faculty who recognized the importance of maintaining an ethical perspective within the very complex health care system. This information is vital to professional nursing practice and absolutely essential for nurses in advanced practice, management, or educational roles.

Finally, **Unit IV, Application of Theory in Nursing**, explains how theories are applied in nursing. Separate chapters cover nursing practice, nursing research, nursing administration and management, and nursing education. These chapters include many specific examples for the application of theory and are intended to be a practical guide for theory use. The heightened development of practice theories and EBP guidelines are critical to theory application in nursing today, so these areas have been expanded. The unit concludes with a chapter that discusses some of the future issues in theory within the discipline.

Key Features

In addition to numerous tables and boxes that highlight and summarize important information, *Theoretical Basis for Nursing* contains case studies, learning activities, exemplars, and illustrations that help students visualize various concepts. New to this edition is a special boxed feature in most chapters that highlights how a topic is outlined in the American Association of Colleges of Nursing (AACN's) *The Essentials of Master's Education in Nursing* or *The Essentials of Doctoral Education for Advanced Nursing Practice*. Other key features include:

- **Link to Practice**: All chapters include at least one "Link to Practice" box, which presents useful information or clinically related examples related to the subject being discussed. The intent is to give additional tools or resources that can be used by nurses to apply the content in their own practice or research.
- **Case Studies**: At the end of Chapter 1 and the beginning of Chapters 2 to 23, case studies help the reader understand how the content in the chapter relates to the everyday experience of the nurse, whether in practice, research, or other aspects of nursing.
- **Learning Activities**: At the end of each chapter, learning activities pose critical thinking questions, propose individual and group projects related to topics covered in the chapter, and stimulate classroom discussion.
- **Exemplars**: In five chapters, an exemplar discusses a scholarly study from the perspectives of concept analysis (Chapter 3); theory development (Chapter 4); theory analysis and evaluation (Chapter 5); middle range theory development (Chapter 10); and theory generation via research, theory testing via research, and use of a theory as the conceptual framework for a research study (Chapter 20).
- **Illustrations**: Diagrams and models are included throughout the book to help the reader better understand the many different theories presented.

New to This Edition

- New Chapter 16, *Ethical Theories and Principles*
- Detailed section on Complexity Science and Complex Adaptive Systems in Chapter 13.
- More detailed explanation of EBP, situation-specific theories, and their relationship to theory in nursing
- Numerous recent examples of application of theories in nursing practice, nursing research, leadership/administration, and education
- Enhanced instructional support, focusing on activities and information directed toward online learning

Student Resources Available on thePoint

- **Literature Assessment Activity** provides an interactive tool featuring journal articles along with critical thinking questions that will encourage students to engage with the literature. Students can print or e-mail their responses to their instructor.
- **Case Studies** with applicable questions guide students in understanding how the various theories link to nursing practice.

- **Learning Objectives** for each chapter help focus the student on outcomes.
- **Internet Resources** provide live web links to pertinent sites so that students can further their study and understanding of the various theories.
- **Journal Articles** for each chapter offer opportunities to gain more knowledge and understanding of the chapter content.

Instructor Resources Available on thePoint

- **Instructor's Guide** includes application-level discussion questions and classroom/online activities that Melanie McEwen uses in her own teaching!
- **Strategies for Effective Teaching of Nursing Theory** provide ideas for instructors to help make the nursing theory class come alive.
- **Test Generator Questions** provide multiple-choice questions that can be used for testing general content knowledge.
- **PowerPoints with audience response (Iclicker) questions**, based on the ones used by Melanie McEwen in her own classroom, help highlight important points to enhance the classroom experience.
- **Case Studies** with questions, answers, and related activities offer opportunities for instructors to make the student case studies an exciting, fun, and rewarding classroom/online experience.
- **Image Bank** provides images from the text that instructors can use to enhance their own presentations.

In summary, the focus of this learning package is on the application of theory rather than on the study, analysis, and critique of grand theorists or a presentation of a specific aspect of theory (e.g., construction or evaluation). It is hoped that practicing nurses, nurse researchers, and nursing scholars, as well as graduate students and theory instructors, will use this book and its accompanying resources to gain a better understanding and appreciation of theory.

Melanie McEwen, PhD, RN, CNE, ANEF
Evelyn M. Wills, PhD, RN

ACKNOWLEDGMENTS

Our heartfelt thanks to Senior Development Editor, Michael Kerns, and Editorial Coordinator, Tim Rinehart, for their assistance, patience, and persistence in helping us complete this project. They made a difficult task seem easy! We also want to thank Senior Acquisitions Editor, Christina Burns, and Helen Kogut, for their support and assistance in getting this project started and help with previous editions. Finally, a huge word of thanks to our contributors who have diligently worked to present the notion of theory in a manner that will engage nursing students and to look for new examples and applications to help make theory fresh and relevant.

CONTENTS

Unit II: Nursing Theories   115

Unit III: Shared Theories Used by Nurses 273

Introduction to Theory

Philosophy, Science, and Nursing

Melanie McEwen

Largely due to the work of nursing scientists, nursing theorists, and nursing scholars over the past five decades, nursing has been recognized as both an emerging profession and an academic discipline. Crucial to the attainment of this distinction have been numerous discussions regarding the phenomena of concern to nurses and countless efforts to enhance involvement in theory utilization, theory generation, and theory testing to direct research and improve practice.

A review of the nursing literature from the late 1970s until the present shows sporadic discussion of whether nursing is a profession, a science, or an academic discipline. These discussions are sometimes pleading, frequently esoteric, and occasionally confusing. Questions that have been raised include: What defines a profession? What constitutes an academic discipline? What is nursing science? Why is it important for nursing to be seen as a profession or an academic discipline?

Nursing as a Profession

In the past, there has been considerable discussion about whether nursing is a profession or an occupation. This is important for nurses to consider for several reasons. An occupation is a job or a career, whereas a profession is a learned vocation or occupation that has a status of superiority and precedence within a division of work. In general terms, occupations require widely varying levels of training or education, varying levels of skill, and widely variable defined knowledge bases. In short, all professions are occupations, but not all occupations are professions (Finkelman & Kenner, 2016).

Professions are valued by society because the services professionals provide are beneficial for members of the society. Characteristics of a profession include (1) defined and specialized knowledge base, (2) control and authority over training and education, (3) credentialing system or registration to ensure competence, (4) altruistic service to society, (5) a code of ethics, (6) formal training within institutions of higher education, (7) lengthy socialization to the profession, and (8) autonomy (control of professional activities) (Ellis & Hartley, 2012; Finkelman & Kenner, 2016;

Rutty, 1998). Professions must have a group of scholars, investigators, or researchers who work to continually advance the knowledge of the profession with the goal of improving practice. Finally, professionals are responsible and accountable to the public for their work (Hood, 2014). Traditionally, professions have included the clergy, law, and medicine.

Until near the end of the 20th century, nursing was viewed as an occupation rather than a profession. Nursing has had difficulty being deemed a profession because many of the services provided by nurses have been perceived as an extension of those offered by wives and mothers. Additionally, historically, nursing has been seen as subservient to medicine, and nurses have delayed in identifying and organizing professional knowledge. Furthermore, education for nurses is not yet standardized, and the three-tier entry-level system (diploma, associate degree, and bachelor's degree) into practice that persists has hindered professionalization because a college education is not yet a requirement. Finally, autonomy in practice is incomplete because nursing is still dependent on medicine to direct much of its practice.

On the other hand, many of the characteristics of a profession can be observed in nursing. Indeed, nursing has a social mandate to provide health care for clients at different points in the health–illness continuum. There is a growing knowledge base, authority over education, altruistic service, a code of ethics, and registration requirements for practice. Although the debate is not closed, it can be successfully argued that nursing is an aspiring, evolving profession (Finkelman & Kenner, 2016; Hood, 2014; Judd & Sitzman, 2014). See Link to Practice 1-1 for more information on the future of nursing as a profession.

Nursing as an Academic Discipline

Disciplines are distinctions between bodies of knowledge found in academic settings. A *discipline* is "a branch of knowledge ordered through the theories and methods evolving from more than one worldview of the phenomenon of concern" (Parse, 1997, p. 74). It has also been termed a field of inquiry characterized by a unique perspective and a distinct way of viewing phenomena (Fawcett, 2012; Rodgers, 2015).

Viewed another way, a discipline is a branch of educational instruction or a department of learning or knowledge. Institutions of higher education are organized around disciplines into colleges, schools, and departments (e.g., business administration, chemistry, history, and engineering).

Disciplines are organized by structure and tradition. The structure of the discipline provides organization and determines the amount, relationship, and ratio of each type of knowledge that comprises the discipline. The tradition of the discipline provides the content, which includes ethical, personal, esthetic, and scientific knowledge (Northrup et al., 2004; Risjord, 2010). Characteristics of disciplines include (1) a distinct perspective and syntax, (2) determination of what phenomena are of interest, (3) determination of the context in which the phenomena are viewed, (4) determination of what questions to ask, (5) determination of what methods of study are used, and (6) determination of what evidence is proof (Donaldson & Crowley, 1978).

Knowledge development within a discipline proceeds from several philosophical and scientific perspectives or worldviews (Litchfield & Jónsdóttir, 2008; Newman, Sime, & Corcoran-Perry, 1991; Risjord, 2010; Rodgers, 2015). In some cases, these worldviews may serve to divide or segregate members of a discipline. For example, in psychology, practitioners might consider themselves behaviorists, Freudians, or any one of a number of other divisions.

Link to Practice 1-1

The Future of Nursing

The Institute of Medicine (IOM, 2011) issued a series of sweeping recommendations directed to the nursing profession. The IOM explained their "vision" is to make quality, patient-centered care accessible for all Americans. Recommendations included a three-pronged approach to meeting the goal.

The first "message" was directed toward transformation of practice and precipitated the notion that nurses should be able to practice to the full extent of their education. Indeed, the IOM advocated for removal of regulatory, policy, and financial barriers to practice to ensure that "current and future generations of nurses can deliver safe, quality, patient-centered care across all settings, especially in such areas as primary care and community and public health" (p. 30).

A second key message related to the transformation of nursing education. In this regard, the IOM promotes "seamless academic progression" (p. 30), which includes a goal to increase the number and percentage of nurses who enter the workforce with a baccalaureate degree or who progress to the degree early in their career. Specifically, they recommend that 80% of registered nurses (RNs) be bachelor of science in nursing (BSN) prepared by 2020. Last, the IOM advocated that nurses be full partners with physicians and other health professionals in the attempt to redesign health care in the United States.

These "messages" are critical to the future of nursing as a profession. Indeed, standardization of entry level into practice at the BSN level, coupled with promotion of advanced education and independent practice, and inclusion as "leaders" in the health care transformation process, will help solidify nursing as a true profession.

An update (IOM, 2016) indicated that there has been "significant progress" (p. 50) toward reducing APRN scope of practices issues from a national perspective, as more states now allow nurse practitioners (NPs) full practice authority. Furthermore, although there has been some progress with expansion of the percentage of RNs with a BSN (from 49% to 51%), there is still much to do to meet the goal of 80%. Finally, the IOM concluded that data are lacking on efforts to develop the skills and competencies nurses need for leadership. The report reinforced the goal for nurses to seek "leadership positions in order to contribute their unique perspective and expertise on such issues as health care delivery, quality, and safety" (p. 149).

Several ways of classifying academic disciplines have been proposed. For instance, they may be divided into the basic sciences (physics, biology, chemistry, sociology, anthropology) and the humanities (philosophy, ethics, history, fine arts). In this classification scheme, it is arguable that nursing has characteristics of both.

Distinctions may also be made between academic disciplines (e.g., physics, physiology, sociology, mathematics, history, philosophy) and professional disciplines (e.g., medicine, law, nursing, social work). In this classification scheme, the academic disciplines aim to "know," and their theories are descriptive in nature. Research in academic disciplines is both basic and applied. Conversely, the professional disciplines are practical in nature, and their research tends to be more prescriptive and descriptive (Donaldson & Crowley, 1978).

Box 1-1	Theory and the American Association of Colleges of Nursing Essentials

"The scientific foundation of nursing practice has expanded and includes a focus on both the natural and social sciences. These sciences that provide a foundation for nursing practice include human biology, genomics, the psychosocial sciences as well as the science of complex organizational structures" (American Association of Colleges of Nursing, 2006, p. 9).

Nursing's knowledge base draws from many disciplines. In the past, nursing depended heavily on physiology, sociology, psychology, and medicine to provide academic standing and to inform practice (Box 1-1). In recent decades, however, nursing has been seeking what is unique to nursing and developing those aspects into an academic discipline (Parse, 2015). Areas that identify nursing as a distinct discipline are as follows:

- An identifiable philosophy
- At least one conceptual framework (perspective) for delineation of what can be defined as nursing
- Acceptable methodologic approaches for the pursuit and development of knowledge (Oldnall, 1995)

To begin the quest to validate nursing as both a profession and an academic discipline, this chapter provides an overview of the concepts of science and philosophy. It examines the schools of philosophical thought that have influenced nursing and explores the epistemology of nursing to explain why recognizing the multiple "ways of knowing" is critical in the quest for development and application of theory in nursing. Finally, this chapter presents issues related to how philosophical worldviews affect knowledge development through research. This chapter concludes with a case study that depicts how "the ways of knowing" in nursing are used on a day-to-day, even moment-by-moment, basis by all practicing nurses.

Introduction to Science and Philosophy

Science is concerned with causality (cause and effect). The scientific approach to understanding reality is characterized by observation, verifiability, and experience; hypothesis testing and experimentation are considered scientific methods. In contrast, *philosophy* is concerned with the purpose of human life, the nature of being and reality, and the theory and limits of knowledge. Intuition, introspection, and reasoning are examples of philosophical methodologies. Science and philosophy share the common goal of increasing knowledge (Fawcett, 2012; Polifroni, 2015; Silva, 1977). The science of any discipline is tied to its philosophy, which provides the basis for understanding and developing theories for science (Gustafsson, 2002; Morse, 2017; Silva & Rothbart, 1984).

Overview of Science

Science is both a process and a product. Parse (1997) defines science as the "theoretical explanation of the subject of inquiry and the methodological process of sustaining knowledge in a discipline" (p. 74). Science has also been described as a way of explaining

Box 1-2	Characteristics of Science

1. Science must show a certain coherence.
2. Science is concerned with definite fields of knowledge.
3. Science is preferably expressed in universal statements.
4. The statements of science must be true or probably true.
5. The statements of science must be logically ordered.
6. Science must explain its investigations and arguments.

Source: Silva (1977).

observed phenomena as well as a system of gathering, verifying, and systematizing information about reality (Streubert & Carpenter, 2011). As a process, science is characterized by systematic inquiry that relies heavily on empirical observations of the natural world. As a product, it has been defined as empirical knowledge that is grounded and tested in experience and is the result of investigative efforts. Furthermore, science is conceived as being the consensual, informed opinion about the natural world, including human behavior and social action (Gortner & Schultz, 1988).

Science has come to represent knowledge, and it is generated by activities that combine advancement of knowledge (research) and explanation for knowledge (theory) (Powers & Knapp, 2011). Citing Van Laer, Silva (1977) lists six characteristics of science (Box 1-2).

Science has been classified in several ways. These include pure or basic science, natural science, human or social science, and applied or practice science. The classifications are not mutually exclusive and are open to interpretation based on philosophical orientation. Table 1-1 lists examples of a number of sciences by this manner of classification.

Some sciences defy classification. For example, computer science is arguably applied or perhaps pure. Law is certainly a practice science, but it is also a social science. Psychology might be a basic science, a human science, or an applied science, depending on what aspect of psychology one is referring to.

There are significant differences between the human and natural sciences. Human sciences refer to the fields of psychology, anthropology, and sociology and may even extend to economics and political science. These disciplines deal with various aspects of humans and human interactions. Natural sciences, on the other hand, are concentrated on elements found in nature that do not relate to the totality of the individual.

Table 1-1 Classifications of Science

Classification	Examples
Natural sciences	Chemistry, physics, biology, physiology, geology, meteorology
Basic or pure sciences	Mathematics, logic, chemistry, physics, English (language)
Human or social sciences	Psychology, anthropology, sociology, economics, political science, history, religion
Practice or applied sciences	Architecture, engineering, medicine, pharmacology, law

There are inherent differences between the human and natural sciences that make the research techniques of the natural sciences (e.g., laboratory experimentation) improper or potentially problematic for human sciences (Gortner & Schultz, 1988).

It has been posited that although nursing draws on the basic and pure sciences (e.g., physiology and chemistry) and has many characteristics of social sciences, it is without question an applied or practice science. However, it is important to note that it is also synthesized, in that it draws on the knowledge of other established disciplines—including other practice disciplines (Dahnke & Dreher, 2016; Holzemer, 2007; Risjord, 2010).

Overview of Philosophy

Within any discipline, both scholars and students should be aware of the philosophical orientations that are the basis for developing theory and advancing knowledge (Dahnke & Dreher, 2016; DiBartolo, 1998; Northrup et al., 2004; Risjord, 2010). Rather than a focus on solving problems or answering questions related to that discipline (which are tasks of the discipline's science), the philosophy of a discipline studies the concepts that structure the thought processes of that discipline with the intent of recognizing and revealing foundations and presuppositions (Blackburn, 2016).

Philosophy has been defined as "a study of problems that are ultimate, abstract, and general. These problems are concerned with the nature of existence, knowledge, morality, reason, and human purpose" (Teichman & Evans, 1999, p. 1). Philosophy tries to discover knowledge and truth and attempts to identify what is valuable and important.

Modern philosophy is usually traced to Rene Descartes, Francis Bacon, Baruch Spinoza, and Immanuel Kant (ca. 1600–1800). Descartes (1596–1650) and Spinoza (1632–1677) were early rationalists. Rationalists believe that reason is superior to experience as a source of knowledge. Rationalists attempt to determine the nature of the world and reality by deduction and stress the importance of mathematical procedures.

Bacon (1561–1626) was an early empiricist. Like rationalists, he supported experimentation and scientific methods for solving problems.

The work of Kant (1724–1804) set the foundation for many later developments in philosophy. Kant believed that knowledge is relative and that the mind plays an active role in knowing. Other philosophers have also influenced nursing and the advance of nursing science. Several are discussed later in the chapter.

Although there is some variation, traditionally, the branches of philosophy include metaphysics (ontology and cosmology), epistemology, logic, esthetics, and ethics or axiology. Political philosophy and philosophy of science are added by some authors (Rutty, 1998; Teichman & Evans, 1999). Table 1-2 summarizes the major branches of philosophy.

Science and Philosophical Schools of Thought

The concept of science as understood in the 21st century is relatively new. In the period of modern science, three philosophies of science (paradigms or worldviews) dominate: rationalism, empiricism, and human science/phenomenology. Rationalism and empiricism are often termed *received view* and human science/phenomenology and related worldviews (i.e., historicism) are considered *perceived view* (Hickman, 2011; Meleis, 2012). These two worldviews dominated theoretical discussion in nursing through the 1990s. More recently, attention has focused on another dominant worldview: "postmodernism" (Meleis, 2012; Reed, 1995).

Table 1-2 Branches of Philosophy	
Branch	**Pursuit**
Metaphysics	Study of the fundamental nature of reality and existence—general theory of reality
Ontology	Study of theory of being (what is or what exists)
Cosmology	Study of the physical universe
Epistemology	Study of knowledge (ways of knowing, nature of truth, and relationship between knowledge and belief)
Logic	Study of principles and methods of reasoning (inference and argument)
Ethics (axiology)	Study of nature of values; right and wrong (moral philosophy)
Esthetics	Study of appreciation of the arts or things beautiful
Philosophy of science	Study of science and scientific practice
Political philosophy	Study of citizen and state

Sources: Blackburn (2016); Teichman and Evans (1999).

Received View (Empiricism, Positivism, Logical Positivism)

Empiricism has its roots in the writings of Francis Bacon, John Locke, and David Hume, who valued observation, perception by senses, and experience as sources of knowledge (Gortner & Schultz, 1988; Powers & Knapp, 2011). Empiricism is founded on the belief that what is experienced is what exists, and its knowledge base requires that these experiences be verified through scientific methodology (Dahnke & Dreher, 2016; Gustafsson, 2002). This knowledge is then passed on to others in the discipline and subsequently built on. The term *received view* or *received knowledge* denotes that individuals learn by being told or receiving knowledge.

Empiricism holds that truth corresponds to observable, reduction, verification, control, and bias-free science. It emphasizes mathematic formulas to explain phenomena and prefers simple dichotomies and classification of concepts. Additionally, everything can be reduced to a scientific formula with little room for interpretation (DiBartolo, 1998; Gortner & Schultz, 1988; Risjord, 2010).

Empiricism focuses on understanding the parts of the whole in an attempt to understand the whole. It strives to explain nature through testing of hypotheses and development of theories. Theories are made to describe, explain, and predict phenomena in nature and to provide understanding of relationships between phenomena. Concepts must be operationalized in the form of propositional statements, thereby making measurement possible. Instrumentation, reliability, and validity are stressed in empirical research methodologies. Once measurement is determined, it is possible to test theories through experimentation or observation, which results in verification or falsification (Cull-Wilby & Pepin, 1987; Suppe & Jacox, 1985).

Positivism is often equated with empiricism. Like empiricism, positivism supports mechanistic, reductionist principles, where the complex can be best understood in terms of its basic components. *Logical positivism* was the dominant empirical philosophy of science between the 1880s and 1950s. Logical positivists recognized only the logical and empirical bases of science and stressed that there is no room for metaphysics, understanding, or meaning within the realm of science (Polifroni, 2015; Risjord, 2010).

Logical positivism maintained that science is value free, independent of the scientist, and obtained using objective methods. The goal of science is to explain, predict, and control. Theories are either true or false, subject to empirical observation, and capable of being reduced to existing scientific theories (Rutty, 1998).

Contemporary Empiricism/Postpositivism

Positivism came under criticism in the 1960s when positivistic logic was deemed faulty (Rutty, 1998). An overreliance on strictly controlled experimentation in artificial settings produced results that indicated that much significant knowledge or information was missed. In recent years, scholars have determined that the positivist view of science is outdated and misleading in that it contributes to overfragmentation in knowledge and theory development (DiBartolo, 1998). It has been observed that positivistic analysis of theories is fundamentally defective due to insistence on analyzing the logically ideal, which results in findings that have little to do with reality. It was maintained that the context of discovery was artificial and that theories and explanations can be understood only within their discovery contexts (Suppe & Jacox, 1985). Also, scientific inquiry is inherently value laden, as even choosing what to investigate and/or what techniques to employ will reflect the values of the researcher.

The current generation of postpositivists accepts the subjective nature of inquiry but still supports rigor and objective study through quantitative research methods. Indeed, it has been observed that modern empiricists or postpositivists are concerned with explanation and prediction of complex phenomena, recognizing contextual variables (Powers & Knapp, 2011; Reed, 2008).

Nursing and Empiricism

As an emerging discipline, nursing has followed established disciplines (e.g., physiology) and the medical model in stressing logical positivism. Early nurse scientists embraced the importance of objectivity, control, fact, and measurement of smaller and smaller parts. Based on this influence, acceptable methods for knowledge generation in nursing have stressed traditional, orthodox, and preferably experimental methods.

Although positivism continues to heavily influence nursing science, that viewpoint has been challenged in recent years (Risjord, 2010). Consequently, postpositivism has become one of the most accepted contemporary worldviews in nursing.

Perceived View (Human Science, Phenomenology, Constructivism, Historicism)

In the late 1960s and early 1970s, several philosophers, including Kuhn, Feyerbend, and Toulmin, challenged the positivist view by arguing that the influence of history on science should be emphasized (Dahnke & Dreher, 2016). The perceived view of science, which may also be referred to as the interpretive view, includes phenomenology, constructivism, and historicism. The interpretive view recognizes that the perceptions of both the subject being studied and the researcher tend to de-emphasize reliance on strict control and experimentation in laboratory settings (Monti & Tingen, 1999).

The perceived view of science centers on descriptions that are derived from collectively lived experiences, interrelatedness, human interpretation, and learned reality, as opposed to artificially invented (i.e., laboratory-based) reality (Rutty, 1998). It is argued that the pursuit of knowledge and truth is naturally historical, contextual, and value laden. Thus, there is no single truth. Rather, knowledge is deemed true if it withstands practical tests of utility and reason (DiBartolo, 1998).

Phenomenology is the study of phenomena and emphasizes the appearance of things as opposed to the things themselves. In phenomenology, *understanding* is the goal of science, with the objective of recognizing the connection between one's experience, values, and perspective. It maintains that each individual's experience is unique, and there are many interpretations of reality. Inquiry begins with individuals and their experiences with phenomena. Perceptions, feelings, values, and the meanings that have come to be attached to things and events are the focus.

For social scientists, the *constructivist* approaches of the perceived view focus on understanding the actions of, and meaning to, individuals. What exists depends on what individuals perceive to exist. Knowledge is subjective and created by individuals. Thus, research methodology entails the investigation of the individual's world. There is an emphasis on subjectivity, multiple truths, trends and patterns, discovery, description, and understanding.

Feminism and critical social theory may also be considered to be perceived view. These philosophical schools of thought recognize the influence of gender, culture, society, and shared history as being essential components of science (Riegel et al., 1992). Critical social theorists contend that reality is dynamic and shaped by social, political, cultural, economic, ethnic, and gender values (Streubert & Carpenter, 2011). Critical social theory and feminist theories will be described in more detail in Chapter 13.

Nursing and Phenomenology/Constructivism/Historicism

Because they examine phenomena within context, phenomenology, as well as other perceived views of philosophy, are conducive to discovery and knowledge development inherent to nursing. Phenomenology is open, variable, and relativistic and based on human experience and personal interpretations. As such, it is an important, guiding paradigm for nursing practice theory and education (DiBartolo, 1998).

In nursing science, the dichotomy of philosophic thought between the received, empirical view of science and the perceived, interpretative view of science has persisted. This may have resulted, in part, because nursing draws heavily both from natural sciences (physiology, biology) and social sciences (psychology, sociology).

Postmodernism (Poststructuralism, Postcolonialism)

Postmodernism began in Europe in the 1960s as a social movement centered on a philosophy that rejects the notion of a single "truth." Although it recognizes the value of science and scientific methods, postmodernism allows for multiple meanings of reality and multiple ways of knowing and interpreting reality (Hood, 2014; Reed, 1995). In postmodernism, knowledge is viewed as uncertain, contextual, and relative. Knowledge development moves from emphasis on identifying a truth or fact in research to discovering practical significance and relevance of research findings (Reed, 1995).

Similar or related constructs and worldviews found in the nursing literature include "deconstruction," "postcolonialism," and, at times, feminist philosophies. In nursing, the postcolonial worldview can be connected to both feminism and critical theory, particularly when considering nursing's historical reliance on medicine (Holmes, Roy, & Perron, 2008; McGibbon, Mulaudzi, Didham, Barton, & Sochan, 2014; Racine, 2009).

Postmodernism has loosened the notions of what counts as knowledge development that have persisted among supporters of qualitative and quantitative research methods. Rather than focusing on a single research methodology, postmodernism promotes use of multiple methods for development of scientific understanding and incorporation of different ways to improve understanding of human nature (Hood, 2014;

Meleis, 2012; Rodgers, 2015). Increasingly, in postmodernism, there is a consensus that synthesis of both research methods can be used at different times to serve different purposes (Hood, 2014; Meleis, 2012; Risjord, Dunbar, & Moloney, 2002).

Criticisms of postmodernism have been made and frequently relate to the perceived reluctance to address error in research. Taken to the extreme as Paley (2005) pointed out, when there is absence of strict control over methodology and interpretation of research, "Nobody can ever be wrong about anything" (p. 107). Chinn and Kramer (2015) echoed the concerns by acknowledging that knowledge development should never be "sloppy." Indeed, although application of various methods in research is legitimate and may be advantageous, research must still be carried out carefully and rigorously.

Nursing and Postmodernism

Postmodernism has been described as a dominant scientific theoretical paradigm in nursing in the late 20th century (Meleis, 2012). As the discipline matures, there has been recognition of the pluralistic nature of nursing and an enhanced understanding that the goal of research is to provide an integrative basis for nursing care (Walker & Avant, 2011).

In terms of scientific methodology, the attention is increasingly on combining multiple methods within a single research project (Chinn & Kramer, 2015). Postmodernism has helped dislodged the authority of a single research paradigm in nursing science by emphasizing the blending or integration of qualitative and quantitative research into a holistic, dynamic model to improve nursing practice. Table 1-3 compares the dominant philosophical views of science in nursing.

Table 1-3 Comparison of the Received, Perceived, and Postmodern Views of Science

Received View of Science—Hard Sciences	Perceived View of Science—Soft Sciences	Postmodernism, Poststructuralism, and Postcolonialism
Empiricism/positivism/logical positivism	Historicism/phenomenology	Macroanalysis
Reality/truth/facts considered acontextual (objective)	Reality/truth/facts considered in context (subjective)	Contextual meaning; narration
Deductive	Inductive	Contextual, political, and structural analysis
Reality/truth/facts considered ahistorical	Reality/truth/facts considered with regard to history	Reality/truth/facts considered with regard to history
Prediction and control	Description and understanding	Metanarrative analysis
One truth	Multiple truths	Different views
Validation and replication	Trends and patterns	Uncovering opposing views
Reductionism	Constructivism/holism	Macrorelationship; microstructures
Quantitative research	Qualitative research methods	Methodologic pluralism methods

Sources: Meleis (2012); Moody (1990).

Nursing Philosophy, Nursing Science, and Philosophy of Science in Nursing

The terms *nursing philosophy*, *nursing science*, and *philosophy of science in nursing* are sometimes used interchangeably. The differences, however, in the general meaning of these concepts are important to recognize.

Nursing Philosophy

Nursing philosophy has been described as "a statement of foundational and universal assumptions, beliefs and principles about the nature of knowledge and thought (epistemology) and about the nature of the entities represented in the metaparadigm (i.e., nursing practice and human health processes [ontology])" (Reed, 1995, p. 76). Nursing philosophy, then, refers to the belief system or worldview of the profession and provides perspectives for practice, scholarship, and research.

No single dominant philosophy has prevailed in the discipline of nursing. Many nursing scholars and nursing theorists have written extensively in an attempt to identify the overriding belief system, but to date, none has been universally successful. Most would agree then that nursing is increasingly recognized as a "multiparadigm discipline" (Powers & Knapp, 2011, p. 129), in which using multiple perspectives or worldviews in a "unified" way is valuable and even necessary for knowledge development (Giuliano, Tyer-Viola, & Lopez, 2005).

Nursing Science

Parse (2016) defined nursing science as "the substantive, discipline-specific knowledge that focuses on the human-universe-health process articulated in the nursing frameworks and theories" (p. 101). To develop and apply the discipline-specific knowledge, nursing science recognizes the relationships of human responses in health and illness and addresses biologic, behavioral, social, and cultural domains. The goal of nursing science is to represent the nature of nursing—to understand it, to explain it, and to use it for the benefit of humankind. It is nursing science that gives direction to the future generation of substantive nursing knowledge, and it is nursing science that provides the knowledge for all aspects of nursing (Holzemer, 2007; Parse, 2016).

Philosophy of Science in Nursing

Philosophy of science in nursing helps to establish the meaning of science through an understanding and examination of nursing concepts, theories, laws, and aims as they relate to nursing practice. It seeks to understand truth; to describe nursing; to examine prediction and causality; to critically relate theories, models, and scientific systems; and to explore determinism and free will (Nyatanga, 2005; Polifroni, 2015).

Knowledge Development and Nursing Science

Development of nursing knowledge reflects the interface between nursing science and research. The ultimate purpose of knowledge development is to improve nursing practice. Approaches to knowledge development have three facets: ontology, epistemology, and methodology. Ontology refers to the study of being: what is or what exists.

Epistemology refers to the study of knowledge or ways of knowing. Methodology is the means of acquiring knowledge (Powers & Knapp, 2011). The following sections discuss nursing epistemology and issues related to methods of acquiring knowledge.

Epistemology

Epistemology is the study of the theory of knowledge. Epistemologic questions include: What do we know? What is the extent of our knowledge? How do we decide whether we know? and What are the criteria of knowledge? (Schultz & Meleis, 1988).

According to Streubert and Carpenter (2011), it is important to understand the way in which nursing knowledge develops to provide a context in which to judge the appropriateness of nursing knowledge and methods that nurses use to develop that knowledge. This in turn will refocus methods for gaining knowledge as well as establishing the legitimacy or quality of the knowledge gained.

Ways of Knowing

In epistemology, there are several basic types of knowledge. These include the following:

- Empirics—the scientific form of knowing. Empirical knowledge comes from observation, testing, and replication.
- Personal knowledge—a priori knowledge. Personal knowledge pertains to knowledge gained from thought alone.
- Intuitive knowledge—includes feelings and hunches. Intuitive knowledge is not guessing but relies on nonconscious pattern recognition and experience.
- Somatic knowledge—knowledge of the body in relation to physical movement. Somatic knowledge includes experiential use of muscles and balance to perform a physical task.
- Metaphysical (spiritual) knowledge—seeking the presence of a higher power. Aspects of spiritual knowing include magic, miracles, psychokinesis, extrasensory perception, and near-death experiences.
- Esthetics—knowledge related to beauty, harmony, and expression. Esthetic knowledge incorporates art, creativity, and values.
- Moral or ethical knowledge—knowledge of what is right and wrong. Values and social and cultural norms of behavior are components of ethical knowledge.

Nursing Epistemology

Nursing epistemology has been defined as "the study of the origins of nursing knowledge, its structure and methods, the patterns of knowing of its members, and the criteria for validating its knowledge claims" (Schultz & Meleis, 1988, p. 217). Like most disciplines, nursing has both scientific knowledge and knowledge that can be termed conventional wisdom (knowledge that has not been empirically tested).

Traditionally, only what stands the test of repeated measures constitutes truth or knowledge. Classical scientific processes (i.e., experimentation), however, are not suitable for creating and describing all types of knowledge. Social sciences, behavioral sciences, and the arts rely on other methods to establish knowledge. Because it has characteristics of social and behavioral sciences, as well as biologic sciences, nursing must rely on multiple ways of knowing.

In a classic work, Carper (1978) identified four fundamental patterns for nursing knowledge: (1) empirics—the science of nursing, (2) esthetics—the art of nursing, (3) personal knowledge in nursing, and (4) ethics—moral knowledge in nursing.

Empirical knowledge is objective, abstract, generally quantifiable, exemplary, discursively formulated, and verifiable. When verified through repeated testing over time, it is formulated into scientific generalizations, laws, theories, and principles that explain and predict (Carper, 1978, 1992). It draws on traditional ideas that can be verified through observation and proved by hypothesis testing.

Empirical knowledge tends to be the most emphasized way of knowing in nursing because there is a need to know how knowledge can be organized into laws and theories for the purpose of describing, explaining, and predicting phenomena of concern to nurses. Most theory development and research efforts are engaged in seeking and generating explanations that are systematic and controllable by factual evidence (Carper, 1978, 1992).

Esthetic knowledge is expressive, subjective, unique, and experiential rather than formal or descriptive. Esthetics includes sensing the meaning of a moment. It is evident through actions, conduct, attitudes, and interactions of the nurse in response to another. It is not expressed in language (Carper, 1978).

Esthetic knowledge relies on perception. It is creative and incorporates empathy and understanding. It is interpretive, contextual, intuitive, and subjective and requires synthesis rather than analysis. Furthermore, esthetics goes beyond what is explained by principles and creates values and meaning to account for variables that cannot be quantitatively formulated (Carper, 1978, 1992).

Personal knowledge refers to the way in which nurses view themselves and the client. Personal knowledge is subjective and promotes wholeness and integrity in personal encounters. Engagement, rather than detachment, is a component of personal knowledge.

Personal knowledge incorporates experience, knowing, encountering, and actualizing the self within the practice. Personal maturity and freedom are components of personal knowledge, which may include spiritual and metaphysical forms of knowing. Because personal knowledge is difficult to express linguistically, it is largely expressed in personality (Carper, 1978, 1992).

Ethics refers to the moral code for nursing and is based on obligation to service and respect for human life. Ethical knowledge occurs as moral dilemmas arise in situations of ambiguity and uncertainty and when consequences are difficult to predict. Ethical knowledge requires rational and deliberate examination and evaluation of what is good, valuable, and desirable as goals, motives, or characteristics (Carper, 1978, 1992). Ethics must address conflicting norms, interests, and principles and provide insight into areas that cannot be tested.

Fawcett, Watson, Neuman, Walkers, and Fitzpatrick (2001) stress that integration of all patterns of knowing is essential for professional nursing practice and that no one pattern should be used in isolation from others. Indeed, they are interrelated and interdependent because there are multiple points of contact between and among them (Carper, 1992). Thus, nurses should view nursing practice from a broadened perspective that places value on ways of knowing beyond the empirical (Silva, Sorrell, & Sorrell, 1995). Table 1-4 summarizes selected characteristics of Carper's patterns of knowing in nursing.

Other Views of Patterns of Knowledge in Nursing

Although Carper's work is considered classic, it is not without critics. Schultz and Meleis (1988) observed that Carper's work did not incorporate practical knowledge into the ways of knowing in nursing. Because of this and other concerns, they described three patterns of knowledge in nursing: clinical, conceptual, and empirical.

Table 1-4 Characteristics of Carper's Patterns of Knowing in Nursing

Pattern of Knowing	Relationship to Nursing	Source or Creation	Source of Validation	Method of Expression	Purpose or Outcome
Empirics	Science of nursing	Direct or indirect observation and measurement	Replication	Facts, models, scientific principles, laws statements, theories, descriptions	Description, explanation, prediction
Esthetics	Art of nursing	Creation of value and meaning, synthesis of abstract and concrete	Appreciation; experience; inspiration; perception of balance, rhythm, proportion, and unity	Appreciation; empathy; esthetic criticism; engaging, intuiting, and envisioning	Move beyond what can be explained, quantitatively formulated, understanding, balance
Personal knowledge	Therapeutic use of self	Engagement, opening, centering, actualizing self	Response, reflection, experience	Empathy, active participation	Promote wholeness and integrity in personal encounters
Ethics	Moral component of nursing	Values clarification, rational and deliberate reasoning, obligation, advocating	Dialogue, justification, universal generalizability	Principles, codes, ethical theories	Evaluation of what is good, valuable, and desirable

Sources: Carper (1978, 1992); Chinn and Kramer (2015).

Clinical knowledge refers to the individual nurse's personal knowledge. It results from using multiple ways of knowing while solving problems during client care provision. Clinical knowledge is manifested in the acts of practicing nurses and results from combining personal knowledge and empirical knowledge. It may also involve intuitive and subjective knowing. Clinical knowledge is communicated retrospectively through publication in journals (Schultz & Meleis, 1988).

Conceptual knowledge is abstracted and generalized beyond personal experience. It explicates patterns revealed in multiple client experiences, which occur in multiple situations, and articulates them as models or theories. In conceptual knowledge, concepts are drafted and relational statements are formulated. Propositional statements are supported by empirical or anecdotal evidence or defended by logical reasoning.

Conceptual knowledge uses knowledge from nursing and other disciplines. It incorporates curiosity, imagination, persistence, and commitment in the accumulation of facts and reliable generalizations that pertain to the discipline of nursing. Conceptual knowledge is communicated in propositional statements (Schultz & Meleis, 1988).

Empirical knowledge results from experimental, historical, or phenomenologic research and is used to justify actions and procedures in practice. The credibility of empirical knowledge rests on the degree to which the researcher has followed procedures accepted by the community of researchers and on the logical, unbiased derivation of conclusions from the evidence. Empirical knowledge is evaluated through systematic review and critique of published research and conference presentations (Schultz & Meleis, 1988).

Chinn and Kramer (2015) also expanded on Carper's patterns of knowing to include "emancipatory knowing"—what they designate as the "praxis of nursing." In their view, emancipatory knowing refers to human's ability to critically examine the current status quo and to determine why it currently exists. This, in turn, supports identification of inequities in social and political institutions and clarification of cultural values and beliefs to improve conditions for all. In this view, emancipatory knowledge is expressed in actions that are directed toward changing existing social structures and establishing practices that are more equitable and favorable to human health and well-being.

Summary of Ways of Knowing in Nursing

For decades, the importance of the multiple ways of knowing has been recognized in the discipline of nursing. If nursing is to achieve a true integration between theory, research, and practice, theory development and research must integrate different sources of knowledge. Kidd and Morrison (1988) state that in nursing, synthesis of theories derived from different sources of knowledge will:

1. Encourage the use of different types of knowledge in practice, education, theory development, and research.
2. Encourage the use of different methodologies in practice and research.
3. Make nursing education more relevant for nurses with different educational backgrounds.
4. Accommodate nurses at different levels of clinical competence.
5. Ultimately promote high-quality client care and client satisfaction.

Research Methodology and Nursing Science

Being heavily influenced by logical empiricism, as nursing began developing as a scientific discipline in the mid-1900s, quantitative methods were used almost exclusively in research. In the 1960s and 1970s, schools of nursing aligned nursing inquiry with scientific inquiry in a desire to bring respect to the academic environment, and nurse researchers and nurse educators valued quantitative research methods over other forms.

A debate over methodology began in the 1980s, however, when some nurse scholars asserted that nursing's ontology (what nursing is) was not being adequately and sufficiently explored using quantitative methods in isolation. Subsequently, qualitative research methods began to be put into use. The assumptions were that qualitative methods showed the phenomena of nursing in ways that were naturalistic and unstructured and not misrepresented (Holzemer, 2007; Rutty, 1998).

The manner in which nursing science is conceptualized determines the priorities for nursing research and provides measures for determining the relevance of various scientific research questions. Therefore, the way in which nursing science is conceptualized also has implications for nursing practice. The philosophical issues regarding methods of research relate back to the debate over the worldviews of received versus perceived views of science versus postmodernism and whether nursing is a practice or applied science, a human science, or some combination. The notion of evidence-based practice has emerged over the last few years, largely in response to these and related concerns. Evidence-based practice as it relates to the theoretical basis of nursing will be examined in Chapter 13.

Nursing as a Practice Science

In early years, the debate focused on whether nursing was a basic science or an applied science. The goal of basic science is the attainment of knowledge. In basic research, the investigator is interested in understanding the problem and produces knowledge for knowledge's sake. It is analytical and the ultimate function is to analyze a conclusion backward to its proper principles.

Conversely, an applied science is one that uses the knowledge of basic sciences for some practical end. Engineering, architecture, and pharmacology are examples. In applied research, the investigator works toward solving problems and producing solutions for the problem. In practice sciences, research is largely clinical and action oriented (Moody, 1990). Thus, as an applied or practical science, nursing requires research that is applied and clinical and that generates and tests theories related to health of human beings within their environments as well as the actions and processes used by nurses in practice.

Nursing as a Human Science

The term *human science* is traced to philosopher Wilhelm Dilthey (1833–1911). Dilthey proposed that the human sciences require concepts, methods, and theories that are fundamentally different from those of the natural sciences. Human sciences study human life by valuing the lived experience of persons and seek to understand life in its matrix of patterns of meaning and values. Some scholars believe that there is a need to approach human sciences differently from conventional empiricism and contend that human experience must be understood in context (Cody & Mitchell, 2002; Polifroni, 2015).

In human sciences, scientists hope to create new knowledge to provide understanding and interpretation of phenomena. In human sciences, knowledge takes the form of descriptive theories regarding the structures, processes, relationships, and traditions that underlie psychological, social, and cultural aspects of reality. Data are interpreted within context to derive meaning and understanding. Humanistic scientists value the subjective component of knowledge. They recognize that humans are not capable of total objectivity and embrace the idea of subjectivity (Streubert & Carpenter, 2011). The purpose of research in human science is to produce descriptions and interpretations to help understand the nature of human experience.

Nursing is sometimes referred to as a human science (Cody & Mitchell, 2002; Polifroni, 2015). Indeed, the discipline has examined issues related to behavior and culture, as well as biology and physiology, and sought to recognize associations among factors that suggest explanatory variables for human health and illness. Thus, it fits the pattern of other humanistic sciences (i.e., anthropology, sociology).

Quantitative Versus Qualitative Methodology Debate

Nursing scholars accept the premise that scientific knowledge is generated from systematic study. The research methodologies and criteria used to justify the acceptance of statements or conclusions as true within the discipline result in conclusions and statements that are appropriate, valid, and reliable for the purpose of the discipline.

The two dominant forms of scientific inquiry have been identified in nursing: (1) empiricism, which objectifies and attempts to quantify experience and may test propositions or hypotheses in controlled experimentation, and (2) phenomenology and other forms of qualitative research (i.e., grounded theory, hermeneutics, historical research, ethnography), which study lived experiences and meanings of events (Gortner & Schultz, 1988; Morse, 2017; Risjord, 2010). Reviews of the scientific status of nursing knowledge usually contrast the positivist–deductive–quantitative approach with the interpretive–inductive–qualitative alternative.

Although nursing theorists and nursing scientists emphasize the importance of sociohistorical contexts and person–environment interactions, they tend to focus on "hard science" and the research process. It has been argued that there is an overvaluation of the empirical/quantitative view because it is seen as "true science" (Tinkle & Beaton, 1983). Indeed, the experimental method is held in the highest regard. A viewpoint has persisted into the 21st century in which scholars assume that descriptive or qualitative research should be performed only where there is little information available or when the science is young. Correlational research may follow and then experimental methods can be used when the two lower ("less rigid" or "less scientific") levels have been explored.

Quantitative Methods

Traditionally, within the "received" or positivistic worldview, science has been uniquely quantitative. The quantitative approach has been justified by its success in measuring, analyzing, replicating, and applying the knowledge gained (Streubert & Carpenter, 2011). According to Wolfer (1993), science should incorporate methodologic principles of objective observation/description, accurate measurement, quantification of variables, mathematical and statistical analysis, experimental methods, and verification through replication whenever possible.

Kidd and Morrison (1988) state that in their haste to prove the credibility of nursing as a profession, nursing scholars have emphasized reductionism and empirical validation through quantitative methodologies, emphasizing hypothesis testing. In this framework, the scientist develops a hypothesis about a phenomenon and seeks to prove or disprove it.

Qualitative Methods

The tradition of using qualitative methods to study human phenomena is grounded in the social sciences. Phenomenology and other methods of qualitative research arose because aspects of human values, culture, and relationships were unable to be described fully using quantitative research methods. It is generally accepted that qualitative research findings answer questions centered on social experience and give meaning to human life. Beginning in the 1970s, nursing scientists were challenged to explain phenomena that defy quantitative measurement, and qualitative approaches, which emphasize the importance of the client's perspective, began to be used in nursing research (Kidd & Morrison, 1988).

Repeatedly, scholars state that nursing research should incorporate means for determining interpretation of the phenomena of concern from the perspective of the client or care recipient. Contrary to the assertions of early scientists, many later nurse scientists believe that qualitative inquiry contains features of good science including theory and observation, logic, precision, clarity, and reproducibility (Monti & Tingen, 1999).

Methodologic Pluralism

In many respects, nursing is still undecided about which methodologic approach (qualitative or quantitative) best demonstrates the essence and uniqueness of nursing because both methods have strengths and limitations. Beck and Harrison (2016), Risjord (2010), and Wood and Haber (2018), among others, believe that the two approaches may be considered complementary and appropriate for nursing as a research-based discipline. Indeed, it is repeatedly argued that both approaches are equally important and even essential for nursing science development.

Although basic philosophical viewpoints have guided and directed research strategies in the past, recently, scholars have called for theoretical and methodologic pluralism in nursing philosophy and nursing science as presented in the discussion on postmodernism. Pluralism of research designs is essential for reflecting the uniqueness of nursing, and multiple approaches to theory development and testing should be encouraged. Because there is no one best method of developing knowledge, it is important to recognize that valuing one standard as exclusive or superior restricts the ability to progress.

Summary

Nursing is an evolving profession, an academic discipline, and a science. As nursing progresses and grows as a profession, some controversy remains on whether to emphasize a humanistic, holistic focus or an objective, scientifically derived means of comprehending reality. What is needed, and is increasingly more evident as nursing matures as a profession, is an open philosophy that ties empirical concepts that are capable of being validated through the senses with theoretical concepts of meaning and value.

It is important that future nursing leaders and novice nurse scientists possess an understanding of nursing's philosophical foundations. The legacy of philosophical positivism continues to drive beliefs in the scientific method and research strategies, but it is time to move forward to face the challenges of the increasingly complex and volatile health care environment.

Key Points

- Nursing can be considered an aspiring or evolving profession.
- Nursing is a professional discipline that draws much of its knowledge base from other disciplines, including psychology, sociology, physiology, and medicine.
- Nursing is an applied or practice science that has been influenced by several philosophical schools of thought or worldviews, including the received view (empiricism, positivism, logical positivism), the perceived view (humanism, phenomenology, constructivism), and postmodernism.
- *Nursing philosophy* refers to the worldview(s) of the profession and provides perspective for practice, scholarship, and research. *Nursing science* is the discipline-specific knowledge that focuses on the human–environment–health process and is articulated in nursing theories and generated through nursing research. *Philosophy of science in nursing* establishes the meaning of science through examination of nursing concepts, theories, and laws as they relate to nursing practice.
- Nursing epistemology (ways of knowing in nursing) has focused on four predominant or "fundamental" ways of knowledge: empirical knowledge, esthetic knowledge, personal knowledge, and ethical knowledge.
- As nursing science has developed, there has been a debate over what research methods to use (i.e., quantitative methods vs. qualitative methods). Increasingly, there has been a call for "methodologic pluralism" to better ensure that research findings are applicable in nursing practice.

Case Study

The following is adapted from a paper written by a graduate student describing an encounter in nursing practice that highlights Carper's (1978) ways of knowing in nursing.

In her work, Carper (1978) identified four patterns of knowing in nursing: empirical knowledge (science of nursing), esthetic knowledge (art of nursing), personal knowledge, and ethical knowledge. Each is essential and depends on the others to make the whole of nursing practice, and it is impossible to state which of the patterns of knowing is most important. If nurses focus exclusively on empirical knowledge, for example, nursing care would become more like medical care. But without an empirical base, the art of nursing is just tradition. Personal knowledge is gained from experience and requires a scientific basis, understanding, and empathy. Finally, the moral component is necessary to determine what is valuable, ethical, and compulsory. Each of these ways of knowing is illustrated in the following scenario.

Mrs. Smith was a 24-year-old primigravida who presented to our unit in early labor. Her husband, and father of her unborn child, had abandoned her 2 months prior to delivery, and she lacked close family support.

I cared for Mrs. Smith throughout her labor and assisted during her delivery. During this process, I taught breathing techniques to ease pain and improve coping. Position changes were encouraged periodically, and assistance was provided as needed. Mrs. Smith's care included continuous fetal monitoring, intravenous hydration, analgesic administration, back rubs, coaching and encouragement, assistance while getting an epidural, straight catheterization as needed, vital sign monitoring per policy, oxytocin administration after delivery, newborn care, and breastfeeding assistance, among many others. All care was explained in detail prior to rendering.

***Empirical knowledge** was clearly utilized in Mrs. Smith's care. Examples would be those practices based on the Association of Women's Health, Obstetric and Neonatal Nurses (AWHONN) evidence-based standards. These include guidelines for fetal heart rate monitoring and interpretation, assessment and management of Mrs. Smith while receiving her epidural analgesia, the assessment and management of side effects secondary to her regional analgesia, and even frequency for monitoring vital signs. Other examples would be assisting Mrs. Smith to an upright position during her second stage of labor to facilitate delivery and delaying nondirected pushing once she was completely dilated.*

***Esthetic knowledge**, or the art of nursing, is displayed in obstetrical nursing daily. Rather than just responding to biologic developments or spoken requests, the whole person was valued and cues were perceived and responded to for the good of the patient. The care I gave Mrs. Smith was holistic; her social, spiritual, psychological, and physical needs were all addressed in a comprehensive and seamless fashion. The empathy conveyed to the patient took into account her unique self and situation, and the care provided was reflexively tailored to her needs. I recognized the profound experience of which I was a part and adapted my actions and attitude to honor the patient and value the larger experience.*

*Many aspects of **personal knowledge** seem intertwined with esthetics, though more emphasis seems to be on the meaningful interaction between the patient and nurse. As above, the patient was cared for as a unique individual. Though secondary to the awesome nature of birth, much of the experience revolved around the powerful interpersonal relationship established. Mrs. Smith was accepted as herself. Though efforts were made by me to manage certain aspects of the experience, Mrs. Smith was allowed control and freedom of expression and reaction. She and I were both committed to the mutual though brief relationship. This knowledge stems from my own personality and ability to accept others, willingness to connect to others, and desire to collaborate with the patient regarding her care and ultimate experience.*

*The **ethical knowledge** of nursing is continuously utilized in nursing care to promote the health and well-being of the patient; and in this circumstance, the unborn child as well. Every decision made must be weighed against desired goals and values, and nurses must strive to act as advocates for each patient. When caring for a patient and an unborn child, there is a constant attempt to do no harm to either, while balancing the care of both. A very common example is the administration of medications for the mother's comfort that can cause sedation and respiratory depression in the neonate. This case involved fewer ethical considerations than many others in obstetrics. These include instances in which physicians do not respond when the nurse feels there is imminent danger and the chain of command must be utilized, or when assistance is required for the care of abortion patients or in other situations that may be in conflict with the nurses moral or religious convictions.*

A close bond was formed while I cared for Mrs. Smith and her baby. Soon after admission, she was holding my hand during contractions and had shared very intimate details of her life, separation, and fears. Though she had shared her financial concerns and had a new baby to provide for, a few weeks after her delivery I received a beautiful gift basket and card. In her note she shared that I had touched her in a way she had never expected and she vowed never to forget me; I've not forgotten her either.

Contributed by Shelli Carter, RN, MSN

Learning Activities

1. Reflect on the previous case study. Think of a situation from personal practice in which multiple ways of knowing were used. Write down the anecdote and share it with classmates.
2. With classmates, discuss whether nursing is a profession or an occupation. What can current and future nurses do to enhance nursing's standing as a profession?
3. Debate with classmates the dominant philosophical schools of thought in nursing (received view, perceived view, postmodernism). Which worldview best encompasses the profession of nursing? Why?

REFERENCES

American Association of Colleges of Nursing. (2006). *The Essentials of Doctoral Education for Advanced Nursing Practice.* Washington, DC: Author.

Beck, C. T., & Harrison, L. (2016). Mixed-methods research in the discipline of nursing. *ANS. Advances in Nursing Science, 39*(3), 224–234.

Blackburn, S. (2016). *The Oxford dictionary of philosophy* (3rd ed.). New York, NY: Oxford University Press.

Carper, B. A. (1978). Fundamental patterns of knowing in nursing. *ANS. Advances in Nursing Science, 1*(1), 13–23.

Carper, B. A. (1992). Philosophical inquiry in nursing: An application. In J. F. Kikuchi & H. Simmons (Eds.), *Philosophic inquiry in nursing* (pp. 71–80). Newbury Park, CA: Sage.

Chinn, P. L., & Kramer, M. K. (2015). *Integrated theory and knowledge development in nursing* (8th ed.). St. Louis, MO: Elsevier.

Cody, W. K., & Mitchell, G. J. (2002). Nursing knowledge and human science revisited: Practical and political considerations. *Nursing Science Quarterly, 15*(1), 4–13.

Cull-Wilby, B. L., & Pepin, J. I. (1987). Towards a coexistence of paradigms in nursing knowledge development. *Journal of Advanced Nursing, 12*(4), 515–521.

Dahnke, M. D., & Dreher, H. M. (2016). *Philosophy of science for nursing practice: Concepts and application* (2nd ed.). New York, NY: Springer Publishing.

DiBartolo, M. C. (1998). Philosophy of science in doctoral nursing education revisited. *Journal of Professional Nursing, 14*(6), 350–360.

Donaldson, S. K., & Crowley, D. M. (1978). The discipline of nursing. *Nursing Outlook, 26*(2), 113–120.

Ellis, J. R., & Hartley, C. L. (2012). *Nursing in today's world: Trends, issues, and management* (10th ed.). Philadelphia, PA: Lippincott Williams & Wilkins.

Fawcett, J. (2012). The future of nursing: How important is discipline-specific knowledge? A conversation with Jacqueline Fawcett. Interview by Dr. Janie Butts and Dr. Karen Rich. *Nursing Science Quarterly, 25*(2), 151–154.

Fawcett, J., Watson, J., Neuman, B., Walkers, P. H., & Fitzpatrick, J. (2001). On nursing theories and evidence. *Journal of Nursing Scholarship, 33*(2), 115–119.

Finkelman, A., & Kenner, C. (2016). *Professional nursing concepts: Competencies for quality leadership* (3rd ed.). Burlington, MA: Jones & Bartlett Learning.

Giuliano, K. K., Tyer-Viola, L., & Lopez, R. P. (2005). Unity of knowledge in the advancement of nursing knowledge. *Nursing Science Quarterly, 18*(3), 243–248.

Gortner, S. R., & Schultz, P. R. (1988). Approaches to nursing science methods. *Image—The Journal of Nursing Scholarship, 20*(1), 22–24.

Gustafsson, B. (2002). The philosophy of science from a nursing-scientific perspective. *Theoria, Journal of Nursing Theory, 11*(2), 3–13.

Hickman, J. S. (2011). An introduction to nursing theory. In J. B. George (Ed.), *Nursing theories: The base for professional nursing practice* (6th ed., pp. 1–22). Upper Saddle River, NJ: Pearson Education.

Holmes, D., Roy, B., & Perron, A. (2008). The use of postcolonialism in the nursing domain: Colonial patronage, conversion, and resistance. *ANS. Advances in Nursing Science, 31*(1), 42–51.

Holzemer, W. L. (2007). Towards understanding nursing science. *Japan Journal of Nursing Science, 4*(1), 57–59.

Hood, L. J. (2014). *Leddy & Pepper's conceptual bases of professional nursing* (8th ed.). Philadelphia, PA: Lippincott Williams & Wilkins.

Institute of Medicine. (2011). *The future of nursing: Leading change, advancing health.* Washington, DC: National Academies Press.

Institute of Medicine. (2016). *Assessing progress on the Institute of Medicine report: The future of nursing.* Washington, DC: National Academies Press.

Judd, D., & Sitzman, K. (2014). *A history of American nursing: Trends and eras* (2nd ed.). Burlington, MA: Jones & Bartlett Learning.

Kidd, P., & Morrison, E. F. (1988). The progression of knowledge in nursing research: A search for meaning. *Image—The Journal of Nursing Scholarship, 20*(4), 222–224.

Litchfield, M. C., & Jónsdóttir, H. (2008). A practice discipline that's here and now. *ANS. Advances in Nursing Science, 31*(1), 79–91.

McGibbon, E., Mulaudzi, F. M., Didham, P., Barton, S., & Sochan, A. (2014). Toward decolonizing nursing: The colonization of nursing and strategies for increasing the counter-narrative. *Nursing Inquiry, 21*(3), 179–191.

Meleis, A. I. (2012). *Theoretical nursing: Development and progress* (5th ed.). Philadelphia, PA: Lippincott Williams & Wilkins.

Monti, E. J., & Tingen, M. S. (1999). Multiple paradigms of nursing science. *ANS. Advances in Nursing Science, 21*(4), 64–80.

Moody, L. E. (1990). *Advancing nursing science through research.* Newbury Park, CA: Sage.

Morse, J. M. (2017). *Analyzing and conceptualizing the theoretical foundations of nursing.* New York, NY: Springer Publishing.

Newman, M. A., Sime, A. M., & Corcoran-Perry, S. A. (1991). The focus of the discipline of nursing. *ANS. Advances in Nursing Science, 14*(1), 1–6.

Northrup, D. T., Tschanz, C. L., Olynyk, V. G., Makaroff, K. L. S., Szabo, J., & Biasio, H. A. (2004). Nursing: Whose discipline is it anyway? *Nursing Science Quarterly, 17*(1), 55–62.

Nyatanga, L. (2005). Nursing and the philosophy of science. 1991. *Nurse Education Today, 25,* 670–674.

Oldnall, A. S. (1995). Nursing as an emerging academic discipline. *Journal of Advanced Nursing, 21,* 605–612.

Paley, J. (2005). Phenomenology as rhetoric. *Nursing Inquiry, 12*(2), 106–116.

Parse, R. R. (1997). The language of nursing knowledge: Saying what we mean. In I. M. King & J. Fawcett (Eds.), *The language of nursing theory and metatheory* (pp. 73–77). Indianapolis, IN: Center Nursing Press.

Parse, R. R. (2015). Nursing: A basic or applied science. *Nursing Science Quarterly, 28*(3), 181–182.

Parse, R. R. (2016). Where have all the nursing theories gone? *Nursing Science Quarterly, 29*(2), 101–102.

Polifroni, E. C. (2015). Philosophy of science: An introduction. In J. B. Butts & K. L. Rich (Eds.), *Philosophies and theories for advanced nursing practice* (2nd ed., pp. 3–18). Burlington, MA: Jones & Bartlett Learning.

Powers, B. A., & Knapp, T. R. (2011). *Dictionary of nursing theory and research* (4th ed.). New York, NY: Springer Publishing.

Racine, L. (2009). Applying Antonio Gramsci's philosophy to postcolonial feminist social and political activism in nursing. *Nursing Philosophy, 10*(3), 180–190.

Reed, P. G. (1995). A treatise on nursing knowledge development in the 21st century: Beyond postmodernism. *ANS. Advances in Nursing Science, 17*(3), 70–84.

Reed, P. G. (2008). Adversity and advancing nursing knowledge. *Nursing Science Quarterly, 21*(2), 133–134.

Riegel, B., Omery, A., Calvillo, E., Elsayed, N. G., Lee, P., Shuler, P., et al. (1992). Moving beyond: A generative philosophy of science. *Image—The Journal of Nursing Scholarship, 24*(2), 115–120.

Risjord, M. W. (2010). *Nursing knowledge: Science, practice, and philosophy.* London, United Kingdom: Wiley-Blackwell.

Risjord, M. W., Dunbar, S. B., & Moloney, M. F. (2002). A new foundation for methodological triangulation. *Journal of Nursing Scholarship, 34*(3), 269–275.

Rodgers, B. L. (2015). The evolution of nursing science. In J. B. Butts & K. L. Rich (Eds.), *Philosophies and theories for advanced nursing practice* (2nd ed., pp. 19–50). Burlington, MA: Jones & Bartlett Learning.

Rutty, J. E. (1998). The nature of philosophy of science, theory and knowledge relating to nursing and professionalism. *Journal of Advanced Nursing, 28*(2), 243–250.

Schultz, P. R., & Meleis, A. I. (1988). Nursing epistemology: Traditions, insights, questions. *Image—The Journal of Nursing Scholarship, 20*(4), 217–221.

Silva, M. C. (1977). Philosophy, science, theory: Interrelationships and implications for nursing research. *Image—The Journal of Nursing Scholarship, 9*(3), 59–63.

Silva, M. C., & Rothbart, D. (1984). An analysis of changing trends of philosophies of science on nursing theory development and testing. *ANS. Advances in Nursing Science, 6*(2), 1–13.

Silva, M. C., Sorrell, J. M., & Sorrell, C. D. (1995). From Carper's patterns of knowing to ways of being: An ontological philosophical shift in nursing. *ANS. Advances in Nursing Science, 18*(1), 1–13.

Streubert, H. J., & Carpenter, D. R. (2011). *Qualitative research in nursing: Advancing the humanistic imperative* (5th ed.). Philadelphia, PA: Lippincott Williams & Wilkins.

Suppe, F., & Jacox, A. (1985). Philosophy of science and the development of nursing theory. In H. H. Werley & J. J. Fitzpatrick (Eds.), *Annual review of nursing research* (pp. 241–267). New York, NY: Springer Publishing.

Teichman, J., & Evans, K. C. (1999). *Philosophy: A beginner's guide* (3rd ed.). Cambridge, MA: Blackwell.

Tinkle, M. B., & Beaton, J. L. (1983). Toward a new view of science: Implications for nursing research. *ANS. Advances in Nursing Science, 5*(2), 27–36.

Walker, L. O., & Avant, K. (2011). *Strategies for theory construction in nursing* (5th ed.). Upper Saddle River, NJ: Pearson Prentice Hall.

Wolfer, J. (1993). Aspects of "reality" and ways of knowing in nursing: In search of an integrating paradigm. *Image—The Journal of Nursing Scholarship, 25*(2), 141–146.

Wood, G. L., & Haber, J. (2018). *Nursing research: Methods and critical appraisal for evidence-based practice* (9th ed.). St. Louis, MO: Elsevier.

2

Overview of Theory in Nursing

Melanie McEwen

Matt Ng has been an emergency room nurse for almost 6 years and recently decided to enroll in a master's degree program to become an acute care nurse practitioner. As he read over the degree requirements, Matt was somewhat bewildered. One of the first courses in his program was entitled Application of Theory in Nursing. He was interested in the courses in advanced pharmacology, advanced physical assessment, and pathophysiology and was excited about the advanced practice clinical courses, but a course that focused on nursing theory did not appear congruent with his goals.

Looking over the syllabus for the theory application course did little to reassure Matt, but he was determined to make the best of the situation and went to the first class with an open mind. The first few class periods were increasingly interesting as the students and instructor discussed the historical evolution of the discipline of nursing and the stages of nursing theory development. As the course progressed, the topics became more relevant to Matt. He learned ways to analyze and evaluate theories, examined a number of different types of theories used by nurses, and completed several assignments, including a concept analysis, an analysis of a middle range nursing theory, and a synthesis paper that examined the use of non-nursing theories in nursing research.

By the end of the semester, Matt was able to recognize the importance of the study of theory. He understood how theoretical principles and concepts affected his current practice and how they would be essential to consider as he continued his studies to become an advanced practice nurse.

When asked about theory, many nurses and nursing students, and often even nursing faculty, will respond with a furrowed brow, a pained expression, and a resounding "ugh." When questioned about their negative response, most will admit that the idea of studying theory is confusing, that they see no practical value, and that theory is, in essence, too theoretical.

Likewise, some nursing scholars believe that nursing theory is practically nonexistent, whereas others recognize that many practitioners have not heard of nursing theory.

Some nurses lament that nurse researchers use theories and frameworks from other disciplines, whereas others believe the notion of nursing theory is outdated and ask why they should bother with theory. Questions and debates about "theory" in nursing abound in the nursing literature.

Myra Levine, one of the pioneer nursing theorists, wrote that "the introduction of the idea of theory in nursing was sadly inept" (Levine, 1995, p. 11). She stated,

> In traditional nursing fashion, early efforts were directed at creating a procedure—a recipe book for prospective theorists—which then could be used to decide what was and was not a theory. And there was always the thread of expectation that the great, grand, global theory would appear and end all speculation. Most of the early theorists really believed they were achieving that.

Levine (1995) went on to explain that every new theory posited new central concepts, definitions, relational statements, and goals for nursing and then attracted a chorus of critics. This resulted in nurses finding themselves confused about the substance and intention of the theories. Indeed, "In early days, theory was expected to be obscure. If it was clearly understandable, it wasn't considered a very good theory" (Levine, 1995, p. 11).

The drive to develop nursing theory has been marked by nursing theory conferences, the proliferation of theoretical and conceptual frameworks for nursing, and the formal teaching of theory development in graduate nursing education. It has resulted in the development of many systems, techniques or processes for theory analysis and evaluation, a fascination with the philosophy of science, and confusion about theory development strategies and division of choice of research methodologies.

There is debate over the types of theories that should be used by nurses. Should they be only nursing theories or can nurses use theories "borrowed" from other disciplines? There is debate over terminology such as *conceptual framework*, *conceptual model*, and *theory*. There have been heated discussions concerning the appropriate level of theory for nurses to develop as well as how, why, where, and when to test, measure, analyze, and evaluate these theories/models/conceptual frameworks. The question has been repeatedly asked: Should nurses adopt a single theory, or do multiple theories serve them best? It is no wonder, then, that nursing students display consternation, bewilderment, and even anxiety when presented with the prospect of studying theory. One premise, however, can be agreed upon: To be useful, a theory must be meaningful and relevant, but above all, it must be understandable. This chapter discusses many of the issues described previously. It presents the rationale for studying and using theory in nursing practice, research, management/administration, and education; gives definitions of key terms; provides an overview of the history of development of theory utilization in nursing; describes the scope of theory and levels of theory; and, finally, introduces the widely accepted nursing metaparadigm.

Overview of Theory

Most scholars agree that it is the unique theories and perspectives used by a discipline that distinguish it from other disciplines. The theories used by members of a profession clarify basic assumptions and values shared by its members and define the nature, outcome, and purpose of practice (Alligood, 2014a; Fawcett, 2012; Rutty, 1998).

Definitions of the term *theory* abound in the nursing literature. At a basic level, theory has been described as a systematic explanation of an event in which constructs and concepts are identified and relationships are proposed and predictions made (Streubert & Carpenter, 2011). Theory has also been defined as a "creative and rigorous structuring of ideas that project a tentative, purposeful and systematic view of phenomena" (Chinn & Kramer, 2015, p. 255). Finally, theory has been called a set of interpretative assumptions, principles, or propositions that help explain or guide action (Young, Taylor, & Renpenning, 2001).

In their classic work, Dickoff and James (1968) state that theory is invented rather than found in or discovered from reality. Furthermore, theories vary according to the number of elements, the characteristics and complexity of the elements, and the kind of relationships between or among the elements.

The Importance of Theory in Nursing

Before the advent of development of nursing theories, nursing was largely subsumed under medicine. Nursing practice was generally prescribed by others and highlighted by traditional, ritualistic tasks with little regard to rationale. The initial work of nursing theorists was aimed at clarifying the complex intellectual and interactional domains that distinguish expert nursing practice from the mere doing of tasks (Omrey, Kasper, & Page, 1995). It was believed that conceptual models and theories could create mechanisms by which nurses would communicate their professional convictions, provide a moral/ethical structure to guide actions, and foster a means of systematic thinking about nursing and its practice (Chinn & Kramer, 2015; Peterson, 2017; Sitzman & Eichelberger, 2011; Ziegler, 2005). The idea that a single, unified model of nursing—a worldview of the discipline—might emerge was encouraged by some (Levine, 1995; Tierney, 1998).

It is widely believed that use of theory offers structure and organization to nursing knowledge and provides a systematic means of collecting data to describe, explain, and predict nursing practice. Use of theory also promotes rational and systematic practice by challenging and validating intuition. Theories make nursing practice more overtly purposeful by stating not only the focus of practice but also specific goals and outcomes. Theories define and clarify nursing and the purpose of nursing practice to distinguish it from other caring professions by setting professional boundaries. Finally, use of a theory in nursing leads to coordinated and less fragmented care (Alligood, 2014a; Chinn & Kramer, 2015; Ziegler, 2005).

Ways in which theories and conceptual models developed by nurses have influenced nursing practice are described by Fawcett (1992), who stated that in nursing they:

- Identify certain standards for nursing practice.
- Identify settings in which nursing practice should occur and the characteristics of what the model's author considers recipients of nursing care.
- Identify distinctive nursing processes and technologies to be used, including parameters for client assessment, labels for client problems, a strategy for planning, a typology of intervention, and criteria for evaluation of intervention outcomes.
- Direct the delivery of nursing services.
- Serve as the basis for clinical information systems, including the admission database, nursing orders, care plan, progress notes, and discharge summary.
- Guide the development of client classification systems.
- Direct quality assurance programs.

Terminology of Theory

In nursing, conceptual models or frameworks detail a network of concepts and describe their relationships, thereby explaining broad nursing phenomena. Theories, according to Young and colleagues (2001), are the narrative that accompanies the conceptual model. These theories typically provide a detailed description of all of the components of the model and outline relationships in the form of propositions. Critical components of the theory or narrative include definitions of the central concepts or constructs; propositions or relational statements; the assumptions on which the framework is based; and the purpose, indications for use, or application. Many conceptual frameworks and theories will also include a schematic drawing or model depicting the overall structure of or interactivity of the components (Chinn & Kramer, 2015).

Some terms may be new to students of theory and others need clarification. Table 2-1 lists definitions for a number of terms that are frequently encountered in writings on theory. Many of these terms will be described in more detail later in the chapter and in subsequent chapters.

Historical Overview: Theory Development in Nursing

Most nursing scholars credit Florence Nightingale with being the first modern nursing theorist. Nightingale was the first to delineate what she considered nursing's goal and practice domain, and she postulated that "to nurse" meant having charge of the personal health of someone. She believed the role of the nurse was seen as placing the client "in the best condition for nature to act upon him" (Hilton, 1997, p. 1211).

Florence Nightingale

Nightingale received her formal training in nursing in Kaiserswerth, Germany, in 1851. Following her renowned service for the British army during the Crimean War, she returned to London and established a school for nurses. According to Nightingale, formal training for nurses was necessary to "teach not only what is to be done, but how to do it." She was the first to advocate the teaching of symptoms and what they indicate. Furthermore, she taught the importance of rationale for actions and stressed the significance of "trained powers of observation and reflection" (Kalisch & Kalisch, 2004, p. 36).

In *Notes on Nursing*, published in 1859, Nightingale proposed basic premises for nursing practice. In her view, nurses were to make astute observations of the sick and their environment, record observations, and develop knowledge about factors that promoted healing. Her framework for nursing emphasized the utility of empirical knowledge, and she believed that knowledge developed and used by nurses should be distinct from medical knowledge. She insisted that trained nurses control and staff nursing schools and manage nursing practice in homes and hospitals (Chinn & Kramer, 2015; Kalisch & Kalisch, 2004).

Stages of Theory Development in Nursing

Subsequent to Nightingale, almost a century passed before other nursing scholars attempted the development of philosophical and theoretical works to describe and define nursing and to guide nursing practice. Kidd and Morrison (1988) described five stages in the development of nursing theory and philosophy: (1) silent knowledge,

Table 2-1 Definitions and Characteristics of Theory Terms and Concepts

Term	Definition and Characteristics
Assumptions	Assumptions are beliefs about phenomena one must accept as true to accept a theory about the phenomena as true. Assumptions may be based on accepted knowledge or personal beliefs and values. Although assumptions may not be susceptible to testing, they can be argued philosophically.
Borrowed or shared theory	A borrowed theory is a theory developed in another discipline that is not adapted to the worldview and practice of nursing.
Concept	Concepts are the elements or components of a phenomenon necessary to understand the phenomenon. They are abstract and derived from impressions the human mind receives about phenomena through sensing the environment.
Conceptual model/ conceptual framework	A conceptual model is a set of interrelated concepts that symbolically represents and conveys a mental image of a phenomenon. Conceptual models of nursing identify concepts and describe their relationships to the phenomena of central concern to the discipline.
Construct	Constructs are the most complex type of concept. They comprise more than one concept and are typically built or constructed by the theorist or philosopher to fit a purpose. The terms *concept* and *construct* are often used interchangeably, but some authors use concept as the more general term—all constructs are concepts, but not all concepts are constructs.
Empirical indicator	Empirical indicators are very specific and concrete identifiers of concepts. They are actual instructions, experimental conditions, and procedures used to observe or measure the concept(s) of a theory.
Epistemology	Epistemology refers to theories of knowledge or how people come to have knowledge; in nursing, it is the study of the origins of nursing knowledge.
Hypotheses	Hypotheses are tentative suggestions that a specific relationship exists between two concepts or propositions. As the hypothesis is repeatedly confirmed, it progresses to an empirical generalization and ultimately to a law.
Knowledge	Knowledge refers to the awareness or perception of reality acquired through insight, learning, or investigation. In a discipline, knowledge is what is collectively seen to be a reasonably accurate understanding of the world as seen by members of the discipline.
Laws	A law is a proposition about the relationship between concepts in a theory that has been repeatedly validated. Laws are highly generalizable. Laws are found primarily in disciplines that deal with observable and measurable phenomena, such as chemistry and physics. Conversely, social and human sciences have few laws.
Metaparadigm	A metaparadigm represents the worldview of a discipline—the global perspective that subsumes more specific views and approaches to the central concepts with which the discipline is concerned. The metaparadigm is the ideology within which the theories, knowledge, and processes for knowing find meaning and coherence. Nursing's metaparadigm is generally thought to consist of the concepts of person, environment, health, and nursing.
Middle range theory	Middle range theory refers to a part of a discipline's concerns related to particular topics. The scope is narrower than that of broad-range or grand theories.
Model	Models are graphic or symbolic representations of phenomena that objectify and present certain perspectives or points of view about nature or function or both. Models may be theoretical (something not directly observable—expressed in language or mathematics symbols) or empirical (replicas of observable reality—e.g., model of an eye).
Ontology	Ontology is concerned with the study of existence and the nature of reality.

(continued)

Table 2-1 Definitions and Characteristics of Theory Terms and Concepts (Continued)	
Term	**Definition and Characteristics**
Paradigm	A paradigm is an organizing framework that contains concepts, theories, assumptions, beliefs, values, and principles that form the way a discipline interprets the subject matter with which it is concerned. It describes work to be done and frames an orientation within which the work will be accomplished. A discipline may have a number of paradigms. The term *paradigm* is associated with Kuhn's *Structure of Scientific Revolutions*.
Phenomena	Phenomena are the designation of an aspect of reality; the phenomena of interest become the subject matter particular to the primary concerns of a discipline.
Philosophy	A philosophy is a statement of beliefs and values about human beings and their world.
Practice or situation-specific theory	A practice or situation-specific theory deals with a limited range of discrete phenomena that are specifically defined and are not expanded to include their link with the broad concerns of a discipline.
Praxis	Praxis is the application of a theory to cases encountered in experience.
Relationship statements	Relationship statements indicate specific relationships between two or more concepts. They may be classified as propositions, hypotheses, laws, axioms, or theorems.
Taxonomy	A taxonomy is a classification scheme for defining or gathering together various phenomena. Taxonomies range in complexity from simple dichotomies to complicated hierarchical structures.
Theory	Theory refers to a set of logically interrelated concepts, statements, propositions, and definitions, which have been derived from philosophical beliefs of scientific data and from which questions or hypotheses can be deduced, tested, and verified. A theory purports to account for or characterize some phenomenon.
Worldview	Worldview is the philosophical frame of reference used by a social or cultural group to describe that group's outlook on and beliefs about reality.

Sources: Alligood (2014b); Blackburn (2016); Chinn and Kramer (2015); Powers and Knapp (2011).

(2) received knowledge, (3) subjective knowledge, (4) procedural knowledge, and (5) constructed knowledge. Table 2-2 gives an overview of characteristics of each of these stages in the development of nursing theory, and each stage is described in the following sections. To contemporize Kidd and Morrison's work, attention will be given to the current decade and a new stage—that of "integrated knowledge."

Silent Knowledge Stage
Recognizing the impact of the poorly trained nurses on the health of soldiers during the Civil War, in 1868, the American Medical Association advocated the formal training of nurses and suggested that schools of nursing be attached to hospitals with instruction being provided by medical staff and resident physicians. The first training school for nurses in the United States was opened in 1872 at the New England Hospital. Three more schools, located in New York, New Haven, and Boston, opened shortly thereafter (Kalisch & Kalisch, 2004). Most schools were under the control of hospitals and superintended by hospital administrators and physicians. Education and practice were based on rules, principles, and traditions that were passed along through an apprenticeship form of education.

There followed rapid growth in the number of hospital-based training programs for nurses, and by 1909, there were more than 1,000 such programs (Kalisch &

Table 2-2 Stages in the Development of Nursing Theory

Stage	Source of Knowledge	Impact on Theory and Research
Silent knowledge	Blind obedience to medical authority	Little attempt to develop theory. Research was limited to collection of epidemiologic data.
Received knowledge	Learning through listening to others	Theories were borrowed from other disciplines. As nurses acquired non-nursing doctoral degrees, they relied on the authority of educators, sociologists, psychologists, physiologists, and anthropologists to provide answers to nursing problems. Research was primarily educational research or sociologic research.
Subjective knowledge	Authority was internalized to foster a new sense of self.	A negative attitude toward borrowed theories and science emerged. Nurse scholars focused on defining nursing and on developing theories about and for nursing. Nursing research focused on the nurse rather than on clients and clinical situations.
Procedural knowledge	Includes both separate and connected knowledge	Proliferation of approaches to theory development. Application of theory in practice was frequently under-emphasized. Emphasis was placed on the procedures used to acquire knowledge, with focused attention to the appropriateness of methodology, the criteria for evolution, and statistical procedures for data analysis.
Constructed knowledge	Combination of different types of knowledge (intuition, reason, and self-knowledge)	Recognition that nursing theory should be based on prior empirical studies, theoretical literature, client reports of clinical experiences and feelings, and the nurse scholar's intuition or related knowledge about the phenomenon of concern
Integrated knowledge	Assimilation and application of "evidence" from nursing and other health care disciplines	Nursing theory will increasingly incorporate information from published literature with enhanced emphasis on clinical application as situation-specific/practice theories and middle range theories.

Source: Kidd and Morrison (1988).

Kalisch, 2004). In these early schools, a meager amount of theory was taught by physicians, and practice was taught by experienced nurses. The curricula contained some anatomy and physiology and occasional lectures on special diseases. Few nursing books were available, and the emphasis was on carrying out physicians' orders. Nursing education and practice focused on the performance of technical skills and application of a few basic principles, such as aseptic technique and principles of mobility. Nurses depended on physicians' diagnosis and orders and as a result largely adhered to the medical model, which views body and mind separately and focuses on cure and treatment of pathologic problems (Donahue, 2011). Hospital administrators saw nurses as inexpensive labor. Nurses were exploited both as students and as experienced workers. They were taught to be submissive and obedient, and they learned to fulfill their responsibilities to physicians without question (Chinn & Kramer, 2015).

Unfortunately, with a few exceptions, this model of nursing education persisted for more than 80 years. One exception was Yale University, which started the first autonomous school of nursing in 1924. At Yale, and in other later collegiate programs, professional training was strengthened by in-depth exposure to the underlying theory of disease as well as the social, psychological, and physical aspects of client welfare. The growth of collegiate programs lagged, however, due to opposition from many physicians who argued that university-educated nurses were overtrained. Hospital schools continued to insist that nursing education meant acquisition of technical skills and that knowledge of theory was unnecessary and might actually handicap the nurse (Donahue, 2011; Judd & Sitzman, 2014; Kalisch & Kalisch, 2004).

Received Knowledge Stage

It was not until after World War II that substantive changes were made in nursing education. During the late 1940s and into the 1950s, serious nursing shortages were fueled by a decline in nursing school enrollments. A 1948 report, *Nursing for the Future*, by Esther Brown, PhD, compared nursing with teaching. Brown noted that the current model of nursing education was central to the problems of the profession and recommended that efforts be made to provide nursing education in universities as opposed to the apprenticeship system that existed in most hospital programs (Donahue, 2011; Kalisch & Kalisch, 2004).

Other factors during this time challenged the tradition of hospital-based training for nurses. One of these factors was a dramatic increase in the number of hospitals resulting from the Hill-Burton Act, which worsened the ongoing and sometimes critical nursing shortage. In addition, professional organizations for nurses were restructured and began to grow. It was also during this time that state licensure testing for registration took effect, and by 1949, 41 states required testing. The registration requirement necessitated that education programs review the content matter they were teaching to determine minimum criteria and some degree of uniformity. In addition, the techniques and processes used in instruction were also reviewed and evaluated (Kalisch & Kalisch, 2004).

Over the next decade, a number of other events occurred that altered nursing education and nursing practice. In 1950, the journal *Nursing Research* was first published. The American Nurses Association (ANA) began a program to encourage nurses to pursue graduate education to study nursing functions and practice. Books on research methods and explicit theories of nursing began to appear. In 1956, the Health Amendments Act authorized funds for financial aid to promote graduate education for full-time study to prepare nurses for administration, supervision, and teaching. These events resulted in a slow but steady increase in graduate nursing education programs.

The first doctoral programs in nursing originated within schools of education at Teachers College of Columbia University (1933) and New York University (1934). But it would be 20 more years before the first doctoral program in nursing began at the University of Pittsburgh (1954) (Kalisch & Kalisch, 2004).

Subjective Knowledge Stage

Until the 1950s, nursing practice was principally derived from social, biologic, and medical theories. With the exceptions of Nightingale's work in the 1850s, nursing theory had its beginnings with the publication of Hildegard Peplau's book in 1952. Peplau described the interpersonal process between the nurse and the client. This started a revolution in nursing, and in the late 1950s and 1960s, a number of nurse theorists emerged seeking to provide an independent conceptual framework for nursing education and practice (Donahue, 2011). The nurse's role came under scrutiny during this decade as nurse leaders debated the nature of nursing practice and theory development.

During the 1960s, the development of nursing theory was heavily influenced by three philosophers, James Dickoff, Patricia James, and Ernestine Wiedenbach, who, in a series of articles, described theory development and the nature of theory for a practice discipline. Other approaches to theory development combined direct observations of practice, insights derived from existing theories and other literature sources, and insights derived from explicit philosophical perspectives about nursing and the nature of health and human experience. Early theories were characterized by a functional view of nursing and health. They attempted to define what nursing is, describe the social purposes nursing serves, explain how nurses function to realize these purposes, and identify parameters and variables that influence illness and health (Chinn & Kramer, 2015).

In the 1960s, a number of nurse leaders (Abdellah, Orlando, Wiedenbach, Hall, Henderson, Levine, and Rogers) developed and published their views of nursing. Their descriptions of nursing and nursing models evolved from their personal, professional, and educational experiences and reflected their perception of ideal nursing practice.

Procedural Knowledge Stage

By the 1970s, the nursing profession viewed itself as a scientific discipline evolving toward a theoretically based practice focusing on the client. In the late 1960s and early 1970s, several nursing theory conferences were held. Also, significantly, in 1972, the National League for Nursing implemented a requirement that the curricula for nursing educational programs be based on conceptual frameworks. During these years, many nursing theorists published their beliefs and ideas about nursing and some developed conceptual models.

During the 1970s, a consensus developed among nursing leaders regarding common elements of nursing. These were the nature of nursing (roles/actions/interventions), the individual recipient of care (client), the context of nurse–client interactions (environment), and health. Nurses debated whether there should be one conceptual model for nursing or several models to describe the relationships among the nurse, client, environment, and health. Books were written for nurses on how to critique, develop, and apply nursing theories. Graduate schools developed courses on analysis and application of theory, and researchers identified nursing theories as conceptual frameworks for their studies. Through the late 1970s and early 1980s, theories moved to characterizing nursing's role from "what nurses do" to "what nursing is." This changed nursing from a context-dependent, reactive position to a context-independent, proactive arena (Chinn & Kramer, 2015).

Although master's programs were growing steadily, doctoral programs grew more slowly, but by 1970, there were 20 such programs. This growth in graduate nursing education allowed nurse scholars to debate ideas, viewpoints, and research methods in the nursing literature. As a result, nurses began to question the ideas that were taken for granted in nursing and the traditional basis in which nursing was practiced.

Constructed Knowledge Stage

During the late 1980s, scholars began to concentrate on theories that provide meaningful foundation for nursing practice. There was a call to develop substance in theory and to focus on nursing concepts grounded in practice and linked to research. The 1990s into the early 21st century saw an increasing emphasis on philosophy and philosophy of science in nursing. Attention shifted from grand theories to middle range theories as well as application of theory in research and practice.

In the 1990s, the idea of evidence-based practice (EBP) was introduced into nursing to address the widespread recognition of the need to move beyond attention given to research per se in order to address the gap in research and practice. The "evidence" is research that has been completed and published (LoBiondo-Wood & Haber, 2014). Ostensibly, EBP promotes employment of theory-based, research-derived evidence to guide nursing practice.

During this period, graduate education in nursing continued to grow rapidly, particularly among programs that produced advanced practice nurses (APNs). A seminal event during this time was the introduction of the doctor of nursing practice (DNP). The DNP was initially proposed by the American Association of Colleges of Nursing (AACN) in 2004 to be the terminal degree for APNs. The impetus for the DNP was based on recognition of the need for expanded competencies due to the increasing complexity of clinical practice, enhanced knowledge to improve nursing practice and outcomes, and promotion of leadership skills (AACN, 2004).

Integrated Knowledge Stage

More recently, development of nursing knowledge shifted to a trend that blends and uses a variety of processes to achieve a given research aim as opposed to adherence to strict, accepted methodologies (Chinn & Kramer, 2015). In the second decade of the 21st century, there has been significant attention to the need to direct nursing knowledge development toward clinical relevance, to address what Risjord (2010) terms the "relevance gap." Indeed, as Risjord states, and virtually all nursing scholars would agree, "The primary goal . . . of nursing research is to produce knowledge that supports practice" (p. 4). But he continues to note that in reality, a significant portion of research supports practice imperfectly, infrequently, and often insignificantly.

In the current stage of knowledge development, considerable focus in nursing science has been on integration of knowledge into practice, largely with increased attention on EBP and translational research (Chinn & Kramer, 2015). Indeed, it is widely accepted that systematic review of research from a variety of health disciplines, often in the form of meta-analyses, should be undertaken to inform practice and policy making in nursing (Melnyk & Fineout-Overholt, 2015; Schmidt & Brown, 2015). Furthermore, this involves or includes application of evidence from across all health-related sciences (i.e., translational research).

Translational research was designated a priority initiative by the National Institutes of Health in 2005 (Powers & Knapp, 2011). The idea of translational research is to close the gap between scientific discovery and translation of research into practice; the intent is to validate evidence in the practice setting (Chinn & Kramer, 2015). Translational research shifts focus to interdisciplinary efforts and integration of the perspectives of different disciplines to "a contemporary movement aimed at producing a concerted multidisciplinary effort to address recognized health disparities and care delivery inadequacies" (Powers & Knapp, 2011, p. 191).

Into the second decade of the 21st century, the number of doctoral programs in the United States continued to grow steadily, and by 2016, there were 128 doctoral programs granting a doctor of philosophy (PhD) in nursing (AACN, 2017a). Furthermore, after a sometimes contentious debate, the DNP gained widespread acceptance, and by 2017, there were 303 programs granting the DNP, with many more being planned (AACN, 2017b).

In this current stage of theory development in nursing, it is anticipated that there will be ongoing interest in EBP and growth of translational research. In this regard, development and application of middle range and practice theories will continue to be stressed, with attention increasing on practical/clinical application and relevance of both research and theory.

Summary of Stages of Nursing Theory Development

A number of events and individuals have had an impact on the development and utilization of theory in nursing practice, research, and education. Table 2-3 provides a summary of significant events.

Table 2-3 Significant Events in Theory Development in Nursing

Event	Year
Nightingale publishes *Notes on Nursing*	1859
American Medical Association advocates formal training for nurses	1868
Teacher's College—Columbia University—Doctorate in Education degree for nursing	1920
Yale University begins the first collegiate school of nursing	1924
Report by Dr. Esther Brown—"Nursing for the Future"	1948
State licensure for registration becomes standard	1949
Nursing Research first published	1950
H. Peplau publishes *Interpersonal Relations in Nursing*	1952
University of Pittsburgh begins the first doctor of philosophy (PhD) program in nursing	1954
Health Amendments Act passes—funds graduate nursing education	1956
Process of theory development discussed among nursing scholars (works published by Abdellah, Henderson, Orlando, Wiedenbach, and others)	1960–1966
First symposium on Theory Development in Nursing (published in *Nursing Research* in 1968)	1967
Symposium Theory Development in Nursing	1968
Dickoff, James, and Wiedenbach—"Theory in a Practice Discipline"	
First Nursing Theory Conference	1969
Second Nursing Theory Conference	1970
Third Nursing Theory Conference	1971
National League for Nursing adopts Requirement for Conceptual Framework for Nursing Curricula	1972
Key articles publish in *Nursing Research* (Hardy—Theories: Components, Development, and Evaluation; Jacox—Theory Construction in Nursing; and Johnson—Development of Theory)	1974
Nurse educator conferences on nursing theory	1975, 1978
Advances in Nursing Science first published	1979
Books written for nurses on how to critique theory, develop theory, and apply nursing theory	1980s
Graduate schools of nursing develop courses on how to analyze and apply theory in nursing	1980s
Research studies in nursing identify nursing theories as frameworks for study	1980s
Publication of numerous books on analysis, application, evaluation, and development of nursing theories	1980s
Philosophy and philosophy of science courses offered in doctoral programs	1990s
Increasing emphasis on middle range and practice theories for nursing	1990s
Nursing literature describes the need to establish interconnections among central nursing concepts	1990s
Introduction of evidence-based practice into nursing	1990s
Philosophy of Nursing first published	1999
Books published describing, analyzing, and discussing application of middle range theory and evidence-based practice	2000s
Introduction of the doctor of nursing practice (DNP)	2004
Growing emphasis on development of situation-specific and middle range theories in nursing	2010+
Attention to theory utilization and development of theories to guide nursing research, practice, education, and administration	2010+
Focus on clinical application of evidence-based practice, practice-based evidence, and translational research	2010+

Sources: Alligood (2014a); Chinn and Kramer (2015); Donahue (2011); Kalisch and Kalisch (2004); Meleis (2012); Moody (1990).

Beginning in the early 1950s, efforts to represent nursing theoretically produced broad conceptualizations of nursing practice. These conceptual models or frameworks proliferated during the 1960s and 1970s. Although the conceptual models were not developed using traditional scientific research processes, they did provide direction for nursing by focusing on a general ideal of practice that served as a guide for research and education. Table 2-4 lists the works of many of the nursing theorists and the titles and year of key theoretical publications. The works of a number of the major theorists are discussed in Chapters 7 through 9. Reference lists and bibliographies outlining application of their work to research, education, and practice are described in those chapters.

Classification of Theories in Nursing

Over the last 40 years, a number of methods for classifying theory in nursing have been described. These include classification based on range/scope or abstractness (grand or macrotheory to practice or situation-specific theory) and type or purpose of the theory (descriptive, predictive, or prescriptive theory). Both of these classification schemes are discussed in the following sections.

Scope of Theory

One method for classification of theories in nursing that has become common is to differentiate theories based on scope, which refers to complexity and degree of abstraction. The scope of a theory includes its level of specificity and the concreteness of its concepts and propositions. This classification scheme typically uses the terms *metatheory, philosophy*, or *worldview* to describe the philosophical basis of the discipline; *grand theory* or *macrotheory* to describe the comprehensive conceptual frameworks; *middle range* or *midrange* theory to describe frameworks that are relatively more focused than the grand theories; and *situation-specific theory*, *practice theory*, or *microtheory* to describe those smallest in scope (Higgins & Moore, 2000; Peterson, 2017; Whall, 2016). Theories differ in complexity and scope along a continuum from practice or situation-specific theories to grand theories. Figure 2-1 compares the scope of nursing theory by level of abstractness.

Metatheory
Metatheory refers to a theory about theory. In nursing, metatheory focuses on broad issues such as the processes of generating knowledge and theory development, and it is a forum for debate within the discipline (Chinn & Kramer, 2015; Powers & Knapp, 2011). Philosophical and methodologic issues at the metatheory or worldview level include identifying the purposes and kinds of theory needed for nursing, developing and analyzing methods for creating nursing theory, and proposing criteria for evaluating theory (Hickman, 2011; Walker & Avant, 2011).

Walker and Avant (2011) presented an overview of historical trends in nursing metatheory. Beginning in the 1960s, metatheory discussions involved nursing as an academic discipline and the relationship of nursing to basic sciences. Later discussions addressed the predominant philosophical worldviews (received view versus perceived view) and methodologic issues related to research (see Chapter 1). Recent metatheoretical issues relate to the philosophy of nursing and address what levels of theory development are needed for nursing practice, research, and education (i.e., grand theory versus middle range and practice theory) and the increasing focus on the philosophical perspectives of critical theory, postmodernism, and feminism.

Table 2-4 Chronology of Publications of Selected Nursing Theorists

Theorist	Year	Title of Theoretical Writings
Florence Nightingale	1859	*Notes on Nursing*
Hildegard Peplau	1952	*Interpersonal Relations in Nursing*
Virginia Henderson	1955	*Principles and Practice of Nursing*, 5th edition
	1966	*The Nature of Nursing: A Definition and Its Implications for Practice, Research, and Education*
	1991	*The Nature of Nursing: Reflections After 25 Years*
Dorothy Johnson	1959	"A Philosophy of Nursing"
	1980	"The Behavioral System Model for Nursing"
Faye Abdellah	1960	*Patient-Centered Approaches to Nursing*
	1968	2nd edition
Ida Jean Orlando	1961	*The Dynamic Nurse–Patient Relationship*
Ernestine Wiedenbach	1964	*Clinical Nursing: A Helping Art*
Lydia E. Hall	1964	*Nursing: What Is It?*
Joyce Travelbee	1966	*Interpersonal Aspects of Nursing*
	1971	2nd edition
Myra E. Levine	1967	*The Four Conservation Principles of Nursing*
	1973	*Introduction to Clinical Nursing*
	1996	"The Conservation Principles of Nursing: A Retrospective"
Martha Rogers	1970	*An Introduction to the Theoretical Basis of Nursing*
	1980	"Nursing: A Science of Unitary Man"
	1983	*Science of Unitary Human Being: A Paradigm for Nursing*
	1989	"Nursing: A Science of Unitary Human Beings"
Dorothea E. Orem	1971	*Nursing: Concepts of Practice*
	1980	2nd edition
	1985	3rd edition
	1991	4th edition
	1995	5th edition
	2001	6th edition
	2011	*Self-Care Science, Nursing Theory and Evidence-Based Practice* (Taylor and Renpenning)
Imogene M. King	1971	*Toward a Theory for Nursing: General Concepts of Human Behavior*
	1981	*A Theory for Nursing: Systems, Concepts, Process*
	1989	"King's General Systems Framework and Theory"
Betty Neuman	1974	"The Betty Neuman Health-Care Systems Model: A Total Person Approach to Patient Problems"
	1982	*The Neuman Systems Model*
	1989	2nd edition

(continued)

Table 2-4 Chronology of Publications of Selected Nursing Theorists (Continued)

Theorist	Year	Title of Theoretical Writings
	1995	3rd edition
	2002	4th edition
	2011	5th edition
Evelyn Adam	1975	*A Conceptual Model for Nursing*
	1980	*To Be a Nurse*
	1991	2nd edition
Callista Roy	1976	*Introduction to Nursing: An Adaptation Model*
	1980	"The Roy Adaptation Model"
	1984	*Introduction to Nursing: An Adaptation Model,* 2nd edition
	1991	*The Roy Adaptation Model*
	1999	2nd edition
	2009	3rd edition
Josephine Paterson and Loretta Zderad	1976	*Humanistic Nursing*
Jean Watson	1979	*Nursing: The Philosophy and Science of Caring*
	1985	*Nursing: Human Science and Human Care*
	1989	*Watson's Philosophy and Theory of Human Caring in Nursing*
	1999	*Human Science and Human Care*
	2006	*Caring Science as Sacred Science*
	2012	*Human Caring Science: A Theory of Nursing,* 2nd edition
Margaret A. Newman	1979	*Theory Development in Nursing*
	1983	*Newman's Health Theory*
	1986	*Health as Expanding Consciousness*
	2000	2nd edition
Madeleine Leininger	1980	*Caring: A Central Focus of Nursing and Health Care Services*
	1988	"Leininger's Theory of Nursing: Cultural Care Diversity and Universality"
	2001	*Culture Care Diversity and Universality*
	2006	2nd edition
	2015	3rd edition (Edited by M. R. McFarland and H. B. Wehbe-Alamah)
Joan Riehl Sisca	1980	*The Riehl Interaction Model*
	1989	2nd edition
Rosemary Parse	1981	*Man-Living-Health: A Theory for Nursing*
	1985	*Man-Living-Health: A Man-Environment Simultaneity Paradigm*
	1987	*Nursing Science: Major Paradigms, Theories, Critiques*
	1989	"Man-Living-Health: A Theory of Nursing"
	1999	*Illuminations: The Human Becoming Theory in Practice and Research*

Table 2-4 Chronology of Publications of Selected Nursing Theorists (Continued)

Theorist	Year	Title of Theoretical Writings
Joyce Fitzpatrick	1983	*A Life Perspective Rhythm Model*
	1989	2nd edition
Helen Erickson et al.	1983	*Modeling and Role Modeling*
Nancy Roper, Winifred Logan, and Alison Tierney	1980	*The Elements of Nursing*
	1985	2nd edition
	1996	*The Elements of Nursing: A Model for Nursing Based on a Model of Living*
	2000	*Roper-Logan-Tierney Model of Nursing*
Patricia Benner and Judith Wrubel	1984	*From Novice to Expert: Excellence and Power in Clinical Nursing Practice*
	1989	*The Primacy of Caring: Stress and Coping in Health and Illness*
Anne Boykin and Savina Schoenhofer	1993	*Nursing as Caring*
	2001	2nd edition
Barbara Artinian	1997	*The Intersystem Model: Integrating Theory and Practice*
	2011	2nd edition
Brendan McCormack and Tanya McCance	2010	*Person-Centred Nursing: Theory and Practice*

Sources: Chinn and Kramer (2015); Hickman (2011); Hilton (1997).

Grand Theories

Grand theories are the most complex and broadest in scope. They attempt to explain broad areas within a discipline and may incorporate numerous other theories. The term *macrotheory* is used by some authors to describe a theory that is broadly conceptualized and is usually applied to a general area of a specific discipline (Higgins & Moore, 2000; Peterson, 2017).

Grand theories are nonspecific and are composed of relatively abstract concepts that lack operational definitions. Their propositions are also abstract and are not generally amenable to testing. Grand theories are developed through thoughtful and insightful appraisal of existing ideas as opposed to empirical research (Fawcett & DeSanto-Madeya, 2013). The majority of the nursing conceptual frameworks (e.g., Orem, Roy, and Rogers) are considered to be grand theories. Chapters 6 through 9 discuss many of the grand nursing theories.

Middle Range Theories

Middle range theory lies between the grand nursing models and more circumscribed, concrete ideas (practice or situation-specific theories). Middle range theories are

Theory	Level of Abstraction
Metatheory	Most abstract
Grand theories	
Middle range theories	
Practice theories	Least abstract

Figure 2-1 Comparison of the scope of nursing theories.

substantively specific and encompass a limited number of concepts and a limited aspect of the real world. They are composed of relatively concrete concepts that can be operationally defined and relatively concrete propositions that may be empirically tested (Higgins & Moore, 2000; Peterson, 2017; Whall, 2016).

A middle range theory may be (1) a description of a particular phenomenon, (2) an explanation of the relationship between phenomena, or (3) a prediction of the effects of one phenomenon or another (Fawcett & DeSanto-Madeya, 2013). Many investigators favor working with propositions and theories characterized as middle range rather than with conceptual frameworks because they provide the basis for generating testable hypotheses related to particular nursing phenomena and to particular client populations (Chinn & Kramer, 2015; Roy, 2014). The number of middle range theories developed and used by nurses has grown significantly over the past two decades. Examples include social support, quality of life, and health promotion. Chapters 10 and 11 describe middle range theory in more detail.

Practice Theories

Practice theories are also called *situation-specific theories, prescriptive theories,* or *microtheories* and are the least complex. Practice theories are more specific than middle range theories and produce specific directions for practice (Higgins & Moore, 2000; Peterson, 2017; Whall, 2016). They contain the fewest concepts and refer to specific, easily defined phenomena. They are narrow in scope, explain a small aspect of reality, and are intended to be prescriptive. They are usually limited to specific populations or fields of practice and often use knowledge from other disciplines. Examples of practice theories developed and used by nurses are theories of postpartum depression, infant bonding, and oncology pain management. Chapters 12 and 18 present additional information on practice theories.

Type or Purpose of Theory

In their seminal work, Dickoff and James (1968) defined theories as intellectual inventions designed to describe, explain, predict, or prescribe phenomena. They described four kinds of theory, each of which builds on the other. These are:

- Factor-isolating theories (descriptive theories)
- Factor-relating theories (explanatory theories)
- Situation-relating theories (predictive theories or promoting or inhibiting theories)
- Situation-producing theories (prescriptive theories)

Dickoff and James (1968) stated that nursing as a profession should go beyond the level of descriptive or explanatory theories and attempt to attain the highest levels—that of situation-relating/predictive and situation-producing/prescriptive theories.

Descriptive (Factor-Isolating) Theories

Descriptive theories are those that describe, observe, and name concepts, properties, and dimensions. Descriptive theory identifies and describes the major concepts of phenomena but does not explain how or why the concepts are related. The purpose of descriptive theory is to provide observation and meaning regarding the phenomena. It is generated and tested by descriptive research techniques including concept analysis, case studies, literature review phenomenology, ethnography, and grounded theory (Young et al., 2001).

Examples of descriptive theories are readily found in the nursing literature. Barkimer (2016), for example, used the process of concept analysis to develop a model of clinical growth for nursing educators. In other works, using grounded theory methodology, Sacks and Volker (2015) developed a theoretical model describing hospice nurses' responses to patient suffering, and El Hussein and Hirst (2016) constructed a theory describing the clinical reasoning processes nurses use to recognize delirium.

Explanatory (Factor-Relating) Theories

Factor-relating theories, or explanatory theories, are those that relate concepts to one another, describe the interrelationships among concepts or propositions, and specify the associations or relationships among some concepts. They attempt to tell *how* or *why* the concepts are related and may deal with cause and effect and correlations or rules that regulate interactions. They are developed by correlational research and increasingly through comprehensive literature review and synthesis. An example of an explanatory theory is the theory of health-related outcomes of resilience in middle adolescents (Scoloveno, 2015). This theory was developed from a correlational research study that surveyed the effects of resilience on hope, well-being, and health-promoting lifestyle in middle adolescents. In other works, comprehensive literature review and synthesis were used by Noviana, Miyazaki, and Ishimaru (2016) to develop a conceptual model for meaning in life and by Lor, Crooks, and Tluczek (2016) to propose a model of person, family, and culture-centered nursing care.

Predictive (Situation-Relating) Theories

Situation-relating theories are achieved when the conditions under which concepts are related are stated and the relational statements are able to describe future outcomes consistently. Situation-relating theories move to prediction of precise relationships between concepts. Experimental research is used to generate and test them in most cases.

Predictive theories are relatively difficult to find in the nursing literature. In one example, Cobb (2012) used a quasi-experimental, model-building approach to predict the relationship between spirituality and health status among adults living with HIV. In another example, Fearon-Lynch and Stover (2015) merged two research-based, extant theories to develop a middle range theory explaining mastery of diabetes self-management.

Another example of a predictive theory in nursing can be found in the caregiving effectiveness model. The process outlining development of this theory was described by Smith and colleagues (2002) and combined numerous steps in theory construction and empirical testing and validation. In the model, caregiving effectiveness is dependent on the interface of a number of factors including the characteristics of the caregiver, interpersonal interactions between the patient and caregiver, and the educational preparedness of the caregiver, combined with adaptive factors, such as economic stability, and the caregiver's own health status and family adaptation and coping mechanisms. The model itself graphically details the interaction of these factors and depicts how they collectively work to impact caregiving effectiveness.

Prescriptive (Situation-Producing) Theories

Situation-producing theories are those that prescribe activities necessary to reach defined goals. Prescriptive theories address nursing therapeutics and consequences of interventions. They include propositions that call for change and predict consequences of nursing interventions. They should describe the prescription, the consequence(s), the type of client, and the conditions (Meleis, 2012).

Prescriptive theories are among the most difficult to identify in the nursing literature. One example is a work by Walling (2006) that presented a "prescriptive theory explaining medical acupuncture" for nurse practitioners. The model describes how acupuncture can be used to reduce stress and enhance well-being. In another example, Auvil-Novak (1997) described the development of a middle range theory of chronotherapeutic intervention for postsurgical pain based on three experimental studies of pain relief among postsurgical clients. The theory uses a time-dependent approach to pain assessment and provides directed nursing interventions to address postoperative pain.

Issues in Theory Development in Nursing

A number of issues related to use of theory in nursing have received significant attention in the literature. The first is the issue of borrowed versus unique theory in nursing. A second issue is nursing's metaparadigm, and a third is the importance of the concept of caring in nursing.

Borrowed Versus Unique Theory in Nursing

Since the 1960s, the question of borrowing—or sharing—theory from other disciplines has been raised in the discussion of nursing theory. The debate over borrowed/shared theory centers in the perceived need for theory unique to nursing discussed by many nursing theorists.

The main premise held by those opposed to borrowed theory is that only theories that are grounded in nursing should guide the actions of the discipline. A second premise that supports the need for unique theory is that any theory that evolves out of the practice arena of nursing is substantially nursing. Although one might "borrow" theory and apply it to the realm of nursing actions, it is transformed into nursing theory because it addresses phenomena within the arena of nursing practice.

Opponents of using borrowed theory believe that nursing knowledge should not be tainted by using theory from physiology, psychology, sociology, and education. Furthermore, they believe "borrowing" requires returning and that the theory is not in essence nursing if concepts are borrowed (Levine, 1995; Risjord, 2010).

Proponents of using borrowed theory in nursing believe that knowledge belongs to the scientific community and to society at large, and it is not the property of individuals or disciplines (Powers & Knapp, 2011). Indeed, these individuals feel that knowledge is not the private domain of one discipline, and the use of knowledge generated by any discipline is not borrowed but shared. Furthermore, shared theory does not lessen nursing scholarship but enhances it (Levine, 1995; Rodgers, 2015).

Furthermore, advocates of borrowed or shared theory believe that, like other applied sciences, nursing depends on the theories from other disciplines for its theoretical foundations. For example, general systems theory is used in nursing, biology, sociology, and engineering. Different theories of stress and adaptation are valuable to nurses, psychologists, and physicians.

In reality, all nursing theories incorporate concepts and theories shared with other disciplines to guide theory development, research, and practice. However, simply adopting concepts or theories from another discipline does not convert them into nursing concepts or theories. It is important, therefore, for theorists, researchers, and practitioners to use concepts from other disciplines appropriately. Emphasis should be placed on redefining and synthesizing the concepts and theories according to a nursing perspective (Fawcett & DeSanto-Madeya, 2013; Rodgers, 2015).

Nursing's Metaparadigm

The most abstract and general component of the structural hierarchy of nursing knowledge is what Kuhn (1974) called the *metaparadigm*. A metaparadigm refers "globally to the subject matter of greatest interest to member of a discipline" (Powers & Knapp, 2011, p. 107). The metaparadigm includes major philosophical orientations or worldviews of a discipline, the conceptual models and theories that guide research and other scholarly activities, and the empirical indicators that operationalize theoretical concepts (Fawcett, 1996). The purpose or function of the metaparadigm is to summarize the intellectual and social missions of the discipline and place boundaries on the subject matter of that discipline (Kim, 1989). Fawcett and DeSanto-Madeya (2013) identified four requirements for a metaparadigm. These are summarized in Box 2-1.

According to Fawcett and DeSanto-Madeya (2013), in the 1970s and early 1980s, a number of nursing scholars identified a growing consensus that the dominant phenomena within the science of nursing revolved around the concepts of man (person), health, environment, and nursing. Fawcett first wrote on the central concepts of nursing in 1978 and formalized them as the metaparadigm of nursing in 1984. This articulation of four metaparadigm concepts (person, health, environment, and nursing) served as an organizing framework around which conceptual development proceeded.

Wagner (1986) examined the nursing metaparadigm in depth. Her sample of 160 doctorally prepared chairpersons, deans, or directors of programs for bachelors of science in nursing revealed that between 94% and 98% of the respondents agreed that the concepts that comprise the nursing metaparadigm are person, health, nursing, and environment. She concluded that these findings indicated a consensus within the discipline of nursing that these are the dominant phenomena within the science. A summary of definitions for each term is presented here.

Person refers to a being composed of physical, intellectual, biochemical, and psychosocial needs; a human energy field; a holistic being in the world; an open system; an integrated whole; an adaptive system; and a being who is greater than the sum of his or her parts (Wagner, 1986). Nursing theories are often most distinguishable from each other by the various ways in which they conceptualize the person or recipient of nursing care. Most nursing models organize data about the individual person as a focus of the nurse's attention, although some nursing theorists have expanded to

---

Box 2-1 | Requirements for a Metaparadigm

1. A metaparadigm must identify a domain that is distinctive from the domains of other disciplines . . . the concepts and propositions represent a unique perspective for inquiry and practice.
2. A metaparadigm must encompass all phenomena of interest to the discipline in a parsimonious manner . . . the concepts and propositions are global and there are no redundancies.
3. A metaparadigm must be perspective-neutral . . . the concepts and propositions do not represent a specific perspective (i.e., a specific paradigm or conceptual model or combination of perspectives).
4. A metaparadigm must be global in scope and substance . . . the concepts and propositions do not reflect particular national, cultural, or ethnic beliefs and values.

Adapted from: Fawcett and DeSanto-Madeya (2013).

include family or community as the focus (Thorne et al., 1998). *Health* is the ability to function independently; successful adaptation to life's stressors; achievement of one's full life potential; and unity of mind, body, and soul (Wagner, 1986). Health has been a phenomenon of central interest to nursing since its inception. Nursing literature indicates great diversity in the explication of health and quality of life (Thorne et al., 1998). Indeed, in a recent work, following a critical appraisal of the works of several nurse theorists, Plummer and Molzahn (2009) suggested replacing the term "health" with "quality of life." They posited that quality of life is a more inclusive notion, as health is often understood in terms of physical status. Alternatively, quality of life better encompasses a holistic perspective, involving physical, psychological, and social well-being, as well as the spiritual and environmental aspects of the human experience.

Environment typically refers to the external elements that affect the person; internal and external conditions that influence the organism; significant others with whom the person interacts; and an open system with boundaries that permit the exchange of matter, energy, and information with human beings (Wagner, 1986). Many nursing theories have a narrow conceptualization of the environment as the immediate surroundings or circumstances of the individual. This view limits understanding by making the environment rigid, static, and natural. A multilayered view of the environment encourages understanding of an individual's perspective and immediate context and incorporates the sociopolitical and economic structures and underlying ideologies that influence reality (Thorne et al., 1998).

Nursing is a science, an art, and a practice discipline and involves caring. Goals of nursing include care of the well, care of the sick, assisting with self-care activities, helping individuals attain their human potential, and discovering and using nature's laws of health. The purposes of nursing care include placing the client in the best condition for nature to restore health, promoting the adaptation of the individual, facilitating the development of an interaction between the nurse and the client in which jointly set goals are met, and promoting harmony between the individual and the environment (Wagner, 1986). Furthermore, nursing practice facilitates, supports, and assists individuals, families, communities, and societies to enhance, maintain, and recover health and to reduce and ameliorate the effects of illness (Thorne et al., 1998).

In addition to these definitions, many grand nursing theorists, and virtually all of the theoretical commentators, incorporate these four terms into their conceptual or theoretical frameworks. Table 2-5 presents theoretical definitions of the metaparadigm concepts from selected nursing conceptual frameworks and other writings.

Relationships Among the Metaparadigm Concepts

The concepts of nursing's metaparadigm have been linked in four propositions identified in the writings of Donaldson and Crowley (1978) and Gortner (1980). These are as follows:

1. Person and health: Nursing is concerned with the principles and laws that govern human processes of living and dying.
2. Person and environment: Nursing is concerned with the patterning of human health experiences within the context of the environment.
3. Health and nursing: Nursing is concerned with the nursing actions or processes that are beneficial to human beings.
4. Person, environment, and health: Nursing is concerned with the human processes of living and dying, recognizing that human beings are in a continuous relationship with their environments (Fawcett & DeSanto-Madeya, 2013, p. 6).

Table 2-5 Selected Theoretical Definitions of the Concepts of Nursing's Metaparadigm

Metaparadigm Concept	Author/Source of Definition	Definition
Person/human being/client	D. Johnson	A behavioral system with patterned, repetitive, and purposeful ways of behaving that link person to the environment
	B. Neuman	A dynamic composite of the interrelationships between physiologic, psychological, sociocultural, developmental, spiritual, and basic structure variables; may be an individual, group, community, or social system
	D. Orem	Are distinguished from other living things by their capacity (1) to reflect upon themselves and their environment, (2) to symbolize what they experience, and (3) to use symbolic creations (ideas, words) in thinking, in communicating, and in guiding efforts to do and to make things that are beneficial for themselves or others
	M. Rogers	An irreducible, indivisible, pan-dimensional energy field identified by pattern and manifesting characteristics that are specific to the whole and that cannot be predicted from knowledge of the parts
Nursing	M. Leininger	A learned humanistic and scientific profession and discipline that is focused on human care phenomena and activities to assist, support, facilitate, or enable individuals or groups to maintain or regain their well-being (or health) in culturally meaningful and beneficial ways, or to help people face handicaps or death
	M. Newman	Caring in the human health experience
	D. Orem	A specific type of human service required whenever the maintenance of continuous self-care requires the use of special techniques and the application of scientific knowledge in providing care or in designing it
	J. Watson	A human science of persons and human health–illness experiences that are mediated by professional, personal, scientific, esthetic, and ethical human care transactions
Health	M. Leininger	A state of well-being that is culturally defined, valued, and practiced and that reflects the ability of individuals (or groups) to perform their daily role activities in culturally expressed, beneficial, and patterned lifeways
	M. Newman	A pattern of evolving, expanding consciousness regardless of the form or direction it takes
	C. Roy	A state and process of being and becoming an integrated and whole person. It is a reflection of adaptation, that is, the interaction of the person and the environment.
	J. Watson	Unity and harmony within the mind, body, and soul. Health is also associated with the degree of congruence between the self as perceived and the self as experienced.
Environment	M. Leininger	The totality of an event, situation, or particular experience that gives meaning to human expressions, interpretations, and social interactions in particular physical, ecologic, sociopolitical, and cultural settings
	B. Neuman	All internal and external factors of influences that surround the client or client system
	M. Rogers	An irreducible, pan-dimensional energy field identified by pattern and integral with the human field
	C. Roy	All conditions, circumstances, and influences that surround and affect the development and behavior of human adaptive systems with particular consideration of person and earth resources

Sources: Johnson (1980); Leininger (1991); Neuman (1995); Newman (1990); Orem (2001); Rogers (1990); Roy and Andrews (1999); Watson (1985).

In addressing how the four concepts meet the requirements for a metaparadigm, Fawcett and DeSanto-Madeya (2013) explain that the first three propositions represent recurrent themes identified in the writings of Nightingale and other nursing scholars. Furthermore, the four concepts and propositions identify the unique focus of the discipline of nursing and encompass all relevant phenomena in a parsimonious manner. Finally, the concepts and propositions are perspective-neutral because they do not reflect a specific paradigm or conceptual model and they do not reflect the beliefs and values of any one country or culture.

Other Viewpoints on Nursing's Metaparadigm

There is some dissension in the acceptance of person/health/environment/nursing as nursing's metaparadigm. Kim (1987, 1989, 2010) identified four domains (client, client–nurse, practice, and environment) as an organizing framework or typology of nursing. In this framework, the most significant difference appears to be in placing health issues (i.e., health care experiences and health care environment) within the client domain and differentiating the nursing practice domain from the client–nurse domain. The latter focuses specifically on interactions between the nurse and the client.

Meleis (2012) maintained that nursing encompasses seven central concepts: interaction, nursing client, transitions, nursing process, environment, nursing therapeutics, and health. Addition of the concepts of interaction, transitions, and nursing process denotes the greatest difference between this framework and the more commonly described person/health/environment/nursing framework. (See Link to Practice 2-1 for another thought on expanding the metaparadigm to include social justice.)

Caring as a Central Construct in the Discipline of Nursing

A final debate that will be discussed in this chapter centers on the place of the concept of caring within the discipline and science of nursing. This debate has been escalating

Link to Practice 2-1

Should Social Justice Be Part of Nursing's Metaparadigm?

Schim, Benkert, Bell, Walker, and Danford (2007) proposed that the construct of "social justice" be added to nursing's metaparadigm. They argued that social justice is interconnected with the four acknowledged metaparadigm concepts of nursing, person, health, and environment. In their model, social justice actually acts as the central, organizational foundation that links the other four concepts, particularly within the context of public health nursing, and more specifically in urban settings.

Using this macroperspective, the goal of nursing is to ensure adequate distribution of resources to benefit those who are marginalized. Suggested strategies to enhance attention to social justice in nursing include shifting to a population health and health promotion/disease prevention perspective; diversifying nursing by recruiting and educating underrepresented minorities into the profession; and engaging in political action at local, state, national, and international levels. They concluded that as a caring profession, nursing should expand efforts with a social justice orientation to help ensure equal access to benefits and protections of society for all.

over the last decade and has been motivated by the perceived urgency of identifying nursing's unique contribution to the health care disciplines and revolves around the defining attributes and roles within the practice of nursing (Thorne et al., 1998).

The concept of caring has occupied a prominent position in nursing literature and has been touted as the essence of nursing by renowned nursing scholars, including Leininger, Watson, and Erickson. Indeed, it has been proposed that nursing be defined as the study of caring in the human health experience (Newman, Sime, & Corcoran-Perry, 1991).

Although some theorists (i.e., Watson, Leininger, and Boykin) have gone so far as to identify caring as the essence of nursing, there is little if any rejection of caring as *a* central concept for nursing, although not necessarily *the* most significant concept. Thorne and colleagues (1998) cited three major areas of contention in the debate about caring in nursing. The first is the diverse views on the nature of caring. These range from caring as a human trait to caring as a therapeutic intervention and differ according to whether the act of caring is conceptualized as being client centered, nurse centered, or both.

A second major issue in the caring debate concerns the use of caring terminology to conceptualize a specialized role. It has been asked whether there is a compelling reason to lay claim to caring as nursing's unique domain when so many professions describe their function as involving caring, and the concept of caring is prominent in the work of many other disciplines (e.g., medicine, social work, and psychology) (Thorne et al., 1998).

A third issue centers on the implications for the future development of the profession that nursing should espouse caring as its unique mandate. It has been observed that nurses should ask themselves if it is politically astute to be the primary interpreters of a construct that is both gendered and devalued (Meadows, 2007; Thorne et al., 1998).

Thus, it is argued by Fawcett (1996) that although caring is included in several conceptualizations of the discipline of nursing, it is not a dominant term in every conceptualization and therefore does not represent a discipline-wide viewpoint. Furthermore, caring is not uniquely a nursing phenomenon, and caring behaviors may not be generalizable across national and cultural boundaries.

Summary

Like Matt Ng, the graduate nursing student described in the opening case study, nurses who are in a position to learn more about theory, and to recognize how and when to apply it, must often be convinced of the relevance of such study to understand the benefits. The study of theory requires exposure to many new concepts, principles, thoughts, and ideas as well as a student who is willing to see how theory plays an important role in nursing practice, research, education, and administration.

Although study and use of theoretical concepts in nursing dates back to Nightingale, little progress in theory development was made until the 1960s. The past five decades, however, have produced significant advancement in theory development for nursing. This chapter has presented an overview of this evolutionary process. In addition, the basic types of theory and purposes of theory were described. Subsequent chapters will explain many of the ideas introduced here to assist professional nurses to understand the relationship among theory, practice, and research and to further develop the discipline, the science, and the profession of nursing.

Key Points

- "Theory" refers to the systematic explanation of events in which constructs and concepts are identified, relationships are proposed, and predictions are made.
- Theory offers structure and organization to nursing knowledge and provides a systematic means of collecting data to describe, explain, and predict nursing practice.
- Florence Nightingale was the first modern nursing theorist; she described what she considered nurses' goals and practice domain to be.
- There has been an evolution of stages of theory development in nursing. Nursing is currently in the "integrated knowledge" stage, which emphasizes EBP and translational research. Theory development increasingly sources meta-analyses, as well as nursing research, and is largely directed toward middle range and situation-specific/practice theories.
- Theories can be classified by scope of level of abstraction (e.g., metatheory, grand theory, middle range theory, and situation-specific theory) or by type or purpose of the theory (e.g., description, explanation, prediction, and prescription).
- Nursing "borrows" or "shares" theories and concepts from other disciplines to guide theory development, research, and practice. It is critical that nurses redefine and synthesize these shared concept and theories according to a nursing perspective.
- The concepts of nursing, person, environment, and health are widely accepted as the dominant phenomena in nursing; they have been identified as nursing's metaparadigm.

Learning Activities

1. Examine early issues of *Nursing Research* (1950s and 1960s) and determine whether theories or theoretical frameworks were used as a basis for research. What types of theories were used? Review current issues to analyze how this has changed.
2. Examine early issues of *American Journal of Nursing* (1900–1950). Determine if and how theories were used in nursing practice. What types of theories were used? Review current issues to analyze how this has changed.
3. Find reports that present middle range or practice theories in the nursing literature. Identify if these theories are descriptive, explanatory, predictive, or prescriptive in nature.
4. Like Matt, the nurse from the opening case study, many nurses initially struggle with recognizing the need to study how "theory" can be important in their practice. With classmates, discuss perceptions, beliefs, and attitudes felt when you learned you were to take a course on "nursing theory." How have your thoughts changed? Why?

REFERENCES

Alligood, M. R. (2014a). Introduction to nursing theory: Its history, significance, and analysis. In M. R. Alligood (Ed.), *Nursing theorists and their work* (8th ed., pp. 2–13). St. Louis, MO: Mosby.

Alligood, M. R. (2014b). *Nursing theorists and their work* (8th ed.). St. Louis, MO: Mosby.

American Association of Colleges of Nursing. (2004). *AACN position statement on the practice doctorate in nursing.* Retrieved from http://www.aacn.nche.edu/dnp/position-statement

American Association of Colleges of Nursing. (2017a). *Nursing program search.* Retrieved from http://www.aacn.nche.edu/membership/nursing-program-search?search=&name=&state=&category_id=9&x=19&y=8

American Association of Colleges of Nursing. (2017b). *DNP fact sheet.* Retrieved from http://www.aacnnursing.org/DNP/Fact-Sheet

Auvil-Novak, S. E. (1997). A middle range theory of chronotherapeutic intervention for postsurgical pain. *Nursing Research, 46*(2), 66–71.

Barkimer, J. (2016). Clinical growth: An evolutionary concept analysis. *ANS. Advances in Nursing Science, 39*(3), E28–E39.

Blackburn, S. (2016). *Oxford dictionary of philosophy* (3rd ed.). New York, NY: Oxford University Press.

Chinn, P. L., & Kramer, M. K. (2015). *Knowledge development in nursing: Theory and process* (9th ed.). St. Louis, MO: Elsevier.

Cobb, R. K. (2012). How well does spirituality predict health status in adults living with HIV-disease: A Neuman systems model study. *Nursing Science Quarterly, 25*(4), 347–355.

Dickoff, J., & James, P. (1968). A theory of theories: A position paper. *Nursing Research, 17*(3), 197–203.

Donahue, M. P. (2011). *Nursing the finest art: An illustrated history* (3rd ed.). St. Louis, MO: Elsevier.

Donaldson, S. K., & Crowley, D. M. (1978). The discipline of nursing. *Nursing Outlook, 26*(2), 113–120.

El Hussein, M., & Hirst, S. (2016). Tracking the footsteps: A constructivist grounded theory of the clinical reasoning processes that registered nurses use to recognize delirium. *Journal of Clinical Nursing, 25,* 381–391.

Fawcett, J. (1992). Contemporary conceptualizations of nursing: Philosophy or science? In J. F. Kikuchi & H. Simmons (Eds.), *Philosophic inquiry in nursing* (pp. 64–70). Newbury Park, CA: Sage.

Fawcett, J. (1996). On the requirements for a metaparadigm: An invitation to dialogue. *Nursing Science Quarterly, 9*(3), 94–97.

Fawcett, J. (2012). The future of nursing: How important is discipline-specific knowledge? A conversation with Jacqueline Fawcett. Interview by Dr. Janie Butts and Dr. Karen Rich. *Nursing Science Quarterly, 25*(2), 151–154.

Fawcett, J., & DeSanto-Madeya, S. (2013). *Contemporary nursing knowledge: Analysis and evaluation of nursing models and theories* (3rd ed.). Philadelphia, PA: Davis.

Fearon-Lynch, J. A., & Stover, C. M. (2015). A middle-range theory of diabetes self-management mastery. *ANS. Advances in Nursing Science, 38*(4), 330–346.

Gortner, S. R. (1980). Nursing science in transition. *Nursing Research, 29*(3), 180–183.

Hickman, J. S. (2011). An introduction to nursing theory. In J. George (Ed.), *Nursing theories: The base for professional nursing practice* (6th ed., pp. 1–22). Upper Saddle River, NJ: Pearson Education.

Higgins, P. A., & Moore, S. M. (2000). Levels of theoretical thinking in nursing. *Nursing Outlook, 48*(4), 179–183.

Hilton, P. A. (1997). Theoretical perspective of nursing: A review of the literature. *Journal of Advanced Nursing, 26*(6), 1211–1220.

Johnson, D. E. (1980). The behavioral system model for nursing. In J. P. Riehl & C. Roy (Eds.), *Conceptual models for nursing practice* (2nd ed., pp. 207–216). New York, NY: Appleton-Century-Crofts.

Judd, D., & Sitzman, K. (2014). *A history of American nursing: Trends and eras* (2nd ed.). Burlington, MA: Jones & Bartlett Learning.

Kalisch, P. A., & Kalisch, B. J. (2004). *The advance of American nursing* (4th ed.). Philadelphia, PA: Lippincott Williams & Wilkins.

Kidd, P., & Morrison, E. F. (1988). The progression of knowledge in nursing: A search for meaning. *Image—The Journal of Nursing Scholarship, 20*(4), 222–224.

Kim, H. S. (1987). Structuring the nursing knowledge system: A typology of four domains. *Scholarly Inquiry for Nursing Practice, 1*(2), 99–110.

Kim, H. S. (1989). Theoretical thinking in nursing: Problems and prospects. *Recent Advances in Nursing, 24,* 106–122.

Kim, H. S. (2010). *The nature of theoretical thinking in nursing* (3rd ed.). New York, NY: Springer Publishing.

Kuhn, T. S. (1974). Second thoughts on paradigms. In F. Suppe (Ed.), *The structure of scientific theories* (pp. 459–482). Urbana, IL: University of Illinois Press.

Leininger, M. (1991). *Culture care diversity and universality: A theory of nursing.* New York, NY: National League for Nursing.

Levine, M. E. (1995). The rhetoric of nursing theory. *Image—The Journal of Nursing Scholarship, 27*(1), 11–14.

LoBiondo-Wood, G., & Haber, J. (2014). *Nursing research: Methods and critical appraisal for evidence-based practice* (8th ed.). St. Louis, MO: Elsevier.

Lor, M., Crooks, N., & Tluczek, A. (2016). A proposed model of person-, family-, and culture-centered nursing care. *Nursing Outlook, 64*(4), 352–366.

Meadows, R. (2007). Beyond caring. *Nursing Administration Quarterly, 31*(2), 158–161.

Meleis, A. I. (2012). *Theoretical nursing: Development and progress* (5th ed.). Philadelphia, PA: Lippincott Williams & Wilkins.

Melnyk, B. M., & Fineout-Overholt, E. (2015). *Evidence-based practice in nursing & healthcare: A guide to best practice* (3rd ed.). Philadelphia, PA: Lippincott Williams & Wilkins.

Moody, L. E. (1990). *Advancing nursing science through research.* Newbury Park, CA: Sage.

Neuman, B. (1995). *The Neuman systems model* (3rd ed.). Norwalk, CT: Appleton & Lange.

Newman, M. A. (1990). Newman's theory of health as praxis. *Nursing Science Quarterly, 3*(1), 37–41.

Newman, M. A., Sime, A. M., & Corcoran-Perry, S. A. (1991). The focus of the discipline of nursing. *ANS. Advances in Nursing Science, 14*(1), 1–6.

Noviana, U., Miyazaki, M., & Ishimaru, M. (2016). Meaning in life: A conceptual model for disaster nursing practice. *International Journal of Nursing Practice, 22*(Suppl. 1), 65–75.

Omrey, A., Kasper, C. E., & Page, G. G. (1995). *In search of nursing science.* Thousand Oaks, CA: Sage.

Orem, D. E. (2001). *Nursing: Concepts of practice* (6th ed.). St. Louis, MO: Mosby.

Peplau, H. (1952). *Interpersonal relations in nursing: A conceptual frame of reference for psychodynamic nursing.* New York, NY: Putnam.

Peterson, S. J. (2017). Introduction to the nature of nursing knowledge. In S. J. Peterson & T. S. Bredow (Eds.), *Middle range theories: Application to nursing research* (4th ed., pp. 3–41). Philadelphia, PA: Wolters Kluwer.

Plummer, M., & Molzahn, A. E. (2009). Quality of life in contemporary nursing theory: A concept analysis. *Nursing Science Quarterly, 22*(2), 134–140.

Powers, B. A., & Knapp, T. R. (2011). *Dictionary of nursing theory and research* (4th ed.). New York, NY: Springer Publishing.

Risjord, M. (2010). *Nursing knowledge: Science, practice, and philosophy.* London, United Kingdom: Wiley-Blackwell.

Rodgers, B. L. (2015). The evolution of nursing science. In J. B. Butts & K. L. Rich (Eds.), *Philosophies and theories for advanced nursing practice* (2nd ed., pp. 19–50). Burlington, MA: Jones & Bartlett Learning.

Rogers, M. E. (1990). Nursing: Science of unitary, irreducible, human beings: Update 1990. In E. A. M. Barrett (Ed.), *Visions of Rogers' science-based nursing* (pp. 5–11). New York, NY: National League for Nursing.

Roy, C. (2014). *Generating middle range theory: From evidence to practice.* New York, NY: Springer Publishing.

Roy, C., & Andrews, H. A. (1999). *The Roy adaptation model* (2nd ed.). Stamford, CT: Appleton & Lange.

Rutty, J. E. (1998). The nature of philosophy of science, theory and knowledge relating to nursing and professionalism. *Journal of Advanced Nursing, 28*(2), 243–250.

Sacks, J. L., & Volker, D. L. (2015). For their patients: A study of hospice nurses' responses to patient suffering. *Journal of Hospice & Palliative Nursing, 17*(6), 490–500.

Schim, S. M., Benkert, R., Bell, S. E., Walker, D. S., & Danford, C. A. (2007). Social justice: Added metaparadigm concept for urban health nursing. *Public Health Nursing, 24*(1), 73–80.

Schmidt, N. A., & Brown, J. M. (2015). *Evidence-based practice for nurses: Appraisal and application of research.* Burlington, MA: Jones & Bartlett Learning.

Scoloveno, R. (2015). A theoretical model of health-related outcomes of resilience in middle adolescents. *Western Journal of Nursing Research, 37*(3), 342–359.

Sitzman, K., & Eichelberger, L. W. (2011). *Understanding the work of nurse theorists: A creative beginning* (2nd ed.). New York, NY: Jones & Bartlett Learning.

Smith, C. E., Pace, K., Kochinda, C., Kleinbeck, S. V. M., Koehler, J., & Popkess-Vawter, S. (2002). Caregiving effectiveness model evolution to a midrange theory of home care: A process for critique and replication. *ANS. Advances in Nursing Science, 25*(1), 50–64.

Streubert, H. J., & Carpenter, D. R. (2011). *Qualitative research in nursing: Advancing the humanistic imperative* (5th ed.). Philadelphia, PA: Lippincott Williams & Wilkins.

Thorne, S., Canam, C., Dahinten, S., Hall, W., Henderson, A., & Kirkham, S. R. (1998). Nursing's metaparadigm concepts: Disimpacting the debates. *Journal of Advanced Nursing, 27*(6), 1257–1268.

Tierney, A. J. (1998). Nursing models: Extant or extinct? *Journal of Advanced Nursing, 28*(1), 77–85.

Wagner, J. (1986). *Nurse scholar's perceptions of nursing's metaparadigm* (Unpublished doctoral dissertation). Ohio State University, Columbus, OH.

Walker, L. O., & Avant, K. C. (2011). *Strategies for theory construction in nursing* (5th ed.). Upper Saddle River, NJ: Prentice-Hall.

Walling, A. (2006). Therapeutic modulation of the psychoneuroimmune system by medical acupuncture creates enhanced feelings of well-being. *Journal of the American Academy of Nurse Practitioners, 18*(4), 135–143.

Watson, J. (1985). *Nursing: Human science and human care*. Norwalk, CT: Appleton-Century-Crofts.

Whall, A. L. (2016). Philosophy of science positions and their importance in cross-national nursing. In J. J. Fitzpatrick & A. L. Whall (Eds.), *Conceptual models of nursing: Global perspective* (5th ed., pp. 8–28). Boston, MA: Pearson.

Young, A., Taylor, S. G., & Renpenning, K. M. (2001). *Connections: Nursing research, theory, and practice*. St. Louis, MO: Mosby.

Ziegler, S. M. (2005). *Theory-directed nursing practice* (2nd ed.). New York, NY: Springer Publishing.

3

Concept Development

Clarifying Meaning of Terms

Evelyn M. Wills and Melanie McEwen

Rebecca Wallis is a certified oncology nurse who is midway through her graduate studies to become an adult nurse practitioner. Recently, she helped care for
Mrs. Janet Benson, a woman in her mid-50s who had undergone a lumpectomy
for breast cancer. Mrs. Benson's pathology report revealed a slow-growing,
noninvasive carcinoma in situ; there were no involved nodes, and further tests
showed no metastasis.

In the hospital, Mrs. Benson progressed well. But after she was discharged and
began radiation, she would frequently weep over things that seemed trivial. Her
husband called Rebecca because he was concerned as this was not Mrs. Benson's
usual behavior. Typically, she was self-contained, stoic, and accepting of life's circumstances, seldom demonstrating excessive emotion. Rebecca set up an appointment with the Bensons. During the consultation, Rebecca asked each to explain
how they felt about Mrs. Benson's cancer. Mr. Benson replied that the change
in his wife's breast was a small matter to him; he was very grateful that she was
getting well. In response to Rebecca's questioning, Mrs. Benson focused on her
sadness and inquired if this was normal in women who had undergone a partial
mastectomy.

Rebecca explained that the reaction was quite common and that oncology
nurses in the region used the term postmastectomy grief (PMG) reaction to describe
it. She told the Bensons how nurses in their facility had worked out a protocol of
nursing therapy for PMG, but it had not been formally tested. In the protocol, the
nurses would request that the oncologist refer the patient to a psychiatric home
health nurse for an assessment. The psychiatric home health nurse would confer
with the oncologist and the nurse practitioner and, if needed, would request a referral to a licensed therapist. Additionally, a group called "Breast Cancer Support"
had been organized in the area by women who had been diagnosed with breast
cancer. In this group, problems, such as sadness, were discussed by women who
had experienced them, and support was given to those who were going through recovery from breast cancer surgery. Rebecca recommended that the Bensons attend
a meeting.

Mrs. Benson's case, and the problem of PMG in general, prompted Rebecca
to seek more information about this reaction of breast cancer patients. Her review

of the literature suggested that the phenomena needed further study to develop the knowledge base for practice. Because of what she had learned in her theoretical foundations course, she realized that she first needed to define and name the problem. To this end, she chose to use one of the concept development strategies she had learned to initiate preparation for a formal research study for her capstone project.

Experienced nurses who are focused on the practical application of evidence-based nursing knowledge demonstrate an inclination toward generalizing what they have learned from a group of clients to other clients with similar problems. This is obvious in the professional discussions of clinical nurses, particularly those educated for advanced practice, who might state, "We see certain phenomenon frequently enough in practice that we have developed clinical protocols or interventions."

These observed phenomena are considered by nurses to be reliable, enduring, and stable features of practical experience, whether or not they have acquired a name and whether or not they have been studied in research (Kim, 2010). Expert practice and enhanced education lead advanced practice nurses to recognize commonalities in phenomena that suggest the need for inquiry. This, in turn, may guide development of clinical hypotheses and testing of interventions. With the current focus on evidence-based practice, clear delineation of the concepts under study in research requires that the linkages among phenomena, concepts, and practice be clarified (Penrod & Hupcey, 2005).

For the nurse who desires to discriminately, formally, and concretely examine a phenomenon in depth, such as described earlier, the most logical place to start is by defining the phenomenon or concept for further study. This is not an easy task, however, and significant time, research, and effort must be made to adequately define nursing concepts. To simplify the process, a number of strategies and methods for concept analysis, concept development, and concept clarification have been proposed and used by nursing scholars for many years.

The rationale for concept development and several methods commonly used by nurses are discussed in this chapter. This will allow expert nurse clinicians and advanced practice nurses to develop or clarify meanings for the phenomena encountered in practice. The outcome can then serve as the basis for further development of theory for research and practice by master's- and doctorally prepared nurses (Box 3-1).

The Concept of "Concept"

Concepts are terms that refer to phenomena that occur in nature or in thought. *Concept* has been defined as an abstract term derived from particular attributes (Kerlinger, 1986) and "a symbolic statement describing a phenomenon or a class of phenomena" (Kim, 2010, p. 22). Concepts may be abstract (e.g., hope, love, desire)

Box 3-1	Theory and American Association of Colleges of Nursing Essentials

"The master's-prepared nurse applies and integrates broad, organizational, patient centered, and culturally responsive concepts into daily practice" (American Association of Colleges of Nursing, 2011, p. 25).

or relatively concrete (e.g., airplane, body temperature, pain). Concepts are formulated in words that enable people to communicate their meanings about realities in the world (Cutcliffe & McKenna, 2005; Kim, 2010; Penrod & Hupcey, 2005) and give meaning to phenomena that can directly or indirectly be seen, heard, tasted, smelled, or touched (Fawcett, 1999). A concept may be a word (e.g., grief, empathy, power, pain), two words (e.g., job satisfaction, need fulfillment, role strain), or a phrase (e.g., maternal role attachment, biomarkers of preterm labor, health-promoting behaviors). Finally, when they are operationalized, concepts become variables used in hypotheses to be tested in research.

Concepts have been compared to bricks in a wall that lend structure to science (Hardy, 1973). Chinn and Kramer (2015) believe that concepts are more than terms, and constructing conceptual meaning is a vital approach to theory building in which mental constructions or ideas are used to represent experiences. Similarly, Parse (2006) agrees that formal study of concepts enhances knowledge development for nursing through naming, creating, and confirming the phenomena of interest.

Although it was once thought that concepts could be defined once and for all, that idea has been disputed (Penrod & Hupcey, 2005; Rodgers & Knafl, 2000). Theorists now understand that conceptual meaning is created by scholars to assist in imparting the meaning to their readers and, ultimately, to benefit the discipline. Conceptual fluidity and dependence on the context is common in writings on concept analysis in the nursing literature (Duncan, Cloutier, & Bailey, 2007; Penrod & Hupcey, 2005). Furthermore, Risjord (2009) suggested that there are two forms of concept analysis, theoretical and colloquial, each with its own purpose and evidence, although the two can and often must be used together. Therefore, it is critical that scholars and researchers define concepts clearly and distinctly so that their readers may thoroughly and accurately comprehend their work. Because conceptual meanings are dynamic, they should be defined for each specific use the writer or researcher makes of the term. Indeed, concepts are defined and their meanings are understood only within the framework of the theory of which they are a part (Hardy, 1973).

Types of Concepts

Concepts explicate the subject matter of the theories of a discipline. For example, concepts from psychology include personality, intelligence, and cognition; concepts from biology include cell, species, and protoplasm (Jacox, 1974). Dubin (1978) explained the differences between various types of concepts, characterizing them as enumerative, associative, relational, statistical, and summative. Table 3-1 shows characteristics and examples of each of these types of concepts.

In nursing, concepts have been borrowed or derived from other disciplines (e.g., adaptation, culture, homeostasis) as well as developed directly from nursing practice and research (e.g., maternal–infant bonding, health-promoting behaviors, breastfeeding attrition). In nursing literature, concepts have been categorized in several ways. For example, they have been described as concrete or abstract, variable or nonvariable (Hardy, 1973), and as operationally or theoretically defined.

Abstract Versus Concrete Concepts

Concepts may be viewed on a continuum from concrete (specific) to abstract (general). At one end of the continuum are concrete concepts, which have simple, directly observable empirical referents that can be seen, felt, or heard (e.g., a chair, the color red, jazz music). Concrete concepts are limited by time and space and are observable in reality.

Table 3-1 Types of Concepts

Concept	Characteristics	Examples
Enumerative concepts	Are always present and universal	Age, height, weight
Associative concepts	Exist only in some conditions within a phenomenon; may have a zero value	Income, presence of disease, anxiety
Relational concepts	Can be understood only through the combination or interaction of two or more enumerative or associative concepts	Elderly (must combine concepts of age and longevity), mother (must combine man, woman, and birth)
Statistical concepts	Relate the property of one thing in terms of its distribution in the population rate	Average blood pressure, HIV/AIDS prevalence rate
Summative concepts	Represent an entire complex entity of a phenomenon; are complex and not measurable	Nursing, health, and environment

Source: Dubin (1978).

At the other end of the continuum are abstract concepts (e.g., art, social support, personality, role). These are not clearly observable directly or indirectly and must be defined in terms of observable concepts (Jacox, 1974). Abstract concepts are independent of time and space. The more abstract a concept is, the more it transcends time and geography (Meleis, 2012).

Some concepts are formed from direct experiences with reality, whereas others are formed from indirect experiences. Relatively concrete or "empirical" concepts are formed from direct observations of objects, properties, or events. Concepts describing objects (e.g., desk or dog) or properties (e.g., cold, hard) are more empirical because the object or property that represents the idea (the empirical indicator) can be directly observed. Slightly more abstract properties, such as height, weight, and gender, can also be observed or measured.

As concepts become more abstract, their empirical indicators become less concrete and less directly measurable, and assessment of abstract concepts increasingly depends on indirect measures. For example, cardiovascular fitness, social support, and self-esteem are not directly observable properties or objects. To study these and similar concepts, their empirical referents must be defined and means must be identified or developed to measure them.

Variable (Continuous) Versus Nonvariable (Discrete) Concepts

Concepts may be categorized as variable or nonvariable (Hardy, 1973). Concepts that describe phenomena according to some dimensions of the phenomena are termed *variables*. A discrete (noninterval level) concept identifies categories or classes of characteristics. Discrete concepts include gender, ethnic background, religion, and marital status. Discrete variables can be single variable categories that may be answered as "yes" or "no" (e.g., either one is pregnant or not pregnant; one is a nurse or is not a nurse) or fits into a predefined category (e.g., religion, marital status, educational attainment).

Continuous (variable) concepts permit classification of dimension or graduation of phenomena on a continuum (e.g., blood pressure, pain) (Hardin, 2014). Variable concepts include quality of life, health-promoting behaviors, and cultural identity.

An examination of nursing research will lead to numerous examples of continuous or variable concepts that have been being studied. These include the concepts of hope, quality of life, resilience, and grief. In each case, the concept was defined operationally and measured by tools, scales, or some other indicator to show where the respondent's level of the variable fell relative to others or relative to a predefined norm.

Theoretically Versus Operationally Defined Concepts

Concepts may be theoretically or operationally defined. A theoretical definition gives meaning to a term in context of a theory and permits any reader to assess the validity of the definition. The operational definition tells how the concept is linked to concrete situations and describes a set of procedures that will be performed to assign a value for the concept. Operational definitions permit the concept to be measured and allow hypotheses to be tested. Thus, operational definitions form the bridge between the theory and the empirical world (Hardy, 1973). Examples of theoretically and operationally defined concepts are shown in Table 3-2.

Table 3-2 Examples of Theoretically and Operationally Defined Concepts

Concept	Theoretical Definition	Operational Definition	Source
Binge eating	"Consuming a large amount of food in a short period of time while experiencing loss of control over eating" (p. 7)	Binge eating was determined to be "consuming an amount of food that is definitely greater than what most people would eat within a two hour period" (p. 8). Responses to four open-ended questions and demographics	Phillips, K. E., Kelly-Weeder, S., & Farrell, K. (2016). Binge eating behavior in college students: What is a binge? *Applied Nursing Research*, 9, 7–11.
Health literacy	"The degree in which individuals have the capacity to obtain, process and understand basic health information and services needed to make appropriate health decisions" (p. 94)	Health literacy is measured using the Omaha System's Problem Rating Score for Outcomes Knowledge (p. 96).	Monsen, K. A., Chatterjee, S. B., Timm, J. E., Poulsen, J. K., & McNaughton, D. B. (2015). Factors explaining variability in health literacy outcomes of public health nursing clients. *Public Health Nursing*, 32(2), 94–100.
Health-promoting lifestyle	" . . . activities that encourage or improve overall general health" (p. 328)	Help promotion behaviors were measured by the Health-Promoting Lifestyle Profile II.	Fisher, K., & Kridli, S.A. (2014). The role of motivation and self-efficacy on the practice of health promoting behaviours in the overweight and obese middle-aged American women. *International Journal of Nursing Practice*, 20(4), 327–335.
Emotional intelligence	"The ability to monitor one's own and others' feelings and emotions to discriminate among them and to use this information to guide one's thinking and action" (p. 464)	Emotional intelligence was measured using the Schutte Self-Report Inventory, a 33-item Likert tool which measures perceptions about emotional skills.	Lana, A., Baizan, E. M., Faya-Ornia, G., & Lopez, M. L. (2015). Emotional intelligence and health risk behaviors in nursing students. *The Journal of Nursing Education*, 54(8), 464–467.

Sources of Concepts

When beginning a review of concepts found in nursing practice, research, education, and administration, one may look to several places or sources for relevant concepts. Indeed, the source of nursing concepts may be from the natural world, from research, or derived from other disciplines.

Naturalistic concepts are concepts seen in nature or in nursing practice such as body weight, thermoregulation, hematologic complications, depression, pain, and spirituality. These may be on a continuum from concrete to abstract, and some may be measurable in fact (e.g., body weight and temperature) and others (e.g., pain or spirituality) measurable only indirectly and only in principle.

Research-based concepts are the result of conceptual development that is grounded in research processes. The theorist/researcher studies the realm of interest and identifies themes. Through qualitative, phenomenologic, or grounded theory approaches, the researcher may uncover meanings of the phenomena of interest and their theoretical relationships (Parse, 1999; Rodgers, 2000). Examples include Alzheimer's caregiver stress (Llanque, Savage, Rosenburg, & Caserta, 2016), food insecurity (Schroeder & Smaldone, 2015), joy and happiness (Cottrell, 2016), and chronic disease self-management (Miller, Lasiter, Ellis, & Buelow, 2015).

Existing concepts are the final type of concept. The nursing literature is filled with adapted concepts, more or less well synthesized through derivation from other disciplines. Such concepts include human needs from Maslow's (1954) hierarchy of needs and stress from Selye's (1956) physiologic theory of the stress of life. Theories of bodily function come from the study of physiology (Guyton & Hall, 1996). Borrowed concepts from medicine are clearly seen in clinical practice, especially in critical care areas of institutions. Other existing concepts commonly used in nursing research, administration, and practice are empathy, suffering, abuse, hope, and burnout. Table 3-3 summarizes the three sources of concepts for nursing.

Table 3-3 Sources of Concepts

Concept	Source	Characteristics	Examples From Nursing Literature
Naturalistic concepts	Present in nursing practice	May be defined and developed for use in research and theory development. Often have medical implications as well as nursing use	Body weight, pain, thermoregulation, depression, hematologic complications, circadian dysregulation
Research-based concepts	Developed through qualitative research processes (e.g., grounded theory or existential phenomenology)	Often relate to a nursing specialty	Hope, grief, cultural competence, chronic pain
Existing concepts	Borrowed from other disciplines	Developed for nursing practice but are useful in research and theory	Job satisfaction, quality of life, abuse, adaptation, stress

Sources: Cowles and Rogers (1993); Parse (1999); Verhulst and Schwartz-Barcott (1993); Wang (2000).

Concept Analysis/Concept Development

Concept analysis, concept development, concept synthesis (Walker & Avant, 2011), and other terms refer to the rigorous process of bringing clarity to the definition of the concepts used in science. Concept analysis and concept development are the terms used most commonly in nursing and are generally applied to the process of inquiry that examines concepts for their level of development as revealed by their internal structure, use, representativeness, and relationship to other concepts. Thus, concept analysis/concept development explores the meaning of concepts to promote understanding.

Purposes of Concept Development

Clarifying, recognizing, and defining concepts that describe phenomena is the purpose of concept development or concept analysis. These processes serve as the basis for development of conceptual frameworks, theories, and research studies.

Because a considerable portion of the conceptual basis of nursing theory, research, and practice has been constructed using concepts adopted from other disciplines, reexamination of these concepts for relevance and fit is important. The process of applying "borrowed" or "shared" concepts may have altered their meaning, and it is important to review them for appropriateness of application (Hupcey, Morse, Lenz, & Tasón, 1996). Also, as knowledge is continually developing, new concepts are being introduced and accepted, and concepts are continually being investigated and refined. Furthermore, some concepts are poorly defined with characteristics that have not been described, whereas other concepts that have been defined may present with inconsistency between the definition and its use in research (Morse, Hupcey, Mitcham, & Lenz, 1996).

In summary, concept analysis can be used to evaluate the level of maturity or development of nursing concepts by:

- Identifying gaps in nursing knowledge
- Determining the need to refine or clarify a concept when it appears to have multiple meanings
- Evaluating the adequacy of competing concepts in their relation to other phenomena
- Examining the congruence between the definition of the concept and the way it has been operationalized
- Determining the fit between the definition of the concept and its clinical application (Morse et al., 1996)

Link to Practice 3-1 gives examples of a number of different concepts that have been suggested for development by graduate nursing students. Some of the examples (e.g., "first-time parentitis in the ED" and "normal birth experience reconciliation") were derived from clinical practice, and others (e.g., chemo brain and hoarding) were derived from non-nursing sources. A few (e.g., chemo brain, wholeness, and successful aging) may have already been presented in the nursing literature and even been a component of nursing research, but most have not.

Context for Concept Development

In the course of nursing practice, multiple instances of a problem will be seen as shown in the opening case study. When talking among peers, nurses may clarify a problem so that colleagues can understand the situation. Eventually, the nurse will

Link to Practice 3-1

Student-Generated Examples of Concepts of Interest to Nurses

Like Rebecca, the oncology nurse specialist (ONS) in the opening case study, nurses routinely encounter ideas, concepts, and phenomena in practice. Here are some concepts suggested by graduate students in the past that might be amenable to concept analysis or concept development and ultimately to theory development and research.

Concepts from the literature and other disciplines:

- Chemo brain
- Chronic fatigue
- Denial
- Forgiveness
- Functional status
- Healing
- Hoarding
- Inner strength
- Postdeployment reassimilation
- Second victim
- Successful aging
- Thermoregulation
- Waiting
- Wholeness
- Genetic health promotion

Phenomena from observation in clinical settings:

- First-time parentitis in the emergency department (ED)
- Males are nurturing caregivers
- Normal birth experience reconciliation
- Palliative care in the neonatal intensive care unit (NICU)
- Rally at the end-of-life

develop a term, a word, or a phrase as a name for the problem. This illustrates the starting point for studying a theoretical phenomenon—concept naming.

In refining the phenomenon so that the phenomenon can be studied, the steps of the concept development process are instituted. In this process, instances of the phenomenon are collected, the similarities and differences between the concept being studied and other concepts are reviewed, and those that are material to the use of the concept are extracted and the concept is defined from its existence in nature. Isolating specific information from all the surrounding information (the context) is important, but nurses must see the concept emerging and take note of the context in which the concept occurs.

In the case study at the beginning of the chapter, the nurses recognized the problem of women with breast cancer and their periodic sadness and noted the context in which the phenomenon occurred. It was important to focus on those situations that are relevant. Questions that might be asked to assess the context include: Did the women have unsupportive husbands? Were their lives threatened by nodal involvement and metastasis? What were the previous experiences of the women with disease or injury? What is the history of cancer in the women's families?

Concept Development and Conceptual Frameworks

Once concepts have been identified, named, and developed, the nurse can test them in descriptive studies, particularly qualitative studies to further develop the concept and make explicit its use in real situations. The concept can be analyzed for its relation to many facets of the nursing discipline and the meaning made explicit for the nurse's use in daily work or scholarly endeavors.

Conceptual frameworks are structures that relate concepts together in a meaningful way. Although relationships are posited in conceptual frameworks, frequently neither the direction nor the strength of the relationships is made explicit for use in practice or for testing in a research project. Chapter 4 provides a detailed discussion of the processes used in the development of theories and conceptual frameworks.

Concept Development and Research

A common language is necessary for communicating the meanings of concepts that comprise theories. Theory, research, and practice are linked, and most scholars recognize that they cannot be separated. Researchers relate concepts together into structures that are called models and theories and derive from them testable relationships called hypotheses (Kerlinger, 1986).

Hickman (2011) points out that nursing research, theory, and practice form a cycle and that entry into this cycle may be at any point. Research both precedes theory and is guided by theory. Both theory and research direct practice, and conversely, research and theory are derived from practice situations. Thus, theory, while guiding research, is simultaneously being tested in the research process. The conceptual elements of the theory that guide the research or are being tested by the research are named and defined during concept analysis.

Difficulties with studying a problem in nursing may be related to the exactness with which the terms in use are developed and defined. Poorly defined concepts may lead to faulty construction of research instruments and methods (Morse, 1995). Frequently, a nursing problem does not lend itself precisely to existing terminology. In this situation, the nurse should engage in the effort of concept development. Furthermore, if one cannot successfully define the problem so that other professionals can understand it, concept development is necessary.

Strategies for Concept Analysis and Concept Development

There are multiple methods of constructing meaning for concepts. This can be accomplished through review of research literature, scholarly critique, and thoughtful definition. When a formal or detailed meaning is warranted, however, a more structured method for concept development will need to be used.

In the early 1960s, John Wilson (1963), a social scientist, developed a process for defining concepts to improve communication and comprehension of the meanings of terms in scientific use. Wilson used 11 steps, or techniques, to guide the concept analysis process. A few recent examples, which used Wilson's method of concept development, were discovered in the nursing literature. In one example, Llanque and colleagues (2016) employed a modification of Wilson's method to analyze the concept of Alzheimer's caregiver's stress. Similarly, Lynch and Lobo (2012) used Wilson's method to examine compassion fatigue in family caregivers, and Chee (2014) used Wilson's method to describe "deliberate practice" in the context of clinical simulation in nursing education.

Building on the process presented by Wilson (1963), nurses have published several techniques, methods, and strategies for concept development. Strategies devised by several nurse scholars will be presented briefly in the following sections, and examples of published works using these methods will be provided where available.

Walker and Avant

Walker and Avant first explicated the process of concept analysis for nurses in 1986. Their procedures were based on Wilson's method and clarified his methods so that graduate students could apply them to examine phenomena of interest to nurses. Three different processes were described by Walker and Avant (2011): concept analysis, concept synthesis, and concept derivation.

Concept Analysis
Concept analysis is an approach espoused by Walker and Avant (2011) to clarify the meanings of terms and to define terms (concepts) so that writers and readers share a common language. Concept analysis should be conducted when concepts require clarification or further development to define them for a nurse scholar's purposes, whether that is research, theory development, or practice. This method for concept analysis requires an eight-step approach, as listed in Box 3-2.

Concept Synthesis
Concept synthesis is used when concepts require development based on observation or other forms of evidence. The individual must develop a way to group or order the information about the phenomenon from his or her own viewpoint or theoretical requirement. Methods of synthesizing concepts follow:

1. Qualitative synthesis—relies on sensory data and looking for similarities, differences, and patterns among the data to identify the new concept
2. Quantitative synthesis—requires numerical data to delineate those attributes that belong to the concept and those that do not

---

Box 3-2   Steps in Concept Analysis

1. Select a concept.
2. Determine the aims or purposes of analysis.
3. Identify all the uses of the concept possible.
4. Determine the defining attributes.
5. Identify model case.
6. Identify borderline, related, contrary, invented, and illegitimate cases.
7. Identify antecedents and consequences.
8. Define empirical referents.

Source: Walker and Avant (2011, p. 160).

Box 3-3	Steps in Concept Derivation

1. Become thoroughly familiar with the existing literature related to the topic of interest.
2. Search other fields for new ways of looking at the topic of interest.
3. Select a parent concept or set of concepts from another field to use in the derivation process.
4. Redefine the concept(s) from the parent field in terms of the topic of interest.

Source: Walker and Avant (2011, p. 76).

3. Literary synthesis—involves reviewing a wide range of the literature to acquire new insights about the concept or to find new concepts
4. Mixed methods—use of any of the three methods described together, either sequentially or combined (Walker & Avant, 2011)

Concept Derivation

Concept derivation from Walker and Avant's (2011) perspective is often necessary when there are few concepts currently available to a nurse that explain a problem area. It is applicable when a comparison or analogy can be made between one field or area that is conceptually defined and another that is not. Concept derivation can be helpful in generating new ways of thinking about a phenomenon of interest. A four-step plan for the work of moving likely concepts from disciplines outside nursing into the nursing lexicon has been developed (Box 3-3).

Examples of Concept Analysis Using Walker and Avant's Techniques

Walker and Avant's techniques have been taught for more than three decades in graduate nursing programs, and their method of concept analysis is the most commonly used in nursing. Table 3-4 lists several examples from recent nursing literature. In their most recent edition, Walker and Avant (2011) outline the processes for each of the methods described in depth and provide a number of examples for clarification. The reader is referred to their work, as well as to the examples listed, for more information.

Rodgers

Rodgers first published her evolutionary method for concept analysis in 1989. According to Rodgers (2000), concept analysis is necessary because concepts are dynamic, "fuzzy," and context dependent and possess some pragmatic utility or purpose. Furthermore, because phenomena, needs, and goals change, concepts must be continually refined and variations introduced to achieve a clearer and more useful meaning.

Rodgers (2000) examined two viewpoints or schools of thought regarding concept development and showed that the methods of each differ significantly. She termed these methods "essentialism" and "evolutionary" viewpoints. In her work, she contrasted the essentialist method of concept development as exemplified by Wilson (1963) and Walker and Avant (1995) with concept development using the evolutionary method.

The evolutionary method of concept development is a concurrent task approach. In it, the tasks may be going on all at the same time rather than a sequence of specific steps that are completed before going to the next step. The activities involved in the evolutionary method are listed in Box 3-4.

Table 3-4 Examples of Concept Analyses Using Walker and Avant's Methods

Concept	Reference
Body image disturbance	Rhoten, B. A. (2016). Body image disturbance in adults treated for cancer—a concept analysis. *Journal of Advanced Nursing, 72*(5), 1001–1011.
Concealed pregnancy	Tighe, S. M., & Lalor, J. G. (2015). Concealed pregnancy: A concept analysis. *Journal of Advanced Nursing, 72*(1), 50–61.
Ethical competence	Kulju, K., Stolt, M., Suhonen, R., & Leino-Kilpi, H. (2016). Ethical competence: A concept analysis. *Nursing Ethics, 23*(4), 401–412.
Food insecurity	Schroeder, K., & Smaldone, A. (2015). Food insecurity: A concept analysis. *Nursing Forum, 50*(4), 274–284.
Meaning in work	Lee, S. (2015). A concept analysis of 'Meaning in work' and its implications for nursing. *Journal of Advanced Nursing, 71*(10), 2258–2267.
Nurse–patient interaction	Evans, E. C. (2016). Exploring the nuances of nurse-patient interaction through concept analysis: Impact on patient satisfaction. *Nursing Science Quarterly, 29*(1), 62–70.
Proactive behavior in midwifery	Mestdagh, E., Van Rompaey, B., Beekman, K., Bogaerts, A., & Timmermans, O. (2016). A concept analysis of proactive behavior in midwifery. *Journal of Advanced Nursing, 72*(6), 1236–1250.
Role transition	Barnes, H. (2015). Nurse practitioner role transition: A concept analysis. *Nursing Forum, 50*(3), 137–146.
Survivor in the cancer context	Hebdon, M., Foli, K., & McComb, S. (2015). Survivor in the cancer context: A concept analysis. *Journal of Advanced Nursing, 71*(8), 1774–1786.

Rodgers (2000) defined many terms and explained the process of concept analysis using the evolutionary view. The goal of the concept analysis will, to an extent, determine how the researcher *identifies the concept of interest* and terms and expressions selected. The incorporation of a new term into a nurse's way of viewing a client situation is often a circumstance warranting analysis of a new concept.

The goal of the analysis will also influence *selection of the setting and sample* for data collection. For instance, the setting may be a library and the sample might be literature. The sampling might be time-oriented, say literature from the previous 5 years. In any case, the researcher's goal is to develop a rigorous design consistent with the purpose

Box 3-4   Steps in Rodgers's Process of Concept Analysis

1. Identify the concept and associated terms.
2. Select an appropriate realm (a setting or a sample) for data collection.
3. Collect data to identify the attributes of the concept and the contextual basis of the concept (i.e., interdisciplinary, sociocultural, and temporal variations).
4. Analyze the data regarding the characteristics of the concept.
5. Identify an exemplar of the concept, if appropriate.
6. Identify hypotheses and implications for further development.

Source: Rodgers (2000, p. 85).

of the analysis. The selection of literature from related disciplines might include those that typically use the concept. An exhaustive review includes all the indexed literature using the concept and may be limited by a time frame such as several years.

A randomization process is then used to select the sample across each discipline over time. In *collecting and managing the data*, a discovery approach is preferred. The focus of the data analysis is on identifying the attributes, antecedents, and consequences and related concepts or surrogate terms. The attributes located by this means constitute a "real definition as opposed to a nominal or dictionary definition" (Rodgers, 2000, p. 91).

Rodgers (2000) defines *surrogate terms* as ways of expressing the concept other than by the term of interest. She distinguishes between surrogate terms and *related concepts* by showing that surrogate terms are different words that express the concept, whereas "related concepts are part of a network that provide a background" and "lend significance to the concept of interest" (Rodgers, 2000, p. 92).

Analyzing the data can go on simultaneously with its collection according to Rodgers (2000), or it can be delayed until all the data are collected. The latter is allowed in concept analysis using the evolutionary process because data are currently available rather than being constantly created by the subjects as in qualitative research study. The researcher must beware of considering the data "saturated," that is, redundant, too early.

Identifying an exemplar from the literature, field observation, or interview is important and will provide a clear example of the concept. Examples of real cases are preferred over constructed cases (in contrast to Wilson's [1963] method). The goal is to illustrate the characteristics of the concept in relevant contexts to enhance the clarity and effective application of the concept.

Interpreting the results involves gaining insight on the current status of the concept and generating implications for inquiry based on this status and identified gaps. Interpreting the results may involve interdisciplinary comparison, temporal comparison, and assessment of the social context within which the concept analysis was conducted.

Identifying implications for further development and formal inquiry may be the result. The results of the analysis may direct further inquiry rather than giving the final answer on the meaning of the concept. The implications of this form of research-based concept analysis may yield questions for further research, or hypotheses may be extracted from the findings. The major outcome of the evolutionary method of concept analysis is the generation of further questions for research rather than the static definition of the concept. Table 3-5 lists a number of references for concept analyses using this method. For more information, the reader is referred to Rodgers (2000).

Schwartz-Barcott and Kim

A hybrid model of concept development was initially presented by Schwartz-Barcott and Kim in 1986 and expanded and revised in 1993 and 2000. This method for concept development involves a three-phase process, which is summarized in Table 3-6.

Theoretical Phase

In the theoretical phase, a borrowed concept, an underdeveloped nursing concept, or a concept from clinical practice may be selected. The main consideration is that the concept has relevance for nursing. A clinical encounter may be described in detail to arrive at the concept through analysis. *The literature is searched* broadly and systematically across disciplines that may use the concept. A set of questions that provides inquiry into the essential nature of the concept, the means of clear definition, and ways to enhance its measurability focuses on questions of measurement and definition.

Table 3-5 Examples of Concept Analyses Using Rodgers's Methods

Concept	Reference
Chronic disease self-management	Miller, W., Lasiter, S., Ellis, R. B., & Buelow, J. M. (2015). Chronic disease self-management: A hybrid concept analysis. *Nursing Outlook, 63*(2), 154–161.
Cultural competence	Garneau, A. B., & Pepin, J. (2015). Cultural competence: A constructivist definition. *Journal of Transcultural Nursing, 26*(1), 9–15.
Joy and happiness	Cottrell, L. (2016). Joy and happiness: A simultaneous and evolutionary concept analysis. *Journal of Advanced Nursing, 72*(7), 1506–1517.
Nursing workload	Swiger, P. A., Vance, D. E., & Patrician, P. A. (2016). Nursing workload in the acute-care setting: A concept analysis of nursing workload. *Nursing Outlook, 64*(3), 244–254.
Patient autonomy	Lindberg, C., Fagerström, C., Sivberg, B., & Willman, A. (2014). Concept analysis: Patient autonomy in a caring context. *Journal of Professional Nursing, 70*(10), 2208–2221.
Person-, family-, and culture-centered nursing care	Lor, M., Crooks, N., & Tluczek, A. (2016). A proposed model of person-, family-, and culture-centered nursing care. *Nursing Outlook, 64*(4), 352–366.
Resilient aging	Hicks, M. M., & Conner, N. E. (2014). Resilient ageing: A concept analysis. *Journal of Advanced Nursing, 70*(4), 744–755.
Spiritual care of the child with cancer at the end of life	Petersen, C. L. (2014). Spiritual care of the child with cancer at the end of life: A concept analysis. *Journal of Advanced Nursing, 70*(6), 1243–1253.
Recovery in mental illness	McCauley, C. O., McKenna, H. P., Keeney, S., & McLauhlin, D. F. (2015). Concept analysis of recovery in mental illness in young adulthood. *Journal of Psychiatric and Mental Health Nursing, 22*(8), 579–589.

Meaning and measurement are dealt with. This requires thought for comparing and contrasting the data. *A working definition* is chosen to be used in the final phase. The definition should maintain a nursing perspective.

Fieldwork Phase

In the *fieldwork* phase, the concept is corroborated and refined. The fieldwork phase integrates with the literature phase and expands into a modified qualitative research approach (e.g., participant observation). The steps of this phase are setting the stage, negotiating entry, selecting cases, and collecting and analyzing the data.

Analytical Phase

The final analytical phase includes examination of the details in the light of the literature review. The researcher reviews the findings with the original purpose in view. Three questions guide the final analysis:

1. How much is the concept applicable and important to nursing?
2. Does the initial selection of the concept seem justified?
3. To what extent do the review of literature, theoretical analysis, and empirical findings support the presence and frequency of the concept within the population selected for empirical study? (Schwartz-Barcott & Kim, 2000, p. 147)

Table 3-6 Phases of Schwartz-Barcott and Kim's Hybrid Model of Concept Development

Phase	Activities
Theoretical phase	Select a concept. Review the literature. Determine meaning and measurement. Choose a working definition.
Fieldwork phase	Set the stage. Negotiate entry into a setting. Select cases. Collect and analyze data.
Final analytical phase	Weigh findings. Write report.

Source: Schwartz-Barcott and Kim (2000).

The final step of the process is to *write up the findings*. The work may be reported as either fieldwork or as a concept analysis. Elements the researcher must consider when writing the findings are length of the study, the intended audience, timing, pacing of the authorship process, anticipated length of the manuscript, how much detail of the process to include, and ethics of the interpretation of the analysis (Schwartz-Barcott & Kim, 2000).

Several results can be realized by this type of analysis:

1. The current meaning of the concept can be supported or refined.
2. A different definition than previously used may stand out.
3. The concept may be completely redefined.
4. A new or refined way of measuring the concept may be the result (Schwartz-Barcott & Kim, 1993).

Examples of published reports using this model are listed in Table 3-7.

Table 3-7 Examples of Concept Analyses Using Schwartz-Barcott and Kim's Hybrid Method

Concept	Reference
Breastfeeding	Sherriff, N., Hall, V., & Panton, C. (2014). Engaging and supporting fathers to promote breast feeding: A concept analysis. *Midwifery, 30*(6), 667–677.
Compassion competence	Lee, Y., & Seomun, G. (2016). Development and validation of an instrument to measure nurses' compassion competence. *Applied Nursing Research, 30*, 76–82.
Grief	Zucker, D. M., Dion, K., & McKeever, R. P. (2015). Concept clarification of grief in mothers of children with an addiction. *Journal of Advanced Nursing, 71*(4), 751–767.

Meleis

Meleis (2012) described three strategies to develop conceptual meaning for use in nursing theory, research, and practice. These are concept exploration, concept clarification, and concept analysis.

Concept Exploration

Concept exploration is used when concepts are new and ambiguous in a discipline, when concepts are camouflaged by being embedded in the daily nursing discussion, or when a concept from another discipline is being redesigned for use in nursing. Concept exploration may awaken nurses to a new concept or revitalize the meanings of an overused concept to make it explicit for practice, research, and theory building. The steps Meleis (2012) suggests for this endeavor follow:

1. Identifying the major components and dimensions of the concept
2. Raising appropriate questions about the concept
3. Proposing triggers for continuing the exploration
4. Identifying and defining the advantages to the discipline of continuing the exploration of this concept (p. 373)

Concept Clarification

Concept clarification is used to "refine concepts that have been used in nursing without a clear, shared, and conscious agreement on the properties of meanings attributed to them" (Meleis, 2012, p. 374). Concept clarification is a way to refine existing concepts when they lack clarity for a specific nursing endeavor. The processes involved in concept clarification allow for reduction of ambiguities while critically reviewing the properties. The processes are presented in Box 3-5.

Concept Analysis

Concept analysis, according to Meleis (2012), assumes that the concept has been introduced into nursing literature but is ready to move to the level of development for research. This process implies that the concept will be broken down to its essentials and then reconstructed for its contribution to the nursing lexicon. The goal of the analysis is to bring the concept close to use in research or clinical practice and to ultimately contribute to instrument development and theory testing.

Box 3-5   Process of Concept Clarification

1. Clarify the boundaries of the concept, including what attributes should be included and what should be excluded.
2. Critically review the properties of the concept.
3. Bring to light new dimensions that had not been considered.
4. Compare, contrast, delineate, and differentiate these properties and provide exemplars of the concept.
5. Identify assumptions and philosophical bases about the events that trigger the phenomena and propose questions from a nursing perspective.

Source: Meleis (2012, p. 374).

Table 3-8 Meleis's Processes for Concept Development

Process	Task or Activity
Defining	Creating theoretical and operational definitions that clarify ambiguities, enhance precision, and relate concepts to empirical referents
Differentiating	Sorting in and out similarities and differences between the concept being developed and other like concepts
Delineating antecedents	Defining the contextual conditions under which the concept is perceived and expected to occur
Delineating consequences	Defining events, situations, or conditions that may result from the concept
Modeling	Defining and identifying exemplars (i.e., clinical referents or research referents) to illustrate some aspect of the concept. Models may be same or like models, or contrary models
Analogizing	Describing the concept through another concept or phenomenon that is similar and has been studied more extensively
Synthesizing	Bringing together findings, meanings, and properties that have been discovered and describing future steps in theorizing

Source: Meleis (2012, pp. 384–386).

Meleis (2012) focused on an integrated approach to concept development, which includes defining, differentiating, delineating antecedents and consequences, modeling, analogizing, and synthesizing. Table 3-8 lists each of these components and presents related activities or tasks to be accomplished for each phase. A few examples using Meleis's strategies were located in the literature. For example, Olsen and Harder (2010) combined Meleis's strategies with Schwartz-Barcott and Kim's to describe "network-focused nursing." Clark and Robinson (2000) used Meleis's earlier work to describe the concept of multiculturalism, and Felten and Hall (2001) used Meleis's strategies to describe the concept of resilience in elderly women.

Morse

In response to concerns that some concepts in the nursing lexicon had been derived and not developed adequately for nursing, or had become overused by those who did not clarify them, Morse (1995) developed a method of concept development to enhance clarity and distinctiveness of nursing concepts. In this method, she used the term "advanced techniques of concept analysis" and described the processes of concept delineation, concept comparison, and concept clarification.

Concept Delineation
Concept delineation is a strategy that requires an extensive literature search and assists in separating two terms that seem closely linked. The concepts are then compared and contrasted to identify commonalities, similarities, and differences such that distinctions may be drawn between the terms (Morse, 1995).

Concept Comparison

Concept comparison clarifies competing concepts, again using an extensive literature review and keeping the literature for each concept separate. Three phases are used in the comparison:

1. Preconditions—the status of the concept in nursing and its use in teaching or clinical practice
2. Process—the type of nursing response to the concept, at what level of consciousness it occurs, and, if it is identified with the client, at what level
3. Outcomes—whether the concept was used to identify process or product, its accuracy in prediction, the client's condition, and the client's experience with the concept (Morse, 1995, pp. 39–41)

Concept Clarification

For Morse (1995), *concept clarification* is used with concepts that are "mature" and have a large body of literature identifying and using them. The concept clarification process requires a "literature review to identify the underlying values and to identify, describe and compare and contrast the attributes of each" (p. 41).

Published reports using Morse's methods for concept development can be found in the nursing literature. For example, Hawkins and Morse (2014) modified the technique to describe the concept of courage as a foundation for care. Other examples of concepts developed by nurse scholars using Morse's techniques are: quality pain management in hospitalized adults (Zoëga, Gunnarsdottir, Wilson, & Gordon, 2016), "crying that heals" (Griffith, Hall, & Fields, 2011), and rest (Bernhofer, 2016).

Penrod and Hupcey

Penrod and Hupcey (2005) built on Morse's method and termed their method "principle-based concept analysis." Explaining their intent to "determine and evaluate the state of the science surrounding the concept" (p. 405) and "produce evidence that reveals scholars' best estimate of 'probable truth' in the scientific literature" (p. 406), they outlined four principles for their method: epistemologic, pragmatic, linguistic, and logical (Box 3-6).

Box 3-6   Four Principles of Concept Analysis

Epistemologic principle is based on the question "Is the concept clearly defined and well differentiated from other concepts?" (p. 405).

Pragmatic principle, in which the question to be answered is "Is the concept applicable and useful within the scientific realm or inquiry? Has it been operationalized?" In this principle, they believe that an operationalized concept has achieved a level of maturity (p. 405).

Linguistic principle asks, "Is the concept used consistently and appropriately within context?" (p. 406). Similarly to Morse and to Rodgers, they find that context or lack of context is a factor important in this type of analysis (p. 406).

Logical principle applies the question "Does the concept hold its boundaries through theoretical integration with other concepts?" (p. 406). The authors require that the concept not be blurred with respect to other concepts but that it remains logically clear and distinct.

Source: Penrod and Hupcey (2005, pp. 405–406).

Penrod and Hupcey (2005) explain that in their method of concept analysis, the findings "are summarized as a theoretical definition that integrates an evaluative summary of each of the criteria posed by the four over-arching principles." To do this, the researcher must consider three issues: (1) selection of appropriate disciplinary literature for review, (2) assurance of the adequacy and appropriateness of the sample derived from the literature, and (3) employment of "within- and across-discipline analytic techniques." They have elucidated that this advanced level of concept development seems to be more relevant to the research endeavor, as it is a research-based concept analysis.

Despite being developed relatively recently, examples of published works using Penrod and Hupcey's (2005) method for concept analysis can be found. For example, Lindauer and Harvath (2014) used a hybrid of Penrod and Hupcey's principle-based method to analyze the concept of predeath grief in the context of family care giving with a dementia victim, and Watson (2015) used the principle-based method of Penrod and Hupcey to analyze the concept of wrong site surgery. Lastly, Mikkelsen and Frederiksen (2011) analyzed the concept of "family-centered care" of hospitalized children using Penrod and Hupcey's method.

Comparison of Models for Concept Development

The nursing literature contains several comparisons and critiques of the various models and methods for concept development/concept analysis. Indeed, Hupcey and colleagues (1996) and Morse and colleagues (1996) provided a detailed and well-researched comparison of the techniques presented by Walker and Avant (1983), Schwartz-Barcott and Kim (1993), and Rodgers (1989). Strengths and weaknesses of each method were described in their papers. More recently, Duncan and colleagues (2007) and Weaver and Mitcham (2008) reviewed the history of concept analysis comparing the major methods in common use. Finally, Risjord (2009) reexamined the philosophical basis and intent of concept analysis and concluded that rather than *preceding* theory development, it must be a *part of* theory development. Table 3-9 compares the various formats for concept development/concept analysis described earlier.

Summary

Rebecca Wallis, the nurse from the opening case study, identified a new phenomenon that was pertinent to her practice of oncology nursing and decided to develop the concept more fully. By applying techniques of concept analysis to the PMG reaction, she began the process of formulating information on this concept that could ultimately be used by other nurses in practice or research.

The process of developing concepts includes reviewing the nurse's area of interest, examining the phenomena closely, pondering the terms that are relevant and that fit together with reality, and operationalizing the concept for practice, research, or educational use. Whether advanced practice nurses or nursing scholars elect to use the methods proposed by Wilson (1963), Walker and Avant (2011), Morse (1995), Rodgers (2000), Schwartz-Barcott and Kim (2000), Meleis (2012), Penrod and Hupcey (2005), or a combination, it is clear that the process of developing, clarifying, comparing and contrasting, and integrating well-derived and defined concepts is necessary for theory development and to guide research studies. This will, in turn, ultimately benefit practice. Chapter 4 builds on the process of concept development by describing the processes used to link concepts to form relationship statements and to construct conceptual models, frameworks, and theories.

Table 3-9 Comparison of Selected Methods of Concept Development

Author(s)	Method	Purpose	No. of Steps	Constructed Cases	Other Factors/Steps
Walker and Avant	Concept analysis	Clarify meaning of terms	8	Model, borderline, related, contrary	Identify empirical referents and defining attributes; delineate antecedents and consequences
Rodgers	Evolutionary concept analysis	Refine and clarify concepts for use in research and practice	5	Model only (identified—not constructed)	Identify appropriate realm (setting and sample); analyze data about characteristics, conduct interdisciplinary or temporal comparisons; identify hypotheses and implications for further study
Schwartz-Barcott and Kim	Hybrid model of concept development	Support or refine the meaning of a concept and/or develop a new or refined way to measure a concept	3 phases	Model case, contrary case	Develop working definitions, search literature, participant observation, collect and analyze data, write findings
Meleis	Concept development	Define concepts theoretically and operationally, clarify ambiguities, relate concepts to empirical referents	7	Same or like models; contrary models	Define concept, use an analogy to describe a similar concept, synthesize findings; differentiate similarities and differences between like concepts; delineate antecedents and consequences
Morse	Concept comparison	Clarifies the meaning of competing concepts	3 phases	Not specified	Use extensive literature review to examine and describe preconditions (status of use of the concepts in teaching or practice), process, and outcomes of use of the concept
Penrod and Hupcey	Principle-based concept analysis	Concept analysis	4 phases based on principles	Not specified	Sampling within bodies of large multidisciplinary literature yields a theoretically based scientific definition

Key Points

- A concept is a symbolic statement that describes a phenomenon or a class of phenomena.
- There are many different ways to explain or classify concepts (e.g., abstract vs. concrete and variable vs. discrete).
- Concepts used in nursing practice, research, education, and administration can come from the natural world (e.g., biology and environment), from research, or from other disciplines.

- Concept analysis/concept development refers to the rigorous process of bringing clarity to the definition of the concepts used in nursing science.
- When theoretically and operationally defined, the concepts can be readily applied in nursing practice, research, education, and administration.
- Several methods for concept analysis/concept development have been described in the nursing literature.

CONCEPT ANALYSIS EXEMPLAR

The following is an outline delineating the steps of a concept analysis using Rodgers's (2000) evolutionary method.

Barkimer, J. (2016). Clinical growth: An evolutionary concept analysis. *Advances in Nursing Science, 39*(3), E28–E29.

1. *Identify the concept and associated terms.*

Concept: Clinical growth

Associated terms: student preparedness, student growth, student development, clinical learning, student learning, student experiences

2. *Select an appropriate realm (setting) for data collection.*

The realm for the study was a search of the Cumulative Index to Nursing and Allied Health Literature (CINAHL), Health Science in ProQuest, Cochrane Library, MEDLINE, PubMed, Ovid, Web of Science, ERIC, and PsycINFO between 2004 and 2015.

3. *Identify the attributes of the concept and the contextual basis of the concept.*

Attributes of clinical growth:

a. Higher level thinking
b. Socialization
c. Skill development
d. Self-reflection
e. Self-investment
f. Interpersonal communication
g. Linking theory to practice

4. *Specify the characteristics of the concept.*

Antecedents:

a. Having a quality educator
b. Supportive environment
c. Intrinsic characteristics

Consequences: Five themes were presented.

a. Lifelong learning
b. Transition toward autonomy
c. Personal growth
d. Competency
e. Confidence

5. *Identify an exemplar of the concept.*

An exemplar case study was presented:

It described a senior-level nursing student who was completing his pediatric rotation. Each of the critical attributes (e.g., quality educator, self-investment, socialization) were present. The resulting consequences included personal growth, competency, and confidence.

6. *Identify hypotheses and implications for development.*

For further study and application, the author suggested:

Development of a clinical performance evaluation tool based on the identified critical attributes to facilitate student-entered learning

Learning Activities

1. Collect and review several of the concept analyses mentioned in the chapter. How are they operationalized? How can they be used for research? In what form(s) of research would you expect to see the concepts you have chosen used?
2. Review the different methods for concept development presented. How are the methods alike? How are they different? Which method appears to be the most likely to reveal a concept suited to the process that the author desires?
3. Consider a phenomenon you have observed in your practice that might be appropriate for further development. Discuss the phenomenon with colleagues and try to name it and determine how you might develop it further.

REFERENCES

American Association of Colleges of Nursing. (2011). *The essentials of master's education in nursing.* Retrieved from http://www.aacn.nche.edu/education-resources/MastersEssentials11.pdf

Bernhofer, E. (2016). Investigating the concept of rest for research and practice. *Journal of Advanced Nursing, 72*(5), 1012–1022.

Chee, J. (2014). Clinical simulation using deliberate practice in nursing education: A Wilsonian concept analysis. *Nurse Education in Practice, 14*(3), 247–252.

Chinn, P. L., & Kramer, M. K. (2015). *Integrated theory and knowledge development in nursing* (9th ed.). St. Louis, MO: Elsevier.

Clark, C., & Robinson, T. (2000). Multiculturalism as a concept in nursing. *Journal of National Black Nurses' Association, 11*(2), 39–43.

Cottrell, L. (2016). Joy and happiness: A simultaneous and evolutionary concept analysis. *Journal of Advanced Nursing, 72*(7), 1506–1517.

Cowles, K. V., & Rogers, B. L. (1993). The concept of grief: An evolutionary perspective. In B. L. Rogers & K. A. Knafl (Eds.), *Concept development in nursing: Foundations, techniques, and applications* (pp. 93–106). Philadelphia, PA: Saunders.

Cutcliffe, J. R., & McKenna, H. P. (2005). *The essential concepts of nursing: Building blocks for practice.* London, United Kingdom: Elsevier.

Dubin, R. (1978). *Theory building.* New York, NY: Free Press.

Duncan, C., Cloutier, J. D., & Bailey, P. H. (2007). Concept analysis: The importance of differentiating the ontological focus. *Journal of Advanced Nursing, 58*(3), 293–300.

Fawcett, J. (1999). *The relationship of theory and research* (3rd ed.). Philadelphia, PA: Davis.

Felten, B. S., & Hall, J. M. (2001). Conceptualizing resilience in women older than 85: Overcoming adversity from illness or loss. *Journal of Gerontological Nursing, 27*(11), 46–53.

Griffith, M. B., Hall, J. M., & Fields, B. (2011). Crying that heals: Concept evaluation. *Journal of Holistic Nursing, 29*(3), 167–179.

Guyton, A. C., & Hall, J. E. (1996). *Textbook of medical physiology* (9th ed.). Philadelphia, PA: Saunders.

Hardin, S. R. (2014). Theory development process. In M. R. Alligood (Ed.), *Nursing theorists and their work* (8th ed., pp. 23–37). St. Louis, MO: Mosby.

Hardy, M. E. (1973). Theories: Components, development, evaluation. *Nursing Research, 23*(2), 100–107.

Hawkins, S. F., & Morse, J. (2014). The praxis of courage as a foundation for care. *Journal of Nursing Scholarship, 46*(4), 263–270.

Hickman, J. S. (2011). An introduction to nursing theory. In J. George (Ed.), *Nursing theories: The base for professional nursing practice* (6th ed., pp. 1–22). Upper Saddle River, NJ: Pearson Education.

Hupcey, J. E., Morse, J. M., Lenz, E. R., & Tasón, M. C. (1996). Wilsonian methods of concept analysis: A critique. *Scholarly Inquiry for Nursing Practice, 10*(3), 185–210.

Jacox, A. K. (1974). Theory construction in nursing: An overview. *Nursing Research, 23*(1), 4–13.

Kerlinger, F. N. (1986). *Foundations of behavioral research* (3rd ed.). New York, NY: Holt, Rinehart & Winston.

Kim, H. S. (2010). *The nature of theoretical thinking in nursing* (3rd ed.). New York, NY: Springer Publishing.

Lindauer, A., & Harvath, T. A. (2014). Pre-death grief in the context of dementia caregiving: A concept analysis. *Journal of Advanced Nursing, 70*(10), 2196–2207.

Llanque, S., Savage, L., Rosenburg, N., & Caserta, M. (2016). Concept analysis: Alzheimer's caregiver stress. *Nursing Forum, 51*(1), 21–31.

Lynch, S. H., & Lobo, M. L. (2012). Compassion fatigue in family caregivers: A Wilsonian concept analysis. *Journal of Advanced Nursing, 68*(9), 2125–2134.

Maslow, A. H. (1954). *Motivation and personality*. New York, NY: Harper.

Meleis, A. I. (2012). *Theoretical nursing: Development and progress* (4th ed.). Philadelphia, PA: Lippincott Williams & Wilkins.

Mikkelsen, G., & Frederiksen, K. (2011). Family-centred care of children in hospital—a concept analysis. *Journal of Advanced Nursing, 67*(5), 1152–1162.

Miller, W. R., Lasiter, S., Ellis, R. B., & Buelow, J. M. (2015). Chronic disease self-management: A hybrid concept analysis. *Nursing Outlook, 63*(2), 154–161.

Morse, J. M. (1995). Exploring the theoretical basis of nursing using advanced techniques of concept analysis. *ANS. Advances in Nursing Science, 17*(3), 31–46.

Morse, J. M., Hupcey, J. E., Mitcham, C., & Lenz, E. R. (1996). Concept analysis in nursing research: A critical appraisal. *Scholarly Inquiry for Nursing Practice, 10*(3), 253–277.

Olsen, P. R., & Harder, I. (2010). Network-focused nursing development of a new concept. *ANS. Advances in Nursing Science, 33*(4), 272–284.

Parse, R. R. (1999). *Hope: An international human becoming perspective*. Sudbury, MA: Jones & Bartlett Learning.

Parse, R. R. (2006). Concept inventing: Continuing clarification. *Nursing Science Quarterly, 19*(4), 289.

Penrod, J., & Hupcey, J. E. (2005). Enhancing methodological clarity: Principle-based concept analysis. *Journal of Advanced Nursing, 50*(4), 403–409.

Risjord, M. (2009). Rethinking concept analysis. *Journal of Advanced Nursing, 65*(3), 684–691.

Rodgers, B. L. (1989). Concept analysis and the development of nursing knowledge: The evolutionary cycle. *Journal of Advanced Nursing, 14*(4), 330–335.

Rodgers, B. L. (2000). Concept analysis: An evolutionary view. In B. L. Rodgers & K. A. Knafl (Eds.), *Concept development in nursing: Foundations, techniques, and applications* (2nd ed., pp. 77–102). Philadelphia, PA: Saunders.

Rodgers, B. L., & Knafl, K. A. (2000). *Concept development in nursing: Foundations, techniques, and applications* (2nd ed.). Philadelphia, PA: Saunders.

Schroeder, K., & Smaldone, A. (2015). Food insecurity: A concept analysis. *Nursing Forum, 50*(4), 274–284.

Schwartz-Barcott, D., & Kim, H. S. (1986). A hybrid model for concept development. In P. L. Chinn (Ed.), *Nursing research methodology: Issues and implementation* (pp. 91–101). Rockville, MD: Aspen.

Schwartz-Barcott, D., & Kim, H. S. (1993). An expansion and elaboration of the hybrid model of concept development. In B. L. Rodgers & K. A. Knafl (Eds.), *Concept development in nursing: Foundations, techniques, and applications* (pp. 107–133). Philadelphia, PA: Saunders.

Schwartz-Barcott, D., & Kim, H. S. (2000). An expansion and elaboration of the hybrid model of concept development. In B. L. Rodgers & K. A. Knafl (Eds.), *Concept development in nursing: Foundations, techniques, and applications* (2nd ed., pp. 129–160). Philadelphia, PA: Saunders.

Selye, H. (1956). *The stress of life*. New York, NY: McGraw-Hill.

Verhulst, G., & Schwartz-Barcott, D. (1993). A concept analysis of withdrawal: Application of the hybrid model of concept development. In B. L. Rogers & K. A. Knafl (Eds.), *Concept development in nursing: Foundations, techniques, and applications* (pp. 135–158). Philadelphia, PA: Saunders.

Walker, L. O., & Avant, K. (1983). *Strategies for theory construction in nursing*. Norwalk, CT: Appleton & Lange.

Walker, L. O., & Avant, K. (1995). *Strategies for theory construction in nursing* (3rd ed.). Norwalk, CT: Appleton & Lange.

Walker, L. O., & Avant, K. (2011). *Strategies for theory construction in nursing* (5th ed.). Upper Saddle River, NJ: Pearson Education.

Wang, C.-E. H. (2000). Developing a concept of hope from a human science perspective. *Nursing Science Quarterly, 13*(3), 248–251.

Watson, D. S. (2015). Concept analysis: Wrong-site surgery. *AORN Journal, 101*(6), 650–656.

Weaver, K., & Mitcham, C. (2008). Nursing concept analysis in North America: State of the art. *Nursing Philosophy, 9*(3), 180–194.

Wilson, J. (1963). *Thinking with concepts*. Cambridge, United Kingdom: Cambridge University Press.

Zoëga, S., Gunnarsdottir, S., Wilson, M., & Gordon, D. B. (2016). Quality pain management in adult hospitalized patients: A concept evaluation. *Nursing Forum, 51*(1), 3–12.

4

Theory Development

Structuring Conceptual Relationships in Nursing

Melanie McEwen

Jill Watson is enrolled in a master's nursing program and is beginning work on her thesis. As an occupational health nurse at a large telecommunication manufacturing company for the past 7 years, Jill has concentrated much of her practice on health promotion. She has organized numerous health fairs, led countless health help sessions, regularly posted health information on intranet bulletin boards, and provided screening programs for many illnesses. Despite her efforts to improve the health of the workers, many still smoke, are overweight, do not exercise, and have other deleterious lifestyle habits. Realizing that lack of information about health-related issues is not a problem, Jill has focused on trying to understand why people choose not to engage in positive health practices. As a result, she became interested in the concept of motivation.

In one of her early courses in her master's program, Jill completed an analysis of the concept of health motivation. During this exercise, she defined the concept; identified antecedents, consequences, and empirical referents; and developed a number of case studies, including a model case, a related case, and a contrary case.

As her studies progressed, Jill reviewed the literature from nursing, psychology, and sociology on health beliefs and health motivation and discovered several related theories. The Health Belief Model appeared to best explain her impressions of the issues at hand, but the model had not been developed for nursing and did not completely fit her concept of the variables and issues in health motivation. For her thesis, she decided to modify the Health Belief Model to focus on the concept of health motivation and to develop an instrument to measure the variables she had generated in her earlier work.

In nursing, theories are systematic explanations of events in which constructs and concepts are identified; relationships are proposed; and predictions are made to describe, explain, predict, or prescribe practice and research (Dickoff, James, & Wiedenbach, 1968; Streubert & Carpenter, 2011). Without nursing theory, nursing activities and interventions are guided by rote, tradition, some outside authority, or hunches, or they may simply be random.

Theories are not discovered; rather, they are constructed or developed to describe, explain, or understand phenomena or solve nagging problems (e.g., Why don't people apply knowledge of positive health practices?). In the past, nursing leaders saw theory development as a means of clearly establishing nursing as a profession, and throughout the last 50 years, many nursing scholars developed models and theories to guide nursing practice, nursing research, nursing administration and management, and nursing education. As discussed in Chapter 2, these models and theories have been created at different levels (grand, middle range, practice) and for different purposes (description, explanation, prediction, etc.).

Theory development seeks to help the nurse understand practice in a more complete and insightful way and provides a method of identifying and expressing key ideas about the essence of practice. Theories help organize existing knowledge and aid in making new and important discoveries to advance practice (Walker & Avant, 2011). As illustrated earlier in the case study, development and application of nursing theory are essential to revise, update, and refine the practice of nursing and to further advance the profession.

Overview of Theory Development

Several terms related to the creation of theory are found in the nursing literature. Theory construction, theory development, theory building, and theory generation are sometimes used synonymously or interchangeably. In other cases (Cesario, 1997; Walker & Avant, 2011), authors have differentiated the constructs or subsumed one term as a component or process within another. In this chapter, the term *theory development* is used as the global term to refer to the processes and methods used to create, modify, or refine a theory. *Theory construction* is used to describe one of the final steps of theory development in which the components of the theory are organized and linkages specified.

Theory development is a complex, time-consuming process that covers a number of stages or phases from inception of concepts to testing of theoretical propositions through research (Powers & Knapp, 2010). In general, the process of theory development begins with one or more concepts that are derived from within a discipline's metatheory or philosophy. These concepts are further refined and related to one another in propositions or statements that can be submitted to empirical testing (Chinn & Kramer, 2015; Peterson, 2017; Reynolds, 1971).

Categorizations of Theory

As described in Chapter 2, theories are often categorized using different criteria. Theories may be grouped based on scope or level of abstraction (grand theory, middle range theory, practice theory), the purpose of the theory, or the source or discipline in which the theory was developed.

Categorization Based on Scope or Level of Abstraction

An overview of "levels of theory" was presented in Chapter 2. In nursing, theories are often viewed based on scope or level of abstraction, where the most global or abstract level is the philosophical, or metatheory level, followed by grand theory, middle range theory, and practice theory. In the early years of nursing theory (1950–1980), theory development was largely at the metatheory and grand theory levels. Recently, however, there has been a significant shift with recognition of the need to focus more on middle range and practice (situation-specific) theories that are more relevant to nursing practice and more amenable to testing through research. The following sections will review and expand on each level of theory.

Philosophy, Worldview, or Metatheory

Metatheory refers to the philosophical and methodologic questions related to developing a theoretical base for nursing. It has also been termed "worldview" by some (Hickman, 2011). According to Walker and Avant (2011), metatheory deals with the processes of generating knowledge and debating broad issues related to the nature of theory, types of theory needed, and suitable criteria for theory evaluation. Chapter 1 discussed a number of philosophical issues related to a worldview or metatheory in nursing, including epistemology, research methods, and related questions.

Grand Theories

In nursing, grand theories are composed of relatively abstract concepts that are not operationally defined and attempt to explain or describe very comprehensive aspects of human experience and response. Grand theories consist of conceptual frameworks defining broad perspectives for practice and ways of looking at nursing phenomena based on these perspectives. They provide global viewpoints for nursing practice, education, and research, but they are limited because of their generality and abstractness. Indeed, because of their level of abstraction, these theories are often considered to be difficult to apply to the daily practice of nurses and are difficult to test (Hickman, 2011; Higgins & Shirley, 2000; Peterson, 2017; Walker & Avant, 2011).

Early grand nursing theories focused on the nurse–client relationship and the role of the nurse. Later grand theories expanded to more encompassing concepts (holistic perspective, interpersonal relations, social systems, and health). Recent grand theories have attempted to address phenomenologic aspects of nursing (caring, transcultural issues) (Moody, 1990). Chapters 6 to 9 provide an examination of grand nursing theories.

Middle Range Theories

The need for practice disciplines to develop middle range theories was first proposed in the field of sociology in the 1960s. In nursing, development of middle range theory is growing to fill the gaps between grand nursing theories and nursing practice.

Compared to grand theories, middle range theories contain fewer concepts and are limited in scope. Within the scope of middle range theories, however, some degree of generalization is possible across specialty areas and settings. Propositions are clear, and testable hypotheses can be derived. Middle range theories cover such concepts as pain, symptom management, cultural issues, and health promotion (Higgins & Shirley, 2000; Peterson, 2017; Walker & Avant, 2011). Chapters 10 and 11 provide a detailed discussion of middle range theories and their application in nursing.

Practice Theories

Practice theories (microtheories, situation-specific, or prescriptive theories) explain prescriptions or modalities for practice. The essence of practice theory is a defined or identified goal and descriptions of interventions or activities to achieve this goal (Walker & Avant, 2011). Practice theories can cover particular elements of a specialty, such as oncology nursing, obstetric nursing, or operating room nursing, or they may relate to another aspect of nursing, such as nursing administration or nursing education. Such theories typically describe specific elements of nursing care, such as cancer pain relief, or a specific experience, such as dying and end-of-life care.

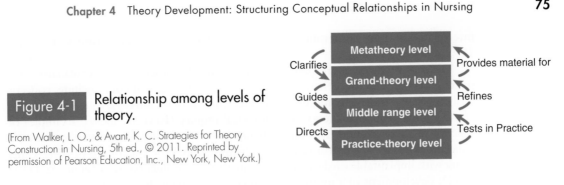

Figure 4-1   Relationship among levels of theory.

(From Walker, L. O., & Avant, K. C. Strategies for Theory Construction in Nursing, 5th ed., © 2011. Reprinted by permission of Pearson Education, Inc., New York, New York.)

Practice theories contain few concepts, are narrow in scope, and explain a relatively small aspect of reality. They are derived from middle range theories, practice experiences, comprehensive literature reviews, and empirical testing (Peterson, 2017). Furthermore, when the concepts and statements are operationally defined, they may be tested by appropriate research strategies (Higgins & Shirley, 2000). Chapters 12 and 18 cover practice—or situation-specific—theories in more detail.

Relationship Among Levels of Theory in Nursing

Walker and Avant (2011) state that the four levels of theory may be linked in order to direct and focus the discipline of nursing. As they describe, metatheory (worldview or philosophy) clarifies the methodologies and roles for each subsequent level of theory development (grand, middle range, and practice). Each level of theory provides material for further analysis and clarification at the level of metatheory. Grand nursing theories guide the phenomena of concern at the middle range level. Middle range theories assist in refinement of grand theories and direct prescriptions of practice theories. Practice theories are constructed from scientifically based propositions about reality and test the empirical validity of those propositions as they are incorporated into client care (Higgins & Shirley, 2000). Figure 4-1 illustrates the relationships among the levels of theory in nursing.

Categorization Based on Purpose

As discussed in Chapter 2, Dickoff and James (1968) described four kinds of theory: factor-isolating theories (descriptive theories), factor-relating theories (explanatory theories), situation-relating theories (predictive theories), and situation-producing theories (prescriptive theories). Each higher level of theory builds on the lower levels (Dickoff et al., 1968), and each is reviewed and expanded upon in the following sections.

Descriptive Theories

Descriptive theories describe, observe, and name concepts, properties, and dimensions, but they typically do not explain the interrelationships among the concepts or propositions, and they do not indicate how changes in one concept affect other concepts. According to Barnum (1998), descriptive theory is the first and most important level of theory development because it determines what will be perceived as the essence of the phenomenon under study. Subsequent theory development expands or refines those elements and specifies relationships that are determined to be important in the descriptive phase. Thus, it is critical that the most significant constituents of the phenomenon be recognized and named in this earliest phase of theory development.

The two types of descriptive theory are naming and classification. *Naming theories* describe the dimension or characteristics of a phenomenon. *Classification theories* describe dimensions or characteristics of a phenomenon that are structurally interrelated and are sometimes referred to as typologies or taxonomies (Barnum, 1998; Fawcett, 1999).

Descriptive theories are generated and tested by descriptive or explanatory research. Techniques for generating and testing descriptive theory include concept analysis, case studies, comprehensive literature review, surveys, phenomenology, ethnography, grounded theory, and historical inquiry (Fawcett, 1999). Examples of descriptive theory found in recent nursing literature include the development of a conceptual model of "almost normal," which describes the experience of adolescents living with implantable cardioverter defibrillators (phenomenology) (Zeigler & Tilley, 2011); development of a middle range theory describing the process of death imminence awareness by family members (grounded theory) (Baumhover, 2015); and a middle range theory of nursing presence (comprehensive literature review) (McMahon & Christopher, 2011). In other examples, concept analysis was used as the method to develop a theoretical model of food insecurity (Schroeder & Smaldone, 2015) and by Lindauer and Harvath (2014) who proposed a situation-specific theory of predeath grief among caregivers of dementia patients.

Explanatory Theories

Explanatory theory is the second level in theory development. Once phenomena have been identified and named, they can be viewed in relation to other phenomena. Explanatory theories relate concepts to one another and describe and specify some of the associations or interrelations between and among the concepts. Furthermore, explanatory theories attempt to tell how or why the concepts are related and may deal with causality, correlations, and rules that regulate interactions (Barnum, 1998; Dickoff et al., 1968).

Explanatory theories can be developed only after the parts of the phenomena have been identified and tested, and they are generated and tested by correlational research. Correlational research requires collection or measurement of data gathered by observation or self-report instruments that will yield either qualitative or quantitative data (Fawcett, 1999). Explanatory theories may also be generated by processes involving in-depth integrative/systematic and rigorous review of extant research literature. Examples of explanatory theories from recent nursing literature include meta-synthesis of qualitative study data in development of a model describing the experience of cancer among teenagers and young adults (Taylor, Pearce, Gibson, Fern, & Whelan, 2013) and a model of nursing care dependence as experienced by adult patients (Piredda et al., 2015). Similarly, Carr (2014) synthesized findings from three qualitative studies to develop a middle range theory of family vigilance, which describes the day-to-day experiences of family members staying with hospitalized relatives.

Predictive Theories

Predictive theories describe precise relationships between concepts and are the third level of theory development. Predictive theories presuppose the prior existence of the more elementary types of theory. They result after concepts are defined and relational statements are generated and are able to describe future outcomes consistently. Predictive theories include statements of causal or consequential relatedness (Dickoff et al., 1968).

Predictive theories are generated and tested by experimental research involving manipulation of a phenomenon to determine how it affects or changes some dimension or characteristic of another phenomenon (Fawcett, 1999). Different research designs may be used in this process. These include pretest–posttest designs, quasi-experiments, and true experiments. These research studies produce quantifiable data that are statistically analyzed. Metasynthesis of research studies or comprehensive reviews of research can also be the source of predictive theories. Examples of predictive theories include a model describing the health-related outcomes of resilience in adolescents (Scoloveno, 2015), a theory of family interdependence that predicted the relationships between spirituality and psychological well-being among elders and their family caregivers (Kim, Reed, Hayward, Kang, & Koenig, 2011), and a model predicting emotional exhaustion among hemodialysis nurses (Hayes, Douglas, & Bonner, 2014). In an interesting work, Tourangeau (2005) synthesized research literature from multiple sources to propose a theoretical model predicting patient mortality. She identified the following contributing or determining factors to mortality: nurses' staffing, burnout, satisfaction, skill mix, experience, and role support as well as such factors as physician expertise, hospital location, and patient characteristics (e.g., age, gender, comorbidity, socioeconomic status, and chronicity).

Prescriptive Theories

Prescriptive theories are perceived to be the highest level of theory development (Dickoff et al., 1968). Prescriptive theories prescribe activities necessary to reach defined goals. In nursing, prescriptive theories address nursing therapeutics and predict the consequence of interventions (Meleis, 2012). Prescriptive theories have three basic components: (1) specified goals or outcomes, (2) explicit activities to be taken to meet the goal, and (3) a survey list that articulates the conceptual basis of the theory (Dickoff et al., 1968).

According to Dickoff and colleagues (1968), the outcome or goal of a prescriptive theory serves as the norm or standard by which to evaluate activities. The goal must articulate the context of the situation, and this provides the basis for testing to determine whether the goal has been achieved. The specified actions or activities are those nursing interventions that should be taken to realize the goal. The goal will not be realized without the activity, and prescriptions for activities directly affect the goals.

The survey list augments and supplements the prescribed activities. In addition, it serves to prepare for future prescriptive activities. The survey list asks six questions about the prescribed activity that relate to the delineated goal (Box 4-1). In current vernacular, as practice guidelines based on research, evidence-based practice (EBP) consists of many attributes of prescriptive theory. This will be discussed in more detail in Chapter 12.

Examples of prescriptive theory are becoming more common in the literature, enhanced by the expanding volume of nursing research and increasing calls for EBP. In one work, Ade-Oshifogun (2012) presented a research-tested and research-supported model to assist and support clinicians to develop interventions to reduce or minimize truncal obesity in people with chronic obstructive pulmonary disease (COPD). The descriptions of feeding, pelvic floor exercise, therapeutic touch, and latex precautions are only a few of many excellent examples of nursing interventions presented

---

Box 4-1   Survey List of Questions for Prescriptive Theories

1. Who performs the activity? (agency)
2. Who or what is the recipient of the activity? (patiency)
3. In what context is the activity performed? (framework)
4. What is the end point of the activity? (terminus)
5. What is the guiding procedure, technique, or protocol of the activity? (procedure)
6. What is the energy source for the activity? (dynamics)

Source: Dickoff et al. (1968).

by Bulechek, Butcher, Dochterman, and Wagner (2012). Lastly, Finnegan, Shaver, Zenk, Wilkie, and Ferrans (2010) developed the "symptom cluster experience profile" framework to anticipate symptom clusters and derive interventions and clinical practice guidelines among survivors of childhood cancers.

Categorization Based on Source or Discipline

Theories may be classified based on the discipline or source of origin. As briefly discussed in Chapter 1, many of the theories used in nursing are borrowed, shared, or derived from theories developed in other disciplines. Because nursing is a human science and a practice discipline, incorporation of shared theories into practice and modification of them for use and testing are common.

Nurses use theories and concepts from the behavioral sciences, biologic sciences, and sociologic sciences as well as learning theories and organizational and management theories, among others. In many cases, these concepts and theories will overlap. For example, adaptation and stress are concepts found in both the behavioral and biologic sciences, and multiple theories have been developed using these concepts. Additionally, some theories defy placement in one discipline but relate to many. These include such basic concepts as systems theory, change theory, and chaos.

This book discusses a number of theories and concepts organized in terms of sociologic sciences, behavioral sciences, biomedical sciences, administration and management sciences, and learning theories. Table 4-1 presents examples of theories from each of these areas. Although by no means exhaustive, Chapters 13 through 17 provide information on many of the shared theories commonly used in nursing practice, research, education, and administration.

Table 4-1 Shared Theory Used in Nursing Practice and Research

Disciplines	Examples of Theories Used by Nurses
Theories from sociologic sciences	Family systems theory Feminist theory Role theory Critical social theory
Theories from behavioral sciences	Attachment theory Theories of self-determination Lazarus and Folkman's theory of stress, coping, and adaptation Theory of planned behavior
Theories from biomedical sciences	Pain Self-regulation theory Immune function Symptomology Germ theory
Theories from administration and management sciences	Donabedian's quality framework Theories of organizational behavior Models of conflict and conflict resolution Job satisfaction
Learning theories	Bandura's social cognitive learning theory Developmental learning theory Prospect theory

Components of a Theory

A theory has several components, including purpose, concepts and definitions, theoretical statements, structure/linkages and ordering, and assumptions (Chinn & Kramer, 2015; Hardin, 2014; Powers & Knapp, 2010). Creation of conceptual models is also a component of theory development that is promoted to further explain and define relationships, structure, and linkages.

Purpose

The purpose of a theory explains why the theory was formulated and specifies the context and situations in which it should be applied. The purpose might also provide information about the sociopolitical context in which the theory was developed, circumstances that influenced its creation, the theorist's past experiences, settings in which the theory was formulated, and societal trends. The purpose of the theory is usually explicitly described and should be found within the discussion of the theory (Chinn & Kramer, 2015).

Concepts and Conceptual Definitions

Concepts and concept development are described in detail in Chapter 3. Concepts are linguistic labels that are assigned to objects or events and are considered to be the building blocks of theories. The theoretical definition defines the concept in relation to other concepts and permits the description and classification of phenomena. Operationally defined concepts link the concept to the real world and identify empirical referents (indicators) of the concept that will permit observation and measurement (Chinn & Kramer, 2015; Hardin, 2014; Walker & Avant, 2011). Theories should include explicit conceptual definitions to describe and clarify the phenomenon and explain how the concept is expressed in empirical reality.

Theoretical Statements

Once a concept is fully developed and presented, it can be combined with other concepts to create statements to describe the real world. Theoretical statements, or propositions, are statements about the relationship between two or more concepts and are used to connect concepts to devise the theory. Statements must be formulated before explanations or predictions can be made, and development of statements asserting a connection between two or more concepts introduces the possibility of analysis (Hardin, 2014). The several types of theoretical statements include propositions, laws, axioms, empirical generalizations, and hypotheses (Table 4-2).

Theoretical statements can be classified into two groups. The first group consists of statements that claim the *existence* of phenomena referred to by concepts (existence statements). The second group describes *relationships* between concepts (relational statements) (Reynolds, 1971).

Existence Statements

Existence statements and definitions relate to specific concepts and make existence claims about that concept (e.g., that chair is brown or that man is a nurse). Each statement has a concept and is identified by a term that is applied to another object or phenomena. Existence statements serve as adjuncts to relational statements and clarify

Table 4-2 Types of Relationship Statements	
Type of Statement	**Characteristics**
Axioms	Consist of a basic set of statements or propositions that state the general relationship between concepts. Axioms are relatively abstract; therefore, they are not directly observed or measured.
Empirical generalizations	Summarize empirical evidence. Empirical generalizations provide some confidence that the same pattern will be repeated in concrete situations in the future under the same conditions.
Hypotheses	Statements that lack support from empirical research but are selected for study. The source of hypotheses may be a variation of a law or a derivation from an axiomatic theory, or they may be generated by a scientist's intuition (a hunch). All concepts in a hypothesis must be measurable, with operational definitions in concrete situations.
Laws	Well-grounded, with strong empirical support and evidence of empirical regulatory. Laws contain concepts that can be measured or identified in concrete settings.
Propositions	Statements of a constant relationship between two or more concepts or facts.

Sources: Hardy (1973); Jacox (1974); Reynolds (1971).

meanings in the theory. Existence statements are also termed *nonrelational statements* and may be right or wrong depending on the circumstances (Reynolds, 1971).

Relational Statements

Existence statements can only name and classify objects. Knowing the existence of one concept may be used to convey information about the existence of other concepts. Relational statements assert that a relationship exists between the properties of two or more concepts. This relationship is basic to development of theory and is expressed in terms of relational statements that explain, predict, understand, or control.

Like concepts, statements may have different levels of abstraction (theoretical and operational). The more general statements contain theoretically defined concepts. If the theoretical concepts are replaced with operational definitions, then the statement is "operationalized." The two broad groups of relational statements are those that describe an *association* between two concepts and those that describe a *causal relationship* between two concepts (Reynolds, 1971).

Associational or Correlational Relationships. Associational statements describe concepts that occur or exist together (Reynolds, 1971; Walker & Avant, 2011). The nature of the association/correlation may be positive (when one concept occurs or is high, the other concept occurs or is high). For example, as the external temperature rises during the summer, consumption of ice cream increases. An example in human beings is a positive correlation between height and weight—as people get taller, in general, their weight will increase.

The association may be neutral when the occurrence of one concept provides no information about the occurrence of another concept. For example, there is no correlation between gender and scores on a pharmacology examination. Finally, the association may be negative. In this case, when one concept occurs or is high, the other concept is low and vice versa. For example, failure to use condoms regularly is associated with an increase in the occurrence of sexually transmitted infections.

Causal Relationships. In causal relationships, one concept is considered to cause the occurrence of a second concept. For example, as caloric intake increases, weight increases. In scientific research, the concept or variable that is the cause is typically referred to as the independent variable and the variable that is affected is referred to as the dependent variable.

In science, there is often disagreement about whether a relationship is causal or simply highly correlated. A classic example is the relationship between cigarette smoking and lung cancer. As early as the 1940s, an association between smoking and lung cancer was recognized, but not until the 1980s was it determined that smoking actually *caused* lung cancer. Likewise, genetic predisposition is *associated* with development of heart disease; it has not been shown to *cause* heart disease.

Structure and Linkages

Structuring the theory by logical arrangement and specifying linkages of the theoretical concepts and statements is critical to the development of theory. The structure of a theory provides overall form to the theory. Theory structuring includes determination of the order of appearance of relationships, identification of central relationships, and delineation of direction, strength, and quality of relationships (Chinn & Kramer, 2015).

Although theoretical statements assert connections between concepts, the rationale for the stated connections needs to be developed. Theoretical linkages offer a reasoned explanation of why the variables in the theory may be connected in some manner, which brings plausibility to the theory. When developed operationally, linkages contribute to the testability of the theory by specifying how variables are connected. Thus, conceptual arrangement of statements and linkages can lead to hypotheses (Hardin, 2014).

Assumptions

Assumptions are notations that are taken to be true without proof. They are beliefs about a phenomenon that one must accept as true to accept a theory, and although they may not be empirically testable, they can be argued philosophically. The assumptions of a theory are based on what the theorist considers to be adequate empirical evidence to support propositions, on accepted knowledge, or on personal beliefs or values (Jacox, 1974; Powers & Knapp, 2010). Assumptions may be in the form of factual assertions or they may reflect value positions. Factual assumptions are those that are known through experience. Value assumptions assert or imply what is right, or good, or ought to be (Chinn & Kramer, 2015).

In a given theory, assumptions may be implicit or explicit. In many nursing theories, they must be "teased out." Furthermore, it is often difficult to separate assumptions that are implicit or integrated into the narrative of the theory from relationship statements (Powers & Knapp, 2010).

Models

Models are schematic representations of some aspect of reality. Various media are used in construction of models; they may be three-dimensional objects, diagrams, geometric formulas, or words. Empirical models are replicas of observable reality (e.g., a plastic model of a uterus or an eye). Theoretical models represent the real world through language or symbols and directional arrows.

In a classic work, Artinian (1982) described the rationale for creating a theoretical or conceptual model. She determined that models help illustrate the processes through which outcomes occur by specifying the relationships among the variables in graphic form where they can be examined for inconsistency, incompleteness, or errors. By creating a model of the concepts and relationships, it is possible to trace the effect of certain variables on the outcome variable rather than making assertions that each variable under study is related to every other variable. Furthermore, the model depicts a process that starts somewhere and ends at a logical point. Using the model, a person should be able to explain what happened, predict what will happen, and interpret what is happening. Finally, Artinian stated that once a model has been conceptually illustrated, the phenomenon represented can be examined in different settings testing the usefulness and generalizability of the underlying theory. The figure in the exemplar at the end of the chapter shows a model illustrating the relationships between the variables of the perceived access to breast health care in African American women theory.

Theory Development

Several factors are vital for nurses to examine the process of theory development. First, an understanding of the relationship among theory, research, and practice should be recognized. Second, the nurse should be aware that there are various approaches to theory development based on the source of initiation (i.e., practice, theory, or research). Finally, the process of theory development should be understood. Each of these factors is discussed in the following sections.

Relationship Among Theory, Research, and Practice

Many nurses lack a true understanding of the interrelationship among theory, research, and practice and its importance to the continuing development of nursing as a profession (Pryjmachuk, 1996). As early as the 1970s, nursing scholars commented on the relationships among theory, research, and practice. Indeed, at that time, nursing leaders urged that nursing research be combined with theory development to provide a rational basis for practice (Flaskerud, 1984; Moody, 1990).

In applied disciplines such as nursing, practice is based on the theories that are validated through research. Thus, theory, research, and practice affect each other in a reciprocal, cyclical, and interactive way (Hickman, 2011; Marrs & Lowry, 2006) (Figure 4-2).

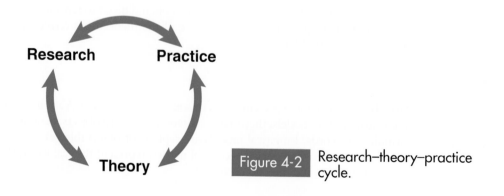

Figure 4-2   Research–theory–practice cycle.

Relationship Between Theory and Research

Research validates and modifies theory. In nursing, theories stimulate nurse scientists to explore significant problems in the field of nursing. In doing so, the potential for the development of nursing knowledge increases (Meleis, 2012). Theories can be used to formulate a set of generalizations to explain relationships among variables. When empirically tested, the results of research can be used to verify, modify, disprove, or support a theoretical proposition.

Relationship Between Theory and Practice

Theory guides practice. One of the primary uses of theory is to contribute insights about nursing practice situations through provision of goals for assessment, diagnosis, and intervention. Likewise, through practice, nursing theory is shaped, and guidelines for practice evolve. Theory renders practice more efficient and more effective, and the ultimate benefit of theory application in nursing is the improvement in client care (Meleis, 2012).

Relationship Between Research and Practice

Research is the key to the development of a discipline. Middle range and practice theories may be tested in practice through clinical research (Hickman, 2011). If individual practitioners are to develop expertise, they must participate in research. In summary, there is a need to encourage nurses to test and refine theories and models to develop their own personal models of practice (Marrs & Lowry, 2006; Pryjmachuk, 1996).

Approaches to Theory Development

Several different approaches may be used to initiate the process of theory development. Meleis (2012) cites four major strategies differentiated by their origin (theory, practice, or research) and by whether sources from outside of nursing were used to develop the theory. These approaches are theory to practice to theory, practice to theory, research to theory, and theory to research to theory. She then proposes employment of an integrated approach to theory development. Table 4-3 summarizes these different approaches.

Theory to Practice to Theory

The theory to practice to theory approach to theory development begins with a theory (typically non-nursing) that describes a phenomenon of interest (Meleis, 2012). This approach assumes that the theory can help describe or explain the phenomenon, but it is not completely congruent with nursing and/or is not directly defined for nursing practice. Thus, the focus of the theory is different from the focus needed for nursing.

Using the theory to practice to theory strategy, the nurse would select a theory that may be used to explain or describe a clinical situation (e.g., adaptation, stress, health beliefs). The nurse could modify concepts and consider relationships between concepts that were not proposed in the original theory. To accomplish this, the nurse would need to (1) have a basic knowledge of the theory; (2) analyze the theory by reducing it into components where each component is defined and evaluated; (3) use assumptions, concepts, and propositions to describe the clinical area; (4) redefine assumptions, concepts, and propositions to reflect nursing; and (5) reconstruct a theory using exemplars representing the redefined assumptions, concepts, and propositions (Meleis, 2012). Examples of a theory to practice to theory strategy include Benner's use of Dreyfus's Model of Skill Acquisition to describe novice to expert

Table 4-3 Strategies for Theory Development			
Origin of Theory	Basis for Development	Type of Theory	Methods for Development
Theory–practice–theory	An existing non-nursing theory that can help describe and explain a phenomenon, but the theory is not complete or not completely developed for nursing	Borrowed or shared theory	Theorist selects a non-nursing theory; analyzes the theory; defines and evaluates each component; and redefines assumptions, concepts, and propositions to reflect nursing.
Practice–theory	Existing theories are not useful in describing the phenomenon of interest; theory is derived from clinical situations.	Grounded theory	Researcher observes phenomenon of interest, analyzes similarities and differences, compares and contrasts responses, and develops concepts and linkages.
Research–theory	Development of theory is based on research; theories evolve from replicated and confirmed research findings.	Scientific theory	Researcher selects a common phenomenon, lists and measures characteristics of the phenomenon in a variety of situations, analyzes the data to determine if there are patterns that need further study, and formalizes patterns as theoretical statements.
Theory–research–theory	Theory drives the research questions; the result of the research informs and modifies the theory.	Theory testing	Theorist defines a theory and determines propositions for testing; the theory is modified, refined, or further developed based on research findings; in some cases, a new theory will be formed.

Source: Meleis (2012).

practice (Benner, 2001) and Roy's use of Helson's Adaptation Theory to describe human responses (Roy & Roberts, 1981). Other examples of theory to practice to theory in recent nursing literature include a work that applied the theory of mastery and organismic integration theory in practice to develop a middle range theory for diabetes self-management mastery (Fearon-Lynch & Stover, 2015) and Davidson's (2010) middle range theory, facilitated sense-making, which supports families of ICU patients. The latter was derived from the work of Karl Weick (2001), an expert in organizational psychology.

Practice to Theory

If no appropriate theory appears to exist to describe or explain a phenomenon, theories may be inductively developed from clinical practice situations. The practice to theory approach is based on the premise that in a given situation, existing theories are not useful in describing the phenomenon of interest. It assumes that the phenomenon is important enough to pursue and that there is a clinical understanding about it that has not been articulated. Furthermore, insight gained from describing the phenomenon has potential for enhancing the understanding of other similar situations through development of a set of propositions (Meleis, 2012).

This strategy is a grounded theory approach, which begins with a question evolving from a practice situation. It relies on observation of new phenomena in a practice situation; development of concepts; and then labeling, describing, and articulating properties of these concepts. To accomplish this, the researcher observes the phenomenon, analyzes similarities and differences, and then compares and contrasts responses. Following this, the researcher may develop concepts and propositional statements and propose linkages (Meleis, 2012). Examples of the practice to theory strategy of theory development include a model of "becoming normal," which describes the emotional process of recovery from stroke (Gallagher, 2011) and a middle range theory of self-care of chronic illness (Riegel, Jaarsma, & Strömberg, 2012). Similarly, Falk-Rafael and Betker (2012) developed the "critical caring theory" following detailed interviews of practice accounts of 25 public health nurses, and Sacks and Volker (2015) created a theory describing hospice nurses' responses to patient suffering following interviews with 22 hospice nurses.

Research to Theory

The research to theory strategy is the most accepted strategy for theory development in nursing, largely due to the early emphasis on empiricism described in Chapter 1. For empiricists, theory development is considered a product of research because theories evolve from replicated and confirmed research findings. The research to theory strategy assumes that there is truth in real life, that the truth can be captured through the senses, and that the truth can be verified (Meleis, 2012). Furthermore, the purpose of scientific theories is to describe, explain, predict, or control a part of the empirical world.

In the research to theory strategy for theory development, the researcher selects a phenomenon that occurs in the discipline and lists characteristics of the phenomenon. A method to measure the characteristics of the phenomenon is developed and implemented in a controlled study. The results of the measurement are analyzed to determine if there are any systematic patterns, and once patterns have been discovered, they are formalized into theoretical statements (Meleis, 2012). Examples of the research to theory strategy from nursing include the development of the middle range theory of family vigilance, which was developed following in-depth review of three ethnographic research studies (Carr, 2014), and "tracking the footsteps" (El Hussein & Hirst, 2016), which describes the clinical reasoning processes used by registered nurses to recognize delirium in acute care settings.

Theory to Research to Theory

In the theory to research to theory approach, theory drives the research questions and the results of the research are used to modify the theory. In this approach, the theorist will begin by defining a theory and determining propositions for testing. If carried through, the research findings may be used to further modify and develop the original theory (Meleis, 2012).

In this process, a theory is selected to explain the phenomenon of interest. The theory is a framework for operational definitions, variables, and statements. Concepts are redefined and operationalized for research. Findings are synthesized and used to modify, refine, or develop the original theory or, in some cases, to create a new theory. The goal is to test, refine, and develop theory and to use theory as a framework for research and theory modification. The researcher/theorist concludes the investigation with a refined, modified, or further developed explanation of the theory (Meleis, 2012). Examples of the theory to research to theory approach from recent nursing literature include a middle range theory of weight management developed from Orem's theory of self-care (Pickett, Peters, & Jarosz, 2014) and Dobratz's (2016) middle range theory of adaptive spirituality (which was derived from Roy's Adaptation Model). Another example is the theory of diversity of human field pattern, which was developed from Martha Rogers's science of unitary human beings using a quantitative research design (Hastings-Tolsma, 2006).

Integrated Approach

An integrated approach to theory development describes an evolutionary process that is particularly useful in addressing complex clinical situations. It requires gathering data from the clinical setting, identifying exemplars, discovering solutions, and recognizing supportive information from other sources (Meleis, 2012).

Integrated theory development is rooted in clinical practice. Practice drives the basic questions and provides opportunities for clinical involvement in research that is designed to answer the questions. In this process for theory development, hunches and conceptual ideas are communicated with other clinicians or participants to allow for critique and further development. Among other strategies, the integrated approach uses skills and tools from clinical practice, various research methods, clinical diaries, descriptive journals, and collegial dialogues in developing a framework or conceptualization (Meleis, 2012).

Process of Theory Development

The process of theory development has been described in some detail by several nursing scholars (Jacox, 1974; Walker & Avant, 2011). Despite slight variations related to terminology and sequencing, the sources are similar in explaining the processes used to develop theory. The three basic steps are concept development, statement/proposition development, and theory construction. Chinn and Kramer (2015) add two additional steps that involve validating, confirming, or testing the theory and applying theory in practice. Each of the steps is described in the following sections, and Table 4-4 summarizes the theory development process.

Concept Development: Creation of Conceptual Meaning

This first step or process of theory development involves creating conceptual meaning. This provides the foundation for theory development and includes specifying,

Table 4-4 Process of Theory Development

Step	Description
Concept development	Specifying, defining, and clarifying the concepts used to describe a phenomenon of interest
Statement development	Formulating and analyzing statements explaining relationships between concepts; also involves determining empirical referents that can validate them
Theory construction	Structuring and contextualizing the components of the theory; includes identifying assumptions and organizing linkages between and among the concepts and statements to form a theoretical structure
Testing theoretical relationships	Validating theoretical relationships through empirical testing
Application of theory in practice	Using research methods to assess how the theory can be applied in practice; research should provide evidence to evaluate the theory's usefulness

defining, and clarifying the concepts used to describe the phenomenon of interest (Jacox, 1974).

Creating conceptual meaning uses mental processes to create mental structures or ideas to be used to represent experience. This produces a tentative definition of the concept(s) and a set of criteria for determining if the concept(s) exists in a particular situation (Chinn & Kramer, 2015). Methods of concept development are described in detail in Chapter 3.

Statement Development: Formulation and Validation of Relational Statements

Relational statements are the skeletons of theory; they are the means by which the theory comes together. The process of formulation and validation of relational statements involves developing the relational statements and determining empirical referents that can validate them.

After a statement has been delineated initially, it should be scrutinized or analyzed. Statement analysis is a process described by Walker and Avant (2011) to thoroughly examine relational statements. Statement analysis classifies statements and examines the relationships between the concepts and helps direct theoretical construction. There are seven steps in the process of statement analysis (Box 4-2). Following the process of statement analysis, the statements are refined and may be operationalized.

Theory Construction: Systematic Organization of the Linkages

The third stage in theory development involves structuring and contextualizing the components of the theory. This includes formulating systematic linkages between and among concepts, which results in a formal, coherent theoretical structure. The format used depends on what is known or assumed to be true about the phenomena in question (Chinn & Kramer, 2015). Aspects of theory construction include identifying and defining the concepts; identifying assumptions; clarifying the context within which the theory is placed; designing relationship statements; and delineating the organization, structure, or relationship among the components.

Theory synthesis is a theory construction strategy developed by Walker and Avant (2011). In theory synthesis, concepts and statements are organized into a network or whole. The purposes of theory synthesis are to represent a phenomenon through an interrelated set of concepts and statements, to describe the factors that precede or influence a particular phenomenon or event, to predict effects that occur after some event, or to put discrete scientific information into a more theoretically organized form.

Theory synthesis can be used to produce a compact, informative graphic representation of research findings on a topic of interest, and synthesized theories may be

---

Box 4-2   Steps in Statement Analysis

1. Select the statement to be analyzed.
2. Simplify the statement.
3. Classify the statement.
4. Examine concepts within the statement for definition and validity.
5. Specify relationship between concepts.
6. Examine the logic.
7. Determine stability.

Source: Walker and Avant (2011).

Box 4-3   Steps in Theory Synthesis

1. Select a topic of interest and specify focal concepts (may be one concept/variable or a framework of several concepts).
2. Conduct a review of the literature to identify related factors and note their relationships. Identify and record relationships indicating whether they are bidirectional, unidirectional, positive, neutral or negative, weak or ambiguous, or strong in support evidence.
3. Organize concepts and relational statements into an integrated representation of the phenomena of interest. Diagrams may be used to express the relationships among the concepts.

Source: Walker and Avant (2011).

---

expressed in several ways such as graphic or model form. The three steps in theory synthesis are summarized in Box 4-3.

Validating and Confirming Theoretical Relationships in Research

Chinn and Kramer (2015) include the process of validating and confirming theoretical relationships as a component of theory development. Validating theoretical relationships involves empirically refining concepts and theoretical relationships, identifying empirical indicators, and testing relationships through empirical methods. In this step, the focus is on correlating the theory with demonstrable experiences and designing research to validate the relationships. Additionally, alternative explanations are considered based on the empirical evidence.

Validation and Application of Theory in Practice

An important final step in theory development identified by Chinn and Kramer (2015) is applying the theory in practice. In this step, research methods are used to assess how the theory can be applied in practice. The theoretical relationships are examined in the practice setting, and results are recorded to determine how well the theory achieves the desired outcomes. The research design should provide evidence of the effect of the interventions on the well-being of recipients of care. Questions to be considered in this step include: Are the theory's goals congruent with practice goals? Is the intended context of the theory congruent with the practice situation? Are explanations of the theory sufficient for use in the nursing situation? Is there research evidence supporting use of the theory? See Link to Practice 4-1 for more information on the process of theory development.

Summary

Jill Watson, the nurse/graduate student introduced in the case study at the beginning of this chapter, was unable to identify a theory or conceptual model that completely met the needs for her study on health motivation. Because of this, she determined that it would be appropriate and feasible to use theory development techniques to revise an existing theory to use in her research project.

Theory development is an important but complex and time-consuming process. This chapter has presented a number of issues related to the process of theory development. These issues included the purpose of developing theory and the components of a theory. Discussion focused on concepts, theoretical statements, assumptions, and model development and explained the relationships among theory, research, and practice. Finally, the process of theory development was presented.

Link to Practice 4-1

Where Do I Begin?

An experienced emergency department (ED) registered nurse wants to conduct a research study on "frequent flyers in the ED" (i.e., patients who return multiple times for the same or similar health problem) and is not sure how to proceed.

Following the guidelines in the chapter, the nurse should begin with developing the concept. For this step, he or she can search the health literature. Has a concept study of "frequent flyers" been published? If not, he or she can perform a formal or informal concept analysis, following one of the strategies presented in Chapter 3. If an analysis of "frequent flyers" has been published, the nurse might use it to set up the next steps—statement development and theory construction.

In the second and third steps, the nurse should continue to search the literature to learn all he or she can about the various aspects of "frequent flyers" and related phenomena. What studies have been published on patients who return to the EDs repeatedly during a short period of time? What characteristics or diagnoses are typically reported? What other factors are usually found? How do they present? How do ED personnel care for them? From this review, the nurse can propose linkages between and among the various concepts/characteristics and draft a conceptual model. This might send him or her back to the literature to search for other, potentially related terms and phenomena. The literature and published studies can also lead him or her to instruments or tools that have been developed to measure some of the concepts and phenomena. Following these steps, the nurse can develop a research study to try to validate and refine the conceptual linkages. Completion and publication of research will contribute to the evidence that can then be used to improve nursing practice.

Key Points

- In nursing, theories are constructed or developed to describe, explain, or understand phenomena to help solve clinical problems or improve practice outcomes.
- Nursing theory can be categorized based on level (grand theory, middle range theory, or practice theory), based on purpose (descriptive theories, explanatory theories, predictive theories, or prescriptive theories), or based on source or background.
- Components of theories include purpose, concepts, definitions, theoretical statements, structure/linkages, assumptions, and often a diagram or model.
- There is a reciprocal relationship among theory, research, and practice that is critical for professional nurses to recognize and understand.
- Several approaches to theory development (e.g., theory to practice to theory, theory to research to theory, practice to theory, and research to theory) are found in the nursing literature.
- The process of theory development often follows these steps: concept development, statement development, theory construction, validation/confirmation of relationships in research, and validation/application of theory in practice.

To further illustrate the process of theory development, a summary report of a theory published in the nursing literature is presented. In the following exemplar, each of the components of the theory is clearly identified. In addition, Chapter 5 expands on the process of theory development by examining the processes of theory analysis and evaluation.

THEORY DEVELOPMENT EXEMPLAR

Garmon, S. C. (2012). Theory of perceived access to breast health care in African American women. *ANS. Advances in Nursing Science, 35*(2), E13–E23.

Garmon developed the perceived access to breast health care in African American women theory to help direct future research studies exploring the relationship between access to care and utilization of preventive services related to breast health care.

Scope of theory: Middle range

Purpose: The perceived access to breast health care in African American women theory was developed to "propose an alternative view of access to breast health care and to demonstrate the importance of testing the relationships between culture, definitions of health, health behaviors, and practices and their influence on the perception of access to breath health care in AAW [African American women]" (p. E16).

Concepts and definitions are listed in the following table.

Concept	Definition
Culture	Combination of age, ethnicity, race, gender, socioeconomic status, religious beliefs, family history, and geographical origin that shapes and guides the values, beliefs, practices, thinking, decisions, and actions of individuals
Health	A state of well-being that is culturally defined, valued, and practiced and that reflects the ability of individuals or groups to perform their daily role activities in a culturally satisfactory way
Health promotion	Behavior(s) aimed at increasing the level of well-being and actualization of health
Health protection	Behavior(s) aimed at decreasing the likelihood of experiencing health problems by active protection or early detection of health problems in the asymptomatic stage
Health behaviors and practices	Culturally guided activities that are performed by an individual to help maintain his or her definition of health and well-being. These include health promotion and disease prevention breast care practices.
Access	The perceived necessity, availability, and appropriateness of breast health care provided by the health care delivery system, which purposes to assist an individual in maintaining his or her cultural definition of health and well-being
Perception of availably of care	Influenced by economic factors such as location of care; fit with time schedules; fit with family; and fit with cultural beliefs, values, and expectations
Perception of necessity of care	Influenced by incorporation of health promotion and disease prevention into definitions of health, symptomatology, and cultural definitions of severity and personal and family priorities
Perception of appropriateness of care	Influenced by fit of the breast health care with cultural values, beliefs, and practices; interactions and relationships with providers of care; and previous experience associated with breast cancer and breast health care

Theoretical Statement and Linkages

1. Culture shapes the definition of health.
2. Perceived access to breast health care is postulated to be a product of three subconcepts: necessity, availability, and appropriateness of care.
3. Health behaviors and practices are a function of the perception of necessity of care, the availably of care, and the appropriateness of care.

4. When (a) the definition of health includes perspectives of health promotion and disease prevention; (b) health behaviors and practices include breast health practices; and (c) access to breast health care is perceived as necessary, available, and appropriate, then breast cancer diagnosis is likely to occur in its early stages.
5. Delayed diagnosis of breast cancer influences cultural beliefs, values, and practices and also reshapes individual definitions of health, health practices, and behaviors.

Model: Garmon's schematic diagram illustrates the main concepts and their interrelationships. It also depicts how perceptions may lead to either early or delayed diagnosis of breast cancer.

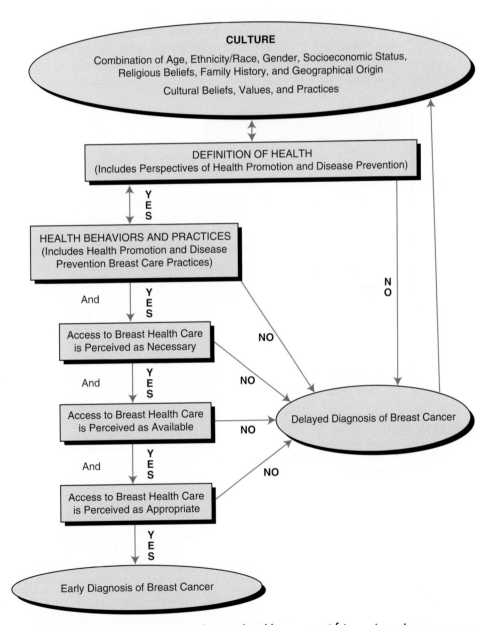

A theory of perceived access to breast health care in African American women (From Garmon, S. C. [2012]. Theory of perceived access to breast health care in African American women. *Advances in Nursing Science,* 35[2], E13–E23).

Assumptions

1. Definitions of health care are shaped by culture and determine an individual's participation in health promotion and disease prevention strategies.
2. Perceived access to necessary care will result in seeking breast health care for health promotion and disease prevention.
3. Seeking breast health care in a health care delivery system with perceived appropriate and available care will result in diagnosis of breast cancer in its early stages.

Implications for Nursing

The theory of perceived access provides nurses with an opportunity for testing the relationships among culture; health definitions; health practices; and perceived necessity, availability, and appropriateness of breast cancer screening. The theory may aid in the discovery of the culturally appropriate approaches for promoting breast health care.

Learning Activities

1. Find an example of a nursing theory in a current book or periodical. Review the theory and classify it based on scope or level of abstraction (grand theory, middle range theory, or practice theory), the purpose of the theory (describe, explain, predict, or control), and the source or discipline in which the theory was developed.
2. Find an example of a middle range nursing theory (see Chapter 10 or 11 for ideas). Following the preceding exemplar, identify the components of the theory (e.g., scope of the theory, purpose, concepts, and definitions).
3. Find an example of a middle range theory that does not contain a model. With classmates, try to create a model that depicts the relationships between and among the concepts. Discuss the challenges posed by this exercise.
4. Jill, the nurse from the opening case study, chose a non-nursing theory to modify to best explain a phenomenon that she had observed in practice. Review the various theories described in the unit on "shared theories" and select one that is applicable to one nursing specialty area. Consider how it might be modified to best reflect advanced nursing practice.

REFERENCES

Ade-Oshifogun, J. B. (2012). Model of functional performance in obese elderly people with chronic obstructive pulmonary disease. *Journal of Nursing Scholarship, 44*(3), 232–241.

Artinian, B. (1982). Conceptual mapping: Development of the strategy. *Western Journal of Nursing Research, 4*(4), 379–393.

Barnum, B. S. (1998). *Nursing theory: Analysis, application, evaluation* (5th ed.). Philadelphia, PA: Lippincott Williams & Wilkins.

Baumhover, N. C. (2015). The process of death imminence awareness by family members of patients in adult critical care. *Dimensions of Critical Care Nursing, 34*(3), 149–160.

Benner, P. (2001). *From novice to expert: Excellence and power in clinical nursing practice.* Upper Saddle River, NJ: Prentice-Hall.

Bulechek, G. M., Butcher, H. K., Dochterman, J. M., & Wagner, C. (2012). *Nursing interventions classification* (6th ed.). St. Louis, MO: Elsevier.

Carr, J. M. (2014). A middle range theory of family vigilance. *Medsurg Nursing, 23*(4), 251–255.

Cesario, S. (1997). The impact of the electronic domain on theory construction. *Journal of Theory Construction and Testing, 1*(2), 60–63.

Chinn, P. L., & Kramer, M. K. (2015). *Integrated theory and knowledge development in nursing* (8th ed.). St. Louis, MO: Elsevier.

Davidson, J. E. (2010). Facilitated sensemaking: A strategy and new middle-range theory to support families of intensive care unit patients. *Critical Care Nurse, 30*(6), 28–39.

Dickoff, J., & James, P. (1968). A theory of theories: A position paper. *Nursing Research, 17*(3), 197–203.

Dickoff, J., James, P., & Wiedenbach, E. (1968). Theory in a practice discipline. II: Practice oriented research. *Nursing Research, 17*(6), 545–554.

Dobratz, M. C. (2016). Building a middle-range theory of adaptive spirituality. *Nursing Science Quarterly, 29*(2), 146–153.

El Hussein, M., & Hirst, S. (2016). Tracking the footsteps: A constructivist grounded theory of the clinical reasoning processes that registered nurses use to recognize delirium. *Journal of Clinical Nursing, 25*(3–4), 381–391.

Falk-Rafael, A., & Betker, C. (2012). The primacy of relationships: A study of public health nursing practice from a critical caring perspective. *ANS. Advances in Nursing Science, 35*(4), 315–332.

Fawcett, J. (1999). *The relationship of theory and research* (3rd ed.). Philadelphia, PA: Davis.

Fearon-Lynch, J. A., & Stover, C. M. (2015). A middle-range theory for diabetes self-management mastery. *Advances in Nursing Science, 38*(4), 330–346.

Finnegan, L., Shaver, J. L., Zenk, S. N., Wilkie, D. J., & Ferrans, C. E. (2010). The symptom cluster experience profile framework. *Oncology Nursing Forum, 37*(6), E377–E386.

Flaskerud, J. H. (1984). Nursing models as conceptual frameworks for research. *Western Journal of Nursing Research, 6*(2), 153–155.

Gallagher, P. (2011). Becoming normal: A grounded theory study on the emotional process of stroke recovery. *Canadian Journal of Neuroscience Nursing, 33*(3), 24–32.

Hardin, S. R. (2014). Theory development process. In M. R. Alligood (Ed.), *Nursing theorists and their work* (8th ed., pp. 23–37). St. Louis, MO: Mosby.

Hardy, M. E. (1973). The nature of theories. In M. E. Hardy (Ed.), *Theoretical foundations for nursing.* New York, NY: MSS Information Systems.

Hastings-Tolsma, M. (2006). Toward a theory of diversity of human field pattern. *Visions, 14*(2), 34–47.

Hayes, B., Douglas, C., & Bonner, A. (2014). Predicting emotional exhaustion among haemodialysis nurses: A structural equation model using Kanter's structural empowerment theory. *Journal of Advanced Nursing, 70*(12), 2897–2909.

Hickman, J. S. (2011). An introduction to nursing theory. In J. B. George (Ed.), *Nursing theories: The base for professional nursing practice* (6th ed., pp. 1–22). Upper Saddle River, NJ: Pearson Education.

Higgins, P. A., & Shirley, M. M. (2000). Levels of theoretical thinking in nursing. *Nursing Outlook, 48*(4), 179–183.

Jacox, A. K. (1974). Theory construction in nursing: An overview. *Nursing Research, 23*(1), 4–13.

Kim, S., Reed, P. G., Hayward, R. D., Kang, Y., & Koenig, H. G. (2011). Spirituality and psychological well-being: Testing a theory of family interdependence among family caregivers and their elders. *Research in Nursing & Health, 34*(2), 103–115.

Lindauer, A., & Harvath, T. A. (2014). Pre-death grief in the context of dementia caregiving: A concept analysis. *Journal of Advanced Nursing, 70*(10), 2196–2207.

Marrs, J., & Lowry, L. W. (2006). Nursing theory and practice: Connecting the dots. *Nursing Science Quarterly, 19*(1), 44–50.

McMahon, M. A., & Christopher, K. A. (2011). Toward a mid-range theory of nursing presence. *Nursing Forum, 46*(2), 71–81.

Meleis, A. I. (2012). *Theoretical nursing: Development and progress* (5th ed.). Philadelphia, PA: Lippincott Williams & Wilkins.

Moody, L. E. (1990). *Advancing nursing science through research.* Newbury Park, CA: Sage.

Peterson, S. J. (2017). Introduction to the nature of nursing knowledge. In S. J. Peterson & T. S. Bredow (Eds.), *Middle range theories: Application to nursing research* (4th ed., pp. 3–34). Philadelphia, PA: Lippincott Williams & Wilkins.

Pickett, S., Peters, R. M., & Jarosz, P. A. (2014). Toward a middle-range theory of weight management. *Nursing Science Quarterly, 27*(3), 242–247.

Piredda, M., Matarese, M., Mastroianni, C., D'Angelo, D., Hammer, M. J., & De Marinis, M. G. (2015). Adult patients' experiences of nursing care dependence. *Journal of Nursing Scholarship, 47*(5), 397–406.

Powers, B. A., & Knapp, T. R. (2010). *Dictionary of nursing theory and research* (4th ed.). New York, NY: Springer Publishing.

Pryjmachuk, S. (1996). A nursing perspective on the interrelationships between theory, research and practice. *Journal of Advanced Nursing, 23*, 679–684.

Reynolds, P. D. (1971). *A primer in theory construction.* Indianapolis, IN: Bobbs-Merrill.

Riegel, B., Jaarsma, T., & Stromberg, A. (2012). A middle-range theory of self-care of chronic illness. *ANS. Advances in Nursing Science, 35*(3), 194–204.

Roy, C., & Roberts, S. (1981). *Theory construction in nursing: An adaptation model.* Englewood Cliffs, NJ: Prentice-Hall.

Sacks, J. L., & Volker, D. L. (2015). A study of hospice nurses' responses to patient suffering. *Journal of Hospice and Palliative Nursing, 17*(06), 490–500.

Schroeder, K., & Smaldone, A. (2015). Food insecurity: A concept analysis. *Nursing Forum, 50*(4), 274–281.

Scoloveno, R. (2015). A theoretical model of health-related outcomes of resilience in middle adolescents. *Western Journal of Nursing Research, 37*(3), 342–359.

Streubert, H. J., & Carpenter, D. R. (2011). *Qualitative research in nursing: Advancing the humanistic imperative* (5th ed.). Philadelphia, PA: Lippincott Williams & Wilkins.

Taylor, R. M., Pearce, S., Gibson, F., Fern, L., & Whelan, J. (2013). Developing a conceptual model of teenage and young adult experiences of cancer through meta-synthesis. *International Journal of Nursing Studies, 50*(6), 832–846.

Tourangeau, A. E. (2005). A theoretical model of the determinants of mortality. *ANS. Advances in Nursing Science, 28*(1), 58–69.

Walker, L. O., & Avant, K. C. (2011). *Strategies for theory construction in nursing* (5th ed.). Upper Saddle River, NJ: Prentice-Hall.

Weick, K. E. (2001). *Making sense of the organization.* London, United Kingdom: Blackwell.

Zeigler, V. I., & Tilley, D. S. (2011). Almost normal: A practice-oriented conceptual model of adolescent living with implantable cardioverter defibrillators. *Journal of Theory Construction & Testing, 14*(1), 23–27.

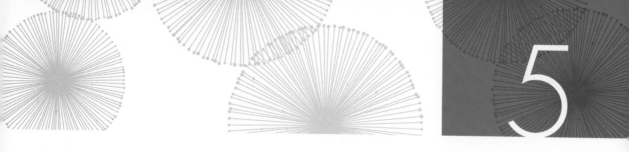

Theory Analysis and Evaluation

Melanie McEwen

Jerry Thompson is nearing completion of his master's degree in nursing leadership. He is currently a case manager for a home health agency, and his goal is to become an agency director after he completes his degree. For his research application project, Jerry wants to compare the effectiveness of health teaching in the hospital setting with the effectiveness of health teaching in the home setting. He has identified several areas to examine. These include the quality and type of health information provided, professional competencies of the nurses providing the information, the client's support system, and environmental resources. Outcome variables he will measure focus on utilization of health care (e.g., length of time on home health service, hospital readmissions, development of complications).

As his research project began to take shape, Jerry realized he needed a conceptual framework to help him set it up and organize it. His advisor suggested Pender's Health Promotion Model. To determine if the model would be appropriate for his study, Jerry obtained the latest edition of Pender's book (Pender, Murdaugh, & Parsons, 2015), which described the model in depth. He then read commentaries in nursing theory books that analyzed Pender's work and completed a literature search to find examples of research studies using the Health Promotion Model as a conceptual framework. After he had compiled the information, Jerry summarized his findings by using Whall's (2016) criteria for analysis and evaluation of middle range theories.

This exercise helped Jerry gain insight into the major concepts of the model and let him examine its important assumptions and linkages. From the evaluation, he determined that the model would be appropriate for use as the conceptual framework for his research study.

As nurses began to participate in the processes of theory development in the 1960s, they realized that there was a corresponding need to identify criteria or develop mechanisms to determine if those theories served their intended purpose. As a result, the first method to describe, analyze, and critique theory was published in 1968. Over the following decades, a number of methods or techniques for theory evaluation were proposed. A general understanding of these methods will help nurses select an evaluation method for theory, which is appropriate to the stage of theory development and for the intended application of the theory (research, practice, administration, or education). This will, in turn, help ensure that the theory is valid and is being used correctly. It will also provide information for developing and testing new theories by identifying gaps and inconsistencies.

Definition and Purpose of Theory Evaluation

Theory evaluation has been defined as the process of systematically examining a theory. Criteria for this process are variable, but they generally include examination of the theory's origins, meaning, logical adequacy, usefulness, generalizability, and testability. Theory evaluation does not generate new information outside the confines of the theory, but it often leads to new insights about the theory being examined.

In short, theory evaluation identifies a theory's degree of usefulness to guide practice, research, education, and administration. Such evaluation gives insight into relationships among concepts and their linkages to each other and allows the reviewer to determine the strengths and weaknesses of a theory. It also assists in identifying the need for additional theory development or refinement. Finally, theory evaluation provides a systematic, objective way of examining a theory that may lead to new insights and new formulations that will add to the body of knowledge and thereby affects practice or research (Walker & Avant, 2011). The ultimate goal of theory evaluation is to determine the potential contribution of the theory to scientific knowledge.

In nursing practice, theory evaluation may provide a clinician with additional knowledge about the soundness of the theory. It also helps identify which theoretical relationships are supported by research, provides guidelines for the choice of appropriate interventions, and gives some indication of their efficacy. In research, theory evaluation helps clarify the form and structure of a theory being tested or will allow the researcher to determine the relevance of the content of a theory for use as a conceptual framework, as described in the case study. Evaluation will also identify inconsistencies and gaps in the theory when used in practice or research (Walker & Avant, 2011). See Link to Practice 5-1 for another example.

Link to Practice 5-1

The Synergy Model for Patient Care

The Synergy Model for Care was developed by the American Association of Critical-Care Nurses (AACN) to be used as the basis for the AACN's certification examination (Curley, 1998). Although the model was explicitly designed to be used to direct nursing care for critically ill patients in the acute care settings (practice), it has also been used in numerous research studies as well as in many different types of settings and for varying types of patients.

When considering its original intended purpose, what processes or methods might a nurse use to determine the Synergy Model's suitability for:

- Directing nursing practice in a high school or occupational health setting?
- Working with elders in a long-term care facility?
- Planning care for a home-based hospice patient?
- Guiding a research study in a pediatric hospital?

Various methods have been outlined to assist with this process. The methods are described by several overlapping terms or terms that are used in different ways by different authors. For example, theory analysis, theory description, theory evaluation, and theory critique all describe the process of critically reviewing a theory to assess its relevance and applicability to nursing practice, research, education, and administration. In this chapter, "theory evaluation" is used as a global term to discuss the process of reviewing theory.

Theory evaluation has been described as a single-phase process (theory analysis) by Alligood (2014a) as well as Hardy (1974) (theory evaluation), a two-phase process (theory analysis and theory critique/evaluation) by Fawcett and DeSanto-Madeya (2013) and Duffey and Muhlenkamp (1974), or a three-phase process (theory description, theory analysis, and theory critique/evaluation) by scholars including Meleis (2012) and Moody (1990). It should be noted that the methods are similar whether they describe one, two, or three phases. A three-phase process is outlined briefly in the following section. Later sections provide more detailed discussions of each phase.

Theory Description

Theory description is the initial step in the evaluation process. In theory description, the works of a theorist are reviewed with a focus on the historical context of the theory (Hickman, 2011). In addition, related works by others are examined to gain a clear understanding of the structural and functional components of the theory. The structural components include assumptions, concepts, and propositions. The functional components consist of the concepts of the theory and how they are used to describe, explain, predict, or control (Meleis, 2012; Moody, 1990).

Theory Analysis

Theory analysis is the second phase of the evaluation process. It refers to a systematic process of objectively examining the content, structure, and function of a theory. Theory analysis is conducted if the theory or framework has potential for being useful in practice, research, administration, or education. Theory analysis is a nonjudgmental, detailed examination of a theory, the main aim of which is to understand the theory (Fawcett & DeSanto-Madeya, 2013; Meleis, 2012).

Theory Evaluation

Theory evaluation, or theory critique, is the final step of the process. Evaluation follows analysis and assesses the theory's potential contribution to the discipline's knowledge base (Fawcett & DeSanto-Madeya, 2013; Walker & Avant, 2011). In theory evaluation, critical reflection involves ascertaining how well a theory serves its purpose, with the process of evaluation resulting in a decision or action about use of the theory (Chinn & Kramer, 2015). This includes consideration of how the theory is used to direct nursing practice and interventions and whether or not it contributes to favorable outcomes (Hickman, 2011).

Historical Overview of Theory Analysis and Evaluation

Since the late 1960s, a number of nursing scholars have published systems or methods for theory analysis/evaluation. Table 5-1 provides a list of these works. Basic components of the processes described by each are presented in the following sections.

Table 5-1 Publications of Methods for Nursing Theory Analysis and Evaluation

Nursing Scholar	Dates of Publications	Techniques Described (Most Recent Publication)
Rosemary Ellis	1968	Characteristics of significant theories
Margaret Hardy	1974, 1978	Theory evaluation
Mary Duffey and Ann Muhlenkamp	1974	Theory analysis and theory evaluation
Barbara Barnum (Stevens)	1979, 1984, 1990, 1994, 1998	Theory evaluation—internal criticism, external criticism
Lorraine Walker and Kay Avant	1983, 1988, 1995, 2005, 2011	Theory analysis
Jacqueline Fawcett and DeSanto-Madeya	1980, 1993, 1995, 2000, 2005, 2013	Theory (conceptual framework) analysis and theory (conceptual framework) evaluation
Peggy Chinn and Maeona Kramer (Jacobs)	1983, 1987, 1991, 1995, 1999, 2004, 2008, 2011, 2015	Theory description and critical reflection
Afaf Meleis	1985, 1991, 1997, 2007, 2012	Theory description, theory analysis, theory critique
Joyce Fitzpatrick and Ann Whall	1989, 1996, 2005, 2016	Analysis and evaluation of practice theory, middle range theory, and nursing models
Sharon Dudley-Brown	1997	Theory evaluation

It should be noted that most of the processes/methods for theory analysis and theory evaluation were implicitly or explicitly developed to review grand nursing theories and conceptual frameworks. Only in recent years have the processes and methods been applied to middle range theories and, rarely, practice theories. This observation, however, does not negate the need for analysis and evaluation (whether formal or informal) of middle range and practice theories. Furthermore, the processes should be applicable to all levels of theory.

Characteristics of Significant Theories: Ellis

Probably the first nursing scholar to document criteria for analyzing theories for use by nurses was Rosemary Ellis. Although not specifically describing a process or method of theory analysis or evaluation, Ellis (1968) identified characteristics of significant theories. The characteristics she specified were scope, complexity, testability, usefulness, implicit values of the theorist, information generation, and meaningful terminology. Her discussion of these characteristics produced the foundation on which later writers developed their criteria.

Theory Evaluation: Hardy

A few years after Ellis, Margaret Hardy (1974) wrote that theory should be evaluated according to certain universal standards. In her writings, Hardy provided a more detailed description of criteria for theory evaluation and presented personal insight on the processes needed. Criteria or standards she suggested for theory evaluation were as follows:

- Meaning and logical adequacy
- Operational and empirical adequacy
- Testability
- Generality
- Contribution to understanding
- Predictability
- Pragmatic adequacy

In a later work, Hardy (1978) discussed logical adequacy (diagramming) and stated that because a theory is a set of interrelated concepts and statements, its structure can be analyzed for internal consistency by examining the syntax of the theory as well as its content. Diagramming involves identifying all major theoretical terms (concepts, constructs, operational definitions, and referents). Once identified, each component can be represented by a symbol, and a model may be drawn illustrating relationships or linkages between or among the terms. These linkages should specify the direction, the type of relationship (whether positive or negative), and the form of the relationship.

According to Hardy (1974), empirical adequacy is the single most important criterion for evaluating a theory applied in practice. Assessing empirical adequacy requires reviewing literature and critically reading relevant research; it is necessary to determine if hypotheses testing the theory are clearly deduced from the theory. The entire body of relevant studies should be evaluated in terms of the extent to which it supports the theory or a part of the theory. Finally, the criteria of usefulness and significance refer to the theory's use in controlling, altering, or manipulating major variables and conditions specified by the theory to realize a desired outcome.

Theory Analysis and Theory Evaluation: Duffey and Muhlenkamp

Writing at approximately the same time as Hardy, Duffey and Muhlenkamp (1974) published a two-phase approach to critically examining nursing theory. Theory analysis was the first phase, for which they posited four questions for examination. For theory evaluation, they suggested six additional questions (Box 5-1).

Box 5-1	Questions for Theory Analysis and Theory Evaluation: Duffey and Muhlenkamp

Theory Analysis

1. What is the origin of the problem(s) with which the theory is concerned?
2. What methods were used in theory development (induction, deduction, synthesis)?
3. What is the character of the subject matter dealt with by the theory?
4. What kind of outcomes of testing propositions is generated by the theory?

Theory Evaluation

1. Does the theory generate testable hypotheses?
2. Does the theory guide practice or can it be used as a body of knowledge?
3. Is the theory complete in terms of subject matter and perspective?
4. Are the biases or values underlying the theory made explicit?
5. Are the relationships among the propositions made explicit?
6. Is the theory parsimonious?

Box 5-2   Theory Evaluation Criteria: Barnum

Internal Criticism

Clarity
Consistency
Adequacy
Logical development
Level of theory development

External Criticism

Reality convergence (how the theory relates to the real world)
Utility
Significance
Discrimination (differentiation between nursing and other health professions)
Scope
Complexity

Theory Evaluation: Barnum

Barbara Barnum (Stevens) first published her ideas for theory evaluation in 1979. Subsequent editions were published in 1984, 1990, 1994, and 1998. Barnum suggested a method of theory evaluation that differentiates internal and external criticisms. Internal criticism examines how the components of the theory fit with each other; external criticism examines how a theory relates to the extant world. Box 5-2 lists points to be examined for both.

Theory Analysis: Walker and Avant

Lorraine Walker and Kay Avant first presented their detailed methods for theory analysis in 1983. Their work was subsequently revised in 1988, 1995, 2005, and 2011. Building on a multiphase background of concept and statement development, which involves concept and statement analysis, synthesis, and derivation, they expanded the processes to include theory analysis. Table 5-2 gives a brief synopsis of the process of theory analysis they propose.

Theory Analysis and Evaluation: Fawcett

Jacqueline Fawcett (Fawcett, 1980, 1993, 1995, 2000, 2005; Fawcett & DeSanto-Madeya, 2013) used a two-phase process for analysis and evaluation of theories and conceptual frameworks. In her writings, she noted that analysis is a nonjudgmental, detailed examination of a theory. In Fawcett's most recent work (Fawcett & DeSanto-Madeya, 2013), components of the analysis process include the theory's origins, unique focus, and content. The theory's "origins" refers to the historical evolution of the model/theory, the author's motivation, philosophical assumptions about nursing, the author's inclusion of works of nursing and non-nursing scholars, and the worldview reflected by the model.

The unique focus refers to distinctive views of the metaparadigm concepts, different problems in nurse–patient situations or interactions, and differences in modes of nursing interventions. She notes that theories can be categorized as developmental, systems, interaction, needs, client-focused, person–environment interaction–focused,

Table 5-2 Theory Analysis: Walker and Avant

Step	Questions or Tasks
Determine the origins of the theory.	Identify the basis of the original development of the theory. Why was it developed? Was the process of development inductive or deductive? Is there evidence to support or refute the theory?
Examine the meaning of the theory.	Identify concepts. Examine definitions and their use (theoretical and operational definitions). Identify statements. Examine relationships.
Analyze the logical adequacy of the theory.	Determine if scientists agree on predictive ability of the theory. Determine if the content makes sense. Identify any logical fallacies.
Determine the usefulness of the theory.	Is the theory practical and helpful to nursing? Does it contribute to understanding and predicting outcomes?
Define the degree of generalizability.	Is the theory highly generalizable or specific?
Determine if the theory is parsimonious.	Can the theory be stated briefly and simply or is it complex?
Determine the testability of the theory.	Can the theory be supported with empirical data? Can testable hypotheses be generated from the theory?

Source: Walker and Avant (2011).

or nursing therapeutics–focused. The content of the model is examined to analyze the abstract and general concepts and propositions. Fawcett's method of theory analysis specifically identifies whether and how the concepts and propositions of the metaparadigm (nursing, environment, health, and person) are included in the theory. Representative questions to be addressed relative to the content include: "How are human beings defined and described? How is environment defined and described? How is health defined? . . . What is the goal of nursing? . . . and What statements are made about the relations among the four metaparadigm concepts?" (Fawcett & DeSanto-Madeya, 2013, p. 49).

Theory evaluation requires judgments to be made about a theory's significance based on how it satisfies certain criteria (Fawcett & DeSanto-Madeya, 2013). The process of theory evaluation includes review of previously published critiques, research reports, and reports of practical application of the theory. During the process of theory evaluation, the criteria to be examined are the explication of the origins of the theory, the comprehensiveness of the content, its logical congruence, how well it can lead to generation of new theory, and its legitimacy. The legitimacy is determined by reviewing the theory's social utility, social congruence, and social significance. The final step in theory evaluation is to examine the theory's contribution to the discipline of nursing.

Theory Description and Critique: Chinn and Kramer

Peggy Chinn and Maeona Kramer (Jacobs) initially wrote on the processes used to analyze theory in 1983. They used the terms theory description and critical reflection to describe a two-phase process. Theory description has six elements: purpose, concepts, definitions, relationships, structure, and assumptions. Table 5-3 presents these elements and their defining characteristics.

Critical reflection of a theory involves determining how well a theory serves its purpose. Critical reflection analyzes clarity and consistency of the theory as well as its

Table 5-3 Components of Theory Description: Chinn and Kramer	
Component	**Characteristics**
Purpose	The purpose of the theory should be stated explicitly or at least be identifiable in the text of the theory.
Concepts	The concepts of the theory should be linguistically expressed.
Definitions	Meanings of concepts are conveyed in theoretical definitions; these definitions give character to the theory.
Relationships	Concepts are structured into a systematic form that links each concept with others.
Structure	The relationships are linked to form a whole when the ideas of the theory interconnect; structure makes it possible to follow the reasoning of the theory.
Assumptions	Assumptions refer to underlying truths that determine the nature of concepts, definitions, purpose, relationship, and structure; may not be explicitly stated.

Source: Chinn and Kramer (2015).

complexity, generality, accessibility, and importance. In assessing clarity and consistency, Chinn and Kramer's (2015) critical reflection would examine:

- Semantic clarity: Are the concepts defined? Do the concepts establish empirical meaning?
- Semantic consistency: Are the concepts used consistently? Are the concepts congruent with their definitions?
- Structural clarity: Are the connections and reasoning within the theory understandable?
- Structural consistency: Is the structure of the theory consistent in its form?
- Simplicity or complexity: Is the theory simple? Is the theory complex?
- Generality: Does the theory cover a wide scope of experiences and phenomena?
- Accessibility: How accessible is the theory? How well are concepts grounded in empirically identifiable phenomena?
- Importance: How can the theory contribute to nursing practice, research, and education?

Theory Description, Analysis, and Critique: Meleis

According to Meleis (1985, 2007, 2012), there are three stages involved in theory evaluation: theory description, theory analysis, and theory critique. During the process of theory description, the reviewer closely examines the structural and functional components of the theory. The structural components include assumptions (implicit and explicit), concepts, and propositions. The functional assessment considers the anticipated consequence of the theory and its purpose. Components that should be examined are the focus of the theory and how it addresses the client, nursing, health, the nurse–client interactions, environment, nursing problems, and nursing therapeutics.

Theory analysis involves considering important variables that may have influenced the development of the theory. These include the theorist, paradigmatic origins of the theory, and internal dimensions of the theory. During the analysis procedure, Meleis (2012) recommends reviewing external and internal factors that influenced the theorist as well as the theorist's experiential background, educational background, and employment history. Likewise, a reconstruction of the professional and academic networks that surrounded the theorist while the theory was evolving should be examined.

Second, Meleis (2012) argues that careful consideration of use of theories from other fields or paradigms is to be encouraged. To identify the paradigm(s) from which the theory may have evolved, or to recognize other theorists who may have influenced the development of the theory, the reviewer would consider references, educational and experiential background of the theorist, and the sociocultural context of the theory as it was developed.

Finally, internal dimensions of the theory should be analyzed. This will provide information about the rationale on which the theory is built, systems of relationships, content of the theory, goal of the theory, scope of the theory, context of the theory, abstractness of the theory, and method of development.

Critique of a theory may follow analysis, and Meleis (2012) identified five elements to consider in this phase: the relationship between structure and function, diagram of the theory, circle of contagiousness, usefulness, and external components. The relationship between structure and function involves evaluating the theory's clarity and consistency, level of simplicity or complexity, and tautology/teleology. In assessing the tautology of the theory, the reviewer would observe for needless repetition of an idea in different parts of the theory, which Meleis claims will decrease the clarity of the theory. Teleology occurs when definitions of concepts, conditions, and events are described by consequences rather than properties and dimensions; this should be avoided.

Although not all theories contain models graphically or pictorially depicting the structure of the theory, Meleis (2012) states that theories and models are enhanced by visual representation. The reviewer should determine if the model does indeed help clarify linkages among the concepts and propositions and, thereby, enhance clarity of the theory.

The circle of contagiousness refers to whether, and to what extent, the model or theory has been adopted by other experts in the field. In evaluating usefulness, Meleis (2012) suggests analysis of the theory's usefulness in practice, research, education, and administration.

The final component of this method is the review of external components of the theory. These include implicit and explicit personal values of both the theorist and the critic. It also refers to congruence with other professional values as well as with social values. Finally, the critic would determine whether the theory has social significance.

Analysis and Evaluation of Practice Theory, Middle Range Theory, and Nursing Models: Whall

Whall (2016) is the only nurse scholar to explicitly outline three separate criteria for analysis and evaluation for the three levels of nursing theory. In her most recent edition, she noted that middle range and practice theories have achieved status equal to that of nursing conceptual models, but it has only been nursing models that have been systematically examined. Following this observation, she outlined distinct, although similar, criteria for evaluation of all three levels of nursing theory using a three-phase approach that reviews basic considerations, internal analysis and evaluation, and external analysis and evaluation.

According to Whall (2016), practice theory (or microtheory) is produced from practice and deduced from middle range theory as well as from research. Because practice theory is designed for immediate application to practice, questions regarding the fit with empirical data are important in the evaluation process. Operational definitions and descriptions of how to apply practice theory are also important. Internal analysis of practice theory may be accomplished by diagramming the interrelationships of all concepts to detect lapses and inconsistencies in the theory's structure. The assumptions of the theory should be considered in light of historical and current perspectives of nursing. This should include ethical and cultural implications of the theory. External analysis should compare standards of care with the theory and examine nursing research to determine if it supports the theory, is neutral, or is in opposition.

Analysis and evaluation of middle range theory modifies the guidelines used for nursing conceptual models. It examines whether the theory fits with the existing nursing perspective and domains. Propositional statements should be examined to determine if they are causal or associative in nature, to assess their relative importance, and to find missing linkages between concepts. It is suggested that diagramming of the relationships may help identify missing relationships. Concepts should be operationally defined to support empirical adequacy. External analysis refers to congruence with more global theories and other related middle range theories. Examination of ethical, cultural, and social policy implications is crucial.

Whall (2016) believes nursing conceptual models should be assessed from a postmodern or neomodern view. In addition, conceptual models should consider the major paradigm concepts (person, environment, health, and nursing) as well as additional concepts specific to the model. Analysis should examine whether the definitions of the concepts and statements are consistently used throughout the model and whether the interrelationships among the concepts are consistent. Internal analysis considers the assumptions and philosophical basis of the model and looks at the uniformity of discussion throughout the model. External consistency examines the model in relation to views external to the model (i.e., whether the model is being evaluated consistent with other nursing conceptual models and with nursing intervention classification systems). Table 5-4 lists some of the questions for consideration by Whall in analysis and evaluation of all three levels of nursing theory.

Theory Evaluation: Dudley-Brown

One of the most contemporary methods for theory evaluation was presented by Dudley-Brown (1997), who strongly relied on Kuhn's (1977) criteria for theory evaluation. In this method, evaluation should consider accuracy, consistency, fruitfulness, simplicity/complexity, scope, acceptability, and sociocultural utility.

To Dudley-Brown (1997), *accuracy* is essential because the theory should describe nursing as it exists today—not the nursing of the future or of the past. The theory should contain a worldview of nursing consistent with the present reality. *Consistency* relates to the importance of the nursing theory being internally consistent. There should be logical order: Terms, concepts, and statements should be used consistently and defined operationally.

Another criterion Dudley-Brown (1997) identifies for evaluation is *fruitfulness*. For this criterion, the theory should be useful in generating information and significant in contributing to the development of nursing knowledge.

Simplicity/complexity is a fourth criterion for evaluation. Both simple and complex theories are needed. In general, a theory should be balanced and logical. The theory should describe the phenomenon consistently in terms of simplicity or complexity.

Scope is a fifth criterion because theories of both broad and limited scope are needed. Scope should be dependent on the phenomenon and its context. Acceptability refers to the adoption of the theory by others. Theories should be useful in practice, education, research, or administration.

Table 5-4 Criteria for Analysis and Evaluation of Theory: Whall			
Level of Theory	**Basic Considerations**	**Internal Analysis and Evaluation**	**External Analysis and Evaluation**
Practice theory	Can the concepts be operationalized? Are operationalized concepts congruent with empirical data? Do statements lead to directives for nursing care? Are statements sufficient to practice and not contradictory?	Are there gaps or inconsistencies within the theory that may lead to conflicts and difficulties? Are assumptions congruent with nursing's historical perspective? Are assumptions congruent with ethical standards and social policy? Are assumptions in conflict with given cultural groups?	Is the theory produced with existing nursing standards? Is the theory consistent with existing standards of education within nursing? Is the theory related to nursing diagnoses and nursing intervention practices? Is the theory supported by existing research internal and external to nursing?
Middle range theory	What are the definitions and relative importance of major concepts? What is the type and relative importance of major theoretical statements?	What are the assumptions of the theory? What is the relationship of the theory to philosophy of science? Are concepts related/not related via statements? Is there loss of information? Is there internal consistency and congruency of all component parts of the theory? What is the empirical adequacy of the theory? Has the theory been examined in practice and research, and has it held up to this scrutiny?	What is the congruency with related theory and research internal and external to nursing? What is the congruence with the perspective of nursing, the domains, and the persistent questions? What ethical, cultural, and social policy issues are related to the theory?
Nursing models	What are the definitions of person, nursing, health, and environment? What are additional understandings of the metaparadigm concepts? What are the interrelationships among the metaparadigm concepts? What are the descriptions of other concepts found in the model?	What are the underlying assumptions of the model? What are the definitions of other components of the model? What is the relative importance of basic concepts or other components of the model? What are the analyses of internal and external consistency? What are the analyses of adequacy?	Is nursing research based on the model or related to the model? Is nursing education based on the model or related to the model? Is nursing practice based on the model? What is the relationship to existing nursing diagnoses and interventions systems?

Source: Whall (2016).

Sociocultural utility is the final criterion for evaluation. Social congruence encompasses the beliefs, values, and expectations of different cultures. The theory should be measured against the criterion of social utility according to the culture for which it was proposed. Theories proposed for Western societies need to be evaluated for their philosophical and theoretical relevance in other societies and cultures.

Comparisons of Methods

Several authors (Dudley-Brown, 1997; Meleis, 2012; Moody, 1990) have compared many of the theory analysis and evaluation methods described here. A number of similarities can be found between and among all the methods. Table 5-5 provides a list of the methods reviewed and criteria specified by each author. It is important to note

Table 5-5 Comparison of Theory Evaluation Criteria

Evaluation Criteria	Ellis	Hardy	Barnum	Walker and Avant	Fawcett	Chinn and Kramer	Meleis	Whall	Dudley-Brown
Complexity/simplicity	X		X	X	X	X	X		X
Testability	X	X		X	X				
Generality/scope	X	X	X	X	X	X			X
Usefulness	X	X	X	X		X	X		
Contribution to understanding		X	X		X	X			X
Implicit values	X						X		
Information generation	X								
Meaningful terminology (definitions)	X			X	X	X	X	X	
Logical adequacy		X	X	X				X	
Validity/accuracy/ empirical adequacy		X			X			X	X
Predictability/tested		X				X		X	
Origins				X	X		X		
Clarity		X			X	X			
Consistency		X		X	X	X	X	X	
Context				X		X			
Pragmatic adequacy				X			X		
Reality convergence		X							
Discrimination		X							
Metaparadigm concepts					X	X	X		
Assumptions					X	X	X		
Purpose					X	X			
Consequences						X			
Nursing therapeutics interventions					X	X	X		
Method of development						X			
Circle of contagion						X	X	X	
Social/cultural significance					X	X	X	X	
Correspondence to standards/professional values						X	X		

that different authors use different terms for similar concepts; thus, some interpretation of meaning of terms was necessary for the comparison.

As Table 5-5 shows, the most common criteria identified among the theory evaluation methods were an examination of complexity/simplicity (seven of nine) and scope/generality (seven of nine). Other common criteria were inclusion of meaningful terminology, definitions of concepts (six of nine), consistency (six of nine), contribution to understanding (five of nine), usefulness (six of nine), testability (four of nine), logical adequacy (four of nine), and validity/accuracy/empirical adequacy (six of nine). Criteria mentioned in only one or two methods were implicit values of the theorist, information generation, reality convergence, discrimination between nursing and other health professions, consequences, method of development, correspondence to existing standards, origins of the theory, context, pragmatic adequacy, and application of or to nursing therapeutics.

There appears to be an evolution of the processes over the past three decades. Similarities of criteria were evident based on time of initial writing. Ellis (1968), Duffey and Muhlenkamp (1974), and Hardy (1974) were the first nurses to describe the processes of theory evaluation, and their criteria are similar. The methods proposed by Walker and Avant (1983, 1988, 1995, 2005, 2011) are also consistent with those of Hardy and Ellis. Fawcett's model (1980, 1993, 2005) is similar to Chinn and Kramer's (1983, 1987, 1991, 1995) approach and to Barnum's (1984, 1990, 1994) internal criticism criteria. Meleis (1985, 1991, 1997) and Whall (Fitzpatrick & Whall, 1989, 1996) present the most detailed methods. Meleis's (2012) system has three components (description, analysis, and critical reflection), and Whall's (2016) examines three levels of theory. Barnum (1998) and Whall (2016) are similar in that they describe separate internal and external dimensions. The later works of Whall (2016), Meleis (2012), and Dudley-Brown (1997) are similar because they include characteristics of circle of contagion and consideration of social and cultural significance as evaluation criteria.

Most methods for analysis and evaluation were developed and used to review grand nursing theories. Indeed, a literature review resulted in no published report of theory evaluation in nursing beyond those in nursing theory textbooks. Books that focus on analysis and evaluation of grand nursing theories include those by Alligood (2014b), Fawcett & DeSanto-Madeya (2013), Fitzpatrick and Whall (2005, 2016), George (2011), Masters (2015), and M. C. Smith and Parker (2015). Alligood (2014b), M. C. Smith and Parker (2015), Peterson and Bredow (2017), and M. J. Smith and Liehr (2013) also analyze/evaluate selected middle range nursing theories in their works.

Synthesized Method of Theory Evaluation

Following the detailed review and comparison of the many methods for theory analysis and evaluation, a method specifically designed to evaluate middle range and practice theories was developed (Box 5-3). These criteria were synthesized from the works of noted nursing scholars described earlier and are intended to be contemporary and responsive to both recent and anticipated changes in use of theory in nursing practice, research, education, and administration.

Summary

Nurses in clinical practice, as well as graduate students like Jerry Thompson from the case study, should know how to analyze or evaluate a theory to determine if it is reliable and valid and to determine when and how to apply it in practice, research,

Box 5-3 Synthesized Method for Theory Evaluation

Theory Description

What is the purpose of the theory (describe, explain, predict, prescribe)?
What is the scope or level of the theory (grand, middle range, practice/situation specific)?
What are the origins of the theory?
What are the major concepts?
What are the major theoretical propositions?
What are the major assumptions?
Is the context for use described?

Theory Analysis

Are concepts theoretically and operationally defined?
Are statements theoretically and operationally defined?
Are linkages explicit?
Is the theory logically organized?
Is there a model/diagram? Does the model contribute to clarifying the theory?
Are the concepts, statements, and assumptions used consistently?
Are outcomes or consequences stated or predicted?

Theory Evaluation

Is the theory congruent with current nursing standards?
Is the theory congruent with current nursing interventions or therapeutics?
Has the theory been tested empirically? Is it supported by research? Does it appear to
    be accurate/valid?
Is there evidence that the theory has been used by nursing educators, nursing researchers,
    or nursing administrators?
Is the theory relevant socially?
Is the theory relevant cross-culturally?
Does the theory contribute to the discipline of nursing?
What are implications for nursing related to implementation of the theory?

administration, or education. This chapter has presented and analyzed a number of different methods for evaluation of theory. Like many issues in the study of use of theory in nursing, the process of theory evaluation, although important, is often confusing. In addition, with very few exceptions, the methods or techniques were developed and used almost exclusively to analyze and evaluate grand nursing theories. It is hoped that with the current emphasis on development and use of both practice and middle range theories, there will be a concurrent emphasis on the analysis and evaluation of those theories. In this chapter, the most commonly used methods were described in some detail and compared. Following this comparison, a synthesized and simplified method for examination of theory was presented.

Key Points

■ Theory evaluation is the process of systematically examining a theory; the intent of evaluation is to determine how well the theory guides practice, research, education, or administration.
■ The process of theory evaluation typically includes examination of the theory's origins, meaning, logical adequacy, usefulness, generalizability, and testability.

Additional criteria are also considered, depending on which process or technique is being used.

■ Several different methods for theory analysis/theory evaluation have been proposed in the nursing literature.

■ The synthesized method for theory evaluation was derived from other published methods and is intended to be used to evaluate middle range and practice theories.

To further help the reader understand the theory evaluation process, this chapter presents an exemplar of the synthesized method for theory evaluation.

THEORY EVALUATION EXEMPLAR: THEORY OF CHRONIC SORROW

Primary References for the Theory of Chronic Sorrow

Burke, M. L., Eakes, G. G., & Hainsworth, M. A. (1999). Milestones of chronic sorrow: Perspectives of chronically ill and bereaved persons and family caregivers. *Journal of Family Nursing, 5*(4), 374–387.

Eakes, G. G. (1993). Chronic sorrow: A response to living with cancer. *Oncology Nursing Forum, 20*(9), 1327–1334.

Eakes, G. G. (1995). Chronic sorrow: The lived experience of parents of chronically mentally ill individuals. *Archives of Psychiatric Nursing, 9*(2), 77–84.

Eakes, G. G. (2016). Chronic sorrow. In S. J. Peterson & T. S. Bredow (Eds.), *Middle range theories: Application to nursing research* (4th ed., pp. 93–105). Philadelphia, PA: Wolters Kluwer.

Eakes, G. G., Burke, M. L., & Hainsworth, M. A. (1998). Middle-range theory of chronic sorrow. *Image—The Journal of Nursing Scholarship, 30*(2), 179–184.

Schreier, A. M., & Droes, N. S. (2014). Theory of chronic sorrow. In M. R. Alligood (Ed.), *Nursing theorists and their work* (8th ed., pp. 609–625). Maryland Heights, MO: Mosby.

References for Examples of Application of the Theory of Chronic Sorrow in Practice and Research

Bowes, S., Lowes, L., Warner, J., & Gregory, J. W. (2009). Chronic sorrow in parents of children with type 1 diabetes. *Journal of Advanced Nursing, 65*(5), 992–1000.

Glenn, A. D. (2015). Using online health communication to manage chronic sorrow: Mothers of children with rare diseases speak. *Journal of Pediatric Nursing, 30*(1), 17–24.

Gordon, J. (2009). An evidence-based approach for supporting parents experiencing chronic sorrow. *Pediatric Nursing, 35*(2), 115–159.

Hobdell, E. F., Grant, M. L., Valencia, I., Mare, J., Kothare, S. V., Legido, A., et al. (2007). Chronic sorrow and coping in families of children with epilepsy. *The Journal of Neuroscience Nursing, 39*(2), 76–82.

Isaksson, A. K., & Ahlstrom, G. (2008). Managing chronic sorrow: Experiences of patients with multiple sclerosis. *The Journal of Neuroscience Nursing, 40*(3), 180–191.

Joseph, H. A. (2012). Recognizing chronic sorrow in the habitual ED patient. *Journal of Emergency Nursing, 38*(6), 539–540.

Kendall, L. C. (2005). *The experience of living with ongoing loss: Testing the Kendall Chronic Sorrow Instrument* (Unpublished doctoral dissertation). Virginia Commonwealth University, Richmond, VA.

Olwit, C., Musisi, S., Leshabari, S., & Sanyu, I. (2015). Chronic sorrow: Lived experiences of caregivers of patients diagnosed with schizophrenia in Butabika mental Hospital, Kampala, Uganda. *Archives of Psychiatric Nursing, 29*(1), 43–48.

Smith, C. S. (2009). Substance abuse, chronic sorrow, and mothering loss: Relapse triggers among female victims of child abuse. *Journal of Pediatric Nursing, 24*(5), 401–410.

Vitale, S. A., & Falco, C. (2014). Children born prematurely: Risk of parental chronic sorrow. *Journal of Pediatric Nursing, 29*(6), 248–251.

Theory Description

Scope of theory: Middle range

Purpose of theory: Explanatory theory—"to explain the experiences of people across the lifespan who encounter ongoing disparity because of significant loss" (Eakes, Burke, & Hainsworth, 1998, p. 179)

Origins of theory: "Chronic sorrow" appeared in the literature in 1962 to describe recurrent grief experienced by parents of children with disabilities. A number of research projects were conducted in the 1980s and 1990s describing chronic sorrow among various groups with loss situations. The resulting theory of chronic sorrow, therefore, was inductively developed using concept analysis, extensive review of the literature, critical review of research, and validation in 10 qualitative studies of various loss situations (Eakes, 2016; Eakes et al., 1998).

Major concepts: Chronic sorrow, loss experience, disparity, trigger events (milestones), external management methods, internal management methods. All are defined and explained (Schreier & Droes, 2014).

Major theoretical propositions are as follows:

1. Disparity between a desired relationship and an actual relationship or a disparity between current reality and desired reality is created by loss experiences.
2. Trigger events bring the negative disparity into focus or exacerbate the experience of disparity.
3. For individuals with chronic or life-threatening illnesses, chronic sorrow is most often triggered when the individual experiences disparity with accepted norms (social, developmental, or personal).
4. For family caregivers, disparity between the idealized and actual is associated with developmental milestones.
5. For bereaved individuals, disparity from the ideal is created by the absence of a person who was central in the life of the bereaved.

Major assumptions: Not stated

Context for use: "Experienced by individuals across the lifespan"; implied that it may be used in multiple settings and nursing situations

Theory Analysis

Theoretical definitions for major concepts:

Chronic sorrow—the periodic recurrence of permanent, pervasive sadness or other grief-related feelings associated with ongoing disparity resulting from a loss experience

Loss experience—a significant loss, either actual or symbolic, that may be ongoing, with no predictable end, or a more circumscribed single-loss event

Disparity—a gap between the current reality and the desired as a result of a loss experience

Trigger events or milestones—a situation, circumstance, or condition that brings the negative disparity resulting from the loss into focus or exacerbates the disparity

External management methods—interventions provided by professionals to assist individuals to cope with chronic sorrow

Internal management methods—positive personal coping strategies used to deal with the periodic episodes of chronic sorrow

Operational definitions for major concepts: No operational definitions are provided in the original works.

Statements theoretically defined: Theoretical propositions are implicitly stated in the body of the text.

Statements operationally defined: Theoretical propositions are not operationally defined.

Linkages explicit: Linkages are described in the text and explicated in the model.

Logical organization: Theory is logically organized and described in detail.

Model/diagram: A model is provided and assists in explaining linkages of the concepts.

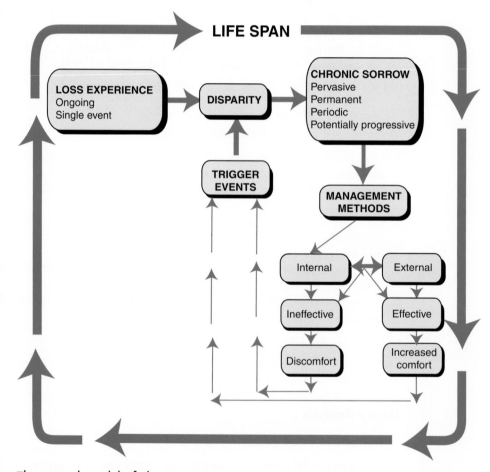

Theoretical model of chronic sorrow.

(Source: Eakes, G. G., Burke, M. L., & Hainsworth, M. A. [1998]. Middle-range theory of chronic sorrow. *Image—The Journal of Nursing Scholarship, 30*[2], 179–184. Used with permission of John Wiley & Sons LTD, Publisher.)

Consistent use of concepts, statements, and assumptions: Concepts and propositions are used consistently. Assumptions are not explicitly addressed.

Predicted or stated outcomes or consequences: Anticipated outcomes are stated in the model.

Theory Evaluation

Congruence with nursing standards: The theory appears congruent with nursing standards. A number of articles were identified in recent nursing literature describing how the construct of chronic sorrow has been identified among various aggregates (Eakes, 2016).

Congruence with current nursing interventions or therapeutics: Literature-based descriptions of application of components of the theory in nursing practice include caring for bereaved persons and family caregivers (Burke, Eakes, & Hainsworth, 1999), a discussion of caring for children with type 1 diabetes (Bowes, Lowes, Warner, & Gregory, 2009), interventions for community nurses to help assist families resolving chronic sorrow (Gordon, 2009), using online health communication to manage chronic sorrow among mothers of children with rare diseases (Glenn, 2015).

Evidence of empirical testing/research support/validity: The theory was derived from multiple research studies and a review of the literature.

The Burke/CCRCS Chronic Sorrow Questionnaire is an interview guide comprising 10 open-ended questions that explore the theory's concepts.

Research using the questionnaire includes investigation of chronic sorrow among cancer patients (Eakes, 1993), chronic sorrow in chronically mentally ill individuals (Eakes, 1995), chronic sorrow in women who were victims of child abuse (Smith, 2009), chronic sorrow in habitual emergency department patients (Joseph, 2012), chronic sorrow and coping in families of children with epilepsy (Hobdell et al., 2007), chronic sorrow among parents of children born prematurely (Vitale & Falco, 2014), and chronic sorrow among patients with multiple sclerosis (Isaksson & Ahlstrom, 2008). Further, a second instrument designed to measure chronic sorrow (Kendall, 2005) has been developed.

Use by nursing educators, nursing researchers, or nursing administrators: The references listed previously indicate that the theory has been used in practice and research. Other studies have cited the work of Eakes and colleagues related to chronic sorrow (Eakes, 2016).

Social relevance: Theory is relevant to individuals, families, and groups, irrespective of age or socioeconomic status.

Transcultural relevance: Theory is potentially relevant across cultures; theorist notes that "relevance for various cultural groups should be explored" (Eakes et al., 1998, p. 184). For example Olwit and team (2015) studied chronic sorrow among caregivers of patients with schizophrenia in a hospital in Uganda.

Contribution to nursing: Authors note that the theory is applicable to different groups, but more study is needed to test the theory and to identify strategies to reduce disparity created by loss (prescriptive interventions). Despite the relative newness of the theory, there is a growing body of nursing literature reporting on use both related to interventions and research (Eakes, 2016).

Conclusions and implications: The theory is useful and appropriate for nurses practicing in a variety of settings. Implications for research were described and implications for education can be inferred. Further development of the theory is warranted to better explicate relationships and operationalize the concepts and propositions to allow testing.

Learning Activities

1. Obtain the original works of two of the nursing scholars whose theory analysis/ evaluation strategies are discussed. Use the strategies to evaluate a recently published middle range nursing theory (see Chapter 11 for examples). How are the conclusions similar? How are they different?
2. For one of the nursing scholars who has published several versions or editions of her work (e.g., Fawcett, Chinn and Kramer, Meleis), obtain a copy of the oldest version and a copy of the most recent version and compare the strategies suggested. Have they changed?
3. Search the literature for examples of published accounts of nursing theory evaluation or theory analysis. Share your findings with classmates.

REFERENCES

Alligood, M. R. (2014a). Introduction to nursing theory: Its history, significance, and analysis. In M. R. Alligood (Ed.), *Nursing theorists and their work* (8th ed., pp. 2–13). St. Louis, MO: Mosby.

Alligood, M. R. (2014b). *Nursing theorists and their work* (8th ed.). St. Louis, MO: Mosby.

Barnum, B. S. (1984). *Nursing theory: Analysis, application, evaluation* (2nd ed.). Boston, MA: Little, Brown.

Barnum, B. S. (1990). *Nursing theory: Analysis, application, evaluation* (3rd ed.). Glenview, IL: Scott, Foresman/Little, Brown Higher Education.

Barnum, B. S. (1994). *Nursing theory: Analysis, application, evaluation* (4th ed.). Philadelphia, PA: Lippincott Williams & Wilkins.

Barnum, B. S. (1998). *Nursing theory: Analysis, application, evaluation* (5th ed.). Philadelphia, PA: Lippincott Williams & Wilkins.

Chinn, P. L., & Jacobs, M. K. (1983). *Theory and nursing: A systematic approach*. St. Louis, MO: Mosby.

Chinn, P. L., & Jacobs, M. K. (1987). *Theory and nursing: A systemic approach* (2nd ed.). St. Louis, MO: Mosby.

Chinn, P. L., & Kramer, M. K. (1991). *Theory and nursing: A systematic approach* (3rd ed.). St. Louis, MO: Mosby.

Chinn, P. L., & Kramer, M. K. (1995). *Theory and nursing: A systematic approach* (4th ed.). St. Louis, MO: Mosby.

Chinn, P. L., & Kramer, M. K. (1999). *Theory and nursing: Integrated knowledge development* (5th ed.). St. Louis, MO: Mosby.

Chinn, P. L., & Kramer, M. K. (2004). *Integrated theory and knowledge development in nursing* (6th ed.). St. Louis, MO: Mosby.

Chinn, P. L., & Kramer, M. K. (2008). *Integrated theory and knowledge development in nursing* (7th ed.). St. Louis, MO: Mosby.

Chinn, P. L., & Kramer, M. K. (2011). *Integrated theory and knowledge development in nursing* (8th ed.). St. Louis, MO: Mosby.

Chinn, P. L., & Kramer, M. K. (2015). *Integrated theory and knowledge development in nursing* (9th ed.). St. Louis, MO: Elsevier.

Curley, M. A. Q. (1998). Patient-nurse synergy: Optimizing patients' outcomes. *American Journal of Critical Care, 7*(1), 64–72.

Dudley-Brown, S. L. (1997). The evaluation of nursing theory: A method for our madness. *International Journal of Nursing Studies, 34*(1), 76–83.

Duffey, M., & Muhlenkamp, A. F. (1974). A framework for theory analysis. *Nursing Outlook, 22*(9), 570–574.

Ellis, R. (1968). Characteristics of significant theories. *Nursing Research, 17*(3), 217–222.

Fawcett, J. (1980). A framework of analysis and evaluation of conceptual models of nursing. *Nurse Educator, 5*(6), 10–14.

Fawcett, J. (1993). *Analysis and evaluation of nursing theories.* Philadelphia, PA: Davis.

Fawcett, J. (1995). *Analysis and evaluation of conceptual models of nursing* (3rd ed.). Philadelphia, PA: Davis.

Fawcett, J. (2000). *Analysis and evaluation of contemporary nursing knowledge: Nursing models and theories.* Philadelphia, PA: Davis.

Fawcett, J. (2005). *Contemporary nursing knowledge: Analysis and evaluation of nursing models and theories* (2nd ed.). Philadelphia, PA: Davis.

Fawcett, J., & DeSanto-Madeya, S. (2013). *Contemporary nursing knowledge: Analysis and evaluation of nursing models and theories* (3rd ed.). Philadelphia, PA: Davis.

Fitzpatrick, J. J., & Whall, A. L. (1989). *Conceptual models of nursing: Analysis and application.* Stamford, CT: Appleton & Lange.

Fitzpatrick, J. J., & Whall, A. L. (1996). *Conceptual models of nursing: Analysis and application* (3rd ed.). Stamford, CT: Appleton & Lange.

Fitzpatrick, J. J., & Whall, A. (2005). *Conceptual models of nursing: Analysis and application* (4th ed.). Upper Saddle River, NJ: Prentice-Hall.

Fitzpatrick, J. J., & Whall, A. (2016). *Conceptual models of nursing: Global perspective* (5th ed.). Boston, MA: Pearson.

George, J. B. (2011). *Nursing theories: The base for professional nursing practice* (6th ed.). Upper Saddle River, NJ: Pearson.

Hardy, M. E. (1974). Theories: Components, development, evaluation. *Nursing Research, 23*, 100–107.

Hardy, M. E. (1978). Perspectives on nursing theory. *ANS. Advances in Nursing Science, 1*(1), 37–48.

Hickman, J. S. (2011). An introduction to nursing theory. In J. B. George (Ed.), *Nursing theories: The base for professional nursing practice* (6th ed., pp. 1–22). Upper Saddle River, NJ: Pearson.

Kuhn, T. S. (1977). Second thoughts on paradigms. In F. Suppe (Ed.), *The structure of scientific theories* (pp. 459–482). Urbana, IL: University of Illinois Press.

Masters, K. (2015). *Nursing theories: A framework for professional practice* (2nd ed.). Burlington, MA: Jones & Bartlett Learning.

Meleis, A. I. (1985). *Theoretical nursing: Development and progress.* Philadelphia, PA: J.B. Lippincott.

Meleis, A. I. (1991). *Theoretical nursing: Development and progress* (2nd ed.). Philadelphia, PA: J.B. Lippincott.

Meleis, A. I. (1997). *Theoretical nursing: Development and progress* (3rd ed.). Philadelphia, PA: J.B. Lippincott.

Meleis, A. I. (2007). *Theoretical nursing: Development and progress* (4th ed.). Philadelphia, PA: Lippincott Williams & Wilkins.

Meleis, A. I. (2012). *Theoretical nursing: Development and progress* (5th ed.). Philadelphia, PA: Lippincott Williams & Wilkins.

Moody, L. E. (1990). *Advancing nursing science through research.* Newbury Park, CA: Sage.

Pender, N. J., Murdaugh, C. L., & Parsons, M. A. (2015). *Health promotion in nursing practice* (7th ed.). Upper Saddle River, NJ: Prentice-Hall.

Peterson, S. J., & Bredow, T. S. (2017). *Middle range theories: Application to nursing research and practice* (4th ed.). Philadelphia, PA: Wolters Kluwer.

Smith, M. C., & Parker, M. E. (2015). *Nursing theories & nursing practice* (4th ed.). Philadelphia, PA: Davis.

Smith, M. J., & Liehr, P. R. (2013). *Middle range theory for nursing* (3rd ed.). New York, NY: Springer Publishing.

Stevens, B. J. (1979). *Nursing theory: Analysis, application, evaluation.* Boston, MA: Little, Brown.

Walker, L. O., & Avant, K. (1983). *Strategies for theory construction in nursing.* Norwalk, CT: Appleton-Century-Crofts.

Walker, L. O., & Avant, K. (1988). *Strategies for theory construction in nursing* (2nd ed.). Norwalk, CT: Appleton & Lange.

Walker, L. O., & Avant, K. (1995). *Strategies for theory construction in nursing* (3rd ed.). Norwalk, CT: Appleton & Lange.

Walker, L. O., & Avant, K. (2005). *Strategies for theory construction in nursing* (4th ed.). Upper Saddle River, NJ: Prentice-Hall.

Walker, L. O., & Avant, K. (2011). *Strategies for theory construction in nursing* (5th ed.). Upper Saddle River, NJ: Prentice-Hall.

Whall, A. L. (2016). Philosophy of science positions and their importance in cross-national nursing. In J. J. Fitzpatrick & A. L. Whall (Eds.), *Conceptual models of nursing: Global perspectives* (5th ed., pp. 8–28). Upper Saddle River, NJ: Prentice-Hall.

Nursing Theories

6

Overview of Grand Nursing Theories

Evelyn M. Wills

Janet Turner works as a nurse on a postsurgical, cardiovascular floor. Because she desires a broader view of nursing knowledge and wants to become an acute care nurse practitioner, she recently began a master's degree program in nursing. The requirements for a course entitled "Theoretical Foundations of Nursing Practice" led Janet to become familiar with some of the many nursing theories. From her readings, she learned about a number of ways to classify theories: grand theory, conceptual model, middle range theory, practice theory, borrowed theory, interactive–integrative model, totality paradigm, and simultaneous action paradigm. She came to the conclusion that there is no consistency among nursing theorists and even questioned their relevance to her practice.

Janet's theory course was conducted via distance learning technology including online classrooms, chats, Twitter, Wikis, and other social media formats. To better understand the material, she consulted with her theory professor and classmates via the Twitter feed and participated in the course's live chat room. Lively online discussions resulted in sharing interesting ways of conceptualizing the grand nursing theories.

As Janet continued to study and work with her professor and classmates, she learned that nursing theories have evolved from several schools of philosophical thought and various scientific traditions. Growing more confident, she considered ways to group or categorize them based on similarities of perspective; thus, she was able to read and analyze the theories more effectively. Ultimately, she selected two to examine further for one of her assignments.

In Chapter 2, the reader was introduced to grand nursing theories and given a brief historical overview of their development. Fawcett and DeSanto-Madeya (2013) distinguish between conceptual models and grand theories, explaining that conceptual models are broad formulations of philosophy based on an attempt to include the whole of nursing reality as the scholar understands it. The concepts and propositions of conceptual models are abstract and not likely to be testable in fact. Grand nursing theories, by contrast, may be derived from conceptual models and are the most complex and widest in scope of the levels of theory; they attempt to explain broad issues within the discipline. Grand theories are composed of relatively abstract concepts and propositions that are less abstract than those of conceptual models and may not be directly amenable to testing (Butts, 2015; Fawcett & DeSanto-Madeya, 2013; Higgins & Moore, 2000). They were developed through thoughtful and insightful appraisal of existing ideas as opposed to empirical research and may provide the basis for scholars to produce innovative middle range or practice theories (Figure 6-1).

The grand nursing theories guide research and assist scholars to integrate the results of numerous diverse investigations so that the findings may be applied to education, practice, further research, and administration. Eun-Ok and Chang (2012), in their review of literature, found support for the idea that grand theories have an important place in nursing, for example, in research and clinical practice. They also found that theorists are further refining concepts and theories. They stated that theories are "essential for our discipline at multiple levels" (p. 162) (Box 6-1). Eun-Ok and Chang also noted that the grand theories provide a background of philosophical reasoning that allows nurse scientists to develop organizing principles for research or practice, sometimes referred to as middle range theory (middle range theories will be discussed in Chapters 10 and 11). One of the most important benefits of invoking theories in education, administration, research, and practice has been the systematization of those domains of nursing activity. Indeed, according to Bachmann, Danuser, and Morin (2015), a theoretical base is essential in that it provides a firm connection between new or adapted knowledge or information and nursing science, thus promoting development of the science.

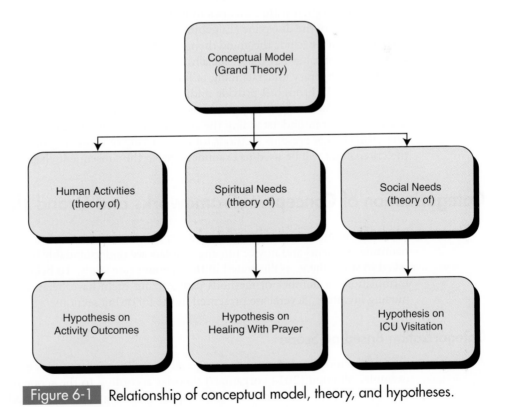

Figure 6-1 Relationship of conceptual model, theory, and hypotheses.

Box 6-1	Nursing Theories and the American Association of Colleges of Nursing Essentials

Essential I of the *Essentials of Master's Education in Nursing* (American Association of Colleges of Nursing [AACN], 2011) specifically notes that "master's-prepared nurses use a variety of theories and frameworks including nursing and ethical theories in the analysis of clinical problems, illness prevention and health promotion strategies" (p. 9). Furthermore, "nursing theories" is listed as one content area to be included in master of science in nursing (MSN) programs.

Advanced practice nurses are more likely to succeed in analyzing research results for evidence-based practice (EBP) when the research fits into a particular theoretical framework. Cody (2003) stated that "nursing theory guided practice can be shown to enhance health and quality of life when it is implemented with strong, well-qualified guidance" (p. 226). Mark, Hughes, and Jones (2004) echoed their beliefs and posited that theory-guided research results not only in greater patient safety but also in more predictable outcomes. These beliefs among nursing scientists provide clear direction that theory-guided research is necessary for evaluating nursing interventions in practice.

Over the last five decades of theory development, review of the health care literature demonstrates that changes in health care, society, and the environment as well as changes in population demographics (e.g., aging, urbanization, and growth of minority populations) led to a need to renew or update existing theories and to develop different theories. Furthermore, contemporary theories, such as complexity science, need to be adapted and adopted within theories to make them more applicable, especially within certain aspects of the discipline (Engebretson & Hickey, 2015). In fact, some theoretical writers would exclude the grand theory–middle range theory–microtheory relationship in favor of value-based and socially attuned constructions of nursing knowledge that fit contemporary understanding of human interactions (Risjord, 2009).

Chapters 7 through 9 provide additional information about some of the more commonly known and widely recognized nursing frameworks and theories. To better assist the reader in understanding the conceptual frameworks and grand nursing theories, this chapter presents methods for categorizing or classifying them and describes the criteria that will be used to examine them in the subsequent chapters.

Categorization of Conceptual Frameworks and Grand Theories

The sheer number and scope of the conceptual frameworks and grand theories are daunting. Students and novice nursing scholars are understandably intimidated when asked to study them, as illustrated in the opening case study. To help understand the formulations, a number of methods categorizing them have been described in the nursing literature. Several are presented in the following sections.

Categorization Based on Scope

One of the most logical ways to categorize grand nursing theories is by scope. For example, Alligood (2014) organized theories according to the scope of the theory. The categories in her work were philosophies, nursing conceptual models, nursing theories, theories, and middle range nursing theories. Pokorny (2014) considered the writings of nursing theorists Peplau; Henderson; Abdellah; Wiedenbach; Hall; Travelbee; Barnard; Adam; Roper, Logan, and Tierney; and Ida Jean (Orlando) Pelletier (hereafter referred to as Orlando) as of historical significance. Alligood considered the works of Nightingale, Watson, Ray, Martinson, Benner, and Katie Eriksson to be philosophies, explaining that those theorists had developed philosophies that were derived through "analysis, reasoning and logical argument" (p. 59). These philosophies may form a basis for professional scholarship and help guide understanding of nursing phenomena.

Alligood (2014) categorized the works of Levine, Rogers, Orem, King, Neuman, Roy, and Johnson as nursing conceptual models. Nursing conceptual models, she explained, "specify a perspective and produce evidence among phenomena specific to the discipline [of nursing]" (p. 203).

Boykin and Schoenhofer; Meleis; Pender; Leininger; Newman; Parse; Helen Erickson, Tomlin, and Swain; and Husted and Husted are classified by Alligood (2014) as nursing theories. She observed that these works are nearly as abstract as conceptual models but apply to nursing practice and form "ways to describe, explain, or predict relationships among the concepts of nursing phenomena" (p. 357). Furthermore, Alligood noted that some of these theories evolved from the more global philosophical frameworks or grand theories.

Categorization Based on Nursing Domains

Meleis (2012) did not categorize according to levels of theory (e.g., grand theory, middle range theory, and practice theory). Rather, she categorized theories based on schools of thought or nursing domains: needs theorists; interaction theorists; outcomes theorists, as they developed in various eras; and, finally, caring/becoming theorists in the current era (Table 6-1).

She further defined each school of thought according to the major influences of that genre. The needs theorists, according to Meleis (2012), are Abdellah, Henderson, and Orem. The interaction theorists are King, Orlando, Paterson and Zderad, Peplau, Travelbee, and Wiedenbach, and the outcome theorists are Johnson, Levine, Rogers, and Roy (Meleis, 2012). She lists the caring/becoming theorists as Watson and Parse. Each school of thought, it was noted, has certain concepts and defining properties.

Meleis (2012) considers areas of agreement among the schools of thought: attention to the client/patient, who requires a nurse to assist in meeting the changes or transitions and wellness experiences of life, and the ideal that nurses have means to assist human beings. Furthermore, the schools of thought share the ideal that nurses' focus is on human beings and on discovering ways to meet health and illness situations.

Categorization Based on Paradigms

A *paradigm* is a worldview or an overall way of looking at a discipline and its science. It is seen as a universal view of life rather than just a model or principle of a theory. Kuhn (1996), a theoretical physicist turned science historian, awakened the scientific community to revolutions in understanding what he called paradigm shifts. Paradigm shifts occur when empirical reality no longer fits the existing theories of science. As an example, he cited Einstein's theory of general relativity, which came about when the extant theories no longer fit the evidence that was being generated regarding matter and energy.

Table 6-1 Meleis's Method of Categorizing Theories

| | Theorist's School | | | |
	Needs	Interaction	Outcome	Caring/Becoming
Focus	Problems, nurse's function	Interaction, illness as experience	Energy, balance, stability, homeostasis, outcomes of care	Human–universe health process, meaning, mutual relations, unitary being
Human being	Set of needs, problems, developmental being	Interacting, set of needs, validated needs, human experience/ meaning	Adaptive, developmental being	Man-living-health, continuously becoming, continuous person/environment relationship
Patient	Needs deficit	Helpless being, human experience/ meaning	Lacks adaptation, systems deficiency	Unique human being, transformation, transcendence, disharmony between spirit–body–mind– soul, sense of incongruence
Orientation	Illness/disease	Illness/disease	Illness/disease	Health, human-becoming: both client and nurse
Nurse's role	Depends on medical practice, begin independent function, fulfills needs requisites	Helping process, self: therapeutic agent, nursing process	External regulatory mechanism	Connect, be present, extract meaning
Decision maker	Health care provider	Health care provider	Health care provider	Mutual between health care provider and client

Source: Meleis (2012).

Recent scientific revolutions in health disciplines have changed the way scientists view human beings and their health. For example, immunotherapy and gene therapy are currently being studied extensively. The human genome has been mapped, and this knowledge has impacted areas of life as varied as ethics, law, pharmacology, and medicine. The impact of these new ideas and research on health care delivery is, in effect, a paradigm shift.

Nursing scientists are finding that the theories that have guided practice in the past are no longer sufficient to explain, predict, or guide current practice. Furthermore, older theories may not be helpful in developing nursing science because scholars working in nursing's new paradigm are finding evidence that distinguishes nursing science from the sciences that nurses have traditionally consulted to explain the discipline, that is, anthropology, biology, chemistry, physics, psychology, sociology, and medicine (Cody, 2000; Newman, 2008). The following sections outline how three modern nursing scholars (Parse, Newman, and Fawcett) have categorized nursing theories based on paradigms or worldviews (Figure 6-2).

Three Categories of Theory (Wills, 2002)

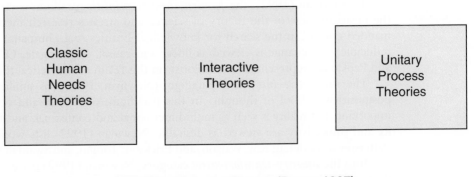

Two Paradigms of Theory (Parse, 1987)

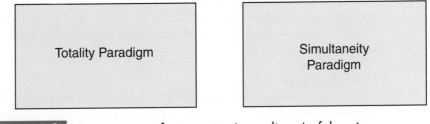

Figure 6-2   Comparison of categories (paradigms) of theories.

Parse's Categorization

Parse (1995) categorized the various nursing theories into two basic paradigms. These she termed the *totality paradigm* and the *simultaneity paradigm*, and she later added the *humanbecoming paradigm* (humanbecoming is all one word) (Parse, 2013). The totality paradigm includes all theoretical perspectives in which humans are biopsychosocial-spiritual beings, adapting to their environment, in whatever way the theory defines environment. The simultaneity paradigm, on the other hand, includes the theoretical perspectives in which humans are identified as unitary beings, which are energy systems in simultaneous, continuous, mutual process with, and embedded in, the universal energy system. Using this classification scheme, the works of Orem, Roy, Johnson, and others would fit within the totality paradigm, and the works of theorists such as Fawcett, Rogers, and Newman are within the simultaneity paradigm. Recently, Parse noted that Rogers's and Newman's theories differed from her current thinking sufficiently that she named a third paradigm. She calls the new paradigm the *humanbecoming* paradigm (Parse, 2013). This new paradigm will be discussed in Chapter 9.

Newman's Categorization

Similarly, Newman (1992) classified nursing theories according to existing philosophical schools but found that nursing paradigms did not neatly fit; therefore, she created three categorizations of theories loosely based on the extant philosophies (i.e., positivism, postpositivism, and humanism). She named the nursing paradigms (1) the particulate–deterministic school, (2) the interactive–integrative school, and (3) the unitary–transformative school. In this classification scheme, the first word in the pair indicates the view of the substance of the theory, and the second word indicates the way in which change occurs.

To Newman (1992), the *particulate–deterministic* paradigm is characterized by the positivist view of the theory of science and stresses research methods that demanded control in the search for knowledge. Entities (e.g., humans) are viewed as reducible, and change is viewed as linear and causal. Nightingale, Orem, Orlando, and Peplau are representative of theorists in this realm of theoretical thinking.

The *interactive–integrative* paradigm (Newman, 1992) has similarities with the postpositivist school of thought. In this paradigm, objectivity and control are still important, but reality is seen as multidimensional and contextual, and both objectivity and subjectivity are viewed as desirable. Newman (1992) lists works of theorists Patterson and Zderad; Roy, Watson, and Erickson; Tomlin; and Swain in this paradigm.

Into the *unitary–transformative* category, Newman (1992) places her works and those of Rogers and Parse. Each of these theorists views humans as unitary beings, which are self-evolving and self-regulating. Humans are embedded in, and constantly and simultaneously interacting with, a universal, self-evolving energy system. These theorists agree that human beings cannot be known by the sum of their parts; rather, they are known by their patterns of energy and ways of being apart and distinct from others.

Fawcett's Categorization

Fawcett and DeSanto-Madeya (2013) simplified Newman's (1992) categorization of theories when they created three categories of worldview based on the treatment of change in each theory. The categories Fawcett and DeSanto-Madeya delineated were (1) reaction, (2) reciprocal interaction, and (3) simultaneous action (Fawcett & DeSanto-Madeya, 2013). Like Newman, they showed that each category coincided with a philosophical tradition.

In describing the *reaction* worldview, Fawcett and DeSanto-Madeya (2013) indicated that these theories classify humans as biopsychosocial-spiritual beings who react to the environment in a causal way. The interaction changes predictably and controllably as humans survive and adapt. They argued that in these theories, phenomena must be objective and observable and may be isolated and measured.

In the *reciprocal interaction* worldview, humans are viewed as holistic, active, and interactive with their environments, with the environments returning interactions (Fawcett, 1993; Fawcett & DeSanto-Madeya, 2013). Fawcett (1993) noted that these theorists viewed reality as multidimensional, dependent on context (i.e., the surrounding conditions), and relative. This means that change is probabilistic (based on chance) and a result of multiple antecedent factors. The reciprocal interaction theories support the study of both objective and subjective phenomena, and both qualitative and quantitative research methods are encouraged, although controlled research methods and inferential statistical techniques are most frequently used to analyze empirical data (Fawcett & DeSanto-Madeya, 2013).

In the third category of grand theories, the *simultaneous action* worldview, Fawcett and DeSanto-Madeya (2013) report that human beings are viewed as unitary, are identified by patterns in mutual rhythmical interchange with their environments, are changing continuously, and are evolving as self-organized fields. She states that in the simultaneous action paradigm, change is in a single direction (unidirectional) and is unpredictable in that beings progress through organization to disorganization on the way to more complex organization. In this paradigm, knowledge and pattern recognition are the phenomena of interest.

Table 6-2 Fawcett's Categorization of Nursing Theories

Paradigm	Characteristics
Reaction	Humans are biopsychosocial-spiritual beings. Humans react to their environment in a causal way. Change is predictable as humans survive and adapt.
Reciprocal interaction	Humans are holistic beings. Humans interact reciprocally with their environment. Reality is multidimensional, contextual, and relative.
Simultaneous action	Humans are unitary beings. Humans and their environment are constantly interacting, changing, and evolving. Change is unidirectional and unpredictable.

This categorization explained the major differences among the many current and past nursing theories and conceptual models (Fawcett, 2005; Fawcett & DeSanto-Madeya, 2013). Table 6-2 summarizes the grand theory categorization scheme. Table 6-3 compares the classification methods of Fawcett and DeSanto-Madeya (2013), Meleis (2012), Newman (1995), and Parse (1995).

Specific Categories of Models and Theories for This Unit

For this book, the conceptual models and grand nursing theories were categorized based on distinctions that are similar to those described by Fawcett and DeSanto-Madeya (2013) and Newman (1992). Chapters 7 through 9 thus present analyses of models and theories according to the following classifications: (1) the human needs

Table 6-3 Classification of Grand Theories by Current Theory Analysts

Theory Analyst	Source	Basis for Typology	Categories
Fawcett	Philosophy	Worldviews	Reaction Reciprocal interaction Simultaneous action
Meleis	Patient care philosophy	Metaparadigm concepts Schools of thought	Nursing clients Human being–environment interactions Interactions Needs, interaction, outcomes, caring
Newman	Paradigm	Philosophical schools	Particulate–deterministic Interactive–integrative Unitary–transformative
Parse	Paradigm	Difference between worldviews	Totality Simultaneity–humanbecoming

Sources: Fawcett (2000, 2005); Fawcett and DeSanto-Madeya (2013); Meleis (2012); Newman (1995); Parse (1995, 2013).

Table 6-4 Categorization of Grand Nursing Theories for Chapters 7–9		
Human Needs	**Models and Theories Interactive Process**	**Unitary Process**
Abdellah	Artinian	Newman
Henderson	Eric on, Tomlin, and Swain	Parse
Johnson	King	Rogers
Nightingale	Levine	
Neuman	Roy	
Orem	Watson	

theories (which relate to Fawcett's reaction category), (2) the interactive theories, and (3) the unitary process theories.

The theories discussed in Chapter 7 are based on a classical needs perspective and are among the earliest theories and models derived for nursing science. They include the works of Nightingale, Henderson, Johnson, and others. In Chapter 8, each of the perspectives has human interactions as the basis of their content, regardless of the era in which they were developed. The works of Roy, Watson, King, and others are also included in Chapter 8. Finally, the unitary process theories are described in Chapter 9. The theorists explained there are Rogers, Newman, and Parse. Table 6-4 summarizes the theories that are presented in Chapters 7 through 9.

Analysis Criteria for Grand Nursing Theories

Describing how models and theories can be employed in nursing practice, research, administration/management, and education necessitates a review of selected elements through theory analysis. Seven criteria were selected for description and analysis of grand theories in this unit. As described in Chapter 5, these seven chosen criteria were among the earliest enumerated by Ellis (1968) and Hardy (1978) and promoted by Walker and Avant (2011) and Fawcett and DeSanto-Madeya (2013).

Complete analysis of each theory was not performed; instead, the presentation of the models and theories in Chapters 7 through 9 is largely descriptive rather than analytical or evaluative. Each theory's ease of interpretation and application is also briefly critiqued. The criteria used for reviewing the grand theories in these three chapters are listed in Box 6-2. Each criterion is also discussed briefly in the following sections.

Background of the Theorist

A review of the background of the theorist is likely to reveal the foundations of the theorist's ideas. The individual's educational experiences, in particular, may be relevant to the development of the theory. At one time, higher education, particularly university education, was open only to the children of financially secure families and often limited to nonminorities. Only in the years after the 1960s were scholarships for students with financial hardships and students of ethnic minorities readily available.

Box 6-2	Review Criteria for Descriptive Analysis of Grand Nursing Theories

Background of the theorist
Philosophical underpinnings of the theory
Major assumptions, concepts, and relationships
Usefulness
Testability
Parsimony
Value in extending nursing science

In addition, nursing graduate programs were not widely available in most parts of the United States before the creation of federal programs in the late 1960s. Because of the limited availability of graduate nursing programs, the majority of the early nursing scholars who developed conceptual models and grand theories received graduate education in disciplines other than nursing. As a result, the earliest nursing models and theories reflected the paradigms that were accepted in the scholar's educative discipline at the time in which they studied or wrote.

The nurse scholar's experience and specialty also influenced the theoretical perspective. For example, Orlando and Peplau were psychiatric nurses who were educated in the first half of the 20th century. Their graduate education in psychology was tempered by the focus of psychology at that time—that of the logical–positivist era, which emphasized reductionistic principles and was mathematically based. Later scholars (e.g., Fawcett, Parse, Fitzpatrick, and Newman) received their doctoral credentials within the discipline of nursing. The writings of these scholars reflect the scientific thought processes, knowledge base, and current thinking of the discipline at the time of their writing as well as their personal perspectives and experiences.

The placement of the author of the model or theory in historical and conceptual perspective promotes understanding of the extant views of science during the time in which the theorist wrote. Only in the most exceptional of cases are scholars not likely to be influenced by the times in which they formulated their work. One exception to this was Rogers. Interestingly, the discipline of nursing was deep in the positivist era in the 1960s when she began her work; the hard sciences (i.e., physics and chemistry), however, had entered the postpositivist era, which posited the idea that change is inherent in a growing discipline. Rogers's (1970) theory did not fit easily into the concurrent paradigm of nursing science of that time and was rejected by many in favor of more intermediate thinking that corresponded to that of the postpositivist thinkers.

Philosophical Underpinnings of the Theory

The background of the scholar most likely contributed heavily to the philosophical basis and paradigmatic origins of the model or theory. Historically, nursing theories of the 1950s and 1960s corresponded to the reaction (Fawcett & DeSanto-Madeya, 2013) worldview. In the late 1960s through the early 1980s, the reciprocal interaction worldviews began to take precedence, and by the 1990s, the unitary process perspectives began to achieve importance, although the earlier paradigms were still influential (Fawcett & DeSanto-Madeya, 2013). It is important to note that most of the scholars who adhered to the interaction worldviews were working and writing in the 1950s, before their ideas achieved general recognition in the profession. The simultaneous action scholars, beginning with Rogers and followed by Parse and Newman, developed their ideas in the 1970s and 1980s and continuously grew their theories as each was influenced by modern thinking and technology.

The fundamental philosophies and the disciplines in which the scholars were educated are reflected in their works. Those educated in the social sciences, for example, incorporated some of the characteristics, concepts, and assumptions of those disciplines in their works. Personal philosophies are also reflected in written views on humans, science, environment, and health. Whether written from the positivist philosophy of science or the postpositivist or modern worldviews, the philosophical viewpoints that form the basis of the works are indicated by the chosen concepts. A component of theory analysis is to point out the underlying philosophy and review the consistency with which the writer demonstrates attention to that background.

Major Assumptions, Concepts, and Relationships

Examination of the major assumptions, concepts, and relationships of the model or theory is vital because they are the substance of the formulation. These components will direct practice, assist with selection of concepts to be studied, and generate collateral theories for the discipline of nursing (Walker & Avant, 2011). Whether the assumptions are spelled out or merely inferred indicates the strength of the theory in elucidating its content. The concepts, carefully defined and explained, along with their derivation, assist the analyst in determining the essence of the model or theory. The relationships between and among the concepts, their strength, and whether they are positive, negative, or neutral indicate the structure of the theory (Walker & Avant, 2011).

Usefulness

Conceptual models and grand theories are reputed not to be particularly useful in directing nursing practice because of their scope and level of abstraction and because they were created through the analytical, logical, and philosophical understandings of a single theorist (Alligood, 2014). The reality is that although many of the conceptual models and grand theories cannot be tested in a single research project, they have been useful in guiding nursing scholarship and practice and in providing the structure from which testable theories may be derived. Grand nursing theories, more often than conceptual models, are likely to provide the basis for concrete theories, with specifically defined concepts and highly derived relationships that may be more easily applied in clinical practice, nursing education, research, or nursing administration (Fawcett & DeSanto-Madeya, 2013).

Testability

To be useful, theories should be disprovable (Shuttleworth, 2008); that is, they can be questioned and tested in the real world through research. Because the major purpose of nursing theory is to guide research, practice, education, and administration, the theory must be subjected to examination. Theories that are capable of being tested make the most reliable guides for scholarly work (Walker & Avant, 2011). Many grand theories are not testable in totality, but they may generate theories that are testable from their conceptual matter, assumptions, or structure. The grand theories that are likely to generate middle range theories and practice theories, as well as theoretical models for research, are those most likely to fulfill the requirement of testability and have the ability to continue to generate new and useful models (Kim, 2006).

Parsimony

Parsimony is a criterion that is important because the more complex the theory, the less easily it is comprehended. Parsimony does not indicate that a theory is simplistic; in fact, often, the more parsimonious the theory, the more depth the theory may have. For example, the standard of parsimony in a theory is Einstein's theory of relativity (Cody, 2012), which can be reduced to the formula $E = mc^2$. Although the theory has only three concepts (E = energy, m = mass, and c^2 = the speed of light squared) (Einstein, 1961), the explanation of this theory is extremely complicated indeed.

Considering the complexity of nurses' primary subjects of interest, human beings in health and illness, it is unlikely that any of the grand nursing theories could ever approximate the mathematical elegance of Einstein's theory of relativity. Parsimonious theoretical constructions, however, provide nurses in research, administration, practice, and education with broad general categories into which to conceptualize problems and therefore may assist in the derivation of methods of problem solving. Indeed, the more elegant and universal a conceptual model or grand theory, the more global it is in contributing to the science of nursing.

Value in Extending Nursing Science

Ultimately, the value of any nursing theory, not just of grand theory, is its ability to extend the discipline and science of nursing. Understanding the nature of human beings and their interaction with the environment, and the impact of this interaction on their health, will help direct holistic and comprehensive nursing interventions that improve health and well-being. Improvement in nursing care is ultimately the reason for formulating theory. Furthermore, the value of the theory in adding to and elaborating nursing science is an important function of grand theory (Fawcett & DeSanto-Madeya, 2013). Questions to be answered when analyzing any theory include: Does the theory generate new knowledge? Can the theory suggest or support new avenues of knowledge generation beyond those that already exist? Does the theory suggest a disciplinary future that is growing and changing? Can the theory assist nurses to respond to the rapid change and growth of health care? (Walker & Avant, 2011).

The Purpose of Critiquing Theories

Critiquing theory is a necessary part of the process when a scholar is selecting a theory for some disciplinary work. Determining whether a grand theory holds promise or value for the effort at hand and whether middle range theories, which are useful in research, practice, education, or administration, can be generated from it is a product of critique.

When a nursing student confronts the overarching ideals of the profession for the first time, it is not at all unlikely that the feeling is complete and overwhelming confusion and even disorientation. As in the case of Janet and her quest for advanced education, frustration was a new feeling to her. Her work in the critical care unit was focused and based on evidence and followed an ordered medical model, whereas the newness of this conceptually based study of theories left her disgruntled. The understanding displayed by her instructor, who had felt similar feelings during her education and who ascribed to the pattern that nurses learn together, was calming and set the stage for Janet to begin to learn the basics of the science of nursing, the theoretical underpinnings of the profession. See Link to Practice 6-1.

Link to Practice 6-1

Janet, the nurse from the opening case study, decided to incorporate a nursing theory into her practice. She consulted with her classmates as to whether they had used theories in this way. One colleague stated that in her baccalaureate program, students were required to use a theory to guide their clinical practicum, and another had been employed in a hospital that based nursing care around the work of a grand nursing theorist. Building on their suggestions and what she learned in her course, Janet used key tenets and ideas from the "human needs" and "interactive process" models in her daily practice, trying out concepts and interventions from some of the theorists as she worked. She found that no matter which major theorist she used, she was able to organize her work more effectively.

It is likely that a nursing student may find it difficult to critique the work of nursing's grand theorists considering the advanced educational attainment of the theorists. Yet, determining the usefulness of the theory to a project is important. The user of the theory must comprehend the paradigm of the theory, believe in the concepts and assumptions from which it is built, and be able to internalize the basic philosophy of the theorist. It is hardly beneficial to attempt to use a theory that one cannot accept or understand or one that seems inappropriate in the current time or place. The choice of a theoretical framework or model must fit with the student's or scholar's personal ideals, and this requires the student or scholar to critique the theory for its value in extending the selected professional work.

One problem that arises among both novice and experienced scholars is combining theories from competing paradigms. Often, the work generated from these efforts is confusing and obfuscating; it does not generate clear results that extend the thinking within either paradigm (Todaro-Franceschi, 2010). Therefore, the conscientious student or scholar selects theories that relate to the same paradigm in science, philosophy, and nursing when combining theories to guide research or practice. Wide reading in the discipline of nursing and the scientific literature of the disciplines from which the theorist has generated ideas will assist in preventing such errors. Theory review and extraction from the grand theories can result in work that satisfies the scholarly impulse in each of us, guides the research process, provides structure for safe and effective practice, and extends the science of nursing.

Summary

Grand theories are global in their application to the discipline of nursing and have been instrumental in helping to develop nursing science. Because of their diversity, their complexity, and their differing worldviews, learning about grand nursing theories can be confusing as illustrated by the experiences of Janet, the student nurse from the opening case study. To help make the study of grand theories more logical and rewarding, this chapter presented several methods for categorizing the grand theories on the basis of scope, basic philosophies, and needs of the discipline. It has also presented the criteria that will be used to describe grand nursing theories in subsequent chapters.

Chapters 7 through 9 discuss many of the grand nursing theories that have been placed into the three defined paradigms of nursing. These analyses are meant to be descriptive to allow the student to choose from different paradigms and the theories contained within them to further their work. The student or scholar must recognize that health care is constantly changing and that some theories may no longer seem applicable, whereas other theories are timeless in their abstraction. Before selecting a theory to guide practice, research, or other endeavors, it is the student's responsibility to obtain and read the theory in its latest iteration by the theorist, read analyses by other scholars in the discipline, and become thoroughly familiar with the theory.

Key Points

- Nursing scholars and nursing leaders have developed philosophies, conceptual frameworks, and grand theories to make the very complex study of nursing clear for both students and practitioners.
- The purpose of theory is to systematize nursing education and practice so that no important element of nursing care is forgotten.
- Reviewing and critiquing nursing theories is important, as nurse scholars, nurse educators, and nurse researchers use theories for the purposes of directing and coordinating practice, education, and research.
- Using nursing theories to guide their work allows practitioners, educators, and researchers to base their work on a system that allows critique of the outcomes of their work.
- Working within a paradigm, rather than combining disparate paradigms, prevents confusion because nursing paradigms relate to paradigms in other sciences.

Learning Activities

1. During an online classroom, debate similarities and differences in the several theoretical categorization schemes put forth by the different theory analysts discussed in this chapter. Which system appears to be the easiest to understand?
2. Does categorizing or classifying grand theories as the writers have done assist in studying and understanding them? Why or why not?
3. With classmates, critique theory-based research articles and decide whether they will yield believable evidence. Do the authors ascribe to the same or similar theoretical worldviews (paradigms)? Do you think that having differing paradigms will make a difference in your group's ability to identify the evidence needed for safe nursing practice?
4. Janet, from the opening case study, practices on a cardiovascular floor and was working toward a degree to become an acute care nurse practitioner. Consider your practice specialty area (i.e. critical care, operating room, pediatrics, labor and delivery, primary care). Which paradigm—human needs, interactive process, or unitary process—best fits that type of nursing and client needs? Explain your answer and compare your thoughts with those of classmates.

REFERENCES

Alligood, M. R. (2014). *Nursing theorists and their work* (8th ed.). St. Louis, MO: Mosby.

American Association of Colleges of Nursing. (2011). *The essentials of master's education in nursing*. Washington, DC: Author.

Bachmann, A. O., Danuser, B., & Morin, D. (2015). Developing a theoretical framework using a nursing perspective to investigate perceived health in the "sandwich generation" group. *Nursing Science Quarterly, 28*(4), 308–318.

Butts, J. B. (2015). Components and levels of abstraction in nursing knowledge. In J. B. Butts & K. L. Rich (Eds.), *Philosophies and theories for advanced nursing practice* (2nd ed., pp. 87–108). Sudbury, MA: Jones & Bartlett Learning.

Cody, W. K. (2000). Paradigm shift or paradigm drift? A meditation on commitment and transcendence. *Nursing Science Quarterly, 13*(2), 93–102.

Cody, W. K. (2003). Nursing theory as a guide to practice. *Nursing Science Quarterly, 16*(3), 225–231.

Cody, W. K. (2012). A brave and startling truth: Parse's humanbecoming school of thought in the context of the contemporary nursing discipline. *Nursing Science Quarterly, 25*(1), 7–10.

Einstein, A. (1961). *Relativity: The special and the general theory.* New York, NY: Crown.

Ellis, R. (1968). Symposium on theory development in nursing. Characteristics of significant theories. *Nursing Research, 17*(3), 217–222.

Engebretson, J. C., & Hickey, J. V. (2015). Complexity science and complex adaptive systems. In J. B. Butts & K. L. Rich (Eds.), *Philosophies and theories for advanced nursing practice* (2nd ed., pp. 113–138). Sudbury, MA: Jones & Bartlett Learning.

Eun-Ok, I., & Chang, S. J. (2012). Current trends in nursing theories. *Journal of Nursing Scholarship, 44*(2), 156–164.

Fawcett, J. (1993). *Analysis and evaluation of nursing theories.* Philadelphia, PA: F.A. Davis.

Fawcett, J. (2000). *Analysis and evaluation of contemporary nursing knowledge: Nursing models and theories.* Philadelphia, PA: F.A. Davis.

Fawcett, J. (2005). *Contemporary nursing knowledge: Analysis and evaluation of nursing models and theories* (2nd ed.). Philadelphia, PA: F.A. Davis.

Fawcett, J., & DeSanto-Madeya, S. (2013). *Contemporary nursing knowledge: Analysis and evaluation of nursing models and theories* (3rd ed.). Philadelphia, PA: F.A. Davis.

Hardy, M. E. (1978). Perspectives on nursing theory. *ANS. Advances in Nursing Science, 1*(1), 27–48.

Higgins, P. A., & Moore, S. M. (2000). Levels of theoretical thinking in nursing. *Nursing Outlook, 48*(4), 179–183.

Kim, H. S. (2006). The concept of holism. In H. S. Kim & I. Kollak (Eds.), *Nursing theories: Conceptual & philosophical foundations* (pp. 89–108). New York, NY: Springer Publishing.

Kuhn, T. S. (1996). *The structure of scientific revolutions* (3rd ed.). Chicago, IL: University of Chicago Press.

Mark, B., Hughes, I., & Jones, C. (2004). The role of theory in improving patient safety and quality health care. *Nursing Outlook, 52*(1), 11–16.

Meleis, A. I. (2012). *Theoretical nursing: Development and progress* (5th ed.). Philadelphia, PA: Lippincott Williams & Wilkins.

Newman, M. A. (1992). Prevailing paradigms in nursing. *Nursing Outlook, 40*(1), 10–13, 32.

Newman, M. A. (1995). *A developing discipline: Selected works of Margaret Newman.* New York, NY: National League for Nursing Press.

Newman, M. A. (2008). *Transforming presence: The difference that nursing makes.* Philadelphia, PA: F.A. Davis.

Parse, R. R. (Ed.). (1995). *Illuminations: The human becoming theory in practice and research.* New York, NY: National League for Nursing Press.

Parse, R. R. (2013). Living quality: A humanbecoming phenomenon. *Nursing Science Quarterly, 26*(2), 111–115.

Pokorny, M. E. (2014). Nursing theorists of historical significance. In M. R. Alligood (Ed.), *Nursing theorists and their work* (8th ed., pp. 42–58). St. Louis, MO: Mosby.

Risjord, M. (2009). *Nursing knowledge: Science, practice, and philosophy.* Ames, IA: Wiley-Blackwell.

Rogers, M. E. (1970). *An introduction to the theoretical basis of nursing.* Philadelphia, PA: F.A. Davis.

Shuttleworth, M. (2008). *Falsifiability.* Retrieved from http://www.explorable.com/falsifiability

Todaro-Franceschi, V. (2010). Two paradigms, different fruit: Mixing apples with oranges. *Visions, 17*(1), 44–51.

Walker, L. O., & Avant, K. (2011). *Strategies for theory construction in nursing* (5th ed.). Upper Saddle River, NJ: Pearson.

7

Grand Nursing Theories Based on Human Needs

Evelyn M. Wills

Donald Crawford is an acute care nurse practitioner who works in an intensive care unit (ICU) who is midway through a doctor of nursing practice (DNP) program. Donald strongly believes that evidence guiding nursing practice should be experiential and measurable, and during his master's program, he devised a way to diagram the disease pathophysiology for many of his patients based on the Neuman Systems Model (Neuman & Fawcett, 2011).

He observed that the model helped predict what would happen next with some patients and helped him define patient's needs, predict outcomes, and prescribe nursing interventions more accurately. In particular, he appreciated how Neuman focused on identification and reduction of stressors through nursing interventions and liked the construct of prevention as intervention. As he continues his graduate studies, Donald plans to expand application of the concepts and principles from Neuman's model. As one component of his DNP project, he is developing a proposal to implement his methods throughout the ICU to help other nurses apply Neuman's model in improving patient care.

The earliest theorists in nursing drew from the dominant worldviews of their time, which were largely related to the medical discoveries from the scientific era of the 1850s through 1940s (Artinian, 1991). During those years, nurses in the United States were seen as handmaidens to doctors, and their practice was guided by disease theories of medical science. Even today, much of nursing science remains based in the positivist era with its focus on disease causality and a desire to produce measurable outcome data. Evidence-based medicine is the current means of enacting the positivist focus on research outcomes for effective clinical therapeutics (Cody, 2013).

In an effort to define the uniqueness of nursing and to distinguish it from medicine, nursing scholars from the 1950s through the 1970s developed a number of nursing theories. In addition to medicine, the majority of these early works were strongly influenced by the needs theories of social scientists (e.g., Maslow). In needs-based theories, clients are typically considered biopsychosocial beings who are the sum of their parts, who are experiencing disease or trauma, and who need nursing care. Furthermore, clients are thought of as mechanistic beings, and if the correct information can be gathered, the cause or source of their problems can be discerned and measured. At that point, interventions can be prescribed that will be effective in meeting their needs (Dickoff, James, & Wiedenbach, 1968). Evidence-based nursing fits with these theories completely and comfortably (Cody, 2013).

The grand theories and models of nursing described in this chapter focus on meeting clients' needs for nursing care. These theories and models, like all personal statements of scholars, have continued to grow and develop over the years; therefore, several sources were consulted for each model. The latest writings of and about the theories were consulted and are presented. As much as possible, the description of the model is either quoted or paraphrased from the original texts. Some needs theorists may have maintained their theories over the years with little change; others updated and adapted theirs to later ideas and methods. Nevertheless, new research has often extended the original work. Students are advised to consult the literature for the newest research using the needs theory of interest.

It should be noted that a concerted attempt was made to ensure that the presentation of the works of all theorists is balanced. Some theories (e.g., Orem and Neuman) are more complex than others, and the body of information is greater for some than for others. As a result, the sections dealing with some theorists are a little longer than others. This does not imply that shorter works are in any way inferior or less important to the discipline.

Finally, all theory analysts, whether novice or expert, will comprehend theories and models from their own perspectives. If the reader is interested in using a model, the most recent edition of the work of the theorist should be obtained and used as the primary source for any project. All further works using the theory or model should come from researchers using the theory in their work. Current research writings are one of the best ways to understand the development of the needs theories.

Florence Nightingale: Nursing: What It Is and What It Is Not

Nightingale's model of nursing was developed before the general acceptance of modern disease theories (i.e., the germ theory) and other theories of medical science. Nightingale knew the germ theory (Beck, 2010), and prior to its wide publication, she had deduced that cleanliness, fresh air, sanitation, comfort, and socialization were necessary to healing. She used her experiences in the Scutari Army Hospital in Turkey and in other hospitals in which she worked to document her ideas on nursing (Beck, 2010; Dossey, 2010a; Small, 1998).

Nightingale was from a wealthy family; yet, she chose to work in the field of nursing, although it was considered a "lowly" occupation. She believed nursing was her call from God, and she determined that the sick deserved civilized care, regardless of their station in life (Nightingale, 1860/1957/1969).

Through her extensive body of work, she changed nursing and health care dramatically. Nightingale's record of letters is voluminous, and several books have been written analyzing them (Attewell, 2012; Dossey, Selanders, Beck, & Attewell, 2005). She wrote many books and reports to federal and worldwide agencies. Books she wrote that are especially important to nurses and nursing include *Notes on*

Nursing: What It Is and What It Is Not (original publication in 1860; reprinted in 1957 and 1969), *Notes on Hospitals* (published in 1863), and *Sick-Nursing and Health-Nursing*, originally published in Hampton's *Nursing of the Sick* (1893) and reprinted in toto in Dossey et al. (2005), to name but a small portion of her great body of works. Much of her work is now available, where once it was kept out of circulation, perhaps because of the sheer volume and perhaps because she originally asked that her papers all be destroyed at her death. She later recanted that request (Bostridge, 2008; Cromwell, 2013).

Background of the Theorist

Nightingale was born on May 12, 1820, in Florence, Italy; her birthday is still honored in many places. She was privately educated in the classical tradition of her time by her father, and from an early age, she was inclined to care for the sick and injured (Bostridge, 2008; Dossey, 2010b). Although her mother wished her to lead a life of social grace, Nightingale preferred productivity, choosing to school herself in the care of the sick. She attended nursing programs in Kaiserswerth, Germany, in 1850 and 1851 (Bostridge, 2008; Dossey, 2010a; Small, 1998), where she completed what was at that time the only formal nursing education available. She worked as the nursing superintendent at the Institution for Care of Sick Gentlewomen in Distressed Circumstances, where she instituted many changes to improve patient care (Cromwell, 2013; Small, 1998).

During the Crimean War, she was urged by Sidney Herbert, Secretary of War for Great Britain, to assist in providing care for wounded soldiers. The dire conditions of British servicemen had resulted in a public outcry that prompted the government to institute changes in the system of medical care (Small, 1998). At Herbert's request, Nightingale and a group of 38 skilled nurses were transported to Turkey to provide nursing care to the soldiers in the hospital at Scutari Army Barracks. There, despite daunting opposition by army physicians, Nightingale instituted a system of care that reportedly cut casualties from 48% to 2% within approximately 2 years (Bostridge, 2008; Dossey, 2010b; Zurakowski, 2005).

Early in her work at the army hospital, Nightingale noted that the majority of soldiers' deaths was caused by transport to the hospital and conditions in the hospital itself. Nightingale found that open sewers and lack of cleanliness, pure water, fresh air, and wholesome food were more often the causes of soldiers' deaths than their wounds; she implemented changes to address these problems (Small, 1998). Although her recommendations were known to be those that would benefit the soldiers, physicians in charge of the hospitals in the Crimea blocked her efforts. Despite this, by her third trip to the Crimea, Nightingale had been appointed the supervisor of all the nurses (Bostridge, 2008; Dossey, 2010b).

At Scutari, she became known as the "lady with the lamp" from her nightly excursions through the wards to review the care of the soldiers (Bostridge, 2008). To prove the value of the work she and the nurses were doing, Nightingale instituted a system of record keeping and adapted a statistical reporting method known as the *polar area diagram* or Coxcomb chart to analyze the data she so rigorously collected (Small, 1998). Thus, Nightingale was the first nurse to collect and analyze evidence that her methods were working.

On her return to England from Turkey, Nightingale worked to reform the Army Medical School, instituted a program of record keeping for government health statistics, and assisted with the public health system in India. The effort for which she is most remembered, however, is the Nightingale School for Nurses at

St. Thomas' Hospital. This school was supported by the Nightingale Fund, which had been instituted by grateful British citizens in honor of her work in the Crimea (Bostridge, 2008; Cromwell, 2013).

Philosophical Underpinnings of the Theory

Nightingale's work is considered a broad philosophy. Zurakowski (2005) indicates it is a "perspective" (p. 21). By contrast, Selanders (2005a) states that her work is a foundational philosophy (p. 66). Dossey (2010b) explains that, in Nightingale's philosophy, "Her basic tenet was healing and secondary to it are the tenets of leadership and global action which are necessary to support healing at its deepest level" (p. 1). Nightingale's work has influenced the nursing profession and nursing education for nearly 160 years. To Nightingale, nursing was the domain of women but was an independent practice in its own right. Nurses were, however, to practice in accord with physicians, whose prescriptions nurses were faithfully to carry out (Nightingale, 1893/1954). Nightingale did not believe that nurses were meant to be subservient to physicians. Rather, she believed that nursing was an independent profession or a calling in its own right. Nightingale's educational model is based on anticipating and meeting the needs of patients and is oriented toward the works a nurse should carry out in meeting those needs. Nightingale's philosophy was inductively derived, abstract yet descriptive in nature, and is classified as a grand theory or philosophy by most nursing writers (Alligood, 2014; Masters, 2015; Selanders, 2005a).

Major Assumptions, Concepts, and Relationships

Nightingale was an educated gentlewoman of the Victorian era. The language she used to write her books—*Notes on Nursing: What It Is and What It Is Not* (1860/1957/1969) and *Sick-Nursing and Health-Nursing* (1893/1954)—was cultured, flowing, logical in format, and elegant in style. She wrote numerous letters, many of which are still available. These were topical, direct and yet abstract, and addressed a plethora of topics, such as personal care of patients and sanitation in army hospitals and communities, to name only a few (Bostridge, 2008; Cromwell, 2013; Dossey, 2010b; Selanders, 2005b).

Nightingale (1860/1957/1969) believed that five points were essential in achieving a healthful house: "pure air, pure water, efficient drainage, cleanliness, and light" (p. 24). She thought buildings should be constructed to admit light to every occupant and to allow the flow of fresh air. Furthermore, she wrote that proper household management makes a difference in healing the ill and that nursing care pertained to the house in which the patient lived and to those who came into contact with the patient as well as to the care of the patient.

Although the metaparadigm concepts had not been so labeled until over 130 years later, Nightingale (1893/1954) addressed them—human, environment, health, and nursing—specifically in her writings. She believed that a healthy environment was essential for healing. For example, noise was harmful and impeded the need of the person for rest, and noises to avoid included caregivers talking within the hearing of the individual, the rustle of the wide skirts (common at the time), fidgeting, asking unnecessary questions, and a heavy tread while walking. Nutritious food, proper beds and bedding, and personal cleanliness were variables Nightingale deemed essential, and she was convinced that social contact was important to healing. Although the germ theory had been proposed, Nightingale's writings do not specifically refer to it. Her ideals of care, however, indicate that she recognized and agreed that cleanliness prevents morbidity (Dossey, 2010b).

Nightingale believed that nurses must make accurate observations of their patients and report the state of the patient to the physician in an orderly manner. She explained that nurses should think critically about the care of the patient and do what was appropriate and necessary to assist the patient to heal. Nursing was seen as a way "to put the constitution in such a state as that it will have no disease, or that it can recover from disease" (Nightingale, 1893/1954, p. 3), which will "put us in the best possible conditions for nature to restore or to preserve health—to prevent or to cure disease or injury" (p. 357). She believed that nursing was an art, whereas medicine was a science, and stated that nurses were to be loyal to the medical plan but not servile. Throughout her writings, Nightingale enumerated tasks that nurses should complete to care for ill individuals, and many of the tasks she outlined are still relevant today (Nightingale, 1860/1957/1969).

Health was defined in her treatise, *Sickness-Nursing and Health-Nursing* (Nightingale, 1893/1954), as "to be well but to be able to use well every power we have" (p. 357). It is apparent throughout that volume that health meant more than the mere absence of disease, a view that placed Nightingale ahead of her time.

Usefulness

Nightingale wrote on hospitals, nursing, and community health in the 19th and into the 20th century, and her works served as the basis of nursing education in Britain and in the United States for over a century. King's College Hospital and St. Thomas' Hospital in London, England, were the initial nursing programs developed by Nightingale, and she maintained a special interest in St. Thomas' Hospital during most of her life (Small, 1998). Nursing programs that used the Nightingale method in the United States included Bellevue Hospital in New York, New Haven Hospital in Connecticut, and Massachusetts Hospital in Boston. Indeed, the influence of Nightingale's methods is felt in nursing programs to the present (Pfettscher, 2014).

A resurgence in attention to Nightingale's philosophy is noteworthy. Jacobs (2001) discussed the attribute of human dignity as a central phenomenon uniting nursing theory and practice—two areas that were extensively treated by Nightingale in her own writings. Cromwell (2013) discussed Nightingale's early feminism and her willingness to fight local and federal authorities to procure humane treatment for British soldiers of the time. She showed how Nightingale continued her works for the British army long after returning from the Bosporus. Many other contemporary writers and researchers have displayed an intense interest in Nightingale's work and its applicability to modern nursing. For example, DeGuzman and Kulbok (2012) used Nightingale's theory to create a framework for nurses to study the impact of "built environment" on health, focusing on vulnerable populations. Similarly, Hegge (2013) explained how Nightingale's focus on the environment is important for nurses to consider when developing interventions for population health. Then, Kagan (2014) abstracted elements of *Notes on Nursing* to apply Nightingale's concepts to identification of determinants of health that need interventions to reduce risk of illnesses—specifically cancer. Nursing educators worldwide continue to use Nightingale's ideals in teaching nurses. These include Adu-Gyamfi and Brenya (2016; Ghana); Haddad and Santos (2011; Portugal); Mackey and Bassendowski (2017; Canada); McDonald (2014; Ireland); and Rahim (2013; Pakistan).

Testability

Nightingale's theory can be the source of testable hypotheses because she treated concrete as well as abstract concepts. Research that is conversant with her ideas of care includes research on noise (Murphy, Bernardo, & Dalton, 2013), environment (Jetha, 2015; Zborowsky, 2014), and spirituality (Tanyi & Werner, 2008). Recently, researchers have written about her statistical work (McDonald, 2010; Rew & Sands, 2010), showing that it stands up to modern thinking as it did in the 19th century. Indeed, research around the globe is still progressing using her work.

Parsimony

In her work, Nightingale succinctly stated what she believed was important in caring for ill individuals. Furthermore, in one small volume, she includes information about nursing care, patient needs, proper buildings in which the sick are to be treated, and the administration of hospitals.

Value in Extending Nursing Science

Nightingale was a noted nurse of her time. She was a consultant who promoted the collection and analyses of health statistics. She was deeply involved in nursing education and promoting the science of public health (Bostridge, 2008; Cromwell, 2013; Small, 1998), hospital administration, community health, and global health (Dossey, 2010b). Nightingale's legacy continues to be important to nursing scholars, and her vast contributions continue to enlighten nursing science. Current Nightingale scholars include Attewell (2012), Bostridge (2008), Cromwell (2013), Dossey et al. (2005), Jacobs (2001), and many others who have contributed to the understanding of her multitudinous works. Nightingale's work was revolutionary for its impact on nursing and health care. Furthermore, her many works continue to present effective guidelines for nurses.

Virginia Henderson: The Principles and Practice of Nursing

Virginia Henderson was a well-known nursing educator and a prolific author. In 1937, Henderson and others created a basic nursing curriculum for the National League for Nursing in which education was "patient centered and organized around nursing problems rather than medical diagnoses" (Henderson, 1991, p. 19). In 1939, she revised Harmer's classic textbook of nursing for its fourth edition and later wrote the fifth edition, incorporating her personal definition of nursing (Henderson, 1991). Although she was retired, she was a frequent visitor to nursing schools well into her 90s. O'Malley (1996) states that Henderson was known as the modern-day mother of nursing. Her work influenced the nursing profession in America and throughout the world.

Background of the Theorist

Henderson was born in Missouri but spent her formative years in Virginia. She received a diploma in nursing from the Army School of Nursing at Walter Reed Hospital in 1921 and worked at the Henry Street Visiting Nurse Service for 2 years after graduation. In 1923, she accepted a position teaching nursing at the Norfolk Protestant

Hospital in Virginia, where she remained for several years. In 1929, Henderson determined that she needed more education and entered Teachers College at Columbia University, where she earned her bachelor's degree in nursing in 1932 and a master's degree in 1934. Subsequently, she joined Columbia as a member of the faculty, where she remained until 1948 (Herrmann, 1998). "Ms. Virginia," as she was known to her friends, died in 1996 at the age of 98 (Allen, 1996). Because of her importance to modern nursing, the Sigma Theta Tau International Nursing Library is named in her honor.

Philosophical Underpinnings of the Theory

Henderson was educated during the empiricist era in medicine and nursing, which focused on patient needs, but she believed that her theoretical ideas grew and matured through her experiences (Henderson, 1991). Henderson was introduced to physiologic principles during her graduate education, and the understanding of these principles was the basis for her patient care (Henderson, 1965, 1991). The theory presents the patient as a sum of parts with biopsychosocial needs, and the patient is neither client nor consumer. Henderson stated that "Thorndike's fundamental needs of man" (Henderson, 1991, p. 16) had an influence on her beliefs.

Although her major clinical experiences were in medical-surgical hospitals, she worked as a visiting nurse in New York City. This experience enlarged Henderson's view to recognize the importance of increasing the patient's independence so that progress after hospitalization would not be delayed (Henderson, 1991). Henderson was a nurse educator, and the major thrust of her theory relates to the education of nurses.

Major Assumptions, Concepts, and Relationships

Henderson's concept of nursing was derived from her practice and education; therefore, her work is inductive. Henderson did not manufacture language to elucidate her theoretical stance; she used correct, scholarly English in all of her writings. She called her definition of nursing her "concept" (Henderson, 1991, pp. 20–21).

Assumptions
The major assumption of the theory is that nurses care for patients until patients can care for themselves once again (Henderson, 1991). She assumes that patients desire to return to health, but this assumption is not explicitly stated. She also assumes that nurses are willing to serve and that "nurses will devote themselves to the patient day and night" (p. 23). A final assumption is that nurses should be educated at the university level in both arts and sciences.

Concepts
The major concepts of the theory relate to the metaparadigm (i.e., nursing, health, patient, and environment). Henderson believed that "the unique function of the nurse is to assist the individual, sick or well, in the performance of those activities contributing to health or its recovery (or to a peaceful death) that he would perform unaided if he had the necessary strength, will or knowledge. And to do this in such a way as to help him gain independence as rapidly as possible" (Henderson, 1991, p. 21). She defined the patient as someone who needs nursing care but did not limit nursing to illness care. She did not define environment, but maintaining a supportive environment is one of the elements of her 14 activities. Health was not explicitly defined, but it is taken to mean balance in all realms of human life. The concept of

> **Box 7-1**   Henderson's 14 Activities for Client Assistance
>
> 1. Breathe normally.
> 2. Eat and drink adequately.
> 3. Eliminate body wastes.
> 4. Move and maintain desirable postures.
> 5. Sleep and rest.
> 6. Select suitable clothes—dress and undress.
> 7. Maintain body temperature within normal range by adjusting clothing and modifying environment.
> 8. Keep the body clean and well groomed and protect the integument.
> 9. Avoid dangers in the environment and avoid injuring others.
> 10. Communicate with others in expressing emotions, needs, fears, or opinions.
> 11. Worship according to one's faith.
> 12. Work in such a way that there is a sense of accomplishment.
> 13. Play or participate in various forms of recreation.
> 14. Learn, discover, or satisfy the curiosity that leads to normal development and health and use the available health facilities.
>
> Source: Henderson (1991, pp. 22–23).

nursing involved the nurse attending to 14 activities that assist the individual toward independence (Box 7-1).

Usefulness

Nursing education has been deeply affected by Henderson's clear vision of the functions of nurses. The principles of Henderson's theory were published in the major nursing textbooks used from the 1930s through the 1960s, and the principles embodied by the 14 activities are still important in evaluating nursing care in the 21st century. Waller-Wise (2013), for example, found that Henderson's theory assisted him in attaining excellence in childbirth education.

Testability

Henderson supported nursing research but believed that it should be clinical research (O'Malley, 1996). Much of the research before her time had been on educational processes and on the profession of nursing itself rather than on the practice and outcomes of nursing, and she worked to change that.

Each of the 14 activities can be the basis for research. Although the statements are not written in testable terms, they may be reformulated into researchable questions. Furthermore, the theory can guide research in any aspect of the individual's care needs. For example, Englebright, Aldrich, and Taylor (2014) used Henderson's model as the framework to help define fundamental nursing care actions for the new electronic health record in a 170-bed community hospital.

Parsimony

Henderson's work is parsimonious in its presentation but complex in its scope. The 14 statements cover the whole of the practice of nursing, and her vision about the nurse's role in patient care (i.e., that the nurse perform for the patient those activities the patient usually performs independently until the patient can again adequately perform them) contributes to that complexity.

Value in Extending Nursing Science

From a historical standpoint, Henderson's concept of nursing enhanced nursing science; this has been particularly important in the area of nursing education. Her contributions to nursing literature extended from the 1930s through the 1990s. Her work has had an international impact on nursing research by strengthening the focus on nursing practice and confirming the value of tested interventions in assisting individuals to regain health. Internationally, researchers continue to direct their work with Virginia Henderson's model as a framework. For example, Scott, Matthews, and Kirwan (2014) found that internationally, Henderson's model was the most often used in evaluating the need for and the practice of nurses. In their reported case study, Younas and Sommer (2015) found Henderson's model "close to realism and applicable to Pakistani context" (p. 443) because of its relevance in developing nursing plans, and Lazenby (2013) argued for the importance of the patient experience using Henderson's model in multiple contexts.

Faye G. Abdellah: Patient-Centered Approaches to Nursing

Faye Abdellah was one of the first nursing theorists. In one of her earliest writings (Abdellah, Beland, Martin, & Matheney, 1960), she referred to the model created by her colleagues and herself as a framework. Her writings spanned the period from 1954 to 1992 and include books, monographs, book chapters, articles, reports, forewords to books, and conference proceedings.

Background of the Theorist

Abdellah earned her bachelor's degree in nursing, master's degree, and doctorate from Columbia University, and she completed additional graduate studies in science at Rutgers University. She served as the chief nurse officer and deputy U.S. Surgeon General, U.S. Public Health Service before retiring in 1993 with the rank of Rear Admiral. She has been awarded many academic honors from both civilian and military sources (Abdellah & Levine, 1994). She retired from her position as dean of the Graduate School of Nursing, Uniformed Services University of the Health Sciences in 2000.

Philosophical Underpinnings of the Theory

Abdellah's patient-centered approach to nursing was developed inductively from her practice and is considered a human needs theory (Abdellah et al., 1960). The theory was created to assist with nursing education and is most applicable to education and practice (Abdellah et al., 1960). Although it was intended to guide care of those in the hospital, it also has relevance for nursing care in community settings.

Major Assumptions, Concepts, and Relationships

The language of Abdellah's framework is readable and clear. Consistent with the decade in which she was writing, she uses the term "she" for nurses and "he" for doctors and patients and refers to the object of nursing as "patient" rather than client or consumer (Abdellah et al., 1960). Interestingly, she was one of the early writers who referred to "nursing diagnosis" (Abdellah et al., 1960, p. 9) during a time when nurses were taught that diagnosis was not a nurse's prerogative.

Assumptions

There are no openly stated assumptions in Abdellah's early work (Abdellah et al., 1960), but in a later work, she added six assumptions. These relate to change and anticipated changes that affect nursing; the need to appreciate the interconnectedness of social enterprises and social problems; the impact of problems such as poverty, racism, pollution, education, and so forth on health and health care delivery; changing nursing education; continuing education for professional nurses; and development of nursing leaders from underserved groups (Abdellah, Beland, Martin, & Matheney, 1973).

Abdellah and colleagues (1960) developed a list of 21 nursing problems (Box 7-2). They also identified 10 steps to identify the client's problems and 10 nursing skills to be used in developing a treatment typology.

According to Abdellah and colleagues (1960), nurses should do the following:

1. Learn to know the patient.
2. Sort out relevant and significant data.
3. Make generalizations about available data in relation to similar nursing problems presented by other patients.

Box 7-2   Abdellah's 21 Nursing Problems

1. To maintain good hygiene and physical comfort
2. To promote optimal activity, exercise, rest, and sleep
3. To promote safety through prevention of accidents, injury, or other trauma and through the prevention of the spread of infection
4. To maintain good body mechanics and prevent and correct deformities
5. To facilitate the maintenance of a supply of oxygen to all body cells
6. To facilitate the maintenance of nutrition of all body cells
7. To facilitate the maintenance of elimination
8. To facilitate the maintenance of fluid and electrolyte balance
9. To recognize the physiologic responses of the body to disease conditions
10. To facilitate the maintenance of regulatory mechanisms and functions
11. To facilitate the maintenance of sensory function
12. To identify and accept positive and negative expressions, feelings, and reactions
13. To identify and accept the interrelatedness of emotions and organic illness
14. To facilitate the maintenance of effective verbal and nonverbal communication
15. To promote the development of productive interpersonal relationships
16. To facilitate progress toward achievement of personal spiritual goals
17. To create and maintain a therapeutic environment
18. To facilitate awareness of self as an individual with varying physical, emotional, and developmental needs
19. To accept the optimum possible goals in light of physical and emotional limitations
20. To use community resources as an aid in resolving problems arising from illness
21. To understand the role of social problems as influencing factors in the cause of illness

Source: Abdellah et al. (1960).

4. Identify the therapeutic plan.
5. Test generalizations with the patient and make additional generalizations.
6. Validate the patient's conclusions about his or her nursing problems.
7. Continue to observe and evaluate the patient over a period of time to identify any attitudes and clues affecting his or her behavior.
8. Explore the patient's and family's reaction to the therapeutic plan and involve them in the plan.
9. Identify how the nurse feels about the patient's nursing problems.
10. Discuss and develop a comprehensive nursing care plan.

Abdellah and colleagues (1960) distinguished between nursing diagnoses and nursing functions. Nursing diagnoses were a determination of the nature and extent of nursing problems presented by individuals receiving nursing care, and nursing functions were nursing activities that contributed to the solution for the same nursing problem. Other concepts central to her work were (1) health care team (a group of health professionals trained at various levels, and often at different institutions, working together to provide health care), (2) professionalization of nursing (requires that nurses identify those nursing problems that depend on the nurse's use of his or her capacities to conceptualize events and make judgments about them), (3) patient (individual who needs nursing care and who is dependent on the health care provider), and (4) nursing (a service to individuals and families and to society, which helps people cope with their health needs) (Abdellah et al., 1960).

Usefulness

The patient-centered approach was constructed to be useful to nursing practice, with the impetus for it being nursing education. Abdellah's publications on nursing education began with her dissertation; her interest in education of nurses continues into the present.

Abdellah also published work on nursing, nursing research, and public policy related to nursing in several international publications. She has been a strong advocate for improving nursing practice through nursing research and has a publication record on nursing research that dates from 1955 to the present. Box 7-3 lists only a few of Abdellah's many publications.

Box 7-3   Examples of Abdellah's Publications

Abdellah, F. G. (1972). Evolution of nursing as a profession: Perspective on manpower development. *International Nursing Review, 19*(3), 219–238.

Abdellah, F. G. (1986). *The nature of nursing science.* In L. H. Nicholl (Ed.), *Perspectives on nursing theory.* Boston, MA: Little, Brown.

Abdellah, F. G. (1987). The federal role in nursing education. *Nursing Outlook, 35*(5), 224–225.

Abdellah, F. G. (1991). Public policy impacting on nursing care of older adults. In E. M. Baines (Ed.), *Perspectives on gerontological nursing.* Newbury Park, CA: Sage.

Abdellah, F. G., Beland, I. L., Martin A., & Matheney, R. V. (1968). *Patient-centered approaches to nursing* (2nd ed.). New York, NY: MacMillan.

Abdellah, F. G., & Levine, E. (1994). *Preparing nursing research for the 21st century: Evolution, methodologies, challenges.* New York, NY: Springer Publishing.

Testability

Abdellah's work is a conceptual model that is not directly testable because there are few stated directional relationships. The model is testable in principle, though, because testable hypotheses can be derived from its conceptual material. One work (Abdellah & Levine, 1957) was identified that described the development of a tool to measure client and personnel satisfaction with nursing care.

Parsimony

Abdellah and colleagues' (1960, 1973) model touches on many factors in nursing but focuses primarily on the perspective of nursing education. It defines 21 nursing problems, 10 steps to identifying client's problems, and 10 nursing skills. Because of its focus and complexity, it is not particularly parsimonious.

Value in Extending Nursing Science

Abdellah's model has contributed to nursing science as an early effort to change nursing education. In the early years of its application, it helped to bring structure and organization to what was often a disorganized collection of lectures and experiences. She categorized nursing problems based on the individual's needs and developed a typology of nursing treatment and nursing skills. Finally, she posited a list of characteristics that described what was distinctly nursing, thereby differentiating the profession from other health professions. Hers was a major contribution to the discipline of nursing, bringing it out of the era of being considered simply an occupation into Nightingale's ideal of becoming a profession.

Dorothea Orem: The Self-Care Deficit Nursing Theory

Dorothea Orem was born in Baltimore, Maryland. She received her diploma in nursing from Providence Hospital School of Nursing in Washington, DC, and her baccalaureate degree in nursing from Catholic University in 1939. In 1945, she also earned her master's degree from Catholic University (Berbiglia & Banfield, 2014).

Background of the Theorist

Orem held a number of positions as private duty nurse, hospital staff nurse, and educator. She was the director of both the School of Nursing and Nursing Service at Detroit's Providence Hospital until 1949, moving from there to Indiana where she served on the Board of Health until 1957. She assumed a role as a faculty member of Catholic University in 1959, later becoming acting dean (Berbiglia & Banfield, 2014).

Orem's interest in nursing theory was piqued when she and a group of colleagues were charged with producing a curriculum for practical nursing for the Department of Health, Education, and Welfare in Washington, DC. After publishing the first book on her theory in 1971, she continued working on her concept of nursing and self-care. She had numerous honorary doctorates and other awards as members of the nursing profession have recognized the value of the self-care deficit theory (Berbiglia & Banfield, 2014). Dr. Orem died in 2007 after a period of failing health. Nurses will remember her as one of the pioneers of nursing theory (Bekel, 2007).

Philosophical Underpinnings of the Theory

Orem (2001) denied that any particular theorist provided the basis for the Self-Care Deficit Nursing Theory (SCDNT). She expressed interest in several theories, although she references only Parsons's Structure of Social Action and von Bertalanffy's System Theory (Orem, 2001). Taylor, Geden, Isaramalai, and Wongvatunyu (2000), however, stated that the ontology of Orem's SCDNT is the school of moderate realism, and its focus is on the person as agent; the SCDNT is a highly developed formalized theoretical system of nursing. Currently, the theory is referred to as Self-Care Science and Nursing Theory (Taylor & Renpenning, 2011). Taylor and Renpenning (2011) make a case for the scientific basis of the life work that was Orem's magnum opus and quote from her works extensively.

Major Assumptions, Concepts, and Relationships

Orem's theory changed to fit the times most notably in the concept of the individual and of the nursing system. The original theory, however, remains largely intact.

Orem (2001) delineated three nested theories: theories of self-care, self-care deficit, and nursing systems (Figure 7-1). The theory of nursing systems is the outer or encompassing theory, which contains the theory of self-care deficit. The theory of self-care is a component of the theory of self-care deficit.

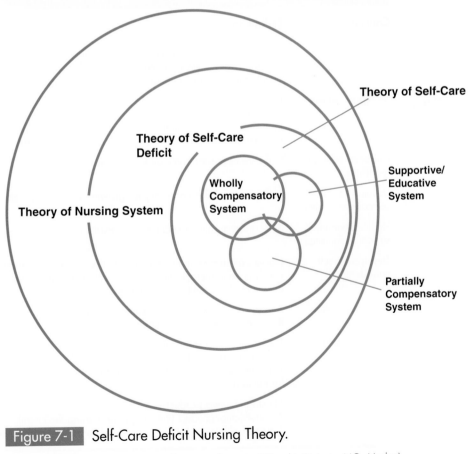

Figure 7-1   Self-Care Deficit Nursing Theory.

(Source: Orem, D. [2001]. *Nursing: Concepts of practice* [6th ed.]. St. Louis, MO: Mosby.)

Concepts

Orem (2001) defined the metaparadigm concepts as follows:

Nursing is seen as an art through which the practitioner of nursing gives specialized assistance to persons with disabilities which makes more than ordinary assistance necessary to meet needs for self-care. The nurse also intelligently participates in the medical care the individual receives from the physician.

Humans are defined as "men, women, and children cared for either singly or as social units," and are the "material object" (p. 8) of nurses and others who provide direct care.

Environment has physical, chemical, and biological features. It includes the family culture and community.

Health is "being structurally and functionally whole or sound" (p. 96). Also, health is a state that encompasses both the health of individuals and of groups, and human health is the ability to reflect on one's self, to symbolize experience, and to communicate with others.

Numerous additional concepts were formulated for Orem's theory; Table 7-1 lists some of the more significant ones.

Table 7-1 Concepts in Orem's Self-Care Deficit Theory

Concept	Definition
Self-care	A human regulatory function that is a deliberate action to supply or ensure the supply of necessary materials needed for continued life, growth, and development and maintenance of human integrity.
Self-care requisites	Part of self-care; expressions of action to be performed by or for individuals in the interest of controlling human or environmental factors that affect human functioning or development. There are three types: universal, developmental, and health deviation self-care requisites.
Universal self-care requisites	Self-care requisites common to all humans.
Developmental self-care requisites	Self-care requisites necessary for growth and development.
Health deviation self-care requisites	Self-care requisites associated with health deficits.
Therapeutic self-care demand	Nurse's assistance in meeting the client's or client dependent's self-care needs is done therapeutically as a result of the client's inability to calculate or to meet therapeutic self-care needs.
Deliberate action	Action knowingly taken with some motivation or some outcome sought by the actor, as self-care or dependent care.
Nursing system	The product of a series of relations between the persons: legitimate nurse and legitimate client. This system is activated when the client's therapeutic self-care demand exceeds available self-care agency, leading to the need for nursing.
Product of nursing	Nursing has two products: An intellectual product (the design for helping the client) A system of care of long or short duration for persons requiring nursing

Source: Orem (1995).

Relationships

An underlying premise of Orem's theory is the belief that humans engage in continuous communication and interchange among themselves and their environments to remain alive and to function. In humans, the power to act deliberately is exercised to identify needs and to make needed judgments. Furthermore, mature human beings experience privations in the form of action in care of self and others involving making life-sustaining and function-regulating actions. Human agency is exercised in discovering, developing, and transmitting to others ways and means to identify needs for, and make inputs into, self and others. Finally, groups of human beings with structured relationships cluster tasks and allocate responsibilities for providing care to group members who experience privations for making required deliberate decisions about self and others (Orem, 2001).

Needs theories, such as Orem's are complex in their application. Over the decades that Orem worked on her theories of nursing, the theory went through several iterations in response to new knowledge and technology. Her continual work indicated that she was aware of the complex nature of patient's needs and of the growing complexity of the health care system. Although this theory is not a complexity theory as such, she does pay tribute in her later writings to the complexity of care for clients/patients in the health care system at that time.

Usefulness

In past years, numerous colleges and schools of nursing base their curricula on the SCDNT. Among them are Illinois Wesleyan University, University of Tennessee at Chattanooga, Anderson College, and University of Toledo (Berbiglia & Banfield, 2014). Hospitals in several areas of the country have based nursing care on Orem's theory, and it has been applied to an ambulatory care setting. Such medical conditions as arthritis or gastrointestinal and renal diseases, and such areas of practice as community nursing, critical care, cultural concepts, maternal–child nursing, medical-surgical nursing, pediatric nursing, perioperative nursing, and renal dialysis, among other specialties have used Orem's theory to structure care (Berbiglia & Banfield, 2014). Orem's SCDNT has received international interest and has been used in many countries including Great Britain, Germany, Japan, the Netherlands, Norway, Sweden, and New Zealand. Moreover, numerous publications define methods for using Orem's SCDNT in practice, research, and education.

Orem was a prolific author and her writings spanned five decades. In addition to her detailed description of her theory through several iterations (Orem, 1971, 1985b, 1991, 1995, 2001), she authored an analysis of hospital nursing service (Orem, 1956) and illustrations for self-care for the rehabilitation client (Orem, 1985a). Further evidence of the usefulness of Orem's work is the International Orem Society, which celebrates the work of Dr. Orem. Their journal, *Self-Care, Dependent-Care & Nursing*, indicates the value to nurses across the globe (Biggs, 2008).

Testability

Many nursing research studies have used Orem's theory as a conceptual framework or as a source of testable hypotheses. Furthermore, over the years, many research studies have tested elements of the theory. The researchers have studied people with diminished self-care agency across age and social groups, in numerous situations, and in many countries. Most research into the SCDNT is descriptive, and the theory has not been subject to testing in its entirety (Berbiglia & Banfield, 2014; Taylor & Renpenning, 2011). Box 7-4 lists some of the recent research studies using the SCDNT.

| Box 7-4 | Orem's Theory in Nursing Research, Practice, and Education |

Green, R. (2013). Application of the self-care deficit nursing theory: The community context. *Self-Care, Dependent-Care & Nursing, 20*(1), 5–15.

Guo, S. H.-M., Lin, Y.-H., Chen, R.-R., Kao, S.-F., & Chang, H.-K. (2013). Development and evaluation of theory-based diabetes support services. *Computers, Informatics, Nursing, 31*(1), 17–26. doi:10.1097/NXN.0b013e318266ca22

Mohammadpour, A., Rahmati, S. N., Khosravan, S., Alami, A., & Akhond, M. (2015). The effect of a supportive educational intervention developed based on Orem's self-care theory on the self-care ability of patients with myocardial infarction: A randomised controlled trial. *Journal of Clinical Nursing, 24*(11–12), 1686–1692.

O'Shaughnessy, M. (2014). Application of Dorothea Orem's theory of self-care to the elderly patient on peritoneal dialysis. *Nephrology Nursing Journal, 41*(5), 495–497.

Pickett, S., Peters, R. M., & Jarosz, P. A. (2014). Toward a middle-range theory of weight management. *Nursing Science Quarterly, 27*(3), 242–247.

Roldan-Merino, J., Lluch-Canut, T., Menarguez-Alcaina, M., Foix-Sanjuan, A., & Haro Abad, J. M. (2014). Psychometric evaluation of a new instrument in Spanish to measure self-care requisites in patients with schizophrenia. *Perspectives in Psychiatric Care, 50*(2), 93–101. doi:10.1111/ppc.12026

Silén, M., & Johansson, L. (2016). Aims and theoretical frameworks in nursing students' bachelor's theses in Sweden: A descriptive study. *Nurse Education Today, 37,* 91–96. doi:10.1016/j.ned.2015.11.020

Tadaura, H., Sato, A., Ueda, E., Ishigaki, H., Saita, T., & Kikuchi, T. (2014). Connecting nursing theory with practice through education based on self-care deficit nursing theory (SCDNT) and utilization of nursing practice. *Self-Care, Dependent-Care & Nursing, 21*(1), 27–29.

Wong, C. L., Ip, W. Y., Choi, K. C., & Lam, L. W. (2015). Examining self-care behaviors and their associated factors among adolescent girls with dysmenorrhea: An application of Orem's self-care deficit nursing theory. *Journal of Nursing Scholarship, 47*(3), 219–227. doi:10.1111/jnu.12134

Parsimony

Orem's (2001) SCDNT is complex. It consists of three nested theories, many presuppositions, and propositions in each of the individual theories. Revisions of the theory from the original (1971) have improved the organization; however, its complexity has increased in response to societal needs throughout the several editions.

Value in Extending Nursing Science

The SCDNT has been the basis for many college and university nursing curricula (Orem, 2001). It has been used in practice situations and extensively in research projects, theses, and dissertations (Taylor, 2011). The practical applicability of the theory is attractive to graduate students because it is perceived as a realistic reflection of nursing practice.

Dorothy Johnson: The Behavioral System Model

Dorothy Johnson began her work on the Behavioral System Model in the late 1950s and wrote into the 1990s. The focus of her model is on needs, the human as a behavioral system, and relief of stress as nursing care.

> Box 7-5   Examples of Johnson's Writings on Nursing Theory
>
> Johnson, D. E. (1959a). A philosophy of nursing. *Nursing Outlook, 7*(4), 198–200.
> Johnson, D. E. (1959b). The nature of a science of nursing. *Nursing Outlook, 7*(5), 291–294.
> Johnson, D. E. (1968). Theory in nursing: Borrowed and unique. *Nursing Research, 17*(3), 206–209.
> Johnson, D. E. (1974). Development of a theory: A requisite for nursing as a primary health profession. *Nursing Research, 23*(5), 372–377.
> Johnson, D. E. (1980). The behavioral system model for nursing. In J. P. Riehl & C. Roy (Eds.), *Conceptual models for nursing practice* (pp. 207–216). New York, NY: Appleton-Century-Crofts.
> Johnson, D. E. (1990). The behavioral system model for nursing. In M. E. Parker (Ed.), *Nursing theories in practice* (pp. 23–32). New York, NY: National League for Nursing Press.

Johnson (1990) reported that her work began as a study of the knowledge that identified nursing while synthesizing content for nursing curricula at the graduate and undergraduate levels. She wanted the curricula to be focused on nursing rather than derived from the knowledge bases of other health care disciplines (Johnson, 1959a, 1959b, 1997). Indeed, she believed that nursing, although relying on the contributions of other sciences, is a discrete science and a unique discipline.

Johnson's model was deductively derived through long study of other theories and applying them to nursing (Johnson, 1997). Her goal was to conceptualize nursing for education of nurses at all levels (Johnson, 1990, 1997), and the model emanated from her practice, study, and teaching experiences.

Although Johnson did not write a book on her theory, she did write several chapters and articles that explained her theoretical framework. Box 7-5 lists a sampling of these writings.

Background of the Theorist

Dorothy Johnson was reared in Savannah, Georgia, and received a bachelor's degree in nursing from Vanderbilt University. She earned a master's degree in public health from Harvard in 1948 and returned to Vanderbilt to begin her teaching career. In 1949, she joined the nursing faculty of the University of California, Los Angeles (UCLA). She retired from UCLA in 1977 and lived in Florida until her death in 1999 (Holaday, 2014).

Philosophical Underpinnings of the Theory

Johnson stated that Nightingale's work inspired her model. Nightingale's philosophical leanings prompted Johnson to consider the person experiencing a disease more important than the disease itself (Johnson, 1990). She reported that she derived portions of her theory from the works of Selye on stress, Grinker's theory of human behavior, and Buckley and Chin on systems theories (Johnson, 1980, 1990).

Major Assumptions, Concepts, and Relationships

Assumptions
Assumptions of Johnson's model are both stated and derived. There are four assumptions about human behavioral subsystems. First is the belief that drives serve as focal

points around which behaviors are organized to achieve specific goals. Second, it is assumed that behavior is differentiated and organized within the prevailing dimensions of set and choice. Third, the specialized parts or subsystems of the behavioral system are structured by dimensions of goal, set, choice, and actions; each has observable behaviors. Finally, interactive and interdependent subsystems tend to achieve and maintain balance between and among subsystems through control and regulatory mechanisms (Grubbs, 1980).

Concepts

Although she adopted concepts from other disciplines, Johnson modified and defined them to apply specifically to nursing situations. This was an evolving process as shown in her writings (Johnson, 1959a, 1959b, 1968, 1974, 1980, 1990).

The metaparadigm concepts are apparent in Johnson's writings. Nursing is seen as "an external regulatory force which acts to preserve the organization and integration of the patient's behavior at an optimal level under those conditions in which the behavior constitutes a threat to physical or social health, or in which illness is found" (Johnson, 1980, p. 214). The concept of human was defined as a behavioral system that strives to make continual adjustments to achieve, maintain, or regain balance to the steady state that is adaptation (Johnson, 1980).

Health is seen as the opposite of illness, and Johnson (1980) defines it as "some degree of regularity and constancy in behavior, the behavioral system reflects adjustments and adaptations that are successful in some way and to some degree . . . adaptation is functionally efficient and effective" (pp. 208, 209). Environment is not directly defined, but it is implied to include all elements of the surroundings of the human system and includes interior stressors. Other concepts defined in Johnson's model are listed in Table 7-2.

Relationships

Johnson (1980) delineated seven subsystems to which the model applied. These are as follows:

1. Attachment or affiliative subsystem—serves the need for security through social inclusion or intimacy
2. Dependency subsystem—behaviors designed to get attention, recognition, and physical assistance
3. Ingestive subsystem—fulfills the need to supply the biologic requirements for food and fluids
4. Eliminative subsystem—functions to excrete wastes
5. Sexual subsystem—serves the biologic requirements of procreation and reproduction
6. Aggressive subsystem—functions in self and social protection and preservation
7. Achievement system—functions to master and control the self or the environment

Finally, there are three functional requirements of humans in Johnson's (1980) model. These are:

1. To be protected from noxious influences with which the person cannot cope
2. To be nurtured through the input of supplies from the environment
3. To be stimulated to enhance growth and prevent stagnation

Table 7-2 Concepts in Johnson's Behavioral System Theory

Concept	Definition
Behavioral system	Man is a system that indicates the state of the system through behaviors
Boundaries	The point that differentiates the interior of the system from the exterior
Function	Consequences or purposes of actions
Functional requirements	Input that the system must receive to survive and develop
Homeostasis	Process of maintaining stability
Instability	State in which the system output of energy depletes the energy needed to maintain stability
Stability	Balance or steady state in maintaining balance of behavior within an acceptable range
Stressor	A stimulus from the internal or external world that results in stress or instability
Structure	The parts of the system that make up the whole
System	That which functions as a whole by virtue of organized independent interaction of its parts
Subsystem	A minisystem maintained in relationship to the entire system when it or the environment is not disturbed
Tension	The system's adjustment to demands, change or growth, or to actual disruptions
Variables	Factors outside the system that influence the system's behavior, but which the system lacks power to change

Source: Grubbs (1980).

Usefulness

That Johnson's model is useful for nursing practice and education has been verified in several articles and chapters. Damus (1980), Dee (1990), and Holaday (1980) described situations in which Johnson's model has been used to direct nursing practice. Other authors have used the theory to apply to various aspects of nursing. For example, Benson (1997) used Johnson's model as a framework to describe the impact of fear of crime on an elder person's health, health-seeking behaviors, and quality of life. Fruehwirth (1989) applied Johnson's model to assess and intervene in a group of caregivers for individuals with Alzheimer disease.

Testability

Parts of Johnson's model have been tested or used to direct nursing research. Indeed, more than 20 research studies have been identified using Johnson's model. Turner-Henson (1992), for example, used Johnson's model as a framework to examine how mothers of chronically ill children perceived the environment (i.e., whether it was supportive, safe, and accessible). Poster, Dee, and Randell (1997) used Johnson's theory as a conceptual framework in a study of client outcome evaluation; they found that the nursing theory made it possible to prescribe nursing care and to distinguish it from medical care. Derdiarian and Schobel (1990) used Johnson's model to develop an assessment tool for individuals with AIDS.

Aspects of Johnson's model have been tested in nursing research. In one study, Derdiarian (1990) examined the relationship between the aggressive/protective subsystem and the other six model subsystems.

Parsimony

Johnson (1980) was able to explicate her entire model in a single short chapter in an edited book. Relatively few concepts are used in the theory, and they are commonly used terms. Additionally, the relationships are clear; therefore, the model is considered to be parsimonious.

Value in Extending Nursing Science

Johnson's model has been used in nursing practice and research to a significant extent. In addition, her work has been used as a curriculum guide for a number of schools of nursing (Grubbs, 1980; Johnson, 1980, 1990), and it has been adapted for use in hospital situations (Dee, 1990). Finally, her work inspired the work of at least two other grand nursing theorists, Betty Neuman and Sister Calista Roy, who were her students.

Betty Neuman: The Neuman Systems Model

Since the 1960s, Betty Neuman has been recognized as a pioneer in the field of nursing, particularly in the area of community mental health. She developed her model while lecturing in community mental health at UCLA and first published it in 1972 under the title "A Model for Teaching the Total Person Approach to Patient Problems" (Neuman & Fawcett, 2011). Since that time, she has been a prolific writer, and her model has been used extensively in colleges of nursing, beginning with Neumann College's baccalaureate nursing program in Aston, Pennsylvania. Numerous other nursing programs have organized their curricula around her model both in the United States and internationally (Neuman & Fawcett, 2011).

The major elements in this review of the Neuman Systems Model are taken from the fifth edition of her book (Neuman & Fawcett, 2011), with references to earlier writings to show development of the model over time. The model was deductively derived and emanated from requests of graduate students who wanted assistance with a broad interpretation of nursing.

Neuman's model uses a systems approach that is focused on the human needs of protection or relief from stress (Neuman & Fawcett, 2011). Neuman believed that the causes of stress can be identified and remedied through nursing interventions. She emphasized the need of humans for dynamic balance that the nurse can provide through identification of problems, mutually agreeing on goals, and using the concept of prevention as intervention. Neuman's model is one of only a few considered prescriptive in nature. The model is universal, abstract, and applicable for individuals from many cultures (Neuman & Fawcett, 2011).

Background of the Theorist

Betty Neuman was born in 1924 on a farm near Lowell, Ohio. In 1947, she earned her nursing diploma from People's Hospital School of Nursing, Akron, Ohio, and moved to California shortly thereafter. She earned a bachelor's degree in nursing from UCLA and also studied psychology and public health. In 1966, she earned a master's degree in mental health and public health consultation, also from UCLA, and then earned her doctorate in clinical psychology in 1985 from Pacific Western University. She worked as a hospital staff nurse, a head nurse, and an industrial nurse and consultant before becoming a nursing instructor. She has taught medical-surgical nursing, critical care, and communicable disease nursing at the University of Southern California Medical Center in Los Angeles and at other colleges in Ohio and West Virginia (Lawson, 2014; Neuman & Fawcett, 2011).

Philosophical Underpinnings of the Theory

Neuman used concepts and theories from a number of disciplines in the development of her theory. In her works, she referred to Chardin and Cornu on wholeness in systems, von Bertalanffy and Lazlo on general systems theory, Selye on stress theory, and Lazarus on stress and coping (Neuman & Fawcett, 2011).

Major Assumptions, Concepts, and Relationships

Concepts

Neuman (Neuman & Fawcett, 2011) adhered to the metaparadigm concepts and has developed numerous additional concepts for her model. In her work, she defined human beings as "client system" . . . "a composite of five interacting variable areas . . . physiological, psychological, sociocultural, developmental, and spiritual" (Neuman & Fawcett, 2011, p. 16). The ring structure is a "basic structure of protective concentric rings, for retention attainment or maintenance of system stability and integrity. . . " (Neuman & Fawcett, 2011, p. 16). Environment to Neuman is a structure of concentric rings representing the three environments, internal, external, and created environments, all of which influence the client's adaptation to stressors. Health is defined as "a continuum; wellness and illness are at opposite ends. . . . Health for the client is equated with optimal system stability that is the best possible wellness state at any given time" (p. 23). "Variances from wellness or varying degrees of system instability are caused by stressor invasion of the normal line of defense" (p. 24). Finally, in the nursing component, the major concern is to maintain client system stability through accurately assessing environmental and other stressors and assisting in client adjustments to maintain optimal wellness. Table 7-3 lists selected additional concepts from Neuman's model, and Figure 7-2 offers a visual representation.

Relationships

Neuman defined five interacting variables: physiologic, psychological, sociocultural, developmental, and spiritual. These five variables function in time to attain, maintain, or retain system stability. The model is based on the client's reaction to stress as it maintains boundaries to protect client stability (Neuman & Fawcett, 2011).

Neuman delineated a three-step nursing process model in which nursing diagnosis (the first step) assumes that the nurse collects an adequate database from which to analyze variances from wellness to make the diagnoses (Neuman & Fawcett, 2011). Nursing goals, which are determined by negotiation with the client, are set in the second step. Appropriate prevention as intervention strategies are decided in that step. The third step, nursing outcomes, is the step in which confirmation of prescriptive change or reformulation of nursing goals is evaluated. The nurse links the client, environment, health, and nursing. The findings feed back into the system as applicable.

Table 7-3 Concepts in Neuman Systems Model

Concept	Definition
Basic structure	Basic survival factors common to human beings; they are located in the central core and represent basic client system energy resources.
Boundary lines	The flexible line of defense is the outer boundary of the client system.
Degree of reaction	The amount of system instability resulting from stressor invasion of the normal line of defense.
Feedback	The process within which matter, energy, and information provides feedback for corrective action to change, enhance, or stabilize the system.
Flexible line of defense	A protective, accordion-like mechanism that surrounds and protects the normal line of defense from invasion by stressors.
Input/output	The matter, energy, and information exchanged between client and environment that is entering or leaving the system at any point in time.
Lines of resistance	Protection factors activated when stressors have penetrated the normal line of defense, causing a reaction symptomatology.
Negentropy	A process of energy conservation that increases organization and complexity, moving the system toward stability or a higher degree of wellness.
Normal line of defense	An adaptational level of health developed over time and considered normal for a particular individual client or system; it becomes a standard for wellness–deviance determination.
Open system	A system in which there is a continuous flow of input and process, output, and feedback. It is a system of organized complexity where all elements are in interaction.
Prevention as intervention	Intervention modes for nursing action and determinants for entry of both client and nurse into the health care system.
Reconstitution	The return and maintenance of system stability, following treatment of stressor reaction, which may result in a higher or lower level of wellness.
Stability	A state of balance or harmony requiring energy exchanges as the client adequately copes with stressors to retain, attain, or maintain an optimal level of health, thus preserving system integrity.
Stressors	Environmental factors, intra-, inter-, and extrapersonal in nature, that have potential for disrupting system stability. A stressor is any phenomenon that might penetrate both the flexible and normal lines of defense, resulting in either a positive or negative outcome.
Wellness/illness	Wellness is the condition in which all system parts and subparts are in harmony with the whole system of the client. Illness indicates disharmony among the parts and subparts of the client system.

Source: Neuman and Fawcett (2011).

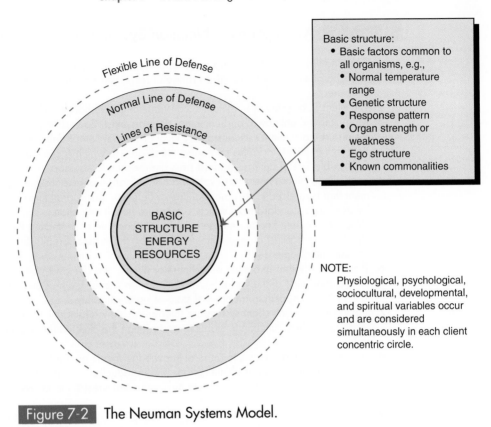

Basic structure:
• Basic factors common to
  all organisms, e.g.,
  • Normal temperature
    range
  • Genetic structure
  • Response pattern
  • Organ strength or
    weakness
  • Ego structure
  • Known commonalities

NOTE:
Physiological, psychological,
sociocultural, developmental,
and spiritual variables occur
and are considered
simultaneously in each client
concentric circle.

Flexible Line of Defense

Normal Line of Defense

Lines of Resistance

BASIC
STRUCTURE
ENERGY
RESOURCES

Figure 7-2   The Neuman Systems Model.

(From Neuman, B., & Fawcett, J. The Neuman Systems Model, 5th ed., © 2011. Reprinted by permission of Pearson Education, Inc., New York, New York.)

A table of prevention as intervention strategies clarifies what comprises the nursing actions to affect this type of intervention. Neuman outlined 10 propositions or assumptions of the model (Box 7-6).

Usefulness

Neuman's model has been used extensively in nursing education and nursing practice. In her latest work, she provides a number of specific examples of the systems processes (Neuman & Fawcett, 2011). The Neuman Systems Model is in place in numerous states of the United States and internationally in countries as diverse as Taiwan and the Netherlands. It reportedly has been initiated to guide nursing practice for the management of patient care in the areas of medicine and surgery, mental health, women's health, pediatric nursing, community as client, and gerontology. Graduate students, in particular, find Neuman's model realistic to define their practice.

Because of its utility and popularity as a model, it has been monitored by a group called the Neuman Systems Model Trustees Group, Inc. This group meets periodically to discuss research and practice related to the model and to promote exchange of information and ideas. Neuman's model is in use as a guide in a plethora of nursing schools at all levels; a partial listing is included in Neuman and Fawcett (2011).

Box 7-6	Assumptions of Neuman Systems Model—a Summary

1. Each individual client or group as an open system is unique, a composite of factors and characteristics within a given range of responses contained within a basic structure.
2. The client as a system is in dynamic, constant energy exchange with the environment.
3. Many known, unknown, and universal stressors exist. Each differs in its potential for disturbing a client's usual stability level or normal line of defense. The interrelationships of client variables can affect the degree to which a client is protected by the flexible line of defense against possible reaction to stressors.
4. Each client/client system has evolved a normal range of responses to the environment that is referred to as a normal line of defense. The normal line of defense can be used as a standard from which to measure health deviation.
5. When the flexible line of defense is no longer capable of protecting the client/ client system against an environmental stressor, the stressor breaks through the normal line of defense.
6. The client, whether in a state of wellness or illness, is a dynamic composite of the interrelationships of the variables. Wellness is on a continuum of available energy to support the system in an optimal state of system stability.
7. Implicit within each client system are internal resistance factors known as lines of resistance, which function to stabilize and realign the client to the usual wellness state.
8. Primary prevention relates to general knowledge that is applied in client assessment and intervention, in identification, and in reduction or mitigation of possible or actual risk factors associated with environmental stressors to prevent possible reaction.
9. Secondary prevention relates to symptomatology following a reaction to stressors, appropriate ranking of intervention priorities, and treatment to reduce their noxious effects.
10. Tertiary prevention relates to the adjustive processes taking place as reconstitution begins and maintenance factors move the client back in a circular manner toward primary prevention.

Testability

Although the Neuman's model is not testable in its entirety, it gives rise to directional hypotheses that are testable in research. As a result, it has been used as a conceptual framework extensively in nursing research, and aspects of the model have been empirically tested. Intermediate theories using the Neuman Systems Model have been developed and are being tested. Box 7-7 lists a few of the many nursing research studies that have used Neuman Systems Model.

Parsimony

Neuman's model is complex, and many parts of the model function in multiple ways. The description of the model's parts can be confusing; therefore, the model is not considered to be parsimonious. Neuman and Fawcett (2011), however, have developed intermediate diagrams to clarify the interactions among parts of the model and to facilitate its use. The definitions are well developed in the latest edition of the model, and the assumptions (propositions), although multileveled, are well organized.

Box 7-7	Examples of Nursing Research Studies Using Neuman Systems Model

Adamson, E. (2014). Caring behaviour of nurses in Malaysia is influenced by spiritual and emotional intelligence, psychological ownership and burnout. *Evidence-Based Nursing, 17*(4), 121. doi:10.1136/eb-2013-101704

Adler, M., & Pietsch, T. (2016). Relationship among smoking, chronic pain, mental health and opioid use in older adults. *Catalyst, Neuman Journal of Student Research and Academic Scholarship, 2*(1), 97–113.

Bachman, A. O., Danuser, B., & Morin, D. (2015). Developing a theoretical framework using a nursing perspective to investigate perceived health in the "sandwich generation" group. *Nursing Science Quarterly, 28*(4), 308–318.

Bauer, J. S. (2014). The use of stress-reducing techniques in nursing education. *Western Journal of Nursing Research, 36*(10), 1386. doi:10.1177/0193945914540097

Phillips, T. M. (2014). Exploration of theoretical models: Postpartum weight retention in African American adolescents. *Nursing Science Quarterly, 27*(4), 308–314.

Willis, D., DeSanto-Madeya, S., Ross, R., Sheehan, D. L., & Fawcett, J. (2015). Spiritual healing in the aftermath of childhood maltreatment: Translating men's lived experiences utilizing nursing conceptual models and theory. *ANS. Advances in Nursing Science, 38*(3), 162–174.

Value in Extending Nursing Science

The Neuman Systems Model has extended nursing science as a needs and causality-focused framework. It appeals to nurses who consider the client to be a holistic individual who reacts to stressors because it predicts the outcomes of interventions to strengthen the lines of defense against stress, which may destabilize the system. Neuman's model is useful not only in the acute critical care area because of the focus on attaining, regaining, and maintaining system stability but also in community health situations because of its focus on prevention as intervention (Neuman & Fawcett, 2011).

Summary

The human needs nursing theories were among the earliest of the nursing theories. In general, these theories followed the philosophical school of thought of the time by considering the person to be a biopsychosocial being and focusing on meeting the individual's needs.

Donald Crawford, the nurse from the opening case study, illustrated how a human needs–based model can be used to help direct client care through anticipating or predicting client needs and determining desirable outcomes. Many other nurses in a variety of settings use these models and theories to direct care for their clients.

It should be noted that succeeding generations of nursing theorists based their models and theories on the works discussed here. Indeed, these theories were building blocks on which the profession of nursing depended during the last half of the 20th century and into the 21st century.

Key Points

- Needs theorists generally come from the positivist school of thought philosophically, and therefore, the theories fit well with medical theories of care.
- The needs theories of nursing work well with the current emphasis on evidence-based practice because of the bias toward experimental science.
- The first nursing theorists mainly focused on the human needs of their patients/clients.
- Florence Nightingale is respected as the mother of modern professional nursing. She brought nursing out of the servant position it held in the 19th century and into the respected professional status it holds currently.
- Virginia Henderson is often seen as the mother of American professional nursing. She was a prolific author and researcher. Her concept of nursing is still used in clinical and community health care.
- Faye Abdellah provided nurses with one of the first academic nursing theories. She was a prolific author and researcher. She categorized nursing problems based on the individual's needs and developed a typology of nursing treatment and nursing skills. Finally, she posited a list of characteristics that described what was distinctly nursing.
- Dorothea Orem provided one of the first theories that gave the patient/client the responsibility for self-care. Her ideas allowed patients to resume more normal lives with respect to their self-care agency.
- Dorothy Johnson was a teacher of nursing at all levels. Her theoretical work inspired many other nurses to become theoretical thinkers.
- Betty Neuman gave nurses the systems model with its lines of defense against stress. She believed that the causes of stress can be identified and remedied through nursing interventions. She developed the concept of prevention as intervention. Neuman's model is one of only a few considered prescriptive in nature.
- The needs theorists' works are still in daily use in education, in clinical nursing, and in clinical nursing research.

Learning Activities

1. Discuss the usefulness of one of the models/theories in this chapter to evidence-based practice. How would you and colleagues present your evidence?
2. Choose one of the models discussed in this chapter and demonstrate its use in the care of a selected client. Write a nursing care plan using the model. Define all elements of the nursing care plan using the language and the assumptions/propositions of the model.
3. Obtain the work of one of the theorists described in this chapter. Outline a research study testing components of the model.
   a. Determine which major concepts or propositions of the model can be tested.
   b. Define the elements of the model to be tested in the research project.
   c. Develop a hypothesis statement that examines the model's propositions in a sample from an acute care or community setting.
4. Donald, the nurse from the opening case study, applied the Neuman Systems Model as a framework for improving patient care in his DNP project. Considering your nursing specialty area, illustrate how one of the theories described in this chapter can be used to more comprehensively provide evidence-based care to your patient population. Discuss your ideas with your classmates.

REFERENCES

Abdellah, F. G., Beland, I. L., Martin, A., & Matheney, R. V. (1960). *Patient-centered approaches to nursing.* New York, NY: MacMillan.

Abdellah, F. G., Beland, I. L., Martin, A., & Matheney, R. V. (1973). *New directions in patient-centered nursing.* New York, NY: MacMillan.

Abdellah, F. G., & Levine, E. (1957). Developing a measure of patient and personnel satisfaction with nursing care. *Nursing Research,* 5(3), 100–108.

Abdellah, F. G., & Levine, E. (1994). *Preparing nursing research for the 21st century: Evolution, methodologies and challenges.* New York, NY: Springer Publishing.

Adu-Gyamfi, S., & Brenya, E. (2016). Nursing in Ghana: A search for Florence Nightingale in an African city. *International Scholarly Research Notices, 2016,* 9754845.

Allen, M. P. (1996). *Tribute to Virginia Avernal Henderson, 1897–1996 from the Interagency Council on Information Resources for Nursing (ICIRN).* Retrieved from http//www.sandiego.edu/nursing/theory/henderson.htm

Alligood, M. R. (2014). *Nursing theorists and their work* (8th ed.). St. Louis, MO: Mosby.

Artinian, N. T. (1991). Philosophy of science and family nursing theory development. In A. L. Whall & J. Fawcett (Eds.), *Family theory development in nursing.* Philadelphia, PA: F.A. Davis.

Attewell, A. (2012). *Illuminating Florence: Finding Nightingale's legacy in your practice.* Indianapolis, IN: Sigma Theta Tau International.

Beck, D. M. (2010). Expanding our Nightingale horizon: Seven recommendations for 21st-century nursing practice. *Journal of Holistic Nursing,* 28(4), 317–326.

Bekel, G. (2007). Dorothea E. Orem—1914–2007. *Nursing Science Quarterly,* 20(4), 302.

Benson, S. (1997). The older adult and fear of crime. *Journal of Gerontological Nursing,* 23(10), 25–31.

Berbiglia, V. A., & Banfield, B. (2014). Dorothea E. Orem: Self-care deficit theory of nursing. In M. R. Alligood (Ed.), *Nursing theorists and their work* (8th ed., pp. 240–257). St. Louis, MO: Mosby.

Biggs, A. (2008). "Toast crumbs"—memories of Dorothea Orem. *Self-Care, Dependent Care & Nursing,* 16(2), 5–6.

Bostridge, M. (2008). *Florence Nightingale: The making of an icon.* New York, NY: Farrar, Straus and Giroux.

Cody, W. K. (Ed.). (2013). *Philosophical and theoretical perspectives for advanced nursing practice* (5th ed.). Burlington, MA: Jones & Bartlett Learning.

Cromwell, J. L. (2013). *Florence Nightingale, feminist.* Jefferson, NC: McFarland.

Damus, K. (1980). An application of the Johnson behavioral system model for nursing practice. In J. P. Riehl & C. Roy (Eds.), *Conceptual models for nursing practice* (2nd ed., pp. 274–289). New York, NY: Appleton-Century-Crofts.

Dee, V. (1990). Implementation of the Johnson model: One hospital's experience. In M. E. Parker (Ed.), *Nursing theories in practice* (pp. 33–44). New York, NY: National League for Nursing Press.

DeGuzman, P. B., & Kulbok, P. A. (2012). Changing health outcomes of vulnerable populations through nursing's influence on neighborhood built environment: A framework for nursing research. *Journal of Nursing Scholarship,* 44(4), 341–348.

Derdiarian, A. K. (1990). The relationships among the subsystems of Johnson's behavioral system model. *Image—The Journal of Nursing Scholarship,* 22(4), 219–225.

Derdiarian, A. K., & Schobel, D. (1990). Comprehensive assessment of AIDS patients using the behavioural systems model for nursing practice instrument. *Journal of Advanced Nursing,* 15(4), 436–446.

Dickoff, J., James, P., & Wiedenbach, E. (1968). Theory in a practice discipline. 1: Practice oriented discipline. *Nursing Research,* 17(5), 415–435.

Dossey, B. M. (2010a). Florence Nightingale: Her Crimean fever and chronic illness. *Journal of Holistic Nursing,* 28(1), 38–53.

Dossey, B. M. (2010b). *Florence Nightingale: Mystic, visionary, healer.* Philadelphia, PA: F.A. Davis.

Dossey, B. M., Selanders, L. C., Beck, D. M., & Attewell, A. (2005). *Florence Nightingale today: Healing, leadership, global action.* Silver Spring, MD: American Nurses Association.

Englebright, J., Aldrich, K., & Taylor, C. R. (2014). Defining and incorporating basic nursing care actions into the electronic health record. *Journal of Nursing Scholarship,* 46(1), 50–57. doi:10.1111/jnu.12057

Fruehwirth, S. E. S. (1989). An application of Johnson's behavioral model: A case study. *Journal of Community Health Nursing,* 6(2), 61–71.

Grubbs, J. (1980). The Johnson behavioral system model. In J. P. Riehl & C. Roy (Eds.), *Conceptual models for nursing practice* (2nd ed., pp. 217–254). New York, NY: Appleton-Century-Crofts.

Haddad, V. C. N., & Santos, T. C. F. (2011). The environmental theory by Florence Nightingale in the reaching of the Nursing School Anna Nery. *Escola Anna Nery Revista de Enfermagen,* 15(4), 765–761.

Hegge, M. (2013). Nightingale's environmental theory. *Nursing Science Quarterly,* 26(3), 211–219.

Henderson, V. (1965). The nature of nursing. *International Nursing Review,* 12(1). Reprinted in E. J. Halloran (Ed.). (1995). *A Virginia Henderson reader: Excellence in nursing* (pp. 213–223). New York, NY: Springer Publishing.

Henderson, V. (1991). *The nature of nursing: Reflections after 25 years.* New York, NY: National League for Nursing Press.

Herrmann, E. K. (Ed.). (1998). *Virginia Avenel Henderson: Signature for nursing.* Indianapolis, IN: Sigma Theta Tau International Center Nursing Press.

Holaday, B. (1980). Implementing the Johnson model for nursing practice. In J. P. Riehl & C. Roy (Eds.), *Conceptual models for nursing practice* (2nd ed., pp. 255–263). New York, NY: Appleton-Century-Crofts.

Holaday, B. (2014). Dorothy E. Johnson: Behavioral System Model. In M.R. Alligood (ed.), *Nursing theorists and their work* (8th ed., pp. 332–356). St. Louis, MO: Mosby.

Jacobs, B. B. (2001). Respect for human dignity: A central phenomenon to philosophically unite nursing theory and practice through consilience of knowledge. *ANS. Advances in Nursing Science,* 24(1), 17–35.

Jetha, Z. A. (2015). Case study: Nursing care in the lance of Florence Nightingale. *i-Manager's Journal on Nursing,* 4(4), 32–36.

Johnson, D. E. (1959a). A philosophy of nursing. *Nursing Outlook,* 7(4), 198–200.

Johnson, D. E. (1959b). The nature of nursing science. *Nursing Outlook,* 7(5), 291–294.

Johnson, D. E. (1968). Theory in nursing: Borrowed and unique. *Nursing Research,* 17(3), 206–209.

Johnson, D. E. (1974). Development of a theory: A requisite for nursing as a primary health profession. *Nursing Research,* 23(5), 372–377. Reprinted in L. H. Nichol (Ed.). (1997). *Perspectives on nursing theory* (3rd ed., pp. 219–225). Philadelphia, PA: Lippincott-Raven.

Johnson, D. E. (1980). The behavioral system model for nursing. In J. P. Riehl & C. Roy (Eds.), *Conceptual models for nursing practice* (2nd ed., pp. 207–216). New York, NY: Appleton-Century-Crofts.

Johnson, D. E. (1990). The behavioral system model for nursing. In M. E. Parker (Ed.), *Nursing theories in practice* (pp. 23–32). New York, NY: National League for Nursing Press.

Johnson, D. E. (1997). Author's comments. In L. H. Nichol (Ed.), *Perspectives on nursing theory* (3rd ed., pp. 225–405). Philadelphia, PA: Lippincott-Raven.

Kagan, S. H. (2014). Florence Nightingale's notes on nursing and the determinants of health. *Cancer Nursing,* 37(6), 478.

Lawson, T. G. (2014). Betty Neuman: Systems model. In M. R. Alligood (Ed.), *Nursing theorists and their work* (8th ed., pp. 281–302). St. Louis, MO: Mosby.

Lazenby, M. (2013). On the humanities of nursing. *Nursing Outlook,* 61(1), e9–e14. doi:10.1016/j.outlook.2012.06.018

Mackey, A., & Bassendowski, S. (2017). The history of evidence-based practice in nursing education and practice. *Journal of Professional Nursing,* 3(1), 51–55.

Masters, K. (2015). *Nursing theories: A framework for professional practice* (2nd ed.). Burlington, MA: Jones & Bartlett.

McDonald, L. (2010). Florence Nightingale: Passionate statistician. *Journal of Holistic Nursing,* 28(1), 92–98.

McDonald, L. (2014). Florence Nightingale and Irish nursing. *Journal of Clinical Nursing, 23*(17–18), 2424–2433. doi:10.1111/jocn.12598

Murphy, G., Bernardo, A., & Dalton, J. (2013). Quiet at night: Implementing a Nightingale principle. *The American Journal of Nursing, 113*(12), 4351.

Neuman, B. M., & Fawcett, J. (2002). *The Neuman systems model* (4th ed.). Upper Saddle River, NJ: Prentice-Hall.

Neuman, B. M., & Fawcett, J. (2011). *The Neuman systems model* (5th ed.). Upper Saddle River, NJ: Pearson.

Nightingale, F. (1893/1954). Sick-nursing and health-nursing. In A. Burdett-Clouts (Ed.), *Women's mission: A series of congress papers of the philanthropic work of women by eminent writers.* New York, NY: Charles Scribner's Sons. Reprinted in L. R. Seymer (Ed.). (1954). *Selected writings of Florence Nightingale.* New York, NY: MacMillan.

Nightingale, F. (1860/1957/1969). *Notes on nursing: What it is and what it is not.* New York, NY: Dover Publications.

O'Malley, J. (1996). A nursing legacy: Virginia Henderson. *Advanced Practice Nursing Quarterly, 2*(2), v–vii.

Orem, D. E. (1956). *Hospital nursing service: An analysis.* Indianapolis, IN: Division of Hospital and Institutional Services, Indiana State Board of Health.

Orem, D. E. (1971). *Nursing: Concepts of practice.* New York, NY: McGraw-Hill.

Orem, D. E. (1985a). A concept of self-care for the rehabilitation client. *Rehabilitation Nursing, 10*, 33–36.

Orem, D. E. (1985b). *Nursing: Concepts of practice* (3rd ed.). New York, NY: McGraw-Hill.

Orem, D. E. (1991). *Nursing: Concepts of practice* (4th ed.). St. Louis, MO: Mosby.

Orem, D. E. (1995). *Nursing: Concepts of practice* (5th ed.). St. Louis, MO: Mosby.

Orem, D. E. (2001). *Nursing: Concepts of practice* (6th ed.). St. Louis, MO: Mosby.

Pfettscher, S. A. (2014). Florence Nightingale: Modern nursing. In M. R. Alligood (Ed.), *Nursing theorists and their work* (8th ed., pp. 60–78). St. Louis, MO: Mosby.

Poster, E. C., Dee, V., & Randell, B. P. (1997). The Johnson behavioral systems model as a framework for patient outcome evaluation. *Journal of the American Psychiatric Nursing Association, 3*(3), 73–80.

Rahim, S. (2013). Clinical application of Nightingale's environmental theory. *Journal on Nursing, 3*(1), 43–46.

Rew, L., & Sands, D. (2010). Reflections: The joy of the research process. *Journal of Holistic Nursing, 28*(1), 99–100.

Scott, P. A., Matthews, A., & Kirwan, M. (2014). What is nursing in the 21st century and what does the 21st century health system require of nursing? *Nursing Philosophy, 15*, 23–34. doi:10.1111/nup.12032

Selanders, L. C. (2005a). Nightingale's foundational philosophy of nursing. In B. M. Dossey, L. C. Selanders, D. M. Beck, & A. Attewell (Eds.), *Florence Nightingale today: Healing, leadership, global action* (pp. 65–79). Silver Spring, MD: American Nurses Association.

Selanders, L. C. (2005b). Social change and leadership: Dynamic forces for nursing. In B. M. Dossey, L. C. Selanders, D. M. Beck, & A. Attewell (Eds.), *Florence Nightingale today: Healing, leadership, global action* (pp. 81–95). Silver Spring, MD: American Nurses Association.

Small, H. (1998). *Florence Nightingale: Avenging angel.* New York, NY: St. Martin's Press.

Tanyi, R. A., & Werner, J. S. (2008). Women's experience of spirituality within end-stage renal disease and hemodialysis. *Clinical Nursing Research, 17*(1), 32–49.

Taylor, S. G. (2011). Moving forward: Ramblings of an antique nurse. *Self-Care, Dependent-Care and Nursing, 16*(1), 61–65.

Taylor, S. G., Geden, E., Isaramalai, S., & Wongvatunyu, S. (2000). Orem's self-care deficit nursing theory: Its philosophic foundation and the state of the science. *Nursing Science Quarterly, 13*(2), 104–110.

Taylor, S. G., & Renpenning, K. (2011). *Self-care science, nursing theory and evidence-based practice.* New York, NY: Springer Publishing.

Turner-Henson, A. (1992). *Chronically ill children's mothers' perceptions of environmental variables* (Unpublished doctoral dissertation). University of Alabama at Birmingham, AL.

Waller-Wise, R. (2013). Utilizing Henderson's nursing theory in childbirth education. *International Journal of Childbirth Education, 28*(2), 30–34.

Younas, A., & Sommer, J. (2015). Integrating nursing theory and process into practice: Virginia's Henderson Need Theory. *International Journal of Caring Sciences, 8*(2), 443–450.

Zborowsky, T. (2014). The legacy of Florence Nightingale's environmental theory: Nursing research focusing on the impact of healthcare environments. *Health Environments Research & Design Journal, 7*(4), 19–34.

Zurakowski, T. L. (2005). Florence Nightingale: Pioneer in nursing knowledge development. In J. J. Fitzpatrick & A. L. Whall (Eds.), *Conceptual models of nursing: Analysis and application* (4th ed., pp. 21–45). Upper Saddle River, NJ: Pearson.

8

Grand Nursing Theories Based on Interactive Process

Evelyn M. Wills

Jean Willowby is a student in a master's of science in nursing program, working to become a pediatric nurse practitioner. For one of her practicum assignments, Jean must incorporate a nursing theory into her clinical work, using the theory as a guide. During an earlier course on theory, she read several nursing theories that focused on interactions between the client and the nurse and between the client and the health care system. She remembered that in the interaction models and theories, human beings are viewed as interacting wholes, and client problems are seen as multifactorial.

The theories that stress human interactions best fit Jean's personal philosophy of nursing because they take into account the complexities of the multitude of factors she believes to be part of clinical nursing practice. Like the perspective taken by interaction model theorists, Jean understands that at times, the results of interventions are unpredictable and that many elements in the client's background and environment have an effect on the outcomes of interventions. She also acknowledges that there are many interactions between clients and their environments, both internal and external, many of which cannot be measured.

To better prepare for the assignment, Jean studied several of the human interaction models and theories, focusing most of her attention on the works of Roy and King. But after discussing her thoughts with her professor, she was referred to the writings of Jean Watson (Watson, 2012). After reviewing the carative factors and the caritas processes, she decided that Watson's Human Caring Science best fit her pediatrics practice and determined that she would learn more about it.

As discussed in Chapter 6, interactive process nursing theories occupy a place between the needs-based theories of the 1950s and 1960s, most of which were philosophically grounded in the positivist school of thought, and the unitary process models, which are grounded in humanist philosophy, which expresses the belief that humans are unitary beings and energy fields in constant interaction with the universal energy field. The interactive theories, in contrast, are grounded in the postpositive schools of philosophy.

The theorists presented in this chapter believe that humans are holistic beings who interact with, and adapt to, situations in which they find themselves. These theorists ascribe to systems theory and agree that there is constant interaction between humans and their environments. In general, human interaction theorists believe that health is a value and that a continuum of health ranges from high-level wellness to illness. They acknowledge, however, that people with chronic illnesses may have healthy lives and live well despite their illnesses.

Nursing models that can be described as interactive process theories include Artinian's Intersystem Model; Erickson, Tomlin, and Swain's Modeling and Role-Modeling; King's Systems Framework and Theory of Goal Attainment; Roy's Adaptation Model; and Watson's Human Caring Science. Each is discussed in this chapter.

An attempt was made to ensure that a balanced approach was used in presenting the works of these theorists. However, some of the theories are quite complex (e.g., those of Erickson, Tomlin, and Swain; King; and Roy), whereas others (e.g., Watson) are quite parsimonious. Additionally, some of the models have been revised repeatedly (e.g., Artinian, King, Roy, and Watson). As a result, the sections dealing with some models are longer or more involved than others, but this does not imply that the works of any of the theorists discussed are more or less important to the discipline than others.

Barbara Artinian: The Intersystem Model

The Intersystem Model was first published in 1983 as the Intersystem Patient-Care Model (Artinian, 1983) and was later expanded to the Intersystem Model (Artinian, 1991). The second edition of Artinian's work was published in 2011, expanded on the previous model, and was renamed the Artinian Intersystem Model (AIM). Its focus is the nursing process using the AIM (Artinian, 2011).

Background of the Theorist

Barbara Artinian received her bachelor's degree from Wheaton College; master's degrees from Case Western Reserve University in Cleveland, Ohio, and the University of California, Los Angeles (UCLA); and her doctorate from the University of Southern California. Influenced by her education as a sociologist, Artinian developed a nursing model that used an intersystems approach and focused on the interactions between client and nurse (Artinian, 2011). She is currently professor emeritus of the School of Nursing at Azusa Pacific University, having taught graduate and undergraduate students in the areas of community health nursing, family theory, nursing theory, and qualitative research methods (Artinian, 2016).

Philosophic Underpinnings of the Theory

Several works were used in developing the components of the model. For example, *sense of coherence* (SOC), a social science construct proposed by Antonovsky, provided grounding for the concept *situational sense of coherence* (SSOC). The SSOC serves as a measure of the integrative potential of clients within the context of situations (Artinian, 2011) (Table 8-1 and Figure 8-1).

Additionally, the model of intrasystem analysis and intersystem interaction developed by Alfred Kuhn was refined by Artinian to explain client–nurse interaction processes in health care situations and for use in developing the nursing plan of care. Finally, the work of Maturana and Varela provided the conceptualization of the person as a perceiving, self-determining, self-regulating human system and explains the patient/client concept of the model (Artinian, 1997a).

Major Assumptions, Concepts, and Relationships

In the Intersystem Model, there is a differentiation between the human as a system (the intrasystem) and the interactive systems of individuals or groups, known as the intersystem (Artinian, 2011). The language of the Intersystem Model is scholarly English, and nonsexist language is used throughout.

Assumptions
A number of major assumptions of the model (Artinian, 1997a) are listed in Box 8-1.

Concepts
The Intersystem Model incorporates nursing's metaparadigm concepts of person, environment, and health and specifies the concept nursing action. Definitions for these concepts are presented in Table 8-2. Person is viewed as a "coherent being who continually strives to make sense of his or her world" (Artinian, 2011, p. 13). The person as an individual has biologic, psychosocial, and spiritual subsystems. Person may also be an aggregate, meaning a group of people, such as a family, community, or other aggregates. Environment includes internal and external environments and specifies developmental environment and situational environment as important to the interaction (Artinian, 2011).

Table 8-1   Relationship Between SOC and SSOC in Artinian's Model

Term	Definition
Sense of coherence (SOC)	The progenitor to the SSOC
Situational sense of coherence (SSOC)	The analytic structure for evaluating the effectiveness of interventions in the plan of care and the current level of health
Comprehensibility	The extent to which one perceives the stimuli present in the situational environment deriving from the internal and external environments as making cognitive sense, in that information is ordered, consistent, structured, and clear, versus disordered random or inexplicable
Meaningfulness	The extent to which one feels that the problem demands posed by the situation are worth investing energy in and are challenges for which meaning or purpose is sought rather than burdens.
Manageability	The extent to which one perceives that resources at one's disposal are adequate to meet the demands posed by stimuli present in the situation.

Source: Artinian (2011).

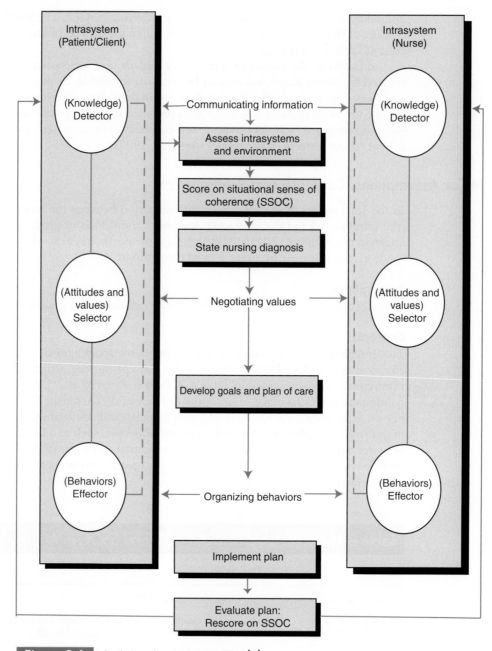

Figure 8-1 Artinian Intersystem Model.

(Republished with permission of John Wiley & Sons, from The Artinian intersystem model, Artinian, B. M., 2nd ed., © 2011; permission conveyed through Copyright Clearance Center, Inc.)

Health is viewed on a multidimensional continuum involving health/disease (Artinian, 2011). The focus is on stability and adaptation, and Artinian developed the concept of SSOC to measure adaptation. Health is defined as "a strong SOC" indicating that the person is confident and events are worth investing in and manageable (Artinian, 2011, p. 16).

Nursing is specified as "nursing action," which is identified by the mutual communication, negotiation, organization, and priorities of both the client and nurse intrasystems.

Box 8-1	Assumptions of Artinian's Intersystem Model

1. The human being exists within a framework of development and change, which is inherent to life.
2. The human's life is a unit of interrelated systems that is viewed as past and potential future.
3. Persons interact with the environment on the biologic level, and the senses are the mode of input from the environment; bodily functions are the mode for output.
4. The person's present can be seen in terms of his past and future.
5. The human spirit is at the center of the person's being, transcending time and affecting all aspects of life.
6. The nurse focuses on all aspects of the total person, systematically noting the interrelations of the systems and the relationships of the systems to time and environment.
7. The nursing process can take place only in the present.

Source: Artinian (1997a).

This is accomplished through intersystem interaction; feedback loops are necessary to produce a mutually determined plan of care (Artinian, 2011). One major innovation of this model is that client spirituality and values are important in the assessment of client needs and within the resulting nursing process.

Relationships

The Intersystem Model consists of two levels: the *intrasystem* and the *intersystem*. The intrasystem applies both to the client and to the nurse and focuses on the individual. The intersystem, by contrast, focuses on the interactions between the nurse and client (Artinian, 2011).

Table 8-2 Concepts of the Intersystem Model

Concept	Definition
Person	A coherent being who continually strives to make sense of his or her world. The person is a system, the subsystems of which are biologic, psychosocial, and spiritual. Subsystem configuration is such that "transactions among the subsystems result in emergent properties at the systemic level" (p. 13).
Environment	The environment has two dimensions: developmental and situational. The developmental environment is "all the events, factors, and influences that affect the system . . . as it passes through its developmental stages" (p. 14). This developmental environment provides the context for other developmental arenas such as the healing environment. Situational environment occurs when the nurse and client interact, and this includes all the details of the encounter.
Health	Health and disease are considered to be a multidimensional continuum. In the Intersystem Model, health is defined as having a strong sense of coherence (SOC) (p. 16).
Nursing	Those actions (interventions) that are needed to resolve concerns and move the client to a higher situational sense of coherence (SSOC). The nurse assesses the client's knowledge (comprehensibility of the problem), the available resources needed to manage the problem (manageability), and the client's motivation to meet the challenges posed by the problem (meaningfulness).

Source: Artinian (2011).

In the intrasystem model, three basic components comprise each intrasystem: the detector, selector, and effector. The detector processes information, the selector compares the situation with the attitudes and values of the individual, and the effector identifies behaviors relevant to the situation (Artinian, 2011).

The first step in an interaction in the intrasystem is to evaluate the detector domain, each person's knowledge of the problem. The detector incorporates knowledge about the internal environment (physical symptoms), social situations, the condition, treatment, and available resources. The selector allows the client and nurse to examine their attitudes and values in choosing a course of action that fits both patient/client and nurse. The effector is the behavioral level in which a response is selected from the repertoire of the behaviors available. This intrasystem level of the model provides the nurse with the capability of progressively clarifying with the client to bring about a mutual plan of care (Artinian, 2011).

The intersystem is seen when client and nurse interact, which occurs when nursing assistance is required (Artinian, 2011). Communication and negotiation between nurse and client lead to developing a plan of care. If the planned intervention is not effective, the determination is made that further assessment is necessary.

SOC and SSOC are the concepts that relate to health. In the intervention phase of the process, "Input is the nurse–client interaction to change the SSOC if it is judged to be low" (Artinian, 1997a, p. 13). Outcomes are scored on the SSOC by changes in knowledge, values and beliefs, and behaviors.

Usefulness

The Intersystem Model is relatively new; nonetheless, examples in nursing literature describing its use in practice and education are available. Indeed, it has been noted that the Glaserian grounded theory method of research as codified by Artinian (1998) for use specifically in nursing research has been used by her students for more than 20 years (McCallin, 2012; McCowan & Artinian, 2011).

Examples from the literature include an investigation by Giske and Artinian (2008) which studied adults aged 80 years and older in a Norwegian hospital who were undergoing gastroenterologic interventions. Findings indicate that participants were concerned with preparing themselves for life after their diagnosis, a difficult period for the participants. Bond and colleagues (2008) and a team lead by Cason (Cason et al., 2008) studied Hispanic students in baccalaureate nursing programs and found multiple barriers and supports. Also, examining educational issues was a work by Cone, Artinian, and West (2011) which looked at student issues in both undergraduate and graduate levels.

In clinical research, Critchley and Ball (2007) studied rheumatology patients using Artinian's descriptive qualitative method, and van Dover and Pfeiffer (2007) studied spiritual care of Christian clients of parish nurses. They developed a theory of spirituality for work in parish nursing. Finally, Vuckovich and Artinian (2005) investigated mental health nurses who administered medications to psychiatric patients and their methods of avoiding coercion.

Testability

The Intersystem Model has not been fully tested. Research studies applying the model primarily involve using grounded theory methodology to examine the meanings of events and the person's reactions to those events in the effort to formulate theories and hypotheses as noted earlier. In addition, the SSOC instrument has been used in research as a self-report instrument (Artinian, 1997b).

Parsimony

The model developed by Artinian (2011) is parsimonious and is explained in a logical and coherent way using two simple diagrams. It is not simplistic, however, and has multiple interacting elements. The more current model has expanded the diagrams to more thoroughly explain the aspects of the model as needed by both graduate and undergraduate students.

Value in Extending Nursing Science

The Intersystem Model has value in guiding education and in implementing practice. Its innovation is attention to the spirituality, goals, and values of both the client and nurse. Nurses use it in diverse clinical settings, such as psychiatric care, acute care, and community nursing. Several chapters, three books by the author and associates, and numerous journal articles have been generated by this model (Artinian, 1997a, 2011; Artinian, Giske, & Cone, 2009; Giske & Cone, 2012; Giske & Artinian, 2008; Treolar & Artinian, 2007).

Helen C. Erickson, Evelyn M. Tomlin, and Mary Ann P. Swain: Modeling and Role-Modeling

Modeling and Role-Modeling (MRM) is considered by its authors to be a theory and a paradigm. They constructed the theory from a multiplicity of resources that explain nurses' interactions with clients.

Background of the Theorists

Helen Erickson earned a diploma in nursing from Saginaw General Hospital in Saginaw, Michigan. She earned a bachelor's degree in nursing, a master's degree in psychiatric nursing, and a doctorate in educational psychology from the University of Michigan. Her career spans positions in nursing practice and education, both in the United States and abroad. She chaired the adult health nursing curriculum in the graduate program at the University of Texas at Austin and was a special assistant to the dean for graduate studies. She is professor emeritus of the University of Texas at Austin (M. E. Erickson, 2014).

Evelyn M. Tomlin was educated at Pasadena City College in Southern California and Los Angeles General Hospital School of Nursing. She received her bachelor's degree in nursing from the University of Southern California and her master's degree from the University of Michigan. She has had varied experiences in practice and education, including medical-surgical nursing, maternity, and pediatric nursing. Tomlin retired as a member of the faculty at the University of Michigan (M. E. Erickson, 2014).

Mary Ann P. Swain was educated in psychology at DePauw University in Greencastle, Indiana, and earned master's and doctoral degrees from the University of Michigan. She taught research methods in psychology at DePauw University and at the University of Michigan. She also served as the director of the doctoral program in nursing at the University of Michigan for a year and assumed the role of chairperson of nursing research from 1977 to 1982. Later, she was professor of nursing research at the University of Michigan and, in 1983, was appointed the associate vice president for academic affairs at the same university. Swain recently retired from her position as a provost for the New York State University system (M. E. Erickson, 2014).

Philosophical Underpinnings of the Theory

A number of theoretical works served as the foundation for MRM. Indeed, MRM is a synthesis of the foundational works of Maslow, Milton Erickson, Piaget, Bowlby, Winnicott, Engel, Lindemann, Selye, Lazarus, and Seligman (M. E. Erickson, 2014).

Philosophically, H. C. Erickson, Tomlin, and Swain (1983) believe "that nursing is a process between the nurse and client and requires an interpersonal and interactive nurse–client relationship" (p. 43). For this reason, their work is considered to be human interaction theory.

Major Assumptions, Concepts, and Relationships

Assumptions

Assumptions about adaptation and nursing are proposed in the MRM theory; the authors state that adaptation "is an innate drive toward holistic health, growth, and development. Self-healing, recovery and renewal, and adaptation are all instinctual despite the aging process or inherent malformations" (H. C. Erickson et al., 1983, p. 47).

When describing nursing, it is assumed that (1) "nursing is the nurturance of holistic self-care"; (2) "nursing is assisting persons holistically to use their adaptive strengths to attain and maintain optimum biopsychosocial-spiritual functioning"; (3) "nursing is helping with self-care to gain optimum health"; and (4) "nursing is an integrated and integrative helping of persons to better care for themselves" (H. C. Erickson et al., 1983, p. 50).

Concepts

The MRM theory contains a detailed set of concepts, and a glossary is provided in their work that assists in its comprehension. Table 8-3 provides definitions for some of the major concepts.

Relationships

The active potential assessment model (APAM) directs nursing assessment in the MRM theory. The APAM is a synthesis of Selye's general adaptation syndrome and Engel's response to stressors (H. C. Erickson et al., 1983). The APAM assists the nurse in predicting a client's potential to cope and is used to assess three states: equilibrium, arousal, and impoverishment. Equilibrium has two facets: adaptive and maladaptive. People in equilibrium have potential for mobilizing resources; those in maladaptive equilibrium have fewer resources.

Both arousal and impoverishment are considered to be states of stress in which mobilizing resources are expected. Persons in impoverishment have diminished or depleted abilities for mobilizing resources. People move between the states as their capacities to meet stress change. The APAM is considered dynamic rather than unidirectional and depends on the person's abilities to mobilize resources. Nursing interventions influence the person's ability to mobilize resources and move from impoverishment to equilibrium within the APAM (H. C. Erickson et al., 1983).

From the data collected, a client model is developed with a description of the functional relationship among the factors. Etiologic factors are analyzed, and possible therapeutic interventions are devised recognizing possible conflicts with treatment plans of other health professionals. Diagnoses and goals are established to complete the planning process (H. C. Erickson et al., 1983).

The success of the process is predicated on nurse's coming to know the client. The five aims of nursing interventions are building trust, promoting the client's

Table 8-3 Major Concepts of the Modeling and Role-Modeling Theory

Concept	Definition
Holism	The idea that "human beings have multiple interacting subsystems including genetic make up and spiritual drive, body, mind, emotion, and spirit are a total unit and act together, affecting and controlling one another interactively" (p. 44).
Health	"The state of physical, mental, and social well-being, not merely the absence of disease or infirmity" (p. 46).
Lifetime growth and development	Lifetime growth and development are continuous processes. When needs are met, growth and development promote health.
Affiliated-individuation	The dependence on support systems while maintaining the independence of the individual.
Adaptation	The individual's response to external and internal stressors in a health- and growth-directed manner. The opposite is maladaptation, which is the taxing of the system when the individual is "unable to engage constructive coping methods or mobilize appropriate resources to contend with the stressor(s)" (p. 47).
Self-care	Knowledge, resources, and action of the client; knowledge considers what has made the client sick, what will make him or her well, and "the mobilization of internal resources, and acquisition of additional resources to gain, maintain, or promote an optimal level of holistic health" (p. 48).
Nursing	"The holistic helping of persons with their self-care activities in relation to their health—an interactive, interpersonal process that nurtures strengths to achieve a state of perceived holistic health" (p. 49).
Modeling	The process by which the nurse seeks to understand the client's unique model of the world.
Role-modeling	The process by which the nurse understands the client's unique model within the context of scientific theories and uses the model to plan interventions that promote health for the client.

Source: H. C. Erickson et al. (1983).

positive orientation, promoting the client's control, affirming and promoting the client's strength, and setting health-directed mutual goals while meeting the client's needs (e.g., biophysical, safety and security, love and belonging, esteem, and self-esteem) (H. C. Erickson et al., 1983; M. E. Erickson, 2014).

Usefulness

The model has been the basis for a series of conferences incorporating MRM into research, practice settings, and curricula. Adherents of the theory state that it has been used in courses or in the curricula of several universities. These include East Carolina University, Greenville, North Carolina; Harding University School of Nursing, Searcy, Arkansas; Metropolitan State University, St. Paul, Minnesota; St. Catherine University School of Nursing, St. Paul, Minnesota; University of Texas at Austin School of Nursing, Austin, Texas; Washtenaw Community College School of Nursing, Ann Arbor, Michigan; and Lamar University Department of Nursing, Beaumont, Texas (M. E. Erickson, 2014).

| Box 8-2 | Examples of Research Studies Using Modeling and Role-Modeling Theory |

Goldstein, L. A. (2013). *Relationships among quality of life, self-care, and affiliated individuation in persons on chronic warfarin therapy* (Doctoral dissertation). University of Texas, Austin, TX. Retrieved from https://repositories.lib.utexas.edu/handle /2152/21865

Gregg, S. R., & Twibell, K. R. (2016). Try-It-On: Experiential learning of holistic stress management in a graduate nursing curriculum. *Journal of Holistic Nursing, 34*(3), 300–308. doi:10.1177/0898010115611788

Koren, M. E., & Papamiditriou, C. (2013). Spirituality of staff nurses: Application of modeling and role modeling theory. *Holistic Nursing Practice, 27*(1), 37–44.

Merryfeather, L. (2015). Passionate scholarship or academic safety: An ethical issue. *Journal of Holistic Nursing, 33*(1), 60–67.

Testability

MRM provides assumptions and relationships that are amenable to testing and have been and continue to be tested in research. The model has been used by nurses who have studied with Erickson, Tomlin, and Swain, and many theses and dissertations have incorporated elements of the model. Box 8-2 lists some of the current works using MRM in research.

Parsimony

The MRM theory is not parsimonious. Its complexity, however, reflects human beings, to whom it applies. MRM incorporates several borrowed theories that are synthesized for use in nursing science. The many linkages among the concepts and multiple levels need to be addressed, and considerable explanation is needed to enhance understanding of the tenets of the theory for nursing practice and for client care activities. However, nurses who use the theory are grateful for the fit it has with their practice.

Value in Extending Nursing Science

In addition to the uses of MRM in nursing education, practice, and research, three middle range nursing theories have been based on MRM. Acton (1997) developed a model describing affiliated-individuation, Irvin and Acton (1996) described caregiver stress, and Rogers (1996) discussed the concept of facilitative affiliation.

MRM theory is used in education, practice, and research. Research has been completed with people of all ages and with those who are suffering from many different health problems. According to those who espouse the theory, its major attraction is that it is practical, reflects the domain of nursing, and is a realistic model for guiding research, practice, and education.

Imogene King: King's Conceptual System and Theory of Goal Attainment and Transactional Process

King's theory evolved from early writings about theory development. In her first book in 1971, she synthesized scholarship from nursing and related disciplines into a theory for nursing (King, 1971). She wrote the Theory of Goal Attainment in 1980.

The most recent edition (King, 1995a) contains further refinements and more de-tailed explanation of the general nursing framework and the theory.

Background of the Theorist

Imogene King graduated from St. John's Hospital School of Nursing in St. Louis, Missouri, with a diploma in nursing in 1945. She received a bachelor of science in nursing education from St. Louis University in 1948 and a master's of science in nurs-ing from the same school in 1957. In 1961, she received the doctor of education de-gree from Teacher's College, Columbia University, in New York (Sieloff & Messmer, 2014). She held a variety of staff nursing, educational, research, and administrative roles throughout her professional life. She worked as a research consultant for the Division of Nursing in the Department of Health, Education, and Welfare for several years before moving to Tampa, Florida, in 1980, assuming the position of professor at the University of South Florida College of Nursing (Sieloff & Messmer, 2014). She remained active in professional organizations for many years. When she died in 2008, her work was widely celebrated by her colleagues (Mensik, 2008; Mitchell, 2008; Smith, Wright, & Fawcet, 2008; Stevens & Messmer, 2008).

Philosophical Underpinnings of the Theory

The von Bertalanffy General Systems Model is acknowledged to be the basis for King's work. She stated that the science of wholeness elucidated in that model gave her hope that the complexity of nursing could be studied "as an organized whole" (King, 1995b, p. 23).

Major Assumptions, Concepts, and Relationships

King's conceptual system and theory contain many concepts and multiple assumptions and relationships. A few of the assumptions, concepts, and relationships are presented in the following sections. The scholar wishing to use King's model or theory is referred to the original writings as both the model and theory are complex (Figure 8-2).

Assumptions

The Theory of Goal Attainment lists several assumptions relating to individuals, nurse–client interactions, and nursing. When describing individuals, the model shows that individuals (1) are social, sentient, rational, reacting beings and (2) are controlling, purposeful, action oriented, and time oriented in their behavior (King, 1995b).

Regarding nurse–client interactions, King (1981) believed that (1) perceptions of the nurse and client influence the interaction process; (2) goals, needs, and values of the nurse and client influence the interaction process; (3) individuals have a right to knowledge about themselves; (4) individuals have a right to participate in decisions that influence their lives, health, and community services; (5) individuals have a right to accept or reject care; and (6) goals of health professionals and goals of recipients of health care may not be congruent.

With regard to nursing, King (1995b) wrote that (1) nursing is the care of human beings; (2) nursing is perceiving, thinking, relating, judging, and acting vis-à-vis the behavior of individuals who come to a health care system; (3) a nursing situation is the immediate environment in which two individuals establish a relationship to cope with situational events; and (4) the goal of nursing is to help individuals and groups attain, maintain, and restore health. If this is not possible, nurses help individuals die with dignity.

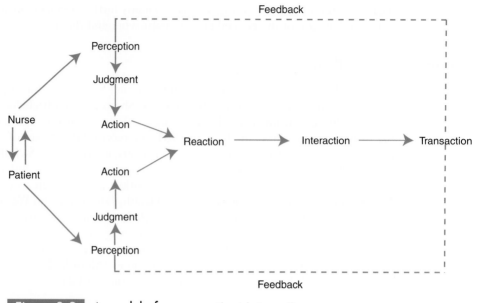

Feedback

Figure 8-2   A model of nurse–patient interactions.

(Source: King, I. M. [1981]. *A theory for nursing: Systems, concepts, process* [p. 61]. Reprinted with permission of Sage Publications.)

Concepts

King's Theory of Goal Attainment defines the metaparadigm concepts of nursing as well as a number of additional concepts. Table 8-4 lists some of the major concepts.

Relationships

The Theory of Goal Attainment encompasses a great many relationships, many of them complex. King organized them into useful propositions that enhance the understanding of the relationships of the theory. A review of some relationships among the theory's concepts follows:

- Nurse and client are purposeful interacting systems.
- Nurse and client perceptions, judgments, and actions, if congruent, lead to goal-directed transactions.
- If perceptual accuracy is present in nurse–client interactions, transactions will occur.
- If nurse and client make transactions, goals will be attained.
- If goals are attained, satisfaction will occur.
- If goals are attained, effective nursing care will occur.
- If transactions are made in nurse–client interactions, growth and development will be enhanced.
- If role expectations and role performance as perceived by nurse and client are congruent, transactions will occur.
- If role conflict is experienced by nurse or client or both, stress in nurse–client interactions will occur.
- If nurses with special knowledge and skills communicate appropriate information to clients, mutual goal setting and goal attainment will occur (King, 1981, pp. 61, 149).

Table 8-4 Major Concepts of the Theory of Goal Attainment

Concept	Definition
Nursing	A process of action, reaction, and interaction whereby nurse and client share information about their perceptions in the nursing situation. The nurse and client share specific goals, problems, and concerns and explore means to achieve a goal.
Health	A dynamic life experience of a human being, which implies continuous adjustment to stressors in the internal and external environment through optimum use of one's resources to achieve maximum potential for daily living.
Individuals	Social beings who are rational and sentient. Humans communicate their thoughts, actions, customs, and beliefs through language. Persons exhibit common characteristics such as the ability to perceive, to think, to feel, to choose between alternative courses of action, to set goals, to select the means to achieve goals, and to make decisions.
Environment	The background for human interactions. It is both external to and internal to the individual.
Perception	The process of human transactions with environment. It involves organizing, interpreting, and transforming information from sensory data and memory.
Communication	A process by which information is given from one person to another, either directly in face-to-face meetings or indirectly. It involves intrapersonal and interpersonal exchanges.
Interaction	A process of perception and communication between person and environment and between person and person represented by verbal and nonverbal behaviors that are goal-directed.
Transaction	A process of interactions in which human beings communicate with the environment to achieve goals that are valued; transactions are goal-directed human behaviors.
Stress	A dynamic state in which a human interacts with the environment to maintain balance for growth, development, and performance; it is the exchange of information between human and environment for regulation and control of stressors.

Source: King (1981).

Usefulness

King's Theory of Goal Attainment has enhanced nursing education. For example, it served as a framework for the baccalaureate program at the Ohio State University School of Nursing, where it determined the content and processes taught at each level of the program (Daubenmire, 1989). Similarly, in Sweden, King's model was used to organize nursing education (Frey, Rooke, Sieloff, Messmer, & Kameoka, 1995). In more recent years, King's model has been useful in nursing education programs in Sweden, Portugal, Canada, and Japan (Sieloff & Messmer, 2014).

King's conceptual system is an organizing guide for nursing practice. In one example, Caceres (2015) used King's Theory of Goal Attainment to explore and expand upon the concept of functional status, concluding that evaluation of functional status is vital and should be incorporated within mutual decision-making processes from the client family's perspective. M. L. Joseph, Laughon, and Bogue (2011) examined the "sustainable adoption of whole-person care" (p. 989) in a Florida hospital guided by

King's Theory of Goal Attainment. Finally, Gemmill and colleagues (2011) assessed nurses' knowledge about and attitudes toward ostomy care using King's Theory of Goal Attainment to guide the research. Their findings explained that it is difficult for staff nurses to maintain their clinical abilities when there are few opportunities. Maintaining currency may require creative teaching interventions, such as simulations.

Testability

Parts of the Theory of Goal Attainment have been tested, and a number of research studies reported in the literature used the model as a conceptual framework. For example, recent research includes a study by L. Joseph (2013) who used King's Theory of Goal Attainment to evaluate the effectiveness of a teaching program to improve accuracy on pediatric growth measurements. In other works, Chacko, Kharde, and Swamy (2013) used King's theory as the framework to assess the efficacy of use of infrared lamps on reducing pain and inflammation due to episiotomy, and Isac, Venkatesaperumal, and D'Sousa (2013) used King's theory to develop and evaluate the efficacy of a nurse-led information desk on assisting patients to manage their sickle cell disease.

Parsimony

The conceptual system and theory were presented together in several versions of King's writings and remain largely as written in 1981. The theory is not parsimonious, having numerous concepts, multiple assumptions, many statements, and many relationships on a number of levels. This complexity, however, mirrors the complexity of human transactions for goal attainment. The model is general and universal and can be the umbrella for many midrange and practice theories.

Value in Extending Nursing Science

In addition to application in practice and research described previously, King's work has been the basis for development of several middle range nursing theories. For example, the Theory of Goal Attainment was used by Rooda (1992) to develop a model for multicultural nursing practice. King's Systems Framework was reportedly used by Alligood and May (2000) to develop a theory of personal system empathy and by Doornbos (2000) to derive a middle range theory of family health.

King's conceptual system and theory have been used internationally in Australia, Brazil, Canada, Pakistan, and Sweden, as well as in numerous university nursing programs in the United States, and have provided a foundation for many research studies. Her work has extended nursing science by its usefulness in education, practice, and research across international boundaries (King, 2001; Sieloff & Messmer, 2014).

Sister Callista Roy: The Roy Adaptation Model

The Roy Adaptation Model (RAM) focuses on the interrelatedness of four adaptive systems. Like many of the models/theories in this unit, it is a deductive theory based on nursing practice. The RAM guides the nurse who is interested in physiologic adaptation as well as the nurse who is interested in psychosocial adaptation.

Background of the Theorist

Sister Callista Roy is a member of the Sisters of Saint Joseph of Carondelet. She received a bachelor of science in nursing from Mount Saint Mary's College in Los Angeles, California, a master's of science in nursing from UCLA, and a master's degree and doctorate in sociology from UCLA (Phillips & Harris, 2014). Roy first proposed the RAM while studying for her master's degree at UCLA, where Dorothy Johnson challenged students to develop conceptual models of nursing (Phillips & Harris, 2014; Roy, 2009). Her work is known internationally; she has presented at conferences in at least 36 countries and throughout the United States. She has received numerous honors and awards for her scholarly and professional work. She was an inaugural inductee into Sigma Theta Tau International's Nurse Researcher hall of fame. In 2007, she was awarded the American Academy of Nursing's Living Legend award. She is currently professor and nurse theorist at Boston College's Connell School of Nursing (Connell School of Nursing, 2016).

Philosophical Underpinnings of the Theory

Johnson's nursing model was the impetus for the development of the RAM. Roy also incorporated concepts from Helson's Adaptation Theory, von Bertalanffy's System Model, Rapoport's System Definition, the stress and adaptation theories of Dohrenrend and Selye, and the Coping Model of Lazarus (Phillips & Harris, 2014).

Major Assumptions, Concepts, and Relationships

Assumptions

In the RAM, assumptions are specified as philosophical, scientific, and cultural (Roy, 2009). Philosophical assumptions include:

- Persons have mutual relationships with the world and God.
- Human meaning is rooted in the omega point convergence of the universe.
- God is intimately revealed in the diversity of creation.
- Persons use human creative abilities of awareness, enlightenment, and faith.
- Persons are accountable for sustaining and transforming the universe (Roy, 2009, p. 31).

Scientific assumptions of the RAM for the 21st century include:

- Systems of matter and energy progress to higher levels of complex self-organization.
- Consciousness and meaning constitute person and environment integration.
- Self and environmental awareness is rooted in thinking and feeling.
- Human decisions account for integration of creative processes.
- Thinking and feeling mediate human action.
- System relationships include acceptance, protection, and fostering interdependence.
- Persons and the earth have common patterns and integral relationships.
- Person and environment transformations are created in human consciousness.
- Integration of human and environment results in adaptation (Roy, 2009, p. 1).

Cultural assumptions include:

- Cultural experiences influence how RAM is expressed.
- A concept central to the culture may influence the RAM to some extent.
- Cultural expressions of the RAM may lead to changes in practice activities such as nursing assessment.
- As RAM evolves within a culture, implications for nursing may differ from experience in the original culture (Roy, 2009, p. 31).

All elements of the model are part of the care of clients and groups. The nurse undertakes a bilevel assessment to accurately define the problem and come to decisions on the plan of care. The process in formulating the nursing plan is intricate and is prescriptive in its objectives.

Concepts
The RAM contains many defined concepts, including the metaparadigm concepts. Table 8-5 lists some of these.

Table 8-5 Major Concepts of the Roy Adaptation Model

Concept	Definition
Environment	Conditions, circumstances, and influences that affect the development and behavior of humans as adaptive systems.
Health	A state and process of being and becoming integrated and whole.
Person	"The human adaptive system" and defined as "a whole with parts that function as a unity for some purpose. Human systems include people groups organizations, communities, and society as a whole" (p. 31).
Goal of nursing	The "promotion of adaptation in each of the four modes" (p. 31).
Adaptation	The "process and outcome whereby thinking and feeling persons as individuals or in groups use conscious awareness and choice to create human and environmental integration" (p. 30).
Focal stimuli	Those stimuli that are the proximate causes of the situation.
Contextual stimuli	All other stimuli in the internal or external environment, which may or may not affect the situation.
Residual stimuli	Those immeasurable and unknowable stimuli that also exist and may affect the situation.
Cognator subsystem	"A major coping process involving four cognitive-emotive channels: perceptual and information processing, learning, judgment, and emotion" (p. 31).
Regulator subsystem	"A basic type of adaptive process that responds automatically through neural, chemical, and endocrine coping channels" (p. 46).
Stabilizer control processes	The structures and processes aimed at system maintenance and involving values and daily activities whereby participants accomplish the primary purpose of the group and contribute to the common purposes of the society.
Innovator control processes	The internal subsystem that involves structures and processes for growth.

Source: Roy and Andrews (1999).

Relationships

Roy's model is composed of four adaptive modes that constitute the specific categories that serve as framework for assessment (Figure 8-3). Through the four modes,
"Responses to and interaction with the client's environment are carried out and adaptation can be observed" (Roy, 2009, pp. 69–72).

They are the:

1. *Physiologic–physical mode*: Physical and chemical processes involved in the
   function and activities of living organisms; the underlying need is physiologic
   integrity: the degree of wholeness achieved through adaptation to changes
   in needs. In groups, this is the manner in which human systems manifest
   adaptation to basic operating resources.
2. *Self-concept–group identity mode*: Focuses on psychological and spiritual
   integrity and a sense of unity, meaning, and purposefulness in the universe.
3. *Role function mode*: Refers to the roles that individuals occupy in society
   fulfilling the need for social integrity; it is knowing who one is, in relation to
   others.
4. *Interdependence mode*: The close relationships of people and their purpose,
   structure, and development, individually and in groups, and the adaptation
   potential of these relationships.

Two subsystems require assessment in the RAM: the regulator and the cognator.
These are coping subsystems that allow the client to adapt and make changes when
stressed. The regulator is the physiologic coping subsystem, and the cognator is the

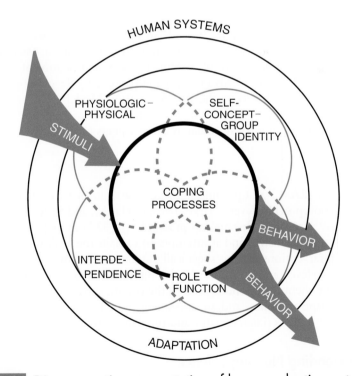

Figure 8-3   Diagrammatic representation of human adaptive systems.

(From Roy, S. C., & Andrews, H. A. The Roy Adaptation Model, 2nd ed., © 1998. Reprinted by permission
of Pearson Education, Inc., New York, New York.)

cognitive–emotive coping subsystem (Roy, 2009). In her writing, Roy (2011a) explained how the four modes work in communities and globally. She stated that "this theoretical work . . . portends well . . . for nurse scholars to meet the challenges . . . for the nursing role in the global community" (Roy, 2011a, p. 350).

Usefulness

The RAM has been used extensively to guide practice and to organize nursing education. International conferences on the RAM have been conducted across the United States and abroad (Roy, 2009). The RAM was adopted as a component of the curricular framework of such widely diverse colleges and departments of nursing as Mount Saint Mary's College Department of Nursing; the University of Texas at Austin School of Nursing; Boston College School of Nursing; and the nurse practitioner program at the University of Miami in Florida. The RAM has also been implemented internationally at the University of Ottawa School of Nursing and in university schools of nursing in Japan and France (Phillips & Harris, 2014).

Several middle range nursing theories derived from the RAM were recently compiled into a book edited by Roy (2014a). These included a middle range theory of coping (Roy, 2014b), a middle range theory of adapting to loss (Dobratz, 2014), and a middle range theory of adapting to chronic health conditions (Buckner & Hayden, 2014). Other examples from the literature are the middle range theory of adaptive spirituality (Dobratz, 2016) and a middle range theory of psychological adaptation (Lévesque, Ricard, Ducharme, Duquette, & Bonin, 1998).

Testability

The RAM is testable. Indeed, an international nursing society specifically focused on researching adaptation nursing, Roy Adaptation Association (RAA), is based in Boston College School of Nursing (Connell School of Nursing, 2016). The goal of the RAA is "to advance nursing practice by developing basic and clinical nursing knowledge based on the Roy Adaptation Model" (RAA, 2016), and the association meets regularly to present research efforts to that end. Box 8-3 lists a few recent examples of nursing research using aspects of the RAM.

Parsimony

The RAM is not parsimonious because of its many elements, systems, structures, and concepts. However, Clarke, Barone, Hanna, and Senesac (2011) state that the RAM is "accessible, elegant and practical" (p. 338) in its presentation. It is complete and comprehensive, and it attempts to explain the reality of the clients so that nursing interventions can be specifically targeted. The nursing assessment is conducted on two levels and is extensive and complex. It requires assessment of the stimuli to which the client is responding and of the coping subsystems. It targets the client in the four adaptive modes, and an assessment must be made to determine how effectively the subsystems (i.e., cognator and regulator) are working.

Value in Extending Nursing Science

The RAM has been a valuable asset in extending nursing science. Phillips and Harris (2014) summarized the impact of the RAM on nursing practice, education, and administration, stating that it has contributed significantly to the science and practice

Box 8-3   Examples of Studies Using the Roy Adaptation Model

Aber, C., Weiss, M., & Fawcett, J. (2013). Contemporary women's adaptation to motherhood: The first 3 to 6 weeks postpartum. *Nursing Science Quarterly, 26*(4), 344–351.

Akyil, R. Ç., & Ergüney, S. (2013). Roy's adaptation model-guided education for adaptation to chronic obstructive pulmonary disease. *Journal of Advanced Nursing, 69*(5), 1063–1075.

Bockwoldt, D., Staffileno, B. A., Coke, L., & Quinn, L. (2016). Perceptions of insulin treatment among African Americans with uncontrolled type 2 diabetes. *Journal of Transcultural Nursing, 27*(2), 172–180.

Buckner, B. S., & Buckner, E. B. (2015). Post-revolution Egypt: The Roy adaptation model in community. *Nursing Science Quarterly, 28*(4), 300–307.

Kaur, H., & Mahal, R. (2013). Development of nursing assessment tool: An application of Roy's adaptation theory. *International Journal of Nursing Education, 5*(1), 60–64.

Perrett, S. E., & Biley, F. C. (2013). A Roy model study of adapting to being HIV positive. *Nursing Science Quarterly, 26*(4), 337–343.

Pullen, L., Modrcin, M. A., McGuire, S. L., Lane, K., Kearnely, M., & Engle, S. (2015). Anger in adolescent communities: How angry are they? *Pediatric Nursing, 41*(3), 135–140.

Seah, X. Y., & Tham, X. C. (2015). Management of bulimia nervosa: A case study with the Roy adaptation model. *Nursing Science Quarterly, 28*(2), 136–141.

of nursing. Indeed, the RAM has generated hundreds of research studies and has contributed to nursing education for more than 35 years (Roy, 2011b). Frederickson (2011) states that chapters of the RAM society are present in such disparate areas such as several countries of South America as well as Japan, thus extending the reach of Roy's principles globally. Indeed, the RAM is used in almost every country in Europe, Asia, South America, and others as well (Clarke et al., 2011). Roy (2011a) states that " . . . the criteria for good . . . is to promote adaptation of individuals and groups; to transform a society to one that promotes dignity, and to sustain and transform the universe" (p. 346).

Jean Watson: Human Caring Science, A Theory of Nursing

Jean Watson's (2012) *Human Caring Science: A Theory of Nursing* is the title of Jean Watson's latest work. It was renamed "to convey a deeper human to human involvement and connection" (p. xi). This theory is one of the newest of nursing's grand theories, having first been completely codified in 1979, revised in 1985 (Watson, 1988), and broadened and advanced several times. Watson (1985) initially called her work a descriptive theory of caring and stated that it was the only theory of nursing to incorporate the spiritual dimension of nursing at the time it was first conceptualized. The theory is both deductive and inductive in its origins and is written at an abstract level of discourse.

It is somewhat difficult to categorize Watson's work with the works of other nursing theorists. It has many characteristics of a human interaction model, although it also incorporates many ideals of the unitary process theories, which are discussed in Chapter 9. Watson has always described the human as a holistic, interactive being and is now explicit in describing the human as an energy field and in explaining health and illness as manifestations of the human pattern (Watson, 2012), two tenets of the unitary process theories. Parse (2014) points out, however, that although theorists profess belief in unitary human beings, other definitions and relationships still separate theories from the interactive process paradigms and the unitary process nursing paradigms. Based on overall considerations, the philosophy and science of caring reflects the interactive process nursing theories.

Background of the Theorist

Jean Watson was born in West Virginia in 1939 and attended Lewis-Gale School of Nursing in Roanoke, Virginia. She earned a bachelor's degree in nursing, master's of science degrees in psychiatric–mental health nursing and sociology and a doctorate in educational psychology and counseling, all from the University of Colorado (Jesse & Alligood, 2014). Watson is an internationally published author, having written many books, book chapters, and articles about the science of human caring (Watson, 1994, 1996, 1999, 2005, 2008, 2012).

Watson was formerly dean of the School of Nursing at the University of Colorado, and she founded and directed the Center for Human Caring at the Health Sciences Center in Denver. She has received numerous awards and honors and is a distinguished professor of nursing and dean emerita at the University of Colorado Denver College of Nursing and Anschutz Medical Center, where she held an endowed chair in Caring Science for 16 years (Jesse & Alligood, 2014). She is a fellow of the American Academy of Nursing and past president of the National League for Nursing, and some of her honors include Fetzer Institute Norman Cousins Award; an International Kellogg Fellowship in Australia; a Fulbright research award in Sweden; and 10 honorary doctoral degrees, including those from Sweden, United Kingdom, Spain, British Columbia and Quebec in Canada, and Japan (Watson Caring Science Institute [WCSI] 2016a). Dr. Watson has been formally designated a "living legend in Nursing" by the American Academy of Nursing (WCSI, 2016a).

Philosophical Underpinnings of the Theory

Watson (1988) noted that she drew parts of her theory from nursing writers, including Nightingale and Rogers. She also used concepts from the works of psychologists Giorgi, Johnson, and Koch as well as concepts from philosophy. She reported being widely read in these disciplines and synthesized a number of diverse concepts from them into nursing as a science of human caring. Watson (2012) further conveys the ideal that changing the title and the use of the words "human caring" and "caring" are meant to convey the ideal of the depth of involvement between humans that is the experience of nurses (p. xi).

Major Assumptions, Concepts, and Relationships

The value system that permeates Watson's Human Caring Science includes a "deep respect for the wonders and mysteries of life" (Watson, 1988, p. 34) and recognition that spiritual and ethical dimensions are major elements of the human care process. Furthermore, she explained that in order to care for humans, there must be a deep responsibility to care for the planet itself (Watson, 2012). A number of assumptions are both stated and implicit in her theory. Additionally, several concepts were defined, refined, and adapted for it. From this, 10 carative factors were developed (Box 8-4).

Box 8-4   Watson's 10 Carative Processes

1. Practicing loving-kindness and equanimity within context of caring consciousness
2. Being authentically present and enabling, and sustaining the deep belief system and subjective life world of self and one-being cared for
3. Cultivating one's own spiritual practices and transpersonal self, going beyond ego-self
4. Developing and sustaining a helping–trusting, authentic, caring relationship
5. Being present to and supportive of the expression of positive and negative feelings
6. Creatively using self and all ways of knowing as part of the caring process; engaging in artistry of caring-healing practices
7. Engaging in genuine teaching–learning experience that attends to wholeness and meaning, attempting to stay within other's frame of reference
8. Creating healing environment at all levels, whereby wholeness, beauty, comfort, dignity, and peace are potentiated
9. Assisting with basic needs, with an intentional caring consciousness, administering "human care essentials" which potentiate alignment of mind-body-spirit, wholeness in all aspects of care
10. Opening and attending to mysterious dimensions of one's life-death; soul care for self and the one-being-cared for; "allowing and being open to miracles"

Source: Watson Caring Science Institute (2016b).

Assumptions

Watson (2012) describes the tenets of human caring science. She proposed that caring and love are universal and mysterious "cosmic forces" that comprise the primal and universal psychic energy. She believes that health professionals make social, moral, and scientific contributions to humankind and that nurses' caring ideal can affect human development. Furthermore, she explained that it is critical in today's society to sustain human caring ideals and a caring ideology in practice, as there has been a proliferation of radical treatment and "cure techniques," often without regard to costs or human considerations. She concluded that human caring goes "beyond objectivism, verification, rigid operations, and definitions, and concern itself more with meaning, relationships, intersubjective and intrasubjective context and patterns"(Watson, 2012, p. 2).

Explicit assumptions that were derived for Watson's (2005) work include:

- An ontologic assumption of oneness, wholeness, unity, relatedness, and connectedness.
- An epistemologic assumption that there are multiple ways of knowing.
- Diversity of knowing assumes all, and various forms of evidence can be included.
- A caring science model makes these diverse perspectives explicitly and directly.
- Moral-metaphysical integration with science evokes spirit; this orientation is not only possible but also necessary for our science, humanity, society-civilization, and world-planet.
- A caring science emergence, founded on new assumptions, makes explicit an expanding unitary, energetic worldview with a relational human caring ethic and ontology as its starting point.

Concepts

Watson (2012) defined three of the four metaparadigm concepts (human, health, and nursing). She coined several other concepts and terms that are integral to

Table 8-6 Major Concepts of the Science of Human Caring

Concept	Definition
Human	"A unique, valued and precious person . . . to be cared for, respected, nurtured, understood, and assisted" (p. 19).
Health	". . . subjective experience . . . unity and harmony with body-mind-spirit. Health is associated with the degree of congruence between the self as perceived and the self as experienced" (p. 60).
Nursing	"A human caring science of persons and human health–illness experiences that are mediated by professional, personal, scientific, esthetic, and ethical human care connections and relationships" (p. 66).
Actual caring moment occasion	"Involves actions and choice both by the nurse and the individual. The moment of coming together in a caring moment occasion presents the two persons with the opportunity to decide how to be in the relationship—what to do with the moment" (p. 71).
Transpersonal caring moment	"Includes the nurse's consciousness, intentionality and unique energetic health presence . . . in which he or she transmits and reflects the person's condition back to that person . . . in a way that allows for the release and flow of his or her intersubjective feelings and thoughts and pent-up energy. . . it opens up shared access to spirit-filled source of infinity" (p. 70).
Phenomenal field	"The totality of human experience (one's being in the world) . . . is the individual's frame of reference that can only be known to that person" (p. 67).
Life	"Human life . . . is defined as spiritually, mentally, emotionally and physically being-in-the-world as a unitary being which is continuous in time and space" (p. 59).
Harmony-disharmony	"Where there is disharmony among the mind, body and soul or between a person and his or her nature and relationship with the larger world/universe, there is a disjunctive between the self as perceived and one's actual experience . . . If there is harmony and unity of mind-body-spirit, then a sense of congruence exists . . . between the self as perceived and the self as experienced by the person" (p. 69).
Time	"The present is more subjectively real and the past is both objectively and subjectively real. The past is prior to, or in a different mode of being, than the present, but it is not clearly distinguishable. Past, present, and future instants merge and fuse" (p. 73).

Source: Watson (2012).

understanding the science of human caring (Table 8-6). Her 10 caritas processes are caring needs specific to human experiences that should be addressed by nurses with their clients in the caring role (Watson, 2012; WCSI, 2016b). The carative processes are listed in Box 8-4.

Relationships

Watson has refined and updated the relationships of the theory, bringing them closer to her current way of understanding human caring and spirituality. Her continued study has involved lengthy examination of her beliefs about caring, spirituality, and human and energy fields (Watson, 2005, 2008). The following are some of the relationships of the theory:

- A transpersonal caring field resides within a unitary field of consciousness and energy that transcends time, space, and physicality.
- A transpersonal caring relationship connotes a spirit-to-spirit unitary connection within a caring moment, honoring the embodied spirit of both practitioner and patient within a unitary field of consciousness.
- A transpersonal caring relationship transcends the ego level of both practitioner and patient, creating a caring field with new possibilities for how to be in the moment.
- The practitioner's authentic intentionality and consciousness of caring has a higher frequency of energy than noncaring consciousness, opening up connections to the universal field of consciousness and greater access to one's inner healer.
- Transpersonal caring is communicated via the practitioner's energetic patterns of consciousness, intentionality, and authentic presence in a caring relationship.
- Caring-healing modalities are often noninvasive, nonintrusive, natural-human, energetic environmental field modalities.
- Transpersonal caring promotes self-knowledge, self-control, and self-healing patterns and possibilities.
- Advanced transpersonal caring modalities draw on multiple ways of knowing and being; they encompass ethical and relational caring, along with those intentional consciousness modalities that are energetic in nature (e.g., form, color, light, sound, touch, vision, scent) that honor wholeness, healing, comfort, balance, harmony, and well-being (Watson, 2005, p. 6).

Usefulness

Watson's works and the Science of Human Caring are used by nurses in diverse settings. For example, Brockopp and colleagues (2011) detail an evidence-based, practice-based practice model grounded in Watson's theory of caring. The 10 carative factors are explicated throughout the hospital to provide a framework for nursing activities in this magnate hospital. The outcomes include 34 research projects, 9 published articles, and 9 funded research studies. Furthermore, the nurses "maintain high levels of work satisfaction, strong retention rates and a large percentage of associate-degree nurses return to school for baccalaureate degrees" (Brockopp et al., 2011, p. 511).

In other examples, Hills and colleagues (2011) developed a text to promote caring science curriculum in nursing, which they called an emancipatory pedagogy for nursing. It is based on Watson's science of caring and explores an alternative method of student evaluation. Lukose (2011) developed a practice model for Watson's theory of caring that "can be used by nurse educators to teach staff nurses and students" (p. 27). Sitzman and Watson (2014) developed methods of implementing Watson's human caring theory, which includes complete instructions in implementing caritas and mindful practices that Sitzman has used for decades in her practice. Sitzman (2015) also determined that all 10 caritas factors were at work with students and validated the possibility and responsibility for educators "to fully address the needs, and facilitate student growth learning and apprehension of caring in the online educational environment" (p. 26). Finally, Link to Practice 8-1 illustrates how Watson's work can be used to help alleviate stress among nurses.

Link to Practice 8-1

Jean Willowby, the nurse from the opening case study, and her preceptor, Allison Manheim, were having coffee one morning in their hospital's cafeteria. During their conversation, Allison told Jean that there appeared to be an increasing number of nurses in the pediatric intensive care unit (PICU) who were taking unscheduled personal days. She explained that the absences seemed to follow the death of a baby or young child and questioned whether the nurses might be experiencing increased levels of stress related to the death of one of their patients. Following the discussion, Jean decided to study the relationship between nurse absenteeism and loss of a patient and to devise a solution for the capstone nursing project required for her program.

Jean's project involved application of Watson's Caritas Processes to work with the PICU nurses to reduce stress. She devised several interventions focused on "caring for one's self" and "caring for each other." She and Allison held both scheduled and impromptu counseling sessions to "develop and sustain helping-trusting and caring relationships." Jean also worked to develop interventions to "create a healing environment" and "align mind-body and spirit" of the nurses. According to the scores on a stress instrument the nurses were asked to complete, Jean found that holding touch therapy sessions—during which the nurses could openly share their personal stories—seemed to be the most useful in stress reduction. Another effective intervention was back and foot massage, combined to listening to soft music, after a shift.

Following implementation of the various caring process interventions, the nurses were able to better tolerate the stressors of the PICU. Furthermore, hospital administrators noted a decrease in unscheduled personal days. These findings were striking enough that Jean was hired after her graduation to continue to develop stress-reduction and caring interventions for all staff.

Testability

Testing of Watson's theory and dissemination of findings are progressing. The science allows both quantitative and qualitative research methods. Indeed, Watson's science of caring has been researched by an extremely large number of nurses. A number of recent research articles are listed in Box 8-5.

Parsimony

Watson's theory is comparatively parsimonious. Although a number of new concepts and terms are defined, there are only 10 carative processes or areas to be addressed by nurses. In addition, there are six "working assumptions" (Watson, 2005, p. 28) and three considerations as to how to frame caring science.

Value in Extending Nursing Science

Watson (2012) explicitly describes the connection between nursing and caring. Her work has been used in education and in practice internationally and in numerous research studies. Collectively, findings present impressive indicators of the value of Watson's theory of caring to the discipline of nursing.

Box 8-5 Examples of Research Using Watson's Model

Arslan-Özkan, I., Okumuş, H., & Buldukoğlu, K. (2014). A randomized controlled trial of the effects of nursing care based on Watson's theory of human caring on distress, self-efficacy and adjustment in infertile women. *Journal of Advanced Nursing, 70*(8), 1801–1812. doi:10.1111/jan.12338.

Berry, D. M., Kaylor, M. B., Church, J., Campbell, K., McMillin, T., & Wamsley, R. (2013). Caritas and job environment: A replication of Persky et al. *Contemporary Nurse, 43*(2), 237–243.

Cooley, S. S., & DeGagne, J. C. (2016). Transformative experience: Developing competence in novice nursing faculty. *The Journal of Nursing Education, 55*(2), 96–100. doi:10.3928/01484834-20160114-07

Derby-Davis, M. J. (2014). Predictors of nursing faculty's job satisfaction and intent to stay in academe. *Journal of Professional Nursing, 30*(1), 19–25. doi:10.1016/j.profnurs.2013.04.001

Lamke, D., Catlin, A., & Mason-Chadd, M. (2014). "Not just a theory": The relationship between Jin Shin Jyutsu® self-care training for nurses and stress, physical health, emotional health, and caring efficacy. *Journal of Holistic Nursing, 32*(4), 278–289. doi:10.1177/0898010114531906

Ozan, Y. D., Okumuş, H., & Lash, A. A. (2015). Implementation of Watson's theory of human caring: A case study. *International Journal of Caring Sciences, 8*(1), 25–35.

Ozkan, I. A., Okumuş, H., Buldukoglu, K., & Watson, J. (2013). A case study based on Watson's theory of human caring: Being an infertile woman in Turkey. *Nursing Science Quarterly, 26*(4), 352–359. doi:10.1177/0894318413500346

Reed, F. M., Fitzgerald, L., & Rae, M. (2016). Mixing methodology, nursing theory and research design for a practice model of district nursing advocacy. *Nurse Researcher, 23*(3), 37–41. doi:10.7748/nr.23.3.37.s8

Rew, L. (2014). Intentional, present and grateful: Holistic nursing research with homeless youths. *Beginnings, 34*(2), 16–20.

Torregosa, M. B., Ynalvez, M. A., & Morin, K. H. (2016). Perceptions matter: Faculty caring, campus racial climate and academic performance. *Journal of Advanced Nursing, 72*(4), 864–877. doi:10.1111/jan.12877

Wicklund Gustin, L., & Wagner, L. (2013). The butterfly effect of caring—clinical nursing teachers' understanding of self-compassion as a source to compassionate care. *Scandinavian Journal of Caring Sciences, 27*(1), 175–183. doi:10.1111/j.1471-6712.2012.01033.x

Summary

The models presented in this chapter all focus on human interactive processes as the basis for nursing care, research, and education. Some of the theories described (e.g., King and Levine) are among the oldest of the grand nursing theories, whereas others (e.g., Watson and Artinian) are among the most recently developed. There is a wide variety of complexity among the models, but each has demonstrated applicability to the discipline, and all are currently used in schools of nursing, hospital clinical and community settings, and nursing research.

Like Jean, the nurse in the case study, nurses in all settings will be able to relate to the perspective described by these theorists. Indeed, the premise that humans are adaptive, holistic beings, in constant interaction with their environment, is easily applied in nursing practice. Some philosophical bases, concepts, assumptions, and relationships (e.g., systems focus, adaptation, goal of nursing, and interaction) are relatively consistently held within the works of this group of theorists, whereas others (e.g., SSOC [Artinian], cognator and regulator subsystems [Roy], and carative processes [Watson]) are unique to just one theory. Evidence-based practice (EBP) fits well with these theories and models because they ascribe to outcomes-based quantitative and to reality-based qualitative research principles.

Nurses studying this group of theories will become aware of how they present and prescribe nursing practice. Many will undoubtedly consider adopting one as a basis for their own professional practice.

Key Points

- The theories in this chapter depend on the ideal that nurses, other health care professionals, and patients are constantly interacting. The environment defined by most of these theorists is also foremost in individuals' interactions.
- The theorists who have developed these theories and models generally include and provide definitions of the four metaparadigm concepts of person, health, environment, and nursing. Several also include spirituality among their concepts.
- Most interactive process theories are practice-based and correspond closely to the work of nurses in clinical practice.
- Several interactive process theories are well suited to and are chosen to guide EBP and research to gather that evidence.
- Several of the theories and models in this group have been used or are being used to guide and structure educational programs in university nursing schools worldwide.

Learning Activities

1. Compare and contrast two of the models or theories presented in this chapter, considering their usefulness in practice, research, education, and/or administration. Share findings with classmates.
2. Select one of the models from this chapter and obtain the original work(s) of the theorist. From the work(s), outline a plan for a research study either using the work as the conceptual framework or testing components of the work.
   a. What concepts, assumptions, or relationships can be studied?
   b. To what population(s) can the work be applied?
   c. What concepts can be used as study variables?
3. Jean, the nurse from the opening case study, determined that Watson's theory best fit her current and future practice as a pediatric nurse practitioner. Review the models presented in this chapter and determine which could best be used to guide your practice. Share you observations with classmates.

REFERENCES

Acton, G. J. (1997). Affiliated-individuation as a mediator of stress and burden in caregivers of adults with dementia. *Journal of Holistic Nursing, 15*(4), 336–357.

Alligood, M. R., & May, B. A. (2000). A nursing theory of personal system empathy: Interpreting a conceptualization of empathy in King's interacting systems. *Nursing Science Quarterly, 13*(3), 243–247.

Artinian, B. M. (1983). Implementation of the intersystem patient-care model in clinical practice. *Journal of Advanced Nursing, 8*(2), 117–124.

Artinian, B. M. (1991). The development of the intersystem model. *Journal of Advanced Nursing, 16,* 194–205.

Artinian, B. M. (1997a). Overview of the intersystem model. In B. M. Artinian & M. M. Conger (Eds.), *The intersystem model: Integrating theory and practice* (pp. 1–17). Thousand Oaks, CA: Sage.

Artinian, B. M. (1997b). Situational sense of coherence. In B. M. Artinian & M. M. Conger (Eds.), *The intersystem model: Integrating theory and practice* (pp. 18–26). Thousand Oaks, CA: Sage.

Artinian, B. M. (1998). Grounded theory research: Its value for nursing. *Nursing Science Quarterly, 11*(1), 5–6.

Artinian, B. M. (2011). Theoretical background of the Artinian intersystem model. In B. M. Artinian, K. S. West, & M. M. Conger (Eds.), *The Artinian intersystem model: Integrating theory and practice for the professional nurse* (2nd ed., pp. 1–66). New York, NY: Springer Publishing.

Artinian, B. M. (2016). *Curriculum vitae.* Retrieved from http://www.apu.edu/faculty/cvs/bartinian.pdf.

Artinian, B. M., Giske, T., & Cone, P. H. (2009). *Glaserian grounded theory in nursing research: Trusting emergence.* New York, NY: Springer Publishing.

Bond, M. L., Gray, J. R., Baxley, S., Cason, C. L., Denke, L., & Moon, M. (2008). Voices of Hispanic students in baccalaureate nursing programs: Are we listening? *Nursing Education Perspectives, 29*(3), 136–142.

Brockopp, D., Schreiber, J., Hill, K., Altpeter, T., Moe, K., & Merritt, S. (2011). A successful evidence-based practice model in an acute care setting. *Oncology Nursing Forum, 38*(5), 509–511.

Buckner, E. B., & Hayden, S. J. (2014). Synthesis of middle range theory of adapting to chronic health conditions: A lifelong process and a common journey. In C. Roy (Ed.), *Generating middle range theory: From evidence to practice* (pp. 207–308). New York, NY: Springer Publishing.

Caceres, B. A. (2015). King's theory of goal attainment: Exploring functional status. *Nursing Science Quarterly, 28*(2), 151–155.

Cason, C., Bond, M. L., Gleason-Wynn, P., Coggin, C., Trevino, E., & Lopez, M. (2008). Perceived barriers and needed supports for today's Hispanic students in the health professions: Voices of seasoned Hispanic health care professionals. *Hispanic Care International, 6*(1), 41–50.

Chacko, J. M., Kharde, S., & Swamy, M. K. (2013). Effectiveness of infrared lamp on reducing pain and inflammation due to episiotomy wound. *International Journal of Nursing Education, 5*(1), 82–85. doi:10.5958/j.0974-9357.5.1020

Clarke, P. N., Barone, S. H., Hanna, D., & Senesac, P. M. (2011). Roy's adaptation model. *Nursing Science Quarterly, 24*(4), 337–344.

Cone, P. H., Artinian, B. M., & West, K. S. (2011). The Artinian intersystem model in nursing school education. In B. M. Artinian, K. S. West, & M. M. Conger (Eds.), *The Artinian intersystem model: Integrating theory and practice for the professional nurse* (2nd ed., pp. 147–172). New York, NY: Springer Publishing.

Connell School of Nursing. (2016). *Sr. Callista Roy. Professor and nurse theorist.* Boston, MA: Author. Retrieved from http://www.bc.edu/bc-web/schools/cson/faculty-research/faculty-directory/sr-callista-roy.html.

Critchley, S., & Ball, E. (2007). Evaluation of the primary/secondary care interface in relation to primary care rheumatology service. *Quality in Primary Care, 15*(1), 33–36.

Daubenmire, M. J. (1989). A baccalaureate nursing curriculum based on King's conceptual framework. In J. Riehl-Sisca (Ed.), *Conceptual models for nursing practice* (3rd ed., pp. 167–178). Norwalk, CT: Appleton & Lange.

Dobratz, M. C. (2014). Synthesis of middle range theory on adapting to loss. In C. Roy (Ed.), *Generating middle range theory: From evidence to practice* (pp. 253–276). New York, NY: Springer Publishing.

Dobratz, M. C. (2016). Building a middle-range theory of adaptive spirituality. *Nursing Science Quarterly, 29*(2), 146–153.

Doornbos, M. M. (2000). King's systems framework and family health: The derivation and testing of a theory. *The Journal of Theory Construction and Testing, 4*(1), 20–26.

Erickson, H. C., Tomlin, E. M., & Swain, M. A. P. (1983). *Modeling and role-modeling: A theory and paradigm for nursing.* Englewood Cliffs, NJ: Prentice-Hall.

Erickson, M. E. (2014). Helen C. Erickson, Evelyn M. Tomlin, Mary Ann P. Swain: Modeling and role-modeling. In M. R. Alligood (Ed.), *Nursing theorists and their work* (8th ed., pp. 496–519). St. Louis, MO: Mosby.

Frederickson, K. (2011). Callista Roy's adaptation model. *Nursing Science Quarterly, 24*(4), 301–303.

Frey, M. A., Rooke, L., Sieloff, C., Messmer, P. R., & Kameoka, T. (1995). King's framework and theory in Japan, Sweden, and the United States. *Image—The Journal of Nursing Scholarship, 27*(2), 127–130.

Gemmill, R., Kravits, K., Oritz, M., Anderson, C., Lai, L., & Grant, M. (2011). What do surgical oncology staff nurses know about colorectal cancer ostomy care? *Journal of Continuing Education in Nursing, 42*(2), 81–88.

Giske, T., & Artinian, B. (2008). Patterns of "balancing between hope and despair" in the diagnostic phase: A grounded theory study of patients on a gastroenterology ward. *Journal of Advanced Nursing, 62*(1), 22–31.

Giske, T., & Cone, P. H. (2012). Opening up to learning spiritual care of patients: A grounded theory study of nursing students. *Journal of Clinical Nursing, 21*(13–14), 2006–2015. doi:10.1111/j.1365- 2702.2011.04054.x

Hills, M., Watson, J., Boykin, A., Touhy, T. A., Smith, M. C., Lewis, S., et al. (2011). *Creating a caring science curriculum: An emancipatory pedagogy for nursing.* New York, NY: Springer Publishing.

Irvin, B. L., & Acton, G. J. (1996). Stress mediation in caregivers of cognitively impaired adults: Theoretical model testing. *Nursing Research, 45*(3), 160–166.

Isac, C., Venkatesaperumal, R., & D'Sousa, M. S. (2013). Conceptual framework for quality care among clients with sickle cell disease through nurse-led information desk. *International Journal of Nursing Education, 5*(1), 39–43. doi:10.5958/j0974-9357.5.1.010

Jesse, D. E., & Alligood, M. R. (2014). Jean Watson: Watson's philosophy and theory of transpersonal caring. In M. R. Alligood (Ed.), *Nursing theorists and their work* (8th ed., pp. 79–97). St. Louis, MO: Mosby.

Joseph, L. (2013). A study to evaluate the effectiveness of planned teaching programme on growth monitoring of children using innovative paediatric growth chart among the third year general nursing and midwifery students in a selected institute in Mangalore. *International Journal of Nursing Education, 5*(1), 103–106.

Joseph, M. L., Laughon, D., & Bogue, R. (2011). An examination of the sustainable adoption of whole person care (WPC). *Journal of Nursing Management, 19*(8), 989–997.

King, I. M. (1971). *Toward a theory for nursing.* New York, NY: Wiley.

King, I. M. (1981). *A theory for nursing, systems, concepts, process.* New York, NY: Wiley.

King, I. M. (1995a). A systems framework for nursing. In M. A. Frey & C. L. Sieloff (Eds.), *Advancing King's systems framework and theory of nursing* (pp. 13–22). Thousand Oaks, CA: Sage.

King, I. M. (1995b). The theory of goal attainment. In M. A. Frey & C. L. Sieloff (Eds.), *Advancing King's systems framework and theory of nursing* (pp. 23–33). Thousand Oaks, CA: Sage.

King, I. M. (2001). Theory of goal attainment. In M. Parker (Ed.), *Nursing theories and nursing practice* (pp. 275–286). Philadelphia, PA: F.A. Davis.

Lévesque, L., Ricard, N., Ducharme, F., Duquette, A., & Bonin, J. (1998). Empirical verification of a theoretical model derived from the Roy adaptation model: Findings from five studies. *Nursing Science Quarterly, 11*(1), 31–39.

Lukose, A. (2011). Developing a practice model for Watson's theory of caring. *Nursing Science Quarterly, 24*(1), 27–30.

McCallin, A. M. (2012). Book review: Artinian, B. M., Giske, T., & Cone, P. H. (2009). Glaserian grounded theory in nursing research: Trusting emergence. *The Grounded Theory Review, 9*(2). Retrieved from http://www.groundedtheoryreview.com/2012/06/25/book-reviewartinian-b-m-giske-t-cone-p-h.

McCowan, D. E., & Artinian, B. M. (2011). An emerging nursing program in a developing country. In B. M. Artinian, K. S. West, & M. M. Conger (Eds.), *The Artinian intersystem model: Integrating theory and practice for the professional nurse* (2nd ed., pp. 173–180). New York, NY: Springer Publishing.

Mensik, J. (2008). Nurses make a difference every day. *Arizona Nurse, 61*(2), 2.

Mitchell, P. H. (2008). President's message: Legends and legacies. *Nursing Outlook, 56*(3), 97–98.

Parse, R. R. (2014). *The humanbecoming paradigm: A transformational worldview.* Pittsburgh, PA: Discovery International.

Phillips, K. D., & Harris, R. (2014). Sister Callista Roy: Adaptation model. In M. R. Alligood (Ed.), *Nursing theorists and their work* (8th ed., pp. 303–330). St. Louis, MO: Mosby.

Rogers, S. (1996). Facilitative affiliation: Nurse–client interactions that enhance healing. *Issues in Mental Health Nursing, 17*(3), 171–184.

Rooda, L. A. (1992). The development of a conceptual model for multicultural nursing. *Journal of Holistic Nursing, 10*(4), 337–347.

Roy, C. (2009). *The Roy adaptation model* (3rd ed.). Upper Saddle River, NJ: Prentice-Hall.

Roy, C. (2011a). Extending the Roy adaptation model to meet changing global needs. *Nursing Science Quarterly, 24*(4), 345–351.

Roy, C. (2011b). Research based on the Roy adaptation model: Last 25 years. *Nursing Science Quarterly, 24*(4), 312–320.

Roy, C. (2014a). *Generating middle range theory: From evidence to practice.* New York, NY: Springer Publishing.

Roy, C. (2014b). Synthesis of a middle range theory of coping. In C. Roy (Ed.), *Generating middle range theory: From evidence to practice* (pp. 211–232). New York, NY: Springer Publishing.

Roy, C., & Andrews, H. A. (1999). *The Roy adaptation model* (2nd ed.). Stamford, CT: Appleton & Lange.

Roy Adaptation Association. (2016). *Welcome/about.* Retrieved from http://www.bc.edu/sites/nurse-theorist/the-roy-adaptation-association1.html/

Sieloff, C. L., & Messmer, P. R. (2014). Imogene M. King: Conceptual system and middle range theory of goal attainment. In M. R. Alligood (Ed.), *Nursing theorists and their work* (8th ed., pp. 258–280). St. Louis, MO: Mosby.

Sitzman, K. (2015). Sense, connect, facilitate: Nurse educator experiences of caring online through Watson's lenses. *International Journal of Human Caring, 19*(3), 25–29.

Sitzman, K., & Watson, J. (2014). *Caring science, mindful practice: Implementing Watson's human caring theory.* New York, NY: Springer Publishing.

Smith, M., Wright, B. W., & Fawcet, J. (2008). In memory: A tribute to two giants of nursing conceptual models and theories. *Visions: Journal of Rogerian Nursing Science, 15*(1), 65–66.

Stevens, K. R., & Messmer, P. R. (2008). In remembrance of Imogene M. King, January 30, 1923–December 24, 2007: Imogene, a pioneer and dear colleague. *Nursing Outlook, 56*(3), 100–101.

Treolar, L., & Artinian, B. M. (2007). Populations affected by disability. In M. Neis & M. McEwen (Eds.), *Community health nursing* (4th ed., pp. 388–418). Philadelphia, PA: Saunders.

van Dover, L., & Pfeiffer, J. B. (2007). Spiritual care in Christian parish nursing. *Journal of Advanced Nursing, 57*(2), 213–221.

Vuckovich, P. K., & Artinian, B. M. (2005). Justifying coercion. *Nursing Ethics, 12*(4), 370–380.

Watson, J. (1985). *The philosophy and science of caring* (Rev. ed.). Boulder, CO: Colorado Associated University Press.

Watson, J. (1988). *Nursing: Human science and human care: A theory of nursing.* New York, NY: National League for Nursing Press.

Watson, J. (Ed.). (1994). *Applying the art and science of human caring.* New York, NY: National League for Nursing Press.

Watson, J. (1996). Nursing, caring-healing paradigm. In D. Pesat (Ed.), *Capsules of comments in psychiatric nursing.* Chicago, IL: Mosby-Year Book.

Watson, J. (1999). *Postmodern nursing and beyond.* Edinburgh, United Kingdom: Churchill Livingstone.

Watson, J. (2005). *Caring science as sacred science.* Philadelphia, PA: F.A. Davis.

Watson, J. (2008). *The philosophy and science of caring.* Boulder, CO: University Press of Colorado.

Watson, J. (2012). *Human caring science: A theory of nursing* (2nd ed.). Sudbury, MA: Jones & Bartlett Learning.

Watson Caring Science Institute. (2016a). *Curriculum vitae.* Retrieved from https://www.watsoncaringscience.org/files/CVs/JeanWatsonCV.pdf.

Watson Caring Science Institute. (2016b). *Core concepts of human caring.* Retrieved from https://www.watsoncaringscience.org/jean-bio/caring-science-theory/.

9

Grand Nursing Theories Based on Unitary Process

Evelyn M. Wills

Kristin Kowalski is a hospice nurse who wishes to expand the scope of her therapeutic practice. She desires to delve more deeply into holistic health care, having
recently completed courses of study in herbal medicine, touch therapy, and holistic
nursing. Kristin is aware that to practice independently, she needs professional credentials that will be widely accepted; therefore, she applied to the graduate program of a nationally ranked nursing school at a large state university.

Because Kristin believes strongly in holistic nursing practice, for her master's
degree, she decided to focus her study of nursing theories on those that look at the
whole person and have a broad, nontraditional view of health. She is particularly
interested in Rosemarie Parse's Humanbecoming Paradigm because this viewpoint
stresses the individual's way of being and becoming healthy and the nurse as an
intersubjective presence.

Kristin is attracted to Parse's idea of true presence and wishes to further explore this
concept as well as the rest of the perspective. She hopes to eventually apply it to her
practice and use it as the research framework for her thesis. For her thesis, Kristin wants
to examine the experiences of nurses who practice therapeutic touch. She desires to
learn their perceptions of how therapeutic touch interventions help their clients. She also
wants to learn more about Parse's research method and hopes to use it for her study.

The term *simultaneity paradigm* was first coined by nursing theorist Rosemarie Parse
(1987) to describe a group of theories that adhered to a unitary process perception
of human beings. This group of theorists believed that humans are unitary beings:
energy systems embedded in the universal energy system. Within this group of theories, human beings are seen as unitary, "Whole, open and free to choose ways of
becoming" (Parse, 1998, p. 6), and health is described as continuous human environmental interchanges (Newman, 1994).

The unitary process nursing model and the work of two of her students are described in this chapter: Science of Unitary Human Beings (Rogers, 1994), Health as Expanding Consciousness (Newman, 1999), and Humanbecoming Paradigm (Parse, 2014). The three are grouped together because they are significantly different in their concepts, assumptions, and propositions when compared to the theories described in Chapters 7 and 8. They are universal in scope and relatively abstract.

The unitary process theories of nursing reflect the newer views of science in their complexity and view the human as energy field, as intentional, as dynamic, limitless, and unpredictable. These are views of humans and their energy fields that place these three theories within the new scientific realm of complexity science (Davidson, Ray, & Turkel, 2011). Rolfe (2015), however, brings us the realization that nursing as a human science relies on engagement with persons and that may include art, science, philosophy, music, and other human endeavors, persons being whole beings. The three theorists, nay, philosophers, Rogers, Newman, and Parse, attest to the necessity for engagement between persons and families experiencing unwanted changes in health and the person who would help them, the nurse.

Martha Rogers: The Science of Unitary and Irreducible Human Beings

Martha Rogers first described her Theory of Unitary Man in 1961, and almost from the first, there has been widespread controversy and debate among nursing theorists and scholars regarding her work (Phillips, 2010, 2016). Prior to Rogers, it was rare that anyone in nursing viewed human beings as anything other than the receivers of care by nurses and physicians. Furthermore, the health care system was organized by specialization, in which nurses and other health providers focused on discrete areas or functions (e.g., a dressing change, medication administration, or health teaching) rather than on the whole person. As a result, it took many professionals working in isolation, none of whom knew the whole person, to care for patients. Rogers's (1970) insistence that the person was a "unitary energy system" in "continuous mutual interaction with the universal energy system" (p. 90) dramatically influenced nursing by encouraging nurses to consider each person as a whole (a unity) when planning and delivering care. Phillips (2013) states that Rogers's "vision was concerned with unitary wholes, a vision she used in creating the science of unitary human beings (SUBH) . . . " (p. 241). A new and dramatically different ideal in health care.

Background of the Theorist

Martha Rogers was born on May 12, 1914 (the anniversary of Florence Nightingale's birth) (Dossey, 2010), in Dallas, Texas. She earned a diploma in nursing from Knoxville General Hospital in 1936 and a bachelor's degree from George Peabody College in Nashville, Tennessee, in 1937. She later received a master's degree in public health nursing from Teachers College, Columbia University in New York, and a master's degree in public health and a doctor of science from The Johns Hopkins University in Baltimore, Maryland (Gunther, 2014).

Rogers became the head of the Division of Nursing of New York University (NYU) in 1954, where she focused on teaching and formulating and elaborating her theory (Hektor, 1989). She was teacher and mentor to an impressive list of nursing scholars and theorists, including Newman and Parse, whose works are described later in the chapter. Rogers continued her work and writing until her death in March 1994.

Philosophical Underpinnings of the Theory

The Science of Unitary and Irreducible Human Beings started as an abstract theory that was synthesized from theories of numerous sciences; therefore, it was deductively derived. She drew from Einstein's Theory of Relativity as well as Heisenberg's Uncertainty Principle to demonstrate the unpredictability of this universe (Caratao-Mojica, 2015). Of particular importance was von Bertalanffy's theory on general systems, which contributed the concepts of entropy and negentropy and posited that open systems are characterized by constant interaction with the environment. The work of Rapoport provided a background on open systems, and the work of Herrick contributed to the premise of evolution of human nature (Rogers, 1994).

Rogers's synthesis of the works of these scientists formed the basis of her proposition that human systems are open systems embedded in larger, open environmental systems. She also brought in other concepts, including the idea that time is unidirectional, that living systems have pattern and organization, and that man is a sentient, thinking being capable of awareness, feeling, and choosing. From all these theories, and from her personal study of nature, Rogers (1970) developed her original Theory of Unitary Man. She continuously refined and elaborated her theory, which she retitled Science of Unitary Humans (Rogers, 1986) and, finally, shortly before her death, the Science of Unitary and Irreducible Human Beings (Rogers, 1994).

Major Assumptions, Concepts, and Relationships

Assumptions

Rogers (1970) presented several assumptions about man. These are as follows:

Man is a unified whole possessing integrity and manifesting characteristics that are more than and different from the sum of his parts (p. 47).

Man and environment are continuously exchanging matter and energy with one another (p. 54).

The life process evolves irreversibly and unidirectionally along the space–time continuum (p. 59).

Pattern and organization identify man and reflect his innovative wholeness (p. 65).

Man is characterized by the capacity for abstraction and imagery, language and thought, sensation, and emotion (p. 73).

Rogers (1990) later revised the term *man* to *human being* to coincide with the request for gender-neutral language in the social sciences and nursing science.

Concepts

In Rogers's work, the unitary human being and the environment are the focus of nursing practice. Other central components are energy fields, openness, pandimensionality, and pattern; these she identified as the "building blocks" (Rogers, 1970, p. 226) of her system. Rogers also derived three other components for the model, which served as a basis of her work. These were based on principles of homeodynamics and were termed *resonancy, helicy,* and *integrality* (Rogers, 1990) (Box 9-1). Definitions of the nursing metaparadigm concepts and other important concepts in Rogers's work are listed in Table 9-1.

Relationships

The Science of Unitary and Irreducible Human Beings is fundamentally abstract; therefore, specifically defined relationships differ from those in more linear theories.

Principles of Homeodynamics Applied in Rogers's Theory

1. Resonancy is continuous change from lower to higher frequency wave patterns in human and environmental fields.
2. Helicy is continuous innovative, unpredictable, increasing diversity of human and environmental field patterns.
3. Integrality is continuous mutual human and environmental field processes.

Source: Rogers (1990, p. 8).

The major components of Rogers's model revolve around the building blocks (energy fields, openness, pattern, and pandimensionality) and the principles of homeodynamics (resonancy, helicy, and integrality). These explain the nature of, and direction of, the interactions between unitary human beings and the environment.

Among the relationships that Rogers posited are that all things are integral in that their energy fields are in continuous mutual process and that pattern is the manifestation of the integrality of each entity and of the environmental energy field

Table 9-1 Central Concepts of Rogers's Science of Unitary Human Beings

Concept	Definition
Human–unitary human beings	"Irreducible, indivisible, multidimensional energy fields identified by pattern and manifesting characteristics that are specific to the whole and which cannot be predicted from the knowledge of the parts" (p. 7).
Health	"Unitary human health signifies an irreducible human field manifestation. It cannot be measured by the parameters of biology or physics or of the social sciences" (p. 10).
Nursing	"The study of unitary, irreducible, indivisible human and environmental fields: people and their world" (p. 6). Nursing is a learned profession that is both a science and an art.
Environmental field	"An irreducible, indivisible, pandimensional energy field identified by pattern and integral with the human field" (p. 7).
Energy field	"The fundamental unit of the living and the non-living. Field is a unifying concept. Energy signifies the dynamic nature of the field; a field is in continuous motion and is infinite" (p. 7).
Openness	Refers to qualities exhibited by open systems; human beings and their environment are open systems.
Pandimensional	"A nonlinear domain without spatial or temporal attributes" (p. 28).
Pattern	"The distinguishing characteristic of an energy field perceived as a single wave" (p. 7).

Source: Rogers (1990).

(Rogers, 1986). Other major relationships within Rogers's (1990) work are contained in the following statements:

> Humans and environment are interrelated in that neither "has an energy field," both are integral energy fields (pp. 6–7).
> Manifestations of pattern emerge out of the human/environmental field mutual process and are continuously innovative (p. 8).
> The group field is irreducible and indivisible to itself and integral with its own environmental field (p. 8).

Nursing is concerned with maintaining and promoting health, preventing illness, and caring for those who are sick or disabled. The purpose of nursing for Rogers (1986) is to help human beings achieve well-being within the potential of each individual, family, or group. Because human energy fields are complex, individualizing nursing services supports simultaneous human and environmental exchange, encouraging health (Rogers, 1990).

Usefulness

Rogers's theory is a synthesis of phenomena that are important to nursing. It is an abstract, unified, and highly derived framework and does not define particular hypotheses or theories. Rather, it provides a worldview from which nurses may derive theories and hypotheses and propose relationships specific to different situations. In essence, the theory allows many options for studying humans as individuals and groups and for studying various situations in health as manifestations of pattern and innovation. Rogers's model stresses the unitary experience and provides an abstract philosophical framework that can guide nursing practice.

Rogers's theory has been evident in nursing education, scholarship, and practice for more than four decades. In education, among other programs, it has guided the nursing curriculum at NYU, where Rogers was head of the Division of Nursing in the 1970s. This resulted in the education of numerous nurses who use her theory in practice internationally (Hektor, 1989). In the area of nursing scholarship, several noted nursing theorists (e.g., Fitzpatrick, 1989; Newman, 1994; Parse, 1998) derived theories from Rogers's work. A number of middle range nursing theories are based on Rogers's work as reported by Fawcett (2015). Among these middle range theories are Health Empowerment Theory (Shearer, 2009), Theory of the Art of Nursing (Alligood, 2002), Theory of Self-Transcendence (Reed, 2014), Theory of Diversity of Human Field Pattern (Hastings-Tolsma, 2006), and Theory of Intentionality (Zahourek, 2005).

In other scholarly works, Barrett (1986, 1989) derived a theory, Power as Knowing Participation in Change, for nursing practice from Rogers's theory. She used several of Rogers's concepts (e.g., energy fields, openness, pattern, and four-dimensionality [now *pandimensionality*]) and the principles of resonancy, helicy, and integrality to form her theory. The Theory of Power as Knowing Participation in Change consists of awareness, choices, freedom to act intentionally, and involvement in creating changes and was tested in research using Barrett's Power as Knowing Participation in Change (PKPIC) tool. Barrett's (1989) theory consequently has been used in research on patterning of pain and power with guided imagery by Fuller, Davis, Servonsky, and Butcher (2012), who examined field patterns in adult substance users in rehab, and Kirton and Morris (2012), who used Barrett's theory to examine adherence to antiretroviral therapy in adults who are infected with HIV. Farren (2010) found in a secondary analysis of data collected using Barrett's PKPIC tool with breast cancer survivors that the dimensions of power (awareness, choices, freedom to act with intention, and involvement in creating change) were responsible for all the variance. Moreover, the breast cancer survivors showed differing intensities of these dimensions.

In clinical settings, Rogerian practitioners employ the visible manifestations of Rogers's science. Madrid, Barrett, and Winstead-Fry (2010), for example, studied the feasibility of using therapeutic touch with patients who were undergoing cerebral angiography. The design was a randomized, single blind clinical pilot study with outcome assessments of blood pressure, pulse, and respirations. The findings of this study were inconclusive, but the researchers followed up with exploration of the reasons and studied the implications. Reed (2008) wrote about nursing time as a dimension of practice, research, and theory. In a nursing educational setting, Malinski and Todaro-Franceschi (2011) studied comeditation to reduce anxiety and facilitate relaxation. Their data from the qualitative study suggested that the participants reported feeling calmer, more relaxed, and balanced and centered after 1 month of practice. Their findings suggest that comeditation may help transform education in nursing programs, most of which have reputations as being stressful to students.

Testability

Because of the model's abstractness, Rogers's (1990) work is not directly testable, but it is testable in principle (Bramlett, 2010). Numerous research studies using Rogers's model have been completed and reported in the nursing literature. A plethora of these studies can be found in *Visions: The Journal of Rogerian Nursing Science.* Madrid and Winstead-Fry (2001) also found in a focused review of literature that from 1990 through 2000, 28 research studies on therapeutic touch were published in peer-reviewed journals, and 18 of them were based on the Science of Unitary Human Beings, typically using Rogers's model as explanation for the underlying processes of therapeutic touch and its relation to energy fields and energy transfer. Examples of some recent nursing studies using Rogers's theory are listed in Box 9-2.

Parsimony

This theory is relatively parsimonious. The model has five key definitions. These, combined with the three principles of homeodynamics and the six assumptions about human beings, are the major elements of the work. Despite its simplicity, however, it is difficult for many nurses to comprehend because the concepts are extremely abstract. Nurses who wish their research and practice to be guided by Rogers's model will benefit from studying with a Rogerian scholar who uses the model regularly.

Value in Extending Nursing Science

Rogers's contributions to nursing have been noted in the nursing literature, and she has had a significant influence on scientific inquiry in professional nursing practice. The major value of Rogers's work has been extending nursing science by challenging traditional ways of thinking about the world and nursing. She moved beyond a focus on such concepts and principles as adaptation, biopsychosocial beings, causal/probabilistic views, and the human-as-sum-of-parts thinking that had been common in nursing science (Parse, 2010; Phillips, 2010, 2013; Rogers, 1990). The contribution to nursing science of the Science of Unitary and Irreducible Human Beings is that it carries nursing into areas that are impossible to study using linear, three-dimensional, and reductionistic methods, now understood as complexity science (Rickles, Hawe, & Schiell, 2007).

> **Box 9-2**   Examples of Research Studies Using Rogers's Theory
>
> Caratoa-Mojica, R. (2015). Being one with the universe: Finding a silver lining in dying. *Nursing Science Quarterly, 28*(3), 229–233. doi:10.1177/0894318415585621
>
> Chang, S. J., Kwak, E. Y., Hahm, B., Seo, S. H., Lee, D. W., & Jang, S. J. (2016). Effects of a meditation program on nurses' power and quality of life. *Nursing Science Quarterly, 29*(3), 227–234. doi:10.1177/0894318416647778
>
> Grumme, V. S., Barry, C. D., Gordon, S. C., & Ray, M. A. (2016). On virtual presence. *ANS. Advances in Nursing Science, 39*(1), 48–59. doi:10.1097/ANS.0000000000000103
>
> Heelan-Fancher, L. (2016a). Improving maternal outcomes: The dynamic role of power in patient advocacy [Abstract]. *Nursing Research, 65*(2), E99.
>
> Heelan-Fancher, L. M. (2016b). Patient advocacy in an obstetric setting. *Nursing Science Quarterly, 29*(4). 316–327. doi:10.1177/0894318416660531
>
> Onieva-Zafra, M. D., García, L. H., & Del Valle, M. G. (2015). Effectiveness of guided imagery relaxation on levels of pain and depression in patients diagnosed with fibromyalgia. *Holistic Nursing Practice, 29*(1), 13–21. doi:10.1097/HNP.0000000000000062
>
> Reis, P. J., & Alligood, M. R. (2014). Prenatal yoga in late pregnancy and optimism, power, and well-being. *Nursing Science Quarterly, 27*(1), 30–36. doi:10.1177/0894318413509706
>
> Smith, M. C., Zahourek, R., Hines, M. E. Engebretson, J., & Wardell, D. W. (2013). Holistic nurses' stories of personal healing. *Journal of Holistic Nursing, 31*(3), 173–187.
>
> Willis, D. G., DeSanto-Madeya, S., & Fawcett, J. (2015). Moving beyond dwelling in suffering: A situation-specific theory of men's healing from childhood maltreatment. *Nursing Science Quarterly, 28*(1), 57–63. doi:10.1177/0894318414558606

Margaret Newman: Health as Expanding Consciousness

Margaret Newman reported that she became interested in theory when asked to speak at a nursing conference in 1978 (George, 2010). She published a theory of health a year later (Newman, 1979) and *Health as Expanding Consciousness* in 1986. She revised this work in 1994 and 1999. Newman has published extensively on her theory and theoretical issues in books, book chapters, and articles (Newman, 1990a, 1990b, 1994, 1995, 1999, 2005, 2008a, 2008b).

Newman's *Health as Expanding Consciousness* is one of the most recent nursing theories; her work builds on the work of Rogers and others. Because of its similarity to Rogers's theory, particularly with regard to its conceptualizations of person, nursing, and the environment, it is included here among the unitary process theories. In 2008, Newman published a new, related work, which she entitled *Transforming Presence: The Difference That Nursing Makes* (Newman, 2008b); in this work, Newman makes the point that the three paradigms are not necessarily contradictory, but "the unitary perspective can include the more particulate view"(p. 15). Just as the theory of relativity may include special cases of more mechanistic theories (p. 15).

Background of the Theorist

As a young woman, Margaret Newman was involved in caring for her mother, who suffered from amyotrophic lateral sclerosis. She explained that it was during this period that she came to know her mother in ways that would have been impossible otherwise (Newman, 1986). This experience led Newman to study nursing, and she enrolled at the University of Tennessee, where she completed her bachelor's degree in 1962. She earned her master's degree from the University of California, San Francisco, in 1964 and a doctorate from NYU in 1971 (Brown & Alligood, 2014).

Newman has served on the faculty at the University of Tennessee (which named her an outstanding alumna), NYU, Pennsylvania State University, and the University of Minnesota. She is currently professor emeritus at the University of Minnesota, Minneapolis. Her work has been recognized internationally, and she has received numerous awards and honors both in the United States and abroad (Jones, 2007).

Philosophical Underpinnings of the Theory

While at NYU, Newman attended seminars taught by Martha Rogers, and she stated that Rogers's Science of Unitary Human Beings was the basis of her theory of Health as Expanding Consciousness. She also noted that, among others, Itzhak Bentov's explanation of the concept of expanding consciousness, Arthur Young's work on pattern recognition, and David Bohm's theory of implicate order brought perspective to her thoughts and ideas (Newman, 2008b).

Major Assumptions, Concepts, and Relationships

Assumptions

As a student of Rogers, Newman believed that "the human is unitary, that is, cannot be divided into parts, and is inseparable from the larger unitary field" (Newman, 1994, p. xviii). She saw humans as open energy systems in continual contact with a universe of open systems (i.e., the environment). Additionally, humans are continuously active in evolving their own pattern of the whole (i.e., health) and are intuitive as well as cognitive and affective beings. She further posited that "persons as individuals, and human beings as a species, are identified by their patterns of consciousness" and that "the person does not possess consciousness—the person is consciousness" (Newman, 1999, p. 33).

In describing health, Newman (1994) explained that health encompasses illness or pathology and that pathologic conditions can be considered manifestations of the pattern of the individual. In addition, the pattern of the individual that eventually manifests itself as pathology is primary and exists prior to structural or functional changes; removal of the pathology in itself will not change the pattern of the individual. Finally, she noted an assumption that changes occur simultaneously and not in linear fashion (Newman, 1994).

Concepts

Newman built on Rogers's definitions for human and environment, but she redefined nursing and health. Health is an essential component of the theory of Health as Expanding Consciousness and is seen as a process of developing awareness of self and the environment together with increasing the ability to perceive alternatives and respond in a variety of ways. Nursing is described as "caring in the human health experience" (Newman, 1994, p. 139). Other central concepts in Newman's theory are pattern, pattern recognition, movement, and time and space. Definitions for these and other concepts specific to the theory are presented in Table 9-2.

Relationships

A fundamental proposition in Newman's model is the idea that health and illness are synthesized as "health." Indeed, the fusion of one state of being (disease) with its opposite (nondisease) results in what can be regarded as health (Newman, 2008b).

Table 9-2 Central Concepts of Newman's Health as Expanding Consciousness

Concept	Definition
Nursing	The act of assisting people to use the power within them to evolve toward higher levels of consciousness. Nursing is directed toward recognizing the patterns of the person in interaction with the environment and accepting the interaction as a process of evolving consciousness. Nursing facilitates the process of pattern recognition by a rhythmic connecting of the nurse with the client for the purpose of illuminating the pattern and discovering the rules of a higher level of organization.
Health	The expanding of consciousness; an evolving pattern of the whole of life. A unitary process; a fluctuating pattern of rhythmic phenomena that includes illness within the pattern of energy. Sickness can "be the shock that reorganizes the relationships of the person's pattern in a more harmonious way" (Newman, 1999, p. 11).
Person	A dynamic pattern of energy and an open system in interaction with the environment. Persons can be defined by their patterns of consciousness.
Consciousness	The information of the system; consciousness refers to the capacity of the system to interact with the environment and includes thinking, feeling, and processing the information embedded in physiologic systems.
Expanding consciousness	The evolving pattern of the whole. Expanding consciousness is the increasing complexity of the living system and is characterized by illumination and pattern recognition resulting in transformation and discovery. Expanding consciousness is health.
Integration via movement	The natural condition of living creatures. Consciousness is expressed in movement, which is the way that the organism interacts with the environment and exerts control over it. Movement patterns reflect and communicate the person's inner pattern and organization. Changes in the person's health patterns may be reflected in changes in their movement rhythms.
Pattern	Relatedness, which is characterized by movement, diversity, and rhythm. Pattern is a scheme, design, or framework and is seen in person–environment interactions. Pattern is recognized on the basis of variation and may not be seen all at once. It is manifest in the way one moves, speaks, talks, and relates with others.
Pattern recognition	The insight or recognition of a principle, realization of a truth, or reconciliation of a duality. Pattern recognition illuminates the possibilities for action and is the key to the process of evolving to a higher level of consciousness.
Time and space	Temporal patterns that are specific to individuals and define their ways of being within their world. Patterns of health may be detected in temporal patterns.

Source: Newman (1999).

To Newman, health is pattern. *Pattern* is information that depicts the whole, and pattern recognition is essential. Pattern recognition involves moving from looking at parts to looking at patterns. Expanding consciousness occurs as a process of pattern recognition (insight) following a synthesis of contradictory events or disturbances in the flow of daily living. Pattern recognition comes from within the observer, and patterns unfold over time and cannot be predicted with certainty. Understanding the meaning of relationships through pattern recognition is important in providing care because patterns are the essence of a unitary view of health.

Newman also wrote of the interrelatedness of time, space, and movement. She explained that time and space have a complementary relationship, and movement is the means by which space and time become reality. Movement is seen as a reflection of consciousness, time is a function of movement, and time is a measure of consciousness (Newman, 2008a). Humans are in a constant state of motion and are constantly changing; movement through time and space gives modern people our unique perception of reality. Constant change is visible currently as technology; for example, smartphones and tablet computers can access e-books and e-libraries, giving people immediate access to high volumes of information. New technology, such as handheld laboratory testing and physical examination technology, is currently being used in clinics and physician and nurse practitioner offices. Such technology gives health professionals and other individuals immediate, conscious, and unrestricted access to information.

Access to information places people in constant contact with the whole world; indeed, instant communications, such as social media, have made it possible for people to respond immediately to a question, concern, or idea. Having information available at their fingertips lessens the need to try to remember telephone numbers and other facts that can be found easily online (Stein & Sanburn, 2013). In these cases, currently expanding consciousness may be more important to them than memory.

Time, space, and movement have all changed in the past few years; indeed, "the person is the center of consciousness with information flow . . . [throughout] the universe" (Newman, 2008b, p. 36). Humans can only expect more and faster change as consciousness expands and our world of knowledge progresses.

Usefulness

Newman (1994) believed that theory must be derived from practice and theory must inform practice. To illustrate this relationship, she proposed a model for practice that she derived from her theory.

Her work has been used by nurses in a number of settings, providing care for different types of clients and for a variety of interventions. For example, Arcari and Flanagan (2015) described the development of a post-master's certificate program in Mind-Body-Spirit nursing certification which was heavily influenced by Newman's Theory of Health as Expanding Consciousness. In another recent example, Sethares and Gramling (2014) described how Newman's theory was used by under graduate nursing students to enhance clinical learning experiences by focusing on student–client partnerships. Stec (2016) also used Newman's theory to describe patterns of relating, knowing, and clinical decision making in a group of senior-level nursing students.

Testability

Newman's theory has been the basis for research projects that have tested parts of the theory (i.e., time and movement) or used it as a framework. Most of the nursing studies using Newman's theory, found in recent literature, were qualitative in nature. In one

Box 9-3	Examples of Research Studies Using Newman's Health as Expanding Consciousness

Ananian, L. (2016). Relationship based care: Exploring the manifestations of health as expanding consciousness within a patient and family centered medical intensive care unit. *Nursing Research, 65*(2), E92–E93.

Bateman, G. C., & Merryfeather, L. (2014). Newman's theory of health as expanding consciousness: A personal evolution. *Nursing Science Quarterly, 27*(1), 57–61.

Condon, B. B. (2014). The living experience of feeling overwhelmed: A Parse research study. *Nursing Science Quarterly, 27*(3), 216–225.

Haney, T., & Tufts, A. (2012). A pilot study using electronic communication in home healthcare: Implications on parental well-being and satisfaction caring for medically fragile children. *Home Healthcare Nurse, 30*(4), 216–224.

Hayes, M. (2015). Life pattern of incarcerated women: The complex and interwoven lives of trauma, mental illness, and substance abuse. *Journal of Forensic Nursing, 11*(4), 214–222.

Rosa, K. C. (2016). Integrative review on the use of Newman praxis relationship in chronic illness. *Nursing Science Quarterly, 29*(3), 211–218.

Stec, M. W. (2016). Health as expanding consciousness: Clinical reasoning in baccalaureate nursing students. *Nursing Science Quarterly, 29*(1), 54–61.

example, MacNeil (2012) used Newman's theory as the framework in a qualitative study of individuals living with hepatitis C. In another example, Brown, Chen, Mitchell, and Province (2007) used a grounded theory approach to study help-seeking by older husbands who were caring for wives with dementia, and Musker (2008) published her work on life transitions in menopausal women. These studies indicate that the ideal of Health as Expanding Consciousness is useful for generating caring interventions in numerous populations.

Box 9-3 lists recent research studies that were conducted using Newman's model.

Parsimony

Newman's model consists of two major concepts: health and consciousness, and thus, it seems parsimonious. Despite this seeming simplicity, however, the theory is one of great complexity (George, 2010). Those who do not comprehend the simultaneity paradigm may wander in its enfolded relationships. The real complexity relates to the nature of the relationships between and among the concepts and to its abstractness.

Value in Extending Nursing Science

The focus of Newman's work is on the person, client, individual, and family. It places the client and nurse as integrated actors in understanding the client's health as consciousness. It also requires the understanding that health and disease are the same and not separate in the life of the individual (Newman, 2008b).

As illustrated by the examples from the literature presented, Newman's model has been successfully used in nursing practice and research. Newman's view can be applied in any setting, and research and practice application are underway to further verify its importance to the discipline (Jones, 2007).

Rosemarie Parse: The Humanbecoming Paradigm

Rosemarie Parse is a noted nursing scholar and prolific author. She first published her theory of nursing, *Man-Living-Health*, in 1981 and has continually revised the work. In 1992, Parse changed the name to the Theory of Humanbecoming. She combined human and becoming into a single word because that is how she sees this phenomenon (Parse, 2014). She is the author of many books and numerous articles. Her works have been translated into Danish, Finnish, French, German, Japanese, Korean, and other languages. She holds that humanbecoming has become a new paradigm, and the adherents to the scholarship of humanbecoming agree (Bournes, 2013; Parse, 2008, 2010, 2013, 2014; Smith, 2010).

Background of the Theorist

Parse was educated at Duquesne University in Pittsburgh, Pennsylvania, and earned her master's and doctoral degrees from the University of Pittsburgh. Some years later, she became dean of the College of Nursing at Duquesne, and she is currently Distinguished Professor emeritus at Loyola University in Chicago, Illinois. She is the founder and editor of *Nursing Science Quarterly* and president of Discovery International, which sponsors international nursing theory conferences. She is also the founder of the Institute of Humanbecoming, where she teaches the ontologic, epistemologic, and methodologic aspects of the Humanbecoming Paradigm. The Humanbecoming Paradigm is honored and acknowledged in colleges of nursing worldwide. She has currently realized that although a student of Martha Rogers, her work has developed into a wholly new paradigm, and she has titled this the Humanbecoming Paradigm (Parse, 2014).

Philosophical Underpinnings of the Theory

Parse synthesized the Humanbecoming Paradigm from principles and concepts from Rogers's work. She also incorporated concepts and principles from existential phenomenologic thought as expressed by Heidegger, Sartre, and Merleau-Ponty (Parse, 2014). The theory comes from her experience in nursing and from a synthesis of theoretical principles of human sciences.

Major Assumptions, Concepts, and Relationships

Assumptions

As with many of the major concepts, the major assumptions of Parse's theory originated with Rogers's Science of Unitary Human Beings and from existential phenomenology. Parse's thinking has brought her to a new ontology. Kuhn (1996) warned the scientific community that when the facts no longer support the current paradigm, the paradigm must change. For the humanbecoming perspective, a new paradigm has ascended. The language comes from the humanbecoming school of thought but has developed beyond that to a newer realm. Assumptions about Humanbecoming Paradigm are shown in Box 9-4.

Parse synthesized the nine assumptions of humanbecoming in four broad statements:

- Humanbecoming is structuring meaning, freely choosing the situation.
- Humanbecoming is configuring rhythmic humanuniverse patterns.

Box 9-4	The Philosophical Assumptions of the Humanbecoming Paradigm

- Humanuniverse is indivisible, unpredictable, and ever-changing.
- Humanuniverse is cocreating reality as a seamless symphony of becoming.
- Humanuniverse is an illimitable mystery with contextually construed pattern preferences.
- Ethos of humanbecoming is dignity.
- Ethos of humanbecoming is august presence, a noble bearing of immanent distinctness.
- Ethos of humanbecoming is embedded with the abiding truths of presence, existence, trust, and worth.
- Living quality is the becoming visible-invisible becoming of the emerging now.
- Living quality is the ever-changing whatness of becoming.
- Living quality is the personal expression of uniqueness.

Source: Parse (2014, pp. 29–30).

- Humanbecoming is cotranscending illimitably with emerging possibilities.
- Humanbecoming is humanuniverse cocreating a seamless symphony (Parse, 2013, p. 113).

Concepts

Parse builds on previous concepts and provides concepts and paradoxes that are found in this paradigm:

- Imaging: explicit–tacit; reflective–prereflective
- Valuing: confirming–not confirming
- Languaging: speaking–being silent; moving–being still
    - Revealing–concealing: disclosing–not disclosing
    - Enabling–limiting: potentiating–restricting
    - Connecting–separating: attending–distracting
- Powering: pushing–resisting; affirming–not affirming; being–nonbeing
- Originating: certainty–uncertainty; conforming–not conforming
- Transforming: familiar–not familiar (Parse, 2013, p. 113)

Relationships

From the major concepts, outlined three principles in the theory. These are updated and meaningful as enduring principles.

1. Structuring meaning is the imaging and valuing of languaging.
2. Configuring rhythmic patterns of relating the revealing–concealing and enabling–limiting of connecting–separating.
3. Cotranscending with the possible is powering and originating of transforming (Parse, 2010, p. 258).

Nurses guide individuals and families in choosing possibilities in changing the health process; this is accomplished by intersubjective participation with the clients. Practice focuses on illuminating meaning, and the nurse acts as a guide to choose possibilities in the changing health experiences (Parse, 2013).

Practitioners using Parse's method do not focus on changing an individual's behavior to fit a defined nursing process and do not attempt to label them with possibly erroneous nursing diagnoses. Rather, they practice from the understanding that the human–universe process involves the nurse's true presence with the person and the family. The nurse "dwells with the rhythms of the person and family" (Parse, 1995, p. 83) as they move through the experience. Nurses taking the time "to be fully present with the patient provides patient and nurse [who are] grounded in the humanbecoming theory [sic]" with meaningful and enlightening experiences (Smith, 2010, p. 216).

Usefulness

Parse's theory has been a guide for nurses all over the world. For example, in practice, McLeod-Sordjan (2013) used Parse's theory to illustrate the concept of "death acceptance." In this work, she described how to promote communication with low-English proficiency patients near the end of life. In other examples, Doucet (2015) described how the humanbecoming model could be applied to caring for a family who had a member with severe dementia, and Hart (2015) used a case study approach to demonstrate how the humanbecoming theory may be used to evaluate long-term care. Finally, Wilson (2016) applied Parse's humanbecoming theory in developing a comprehensive plan of care for a family experiencing the loss of a pregnancy or an infant.

In educational settings, Ursel (2015) used Parse's humanbecoming theory to describe a tool to enhance communication between patients and nursing students, seeking to use the theory to better focus on communicating relevant, timely, and accurate patient information. Several service learning opportunities directed by Parse's theory of humanbecoming were provided to a cohort of nursing students (Condon, Grimsley, Knaack, Pitz, & Stehr, 2015). In this work, theory and practice were creatively and effectively connected to the benefit of both students and various community groups. Finally, Drummond and Oaks (2016) describe how concepts and processes from Parse's theory have been interwoven within the curricula of both undergraduate and graduate programs in one nursing school.

Testability

The humanbecoming perspective is testable in principle, and many concepts that arise from it are being studied as the researchers develop perspectives on the human science of nursing. Research within Parse's method describes the lives, lived experiences, and ways of being of humans differently from research in the more reductionistic models. To study humanbecoming, Parse developed a research method similar to those of existential phenomenologists and derived specific steps that are rigorous and reproducible. The method involves dwelling with the information from the participant's perspective (dialogical engagement) and deriving themes from that data (extraction–synthesis) and then synthesizing the meanings into a relevant whole through heuristic interpretation (Parse, 1987). The inductive research method Parse and others have created is a research strategy that values the lived experiences of humans as they go about their daily lives, cocreating their health in human universe concert. Welch (2004) explored his experience using the method developed by Parse. His comments (Table 9-3) are important to students who wish to develop themselves as researchers within the method.

Parse's method for research, a descriptive phenomenologic method of inquiry, entitled "the Human Becoming Hermeneutic Method" (Barrett, 2002, p. 53), has been selected by nurse scholars in Australia, Canada, Denmark, Finland, Greece, Italy, Japan, South Korea, Sweden, the United Kingdom, and the United States. Baumann (2016) used this method to study how older adults experience suffering, and Doucet (2013) used the method to discover the lived experience of "feeling

Table 9-3 Lessons From a Doctoral Dissertation

Lessons	Writings as He Worked Through the Process	Welch's Actions
Finding a focus for the study	Considered depression incurable and had other preconceived ideas.	Reviewed literature, thought through process. Came to view depression as a time for people to work through difficult times (p. 202).
Locating a philosophical approach to inquiry	Considered several different approaches to phenomenologic inquiry.	Realized the superficiality of his understanding but was unaware of the significance of the differences in the approaches.
Deciding on a phenomenologic position	Found himself at an impasse, different terms, philosophical stances. Read the works of Parse.	Developed a lexicon of terms to understand the world of phenomenology (p. 203).
	Walked in the desert of theoretical confusion and increasing disillusionment with lack of progress in 2 years.	Found humanbecoming method, but his advisors were not familiar with process and terminology of Parse's method.
	Discussion with Parse was a "watershed" in realizing that he needed to review the focus on the study and also his philosophical disposition toward adopting the humanbecoming perspective.	Attended Humanbecoming Institute in Pittsburgh. Dialogued with Parse and other scholars. Parse agreed to assist with dissertation as a second advisor.
Selecting participants for the study	Wanted to include only the best and most appropriate potential participants to tell their stories of taking life day by day.	Realized that his inclination to take only the best candidates would compromise the integrity of the study. Therefore, he decided he had to adhere to the established criteria and remain cognizant of his personal bias.
Engaging the participants	As each participant talked of taking life day by day, I sensed myself moving with the rhythms of their stories (p. 205).	Being with the participants in true presence as they shared their stories was a profound experience (p. 205).
Inadvertently straying from the humanbecoming path	Embracing the art of living humanbecoming was an affirming enterprise; however, learning the art of humanbecoming was difficult (p. 205).	Dr. Parse provided important feedback about the conduct of the first tape and it was subsequently excluded. Came to the understanding of the importance of maintaining rigor (p. 205).
Allowing the voice of the text to be heard	My initial attempts to move the essences of the participants' stories to the language of the researcher and engage in the process of heuristic interpretation could be described only as throwing seed on barren ground (p. 206).	"I realized that the process of abstraction is concept driven; in other words, language is a vehicle for expressing what has already been formulated in the mind's eye. The extraction–synthesis and heuristic interpretation processes of Parse's method were perceived as pathways to new levels of knowing in explicating the participants' lived experiences" (p. 206).

(continued)

	Writings as He Worked	
Table 9-3 Lessons From a Doctoral Dissertation (Continued)		
Lessons	Through the Process	Welch's Actions
Gleaning insights from the journey	**Being comfortable with the uncomfortable:** A willingness to learn from the experienced scholars and a preparedness to move with the rhythms of the humanbecoming school of thought. **Mapping the journey:** The telling of the researchers' experience is an opportunity for other researchers contemplating such endeavors (p. 206). **Rethinking authentic rigor:** Authentic rigor involves more than adhering strictly to an established set of protocols; it also requires the researcher to be the embodiment of humanbecoming. Living the spirit of humanbecoming has to engage in a seamless movement of researcher with participant, researcher with text, and researcher with reader in the process of cocreating new horizons of understanding of the phenomenon under study (p. 206).	"I feel comfortable about testing the boundaries of conventional scientific inquiry. I no longer feel the need to engage in academic debate concerning the primacy of particular research paradigms within the community of scholars. Of importance to me is keeping alive the creative process or inquiry even though at times doing so means being lost in the labyrinthine paths of creative discovery" (p. 207).

Source: Welch (2004). Reprinted by permission of Sage Publications.

at home" in community-dwelling adults. A small sample of the numerous current studies of other aspects of human experience within Parse's Humanbecoming Paradigm are listed in Box 9-5.

Parsimony

Parse's model is parsimonious and artistic, having nine assumptions, which have been synthesized to four working assumptions; four postulates; three principles; and numerous concepts and paradoxes organized together in artful, logical, balanced ways to explain humanbecoming. With careful study, the paradigm lends itself to scholarly research and debate. The paradigm may seem complicated because much of the terminology is unfamiliar to most nurses. Indeed, this is a new and working way of seeing nursing in the real world (Smith, 2010). Students who want to use this model to guide their research and practice might consider contacting Parse and or one of her students for assistance to fully understand this new paradigm.

Value in Extending Nursing Science

The principal value of the Humanbecoming Paradigm is the worldview that sees humans as intentional beings, freely choosing to live within paradoxical ways of being.

Box 9-5	Examples of Current Research Using Parse's Humanbecoming Perspective

Bauman, S. L. (2016). The living experience of suffering: A Parse method study with older adults. *Nursing Science Quarterly, 29*(4), 308–315. doi:10.1177 /0894318416660530

Florczak, K. L. (2016). Power relations: Their embodiment in research. *Nursing Science Quarterly, 29*(3), 192–196. doi:10.1177/0894318416647167

Hawkins, K. (2015). Feeling disrespected: An exploration of the extant literature. *Nursing Science Quarterly, 28*(1), 8–12. doi:10.1177/0894318414558612

Ma, L. (2014). A humanbecoming qualitative descriptive study on quality of life with older adults. *Nursing Science Quarterly, 27*(2), 132–141. doi:10.1177 /0894318414522656

Parse, R. R. (2016). Parsciencing: A basic science mode of inquiry. *Nursing Science Quarterly, 29*(4), 271–274. doi:10.1177/0894318416661103

PetersonLund, R. R. (2013). Living on the edge: A review of the literature. *Nursing Science Quarterly, 26*(4), 303–310. doi:10.1177/0894318413500311

It is a unique way to view health and gives insight into how individuals create their own destiny.

Practice and research in the Humanbecoming Paradigm are quite different from those espoused in the other nursing perspectives. By living true presence with their clients, nurses guide and cocreate ways of being that enable choosing health. The amount of literature depicting use of Parse's work is multiplying rapidly, and support for the Humanbecoming Paradigm is growing.

Summary

The models presented in this chapter are considerably different from those described in the previous chapters. Additionally, significant similarities and differences are evident among these three models. Table 9-4 summarizes some of these by comparing definitions of the metaparadigm concepts. As Table 9-4 shows, the conceptualization of human beings is similar because Rogers heavily influenced both Newman and Parse. On the other hand, Parse was more specific when describing the environment, and Newman was much more explicit in her discussions of health. Perhaps, the greatest difference, however, relates to how they view nurses and nursing. Those wishing to use these theories should study these concepts closely and seek to apply them in their practice and research. When employing the research methods, which are unique, close work with the researchers or their former students will assist the novice researcher to develop the depth of effort that is required (Welch, 2004).

Nurses, such as Kristin from the opening case study, who prefer to view the person as a unitary being and who have a comprehensive view of health often find the theories from the simultaneity paradigm fascinating and helpful. These works have been extremely enlightening and helpful for the discipline of nursing, and all three have many adherents worldwide. A large and growing body of research explores patterns of lived experiences and health perspectives based on them, and the expanding topics of study currently enhance nursing science and will continue to do so into the future.

Table 9-4 Comparison of Concepts Common to the Unitary Process Nursing Theories

Author and Model	Human	Health	Environment	Nursing
Rogers: Unitary Human Beings (Rogers, 1990)	A sentient, unitary being; a multidimensional irreducible energy field known by pattern manifestation, and who cannot be known by the sum of parts.	Signifies an irreducible human field manifestation.	"An irreducible, indivisible, multidimensional energy field identified by pattern . . . integral with the human field" (p. 7).	A learned profession, a science and an art, whose uniqueness lies in concern for human beings.
Newman: Health as Expanding Consciousness (Newman, 1999)	Accepts the definition of human as stated by Rogers.	Health is a unitary process, a fluctuating pattern of rhythmic phenomena. Health includes illness within the pattern of energy.	Universal energy system as in Rogers's Science of Unitary Human Beings.	Assist persons to use innate power to evolve toward a higher level of consciousness. Nurses facilitate pattern recognition in this process.
Parse: Humanbecoming Paradigm (Parse, 2010)	Intentional beings involved with their world, having a fundamental nature of knowing, being present, and open to their world. The unitary human is one who "coparticipates in the universe in creating becoming and who is whole, open, free to choose ways of becoming" (p. 260).	A way of being in the world; it is not a continuum of healthy to ill, nor is it a dichotomy of health or illness, rather it is the living of day-to-day ways of being.	The world, the universe, and those who occupy spaces along with others who freely choose to be in the situation.	Guides humans toward ways of being, finding meaning in situations, and choosing ways of cocreating their own health. Nurses live true presence in the day to day of the person's life.

Key Points

- The simultaneity paradigm is an entirely different and nursing-centered way of studying nursing and humans.
- Martha Rogers and two of her students, Margaret Newman and Rosemarie Parse, have been active in providing education, collaborative communities, and the groundwork for students and nursing scientists who are currently working within the paradigm.
- Newman's Health as Expanding Consciousness is conversant with the current lives of the millennial age. Young people live an age of motion, information, and continuous communication. Expanding consciousness is the hallmark of this generation.
- Parse continues to develop the Humanbecoming Paradigm and frame its research processes. This paradigm offers new ways to understand the human–environment process and new lenses through which nursing care is provided. This paradigm generates considerable nursing-focused research and scholarship.

Learning Activities

1. Select one of the theories described and apply it in developing comprehensive patterns of nursing care for young teenagers who are becoming first-time mothers. How would a nurse practicing in this paradigm care for new mothers and the issues they encounter as they prepare for the birth of their babies. Share findings with classmates.

2. Select two simultaneity paradigm theories and apply them in developing comprehensive patterns of nursing care for the family of an elderly client with Alzheimer disease. Compare the two models for depth of understanding the client and family responses.

3. These three theorists suggest that health—rather than being a dichotomy (health-illness)—is as a way of being, a pattern of consciousness, or a manifestation of the human field. Can you envision health in this way? How would such a belief affect your practice?

4. Two of the theorists, (Newman and Parse) provide art and musical referents in their theories. Can you describe how using art and music might add to the ability of nurses to effectively interact with patients?

5. Kristin, the nurse from the opening case study, determined that Parse's Human-becoming Paradigm best fits her practice of hospice nursing. Reflect on a case or situation from your personal practice or experience. Can you apply one of the theories described in this chapter to the situation? How does the perspective from the theory change how you view the situation? Are nursing interventions the same? Do you anticipate that the care would be more holistic? Why or why not?

REFERENCES

Alligood, M. (2002). A theory of the art of nursing discovered in Rogers' science of unitary human beings. *International Journal for Human Caring, 6*(2), 55–60.

Arcari, P. M., & Flanagan, J. (2015). The development of a mind-body-spirit certification program in nursing. *Journal of Holistic Nursing, 33*(2), 168–176.

Barrett, E. A. M. (1986). Investigation of the principle of helicy: The relationship of human field motion and power. In V. M. Malinski (Ed.), *Explorations on Martha Rogers' science of unitary human beings* (pp. 173–188). Norwalk, CT: Appleton-Century-Crofts.

Barrett, E. A. M. (1989). A nursing theory of power for nursing practice: Derivation from Rogers' paradigm. In J. Riehl-Sisca (Ed.), *Conceptual models for nursing practice* (3rd ed., pp. 207–217). Norwalk, CT: Appleton & Lange.

Barrett, E. A. M. (2002). What is nursing science? *Nursing Science Quarterly, 15*(1), 51–60.

Baumann, S. L. (2016). The living experience of suffering: A Parse method study with older adults. *Nursing Science Quarterly, 29*(4), 308–315.

Bournes, D. A. (2013). Cultivating a spirit of inquiry using a nursing leading-following model. *Nursing Science Quarterly, 26*(2), 182–188.

Bramlett, M. H. (2010). What is nursing? What constitutes the science of unitary human beings? *Visions: The Journal of Rogerian Nursing Science, 17*(1), 6–7.

Brown, J. W., & Alligood, M. R. (2014). Margaret A. Newman: Health as expanding consciousness. In M. R. Alligood (Ed.), *Nursing theorists and their work* (8th ed., pp. 442–463). St. Louis, MO: Mosby.

Brown, J. W., Chen, S., Mitchell, C., & Province, A. (2007). Help-seeking by older husbands caring for wives with dementia. *Journal of Advanced Nursing, 59*(4), 352–360.

Caratao-Mojica, R. (2015). The science of unitary human beings in a creative perspective. *Nursing Science Quarterly, 28*(4), 297–299. doi:10.1177/0894318415599219

Condon, B. B., Grimsley, C., Knaack, L., Pitz, J., & Stehr, H. J. (2015). The art of service learning. *Nursing Science Quarterly, 28*(3), 195–200.

Davidson, A. W., Ray, M. A., & Turkel, M. C. (2011). *Nursing, caring, and complexity science: For human-environment well-being.* New York, NY: Springer Publishing.

Dossey, B. M. (2010). *Florence Nightingale: Mystic, visionary, healer.* Philadelphia, PA: F.A. Davis.

Doucet, T. J. (2013). Feeling at home: A humanbecoming living experience. *Nursing Science Quarterly, 26*(3), 247–256.

Doucet, T. J. (2015). Living the art of humanbecoming with the Smith family. *Nursing Science Quarterly, 28*(2), 122–126.

Drummond, S., & Oaks, G. (2016). A curriculum founded on humanbecoming: Educational endeavoring. *Nursing Science Quarterly, 29*(1), 25–29.

Farren, A. T. (2010). Power in breast cancer survivors: A secondary analysis. *Visions: The Journal of Rogerian Nursing Science, 17*(1), 29–43.

Fawcett, J. (2015). Evolution of the science of unitary human beings: The conceptual system, theory development and research and practice methodologies. *Visions: The Journal of Rogerian Nursing Science, 21*(1), 9–16.

Fitzpatrick, J. J. (1989). A life perspective rhythm model. In J. J. Fitzpatrick & A. L. Whall (Eds.), *Conceptual model of nursing: Analysis and application* (2nd ed., pp. 401–407). Norwalk, CT: Appleton-Century-Crofts.

Fuller, J. M., Davis, B. L., Servonsky, E. J., & Butcher, H. K. (2012). A family field pattern portrait of adult substance users in rehabilitation. *Visions: The Journal of Rogerian Nursing Science, 19*(1), 42–64.

George, J. B. (2010). Health as expanding consciousness: Margaret Newman. In J. B. George (Ed.), *Nursing theories: The base for professional nursing practice* (6th ed., pp. 519–538). Upper Saddle River, NJ: Pearson.

Gunther, M. E. (2014). Martha E. Rogers: Unitary human beings. In M. R. Alligood (Ed.), *Nursing theorists and their work* (8th ed., pp. 220–239). St. Louis, MO: Mosby.

Hart, J. D. (2015). Evaluating long-term care through the human-becoming lens. *Nursing Science Quarterly, 28*(4), 280–283.

Hastings-Tolsma, M. (2006). Toward a theory of diversity of human field pattern. *Visions: The Journal of Rogerian Nursing Science, 14*(2), 34–47.

Hektor, L. M. (1989). Martha E. Rogers: A life history. *Nursing Science Quarterly, 2*(2), 63–73.

Jones, D. (2007). Margaret A. Newman over the years. *Nursing Science Quarterly, 20*(4), 306.

Kirton, C. A., & Morris, D. L. (2012). Knowing participation in change and patient adherence to antiretroviral therapy in HIV infected adults. *Visions: The Journal of Rogerian Nursing Science, 19*(1), 11–25.

Kuhn, T. S. (1996). *The structure of scientific revolutions* (3rd ed.). Chicago, IL: University of Chicago Press.

MacNeil, J. M. (2012). The complexity of living with hepatitis C: A Newman perspective. *Nursing Science Quarterly, 25*(3), 261–266.

Madrid, M. M., Barrett, E. A. M., & Winstead-Fry, P. (2010). A study of the feasibility of introducing therapeutic touch into the operative environment with patients undergoing cerebral angiography. *Journal of Holistic Nursing, 28*(3), 168–174.

Madrid, M. M., & Winstead-Fry, P. (2001). Nursing research on the health patterning modalities of therapeutic touch and imagery. *Nursing Science Quarterly, 14*(3), 187–193.

Malinski, V. M., & Todaro-Franceschi, V. (2011). Exploring co-meditation as a means of reducing anxiety and facilitating relaxation in a nursing school setting. *Journal of Holistic Nursing, 29*(4), 242–248.

McLeod-Sordjan, R. (2013). Human becoming: Death acceptance: Facilitated communication with low-English proficiency patients at end of life. *Journal of Hospice and Palliative Nursing, 15*(7), 390–395.

Musker, K. M. (2008). Life patterns of women transitioning through menopause: A Newman research study. *Nursing Science Quarterly, 21*(4), 330–342.

Newman, M. A. (1979). *Theory development in nursing.* Philadelphia, PA: F.A. Davis.

Newman, M. A. (1986). *Health as expanding consciousness.* St. Louis, MO: Mosby.

Newman, M. A. (1990a). Newman's theory of health as praxis. *Nursing Science Quarterly, 3*(1), 37–41.

Newman, M. A. (1990b). Toward an integrative model of professional practice. *Journal of Professional Nursing, 6,* 167–173.

Newman, M. A. (1994). *Health as expanding consciousness.* New York, NY: National League for Nursing Press.

Newman, M. A. (1995). *A developing discipline: Selected works of Margaret Newman.* New York, NY: National League for Nursing Press.

Newman, M. A. (1999). *Health as expanding consciousness* (2nd ed.). New York, NY: National League for Nursing Press.

Newman, M. A. (2005). Caring in the human health experience. In C. Picard & D. Jones (Eds.), *Giving voice to what we know: Margaret Newman's theory of health as expanding consciousness in nursing practice, research, and education* (pp. 3–9). Sudbury, MA: Jones & Bartlett Learning.

Newman, M. A. (2008a). It's about time. *Nursing Science Quarterly, 21*(3), 225–227.

Newman, M. A. (2008b). *Transforming presence: The difference that nursing makes.* Philadelphia, PA: F.A. Davis.

Parse, R. R. (1981). *Man-living-health: A theory of nursing.* New York, NY: Wiley.

Parse, R. R. (1987). *Nursing science: Major paradigms, theories, and critiques.* Philadelphia, PA: Saunders.

Parse, R. R. (1995). *Illuminations: The human becoming theory in practice and research.* New York, NY: National League for Nursing Press.

Parse, R. R. (1998). *The human becoming school of thought: A perspective for nurses and other health professionals.* Thousand Oaks, CA: Sage.

Parse, R. R. (2008). The human becoming leading following model. *Nursing Science Quarterly, 21*(4), 369–375.

Parse, R. R. (2010). Human dignity: A humanbecoming ethical phenomenon. *Nursing Science Quarterly, 23*(3), 257–262.

Parse, R. R. (2013). Living quality: A humanbecoming phenomenon. *Nursing Science Quarterly, 26*(2), 111–115.

Parse, R. R. (2014). *The humanbecoming paradigm: A transformational worldview.* Pittsburgh, PA: Discovery.

Phillips, J. (2010). Perspectives of Rogers' relative present. *Visions: The Journal of Rogerian Nursing Science, 17*(1), 8–18.

Phillips, J. (2013). Creating an epiphany with Martha E. Rogers. *Nursing Science Quarterly, 26*(3), 241–246. doi:10.1177/0894318413489181

Phillips, J. R. (2016). Rogers' science of unitary human beings: Beyond the frontier of science. *Nursing Science Quarterly, 29*(1), 38–46.

Reed, P. (2008). Nursing time: Research, practice, and theory dimensions. *Nursing Science Quarterly, 21*(3), 222–223.

Reed, P. (2014). Theory of self-transcendence. In M. J. Smith & P. R. Liehr (Eds.), *Middle range theory for nursing* (3rd ed., pp. 109–140). New York, NY: Springer Publishing.

Rickles, D., Hawe, P., & Shiell, A. (2007). A simple guide to chaos and complexity. *Journal of Epidemiology and Community Health, 61,* 933–937. doi:10.1136/jech.2006.054254

Rogers, M. E. (1970). *An introduction to the theoretical basis of nursing.* Philadelphia, PA: F.A. Davis.

Rogers, M. E. (1986). Science of unitary human beings. In V. M. Malinski (Ed.), *Explorations on Martha Rogers' science of unitary human beings* (pp. 3–8). Norwalk, CT: Appleton-Century-Crofts. Reprinted in V. M. Malinski, E. A. M. Barrett, & J. R. Phillips (Eds.). (1994). *Martha E. Rogers: Her life and her work* (pp. 233–238). Philadelphia, PA: F.A. Davis.

Rogers, M. E. (1990). Nursing: Science of unitary, irreducible, human beings: Update 1990. In E. A. M. Barrett (Ed.), *Visions of Rogers' science-based nursing* (pp. 5–11). New York, NY: National League for Nursing Press.

Rogers, M. E. (1994). Nursing science evolves. In M. Madrid & E. A. M. Barrett (Eds.), *Rogers' scientific art of nursing practice* (pp. 3–9). New York, NY: National League for Nursing Press.

Rolfe, G. (2015). Foundations for a human science of nursing: Gadamer, Laing, and the hermeneutics of caring. *Nursing Philosophy, 16*(3), 141–152.

Sethares, K. A., & Gramling, K. L. (2014). Newman's health as expanded consciousness in baccalaureate education. *Nursing Science Quarterly, 27*(4), 302–307.

Shearer, N. (2009). Health empowerment theory as a guide for practice. *Geriatric Nursing, 30*(Suppl. 2), 4–10.

Smith, S. M. (2010). Humanbecoming: Not just a theory—it is a way of being. *Nursing Science Quarterly, 23*(3), 216–219.

Stec, M. W. (2016). Health as expanding consciousness: Clinical reasoning in baccalaureate nursing students. *Nursing Science Quarterly, 29*(1), 54–61.

Stein, J., & Sanburn, J. (2013, May). The new greatest generation: Why millennials will save us all. *Time, 181*(19), 26–32.

Ursel, K. L. (2015). Theory to practice: The humanbecoming leading-following model. *Nursing Science Quarterly, 28*(1), 28–33.

Welch, A. J. (2004). The researcher's reflections on the research process. *Nursing Science Quarterly, 17*(3), 201–207.

Wilson, D. R. (2016). Parse's nursing theory and its application to families experiencing empty arms. *International Journal of Childbirth Education, 31*(2), 29–33.

Zahourek, R. (2005). Intentionality: Evolutionary development in healing: A grounded theory study for holistic nursing. *Journal of Holistic Nursing, 23*(1), 89–109.

10

Introduction to Middle Range Nursing Theories

Melanie McEwen

Annette Cohen is a second-year graduate nursing student interested in starting her major research/scholarship project. For this project, she would like to develop some of her experiences in hospice nursing into a preliminary middle range theory of spiritual health. Annette has studied spiritual needs and spiritual care for many years but believes that the construct of spiritual health is not well understood. She views spiritual health as the result of the interaction of multiple intrinsic values and external variables within a client's experiences, and she believes that it is a significant contributing factor to overall health and well-being.

After reviewing theoretical writings dealing with spiritual nursing care, Annette found a starting point for her work in Jean Watson's Theory of Human Caring (Watson, 2012) because of its emphasis on spirituality and faith. From Watson's (2012) work, she was particularly interested in applying the concepts of "actual caring occasion" and "transpersonal" care. To develop the theory, Annette obtained a copy of Watson's most recent work and performed a comprehensive review of the literature covering theory development and the Theory of Human Caring. She then did an analysis of the concept of spiritual health. Combining the concept analysis and the literature review of Watson's work led to the development of assumptions and formal definitions of related concepts and empirical indicators. After conversing with her instructor, she concluded that her next steps were to construct relational statements and then draw a model depicting the relationships among the concepts that comprise spiritual health.

As discussed in Chapter 2, middle range nursing theories lie between the most abstract theories (grand nursing theories, models, or conceptual frameworks) and more circumscribed, concrete theories (practice theories, situation-specific theories, or microtheories). Compared to grand theories, middle range theories are more specific, have fewer concepts, and encompass a more limited aspect of the real world. Concepts are relatively concrete and can be operationally defined. Propositions are also relatively concrete and may be empirically tested.

The discipline of nursing recognizes middle range theory as one of the contemporary trends in knowledge development, and there is broad acceptance of the need to develop middle range theories to support nursing practice and nursing research (Alligood, 2014; Fitzpatrick, 2014; Kim, 2010; Peterson, 2017). According to Suppe (1996), this call to develop middle range theory is consistent with the third stage of legitimizing the discipline of nursing. The first stage focuses on differentiation of the perspective of the emerging discipline, which is characterized by separation from antecedent disciplines (i.e., medicine) and the establishment of university-based education, which in nursing occurred during the 1950s and 1960s. The second stage is marked by the quest to secure institutional legitimacy and academic autonomy. This stage characterized nursing during the 1970s and through the 1980s, when pursuit of nursing's unique perspective on and clarification of the phenomena of interest to the discipline were stressed. The third stage began in the 1990s and is distinguished by increased attention to substantive knowledge development, which includes development and testing of middle range theories. This stage is expanding and evolving further to include evidence-based practice and situation-specific theories (see Chapter 12).

Middle range theories are increasingly being used in nursing research studies. Many researchers prefer to work with middle range theories rather than grand theories or conceptual frameworks because they provide a better basis for generating testable hypotheses and addressing particular client populations. A review of nursing research journals and dissertation abstracts indicates that nursing research is currently being used in the development and testing of a number of middle range theories, and middle range theories are frequently being used as frameworks for investigation. Furthermore, middle range theories are presently being refined on the basis of research results.

Despite the recent promotion of middle range theories, there is a lack of clarity regarding what constitutes middle range theory in nursing. According to Cody (1999), "It appears that almost any theoretical entity that is more concrete than the broadest of grand theories is considered middle range by someone" (p. 10). Several nursing theory textbooks (e.g., Alligood, 2014; Chinn & Kramer, 2015; Fawcett & DeSanto-Madeya, 2013; M. C. Smith & Parker, 2015) disagree to some extent on which theories should be labeled as middle range. Indeed, some authors list a few of the readily accepted grand theories (e.g., Parse, Newman, Peplau, and Orlando) as middle range. Others consider somewhat more circumscribed theories (e.g., Leininger, Pender, Benner and Erickson, Tomlin, and Swain) to be middle range, although the theory's authors may not agree. In essence, there has been a paucity of discussion on the subject, and therefore, there is little consensus. This issue is discussed in more detail later in the chapter.

Purposes of Middle Range Theory

Middle range theories were first suggested in the discipline of sociology in the 1960s and were introduced to nursing in 1974. Scholars came to believe that middle range theories were useful for emerging disciplines because they are more readily operationalized and addressed through research than are grand theories. More than 15 years elapsed, however, before there was a concerted call for middle range theory development in nursing (Blegen & Tripp-Reimer, 1997; Meleis, 2012).

Development of middle range theories is supported by the frequent critique of the abstract nature of grand theories and the difficulty of their application to practice and research. The function of middle range theories is to describe, explain, or predict phenomena, and, unlike grand theory, they must be explicit and testable. Thus, they are easier to apply in practice situations and to use as frameworks for research studies. In addition, middle range theories have the potential to guide nursing interventions and change conditions of a situation to enhance nursing care. Finally, a major role of middle range theory is to define or refine the substantive component of nursing science and practice (Higgins & Moore, 2000). Indeed, Lenz (1996) noted that practicing nurses are actually using middle range theories but are not consciously aware that they are doing so.

Each middle range theory addresses relatively concrete and specific phenomena by stating what the phenomena are, why they occur, and how they occur. In addition, middle range theories can provide structure for the interpretation of behavior, situations, and events. They support understanding of the connections between diagnosis and outcomes and between interventions and outcomes (Fawcett & DeSanto-Madeya, 2013).

Enhancing the focus on middle range theories in nursing is supported by several factors. These include the observations that middle range theories:

- Are more useful in research than grand theories because of their low level of abstraction and ease of operationalization
- Tend to support prediction better than grand theories due to circumscribed range and specificity of the concepts
- Are more likely to be adopted in practice because their relative simplicity eases the process of developing interventions for identified health problems (Cody, 1999; Peterson, 2017)

Like theory in general, middle range theory has three functions in nursing knowledge development. First, middle range theories are used as theoretical frameworks for research studies. Second, middle range theories are open to use in practice and should be tested by research. Finally, middle range theories can be the scientific end product that expresses nursing knowledge (Suppe, 1996).

Characteristics of Middle Range Theory

Several characteristics identify nursing theories as middle range. First, the principal ideas of middle range theories are relatively simple, straightforward, and general. Second, middle range theories consider a limited number of variables or concepts; they have a particular substantive focus and consider a limited aspect of reality. In addition, they are receptive to empirical testing and can be consolidated into more wide-ranging theories. Third, middle range theories focus primarily on client problems and likely outcomes as well as the effects of nursing interventions on client outcomes. Finally, middle range theories are specific to nursing and may specify an area of practice, age range of the client, nursing actions or interventions, and proposed outcomes (Meleis, 2012; Peterson, 2017).

The more frequently used middle range theories tend to be those that are clearly stated, easy to understand, internally consistent, and coherent. They deal with current nursing perspectives and address socially relevant topics that solve meaningful and persistent problems. In summary, middle range theories for nursing combine postulated relationships between specific, well-defined concepts with the ability to measure or objectively code concepts. Thus, middle range theories contain concepts and statements from which hypotheses may be logically derived and empirically tested, and they can be easily adopted to guide nursing practice. Table 10-1 compares characteristics of grand theory, middle range theory, and practice/situation-specific theory, and characteristics of middle range theory are shown in Box 10-1.

Table 10-1 Characteristics of Grand, Middle Range, and Practice/Situation-Specific Theories

Characteristic	Grand Theories	Middle Range Theories	Practice/Situation-Specific Theories
Complexity/ abstractness, scope	Comprehensive, global viewpoint (all aspects of human experience)	Less comprehensive than grand theories, middle view of reality	Focused on a narrow view of reality, simple and straightforward
Generalizability/ specificity	Nonspecific, general application to the discipline irrespective of setting or specialty area	Some generalizability across settings and specialties, but more specific than grand theories	Linked to special populations or an identified field of practice
Characteristics of concepts	Concepts abstract and not operationally defined	Limited number of concepts that are fairly concrete and may be operationally defined	Single, concrete concept that is operationalized
Characteristics of propositions	Propositions not always explicit	Propositions clearly stated	Propositions defined
Testability	Not generally testable	May generate testable hypotheses	Goals or outcomes defined and testable
Source of development	Developed through thoughtful appraisal and careful consideration over many years	Evolve from grand theories, clinical practice, literature review, and practice guidelines	Derived from practice or deduced from middle range or grand theory

Concepts and Relationships for Middle Range Theory

Middle range theories consist of two or more concepts and a specified relationship between the concepts. Middle range theories address phenomena (concepts) that are toward the middle of a continuum of scope with the metaparadigm concepts (nursing, person, health, environment) at one end and specific concrete actions or events (medication administration, preoperative teaching, electrolyte management, fall prevention) at the other. The concepts should be discrete, observable, and sufficiently abstract to be applied across multiple settings and used with clients with differing problems (Blegen & Tripp-Reimer, 1997). Examples from the nursing literature include theories describing health promotion, comfort, coping, resilience, uncertainty, pain, grief, fatigue, self-care, adaptation, self-transcendence, and transitions (Meleis, 2012; Peterson, 2017; M. J. Smith & Liehr, 2014).

Box 10-1   Characteristics of Middle Range Nursing Theory

Not comprehensive but not narrowly focused
Some generalizations across settings and specialties
Limited number of concepts
Propositions that are clearly stated
May generate testable hypotheses

Middle range theories link discrete and observable phenomena or concepts in relationships statements. In middle range theory, relationships are explicitly stated, and, preferably, they are unidirectional. Relationships can be of several types. The most common are causal relationships that state that a change in the value of one variable or concept is associated with a change in the value of another variable or concept (Peterson, 2017).

Categorizing Middle Range Theory

The question as to which nursing theories are middle range is not clear-cut. Middle range theory is more specific than grand theory but abstract enough to support both generalization and operationalization across a range of populations; this sets it apart from practice or situation-specific theory.

In a well-researched effort to describe the place of middle range theory in nursing, Liehr and Smith (1999) analyzed 22 middle range theories published during the previous decade. These theories were categorized as "high-middle," "middle," and "low-middle" based on their level of abstraction or degree of specificity. In the review, high-middle theories included concepts such as caring, growth and development, self-transcendence, resilience, and psychological adaptation. Middle theories included concepts such as uncertainty in illness, unpleasant symptoms, chronic sorrow, peaceful end of life, cultural brokering, and nurse-expressed empathy. Low-middle theories, those that are closer to practice or situation-specific theories, included hazardous secrets, women's anger, nurse midwifery care, acute pain management, helplessness, and intervention for postsurgical pain.

As mentioned, there is some debate on which theories should be considered middle range. Indeed, some theories *not* termed middle range more appropriately fit the criteria of middle range theory than a grand theory, and some theories that are labeled middle range better fit the criteria of situation-specific or practice theory. Chapter 11 presents a number of middle range nursing theories described in the literature, organized as high, middle, and low theories. It should be noted that the designations are arguably arbitrary and that one theory that is listed here as "high-middle" may be considered by others to be a grand theory. Likewise, another theory listed here as "middle" might be considered by others to be "high-middle" and so forth. Situation-specific theories and their relationship to evidence-based practice are discussed in more detail in Chapter 12.

Development of Middle Range Theory

Several methods for development of middle range theories have been identified in the nursing literature. Middle range theories emerge from combining research and practice and building on the work of others. Sources used to generate middle range theory include literature reviews, qualitative research, field studies, conceptual models, taxonomies of nursing diagnoses and interventions, clinical practice guidelines, theories from other disciplines, and statistical analysis of empirical data (Fawcett & DeSanto-Madeya, 2013; Peterson, 2017). Five approaches for middle range theory generation were identified by Liehr and Smith (1999) (Box 10-2). The following sections present examples describing the source and development process of middle range theories from each of the five approaches listed in Box 10-2.

Box 10-2   Approaches for Middle Range Theory Generation

1. Induction through research and practice
2. Deduction from research and practice or application of grand theories
3. Combination of existing nursing and non-nursing middle range theories
4. Derivation from theories of other disciplines that relate to nursing
5. Derivation from practice guidelines and standards rooted in research

Middle Range Theories Derived From Research and/or Practice

The most common sources for development of middle range nursing theories and models are nursing research and nursing practice. Grounded theory research and other qualitative methods in particular are frequently noted as sources for middle range theory development. Examples of middle range theories derived from qualitative research include the Theory of Family Vigilance (Carr, 2014) (see Nursing Exemplar 1), the Theory of Spiritual Care in Nursing Practice (Burkhart & Hogan, 2017), a theory describing sustaining health in faith community nursing practice (Dyess & Chase, 2012), a theory describing "death imminence awareness" of family member of patients in critical care (Baumhover, 2015), and a theory of career persistence in acute care nurses (Hodges, Troyan, & Keeley, 2010).

Variations of the idea of development of middle range theory from research are fairly common. Theorists report combining qualitative research with literature review, concept analysis, concept synthesis, theory synthesis, and other techniques in the process of developing middle range theory. For example, Murrock and Higgins (2009) explained that they used statement and theory synthesis, along with literature review, to develop "the theory of music, mood and movement to improve health outcomes." In other works, Davidson (2010) developed "facilitated sensemaking" to support families of intensive care unit (ICU) patients following systematic literature review and synthesis, and Eakes, Burke, and Hainsworth developed the middle range Theory of Chronic Sorrow from an extensive review of the literature and data gathered through 10 qualitative research studies (Eakes, 2017).

Identification of middle range theories and models derived primarily from practice is more difficult. One example is the Theory of Unpleasant Symptoms (Lenz, Pugh, Milligan, & Gift, 2017), which was reportedly developed by integrating or melding existing practice and research information about a variety of symptoms. A second example is the Client Experience Model (Holland, Gray, & Pierce, 2011), which was reportedly developed through clinical observations in acute care settings using a practice-to-theory method.

Some models that describe areas of specialty nursing practice report being developed from combination of practice and another source, typically research or standards. One example of this technique is Benoit and Mion's (2012) model for pressure ulcer etiology in critically ill patients, which was constructed from combining a literature review and practice standards. The Omaha System, which is a model for community and home health nursing practice, is a second example. Martin (2005) explained that the conceptual framework for the Omaha System was a combination of practice, research, and literature review.

NURSING EXEMPLAR 1: MIDDLE RANGE THEORY DERIVED FROM RESEARCH/ PRACTICE

The process used to develop a middle range Theory of Family Vigilance was described by Carr (2014). Her purpose was to provide an explanation of "the meanings, patterns and day-to-day experience of family members staying with hospitalized relatives" (p. 251).

Theory Development Process: The *Theory of Family Vigilance* was derived from three ethnographic studies carried out among family members of patients in various units of a large, acute care hospital. The first study among family members of patients in a neurology unit, yielded five "categories of meaning"—commitment to care, resilience, emotional upheaval, dynamic nexus, and transition. Carr (2014) noted that each of these categories of meaning were supported by the findings of the subsequent studies.

Carr (2014) then described how she employed the strategies of concept synthesis and statement synthesis to define and then illustrate the relationships between and among the different defining characteristics of the categories that comprise family vigilance. Finally, through the process of theory synthesis, she constructed the information into a formalized theory.

Middle Range Theory Derived From a Grand Theory

As explained previously, many nursing theorists and scholars agree that grand theories are difficult to apply in research and practice and suggest development of middle range theories derived from them. During the last two decades, several theories developed from grand theories have been published in the nursing literature. One example is a middle range theory of health promotion for preterm infants (Mefford, 2004), which was derived from application of Levine's Conservation Model (see Nursing Exemplar 2). Two examples used Orem's theory. In one, Riegel, Jaarsma, and Strömberg (2012) developed the Theory of Self-Care of Chronic Illness, patterning their notion of self-care from Orem's theory. Similarly, Pickett, Peters, and Jarosz (2014) developed a middle range Theory of Weight Management based on Orem's theory.

In other examples, Hastings-Tolsma (2006) developed the Theory of Diversity of Human Field Pattern from Martha Rogers's Science of Unitary Human Beings. Cazzell (2008) employed the Neuman Systems Model as a basis for the middle range theory of adolescent vulnerability to risk behaviors, and in another work, Polk (1997) cited the work of both Margaret Newman and Martha Rogers as sources contributing to her middle range theory of resilience.

Several middle range theories were found which were developed from the Roy Adaptation Model (RAM). In one example, Dobratz (2011) derived the Theory of Psychological Adaptation in death and dying from a series of studies linked to the RAM, and in a similar example, she synthesized the middle range Theory of Adaptive Spirituality based on 21 published studies in which the RAM examined aspects of spirituality (Dobratz, 2016). In other examples, Hamilton and Bowers (2007) developed

NURSING EXEMPLAR 2: MIDDLE RANGE THEORY DERIVED FROM A GRAND THEORY

Mefford (2004) used Levine's Conservation Model of Nursing to develop a Theory of Health Promotion for Preterm Infants. In this case, Levine's theory was used as a framework for nursing practice for the neonatal intensive care unit (NICU) to ensure that needs of both the infant and family are addressed.

Theory Development Process: To develop the Theory of Health Promotion for Preterm Infants, the theorist first described elements of Levine's Conservation Model internal and external environments, wholeness, and conservation principles (conservation of energy, structural integrity, personal integrity, and social integrity) and applied these concepts in the NICU. She determined a "goal of restoring a state of wholeness, or health" (p. 260) (Figure 10-1).

Following initial development of the theory, its validity was tested in a retrospective study of 235 preterm infants. This study was designed to examine the influence of "consistency nursing care" on the health outcomes of the infants at discharge. Structural equation modeling demonstrated "strong support for the utility of this theory of health promotion . . . as a guide for nursing practice in the NICU" (p. 266). It was noted that the derived middle range theory validated Levine's work.

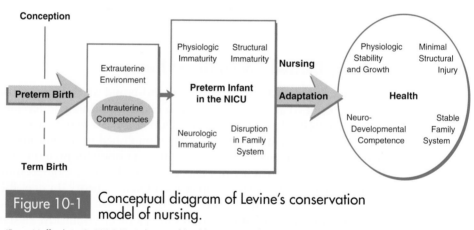

| Figure 10-1 | Conceptual diagram of Levine's conservation model of nursing. |

(From Mefford, L. C. [2004]. A theory of health promotion for preterm infants based on Levine's conservation model of nursing. *Nursing Science Quarterly, 17*[3], 261. Used with permission of Sage Publications, Inc.)

the Theory of Genetic Vulnerability from Roy's work, and Troutman-Jordan (2015) applied the results of a concept analysis within the RAM to develop the Theory of Successful Aging. Finally, Roy (2014) described synthesis of a middle range Theory of Coping using concepts and processes from the RAM.

Middle Range Theory Combining Existing Nursing and Non-Nursing Theories

Combining concepts or elements of multiple theories is common in middle range theory development. In many cases found in recent nursing literature, the authors of a middle range theory reported that they had derived their theory from both nursing

NURSING EXEMPLAR 3: MIDDLE RANGE THEORY COMBINING EXISTING NURSING AND NON-NURSING THEORIES

Dunn (2004) provided an excellent example of combining existing nursing and non-nursing theories in development of a middle range Theory of Adaptation to Chronic Pain. Her intention was to describe coping and pain control in older adults with the purpose of maintaining their quality of life and functional ability.

Theory Development Process: Dunn wrote that the first step in developing her theory was to review and synthesize the theoretical knowledge related to pain in older adults, coping with pain, religious coping, and spirituality. She reported identification of three theoretical models that addressed concepts related to pain control and coping in older adults. These were Melzack and Wall's (1992) Gate Control Theory of Pain, Lazarus and Folkman's (1984) Stress and Coping Theory, and Wallace, Benson, and Wilson's (1971) Relaxation Response. To ensure that the final model was applicable to nursing, she selected the RAM to guide the theory development process.

The second step reported by Dunn was to define assumptions for the theory; these were reportedly based on the assumptions from the four models from which the theory was drawn. Using the process of theoretical substraction, she then took concepts, relational statements, and propositions from the existing theories and arranged them into a diagram to represent the theoretical and operational systems. Finally, the concepts from the Adaptation to Chronic Pain Model were linked to empirical indicators to provide a logical and consistent connection.

and non-nursing theories. For example, Sousa and Zauszniewski (2005) used Orem's Self-Care Theory and Bandura's Self-Efficacy Theory to develop a theory of diabetes self-care management. Similarly, Ulbrich (1999) developed the Theory of Exercise as Self-Care through "triangulation of Orem's self-care deficit theory of nursing, the transtheoretical model of exercise behavior, and characteristics of a population at risk for cardiovascular disease" (p. 65). In another example, Reed (2014) used the philosophic views of Rogers's Science of Unitary Human Beings to relate the nursing perspective to self-transcendence. For this theory, Rogers's work was used as a framework, and it was reportedly combined with concepts and processes from developmental psychologists, including Piaget and Fagan. Finally, Dunn (2004) combined several non-nursing theories with the RAM to develop her middle range Theory of Adaption to Chronic Pain (see Nursing Exemplar 3).

Middle Range Theory Derived From Non-Nursing Disciplines

A significant number of middle range nursing theories are developed from one or more non-nursing theories. Indeed, non-nursing theories, including those from the behavioral sciences, sociology, physiology, and anthropology, appear to be the most common source for theory development, and many examples are evident. Kolcaba's Theory of Comfort, for example, was reportedly derived from a review of literature from medicine, psychiatry, ergonomics, and psychology as well as from nursing literature and history (Dowd, 2014). Role Theory was foundational for both

Meleis's Transitions Theory (Meleis, 2015) and Mercer's Theory of Maternal Role Attainment (Meighan, 2014). In other examples, Benner explained that the Dreyfus Model of Skill Acquisition, developed by a mathematician and a philosopher, was the primary source for her work (Brykczynski, 2014) and Mishel's Uncertainty in Illness Theory incorporated elements of Chaos Theory (Mishel, 2014).

In a work of theory synthesis, Pickering and Phillips (2014) described how their model for elder mistreatment was derived from several sources including Caregiver Burden Theory, theories describing "non-normal caregivers," Transgenerational

NURSING EXEMPLAR 4: MIDDLE RANGE THEORY DERIVED FROM A NON-NURSING DISCIPLINE

Covell (2008) proposed the middle range Theory of Nursing Intellectual Capital to explain the influence of nurses' knowledge, skills, and experience on patient and organizational outcomes.

Theory Development Process: Covell (2008) described using strategies of concept and theory derivation followed by research synthesis to develop and support the theory's propositions. Specifically, she noted how "Intellectual Capital Theory" (ICT) consisted of concepts from economics, accounting, and organizational learning theory. Key concepts or elements from ICT applied to her work were human capital, structural capital, relational capital, social capital, and business performance outcomes.

In applying ICT to nursing, Covell (2008) explained that she followed the steps in Walker and Avant's process of theory derivation to identify and define the theory's major concepts: nursing human capital and nursing structural capital. She also identified two factors within the work environment that influences nursing human capital—specifically nurse staffing and employer support for continuing professional developing. Following this, she proposed relationships among the concepts and illustrated how they influence both patient and organizational outcomes (Figure 10.2).

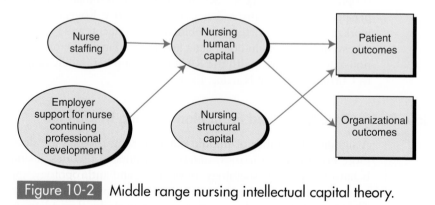

Figure 10-2   Middle range nursing intellectual capital theory.

(From Covell, C. L. [2008]. The middle-range theory of nursing intellectual capital. *Journal of Advanced Nursing, 63*[1], 94–103. Reprinted with permission of John Wiley and Sons.)

Table 10-2 Middle Range Nursing Theories Derived From Behavioral Theories

Theory	Non-Nursing Theory Source(s)
Commitment to Health Theory (Kelly, 2008)	Transtheoretical Model of Behavior Change
Recovery Alliance Theory of Mental Health Nursing (Shanley & Jubb-Shanley, 2007)	Humanistic Philosophy
Health Promotion Model (Pender, Murdaugh, & Parsons, 2015)	Social Learning Theory and Expectancy-Value Theory
Theory of Care-Seeking Behavior (Lauver, 1992)	Health Belief Model and the Theory of Reasoned Action
Medication Adherence Model (Johnson, 2002)	Health Belief Model, Social Learning Theory, the Theory of Reasoned Action, and the Self-Regulation Model
Self-Efficacy in Nursing Theory (Lenz & Shortridge-Baggett, 2002)	Social Learning Theory
Theory of Prenatal Care Access (Phillippi & Roman, 2013)	Lewin's Theory of Human Behavior
Cues to Participation in Prostate Screening (Nivens, Herman, Pweinrich, & Weinrich, 2001)	Health Belief Model, Social Learning Theory
Model for Cross-Cultural Research (Poss, 2001)	Health Belief Model, Theory of Reasoned Action

Transmission of Violence Theory, ecological theory, the Family Caregiving Dynamics Model, and the Phenomenon of Caregiver Dependency. Lastly, Covell (2008) explained how she derived the middle-range Theory of Nursing Intellectual Capital from a number of organizational behavior theories (see Nursing Exemplar 4).

Several middle range nursing theories have been derived from theories or models of behavioral change. Frequently cited are the Health Belief Model (Becker & Maiman, 1975; Rosenstock, 1990), the Theory of Reasoned Action (Ajzen & Fishbein, 1980), and the Social Learning/Social Cognitive Theory (Bandura, 1977, 1986), along with others. Table 10-2 lists some of these middle range theories and gives sources from which the theorist claims derivation of portions of their work.

Middle Range Theory Derived From Practice Guidelines or Standard of Care

Practice guidelines or standards of care appear to be the least common source for middle range theory development, as only a few examples could be found. In one example, the Public Health Nursing Practice Model (K. Smith & Bazini-Barakat, 2003) was developed by "melding of nationally recognized components" (p. 44) of public health nursing (PHN) practice. The identified components were the Standards of PHN practice, the 10 Essential Public Health Services, *Healthy People 2010*'s 10 Leading Health Indicators, and Minnesota's Public Health Interventions Model. In other examples, Good (1998) used clinical guidelines for management of postoperative pain to develop a middle range Theory of Acute Pain Management, and Huth and Moore (1998) used practice standards to develop a Theory of Acute Pain Management in infants and children. Finally, Ruland and Moore (1998) used standards of care to develop the Theory of the Peaceful End of Life from standards of care for terminally ill patients (see Nursing Exemplar 5).

NURSING EXEMPLAR 5: MIDDLE RANGE THEORY DERIVED FROM PRACTICE GUIDELINES OR STANDARD OF CARE

Ruland and Moore (1998) developed the Theory of the Peaceful End of Life from standards of care for terminally ill patients. In this work, the theorists observed that relational statements of the standards needed to be more specifically defined to make them applicable for empirical testing. Because the standards were too specific, they were too detailed to illustrate the major themes succinctly.

Theory Development Process: The first step of the theory development process was to define the theory's assumptions based on the standards of care. The second step was to perform a "statement synthesis," whereby five outcome criteria were developed that contributed to a peaceful end of life (not being in pain, experiencing comfort, experiencing dignity and respect, being at peace, and experiencing closeness to significant others or another caring person). For the third step, conceptual definitions for each of the outcome indicators were determined, and the fourth step involved defining relational statements between the outcome indicators and the nursing interventions. In this step, all process criteria from the standard were examined and combined into "prescriptors" to facilitate the desired outcome. The process of theory synthesis was then used to combine the relational statements into an integrated structure or theory. The final step was to draw a diagram of the relationships as a model (Figure 10-3).

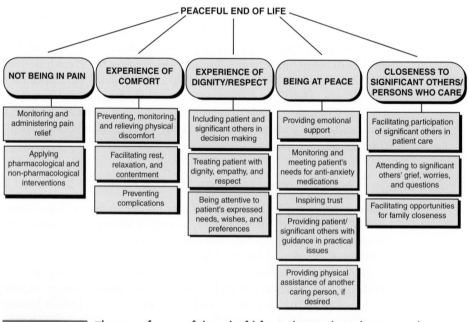

Figure 10-3 **Theory of peaceful end of life: Relationships between the concepts of the theory.**

(Reprinted from Ruland, C. M., & Moore, S. M. [1998]. Theory construction based on standards of care: A proposed theory of the peaceful end of life. *Nursing Outlook, 46*[4], 174. Used with permission from Elsevier.)

Final Thoughts on Middle Range Theory Development

Middle range theories should be "user-friendly" in language and style. They need to be described with practice implications in journals that practicing nurses are likely to read, and the theorists need to identify implications and specific interventions suggested by the theory (Lenz, 1996). Liehr and Smith's (1999) specific recommendations to enhance development and use of middle range theory include:

- Clearly articulate the theory name.
- Succinctly describe approaches used for generating the theory.
- Clarify the conceptual linkages of the theory in a diagrammed model.
- Elucidate the research–practice links of the theory.
- Explain the association between the theory and the discipline of nursing.

Analysis and Evaluation of Middle Range Theory

The move to enhance middle range theory development and use in nursing practice and research necessitates corresponding analysis and critique. Like grand theories and conceptual frameworks, middle range theories should be subject to evaluation. In addition, research guided by middle range theory should be congruent with the philosophical underpinnings of the theory and should be critiqued with regard to more than just the statistical significance of the findings.

Whall (2016) specifically addressed analysis and evaluation of middle range theory. Her criteria modified the guidelines she used for analysis and evaluation of grand nursing theories. The modifications removed explicit review of the metaparadigm concepts, which are assumed to be more implicit than explicit in middle range theory, and added questions regarding the congruence and fit of the middle range theory with the existing nursing perspective and domains. Furthermore, Whall explained that middle range theories should provide specific empirical referents for defined concepts. The ability to operationalize and measure aspects of the theory is extremely important in middle range theory, and operational definitions should be evaluated. Finally, she suggested analysis of middle range theories to assess their congruence with grand theories.

Smith (2014) also proposed a format for evaluation of middle range theories. She suggested evaluation based on three categories: substantive foundations, structural integrity, and functional adequacy. When evaluating substantive foundations, one would determine whether the theory was within the focus of nursing; whether assumptions are specified and congruent with the focus; whether the theory provides substantive description, explanation, or interpretation of a phenomenon that would be considered middle range; and whether the theory is rooted in practice or research experience. Evaluation of structural integrity would determine whether concepts are clearly defined and at the middle range of abstraction, whether the number of concepts is appropriate, and whether the concepts and relationship are logically represented with a model. Evaluation of functional adequacy examines whether the theory can be applied in practice or with various client groups, if empirical indicators have been identified for theoretical concepts, and if there are published examples of use of the theory in practice or research.

Chapter 5 includes a more detailed discussion of analysis and evaluation of middle range theories. In addition, the synthesized method for theory evaluation (see Box 5-3, p. 107) can be used as a guide for analysis and evaluation of middle range theory.

Summary

This chapter has described the current emphasis of nursing theory development, which focuses on efforts to construct, test, refine, and evaluate middle range theories. To help advance the discipline, nurses should be encouraged to write and publish papers that describe middle range theories and report research studies in which a middle range theory has been used. This process of middle range theory generation and refinement will further develop the discipline's substantive knowledge base.

Annette Cohen, the graduate student in the opening case study who was working toward development of a theory of spiritual health, related it to the practice of hospice nursing. Like Annette, nurses in all settings should strive to learn about existing or emerging middle range theories or seek to develop and describe theories that will explain phenomena they observe in practice.

Nursing has the knowledge, skills, manpower, and resources to move beyond delineation of conceptual models and domain concepts to emphasize development and application of middle range theory. Middle range theory holds much promise for the evolution of the discipline's science and practice. But, as Liehr and Smith (1999) pointed out, the challenge is to develop middle range theories that are empirically sound, coherent, meaningful, useful, and illuminating.

Key Points

- Middle range nursing theories were first introduced into nursing in the mid-1970s; their number and use have grown dramatically in the last decade.
- Middle range theories are more specific, have fewer concepts, and encompass a more limited aspect of the real world compared with grand nursing theories; they are also more readily testable in research.
- Middle range theories may be developed through research, practice, or literature synthesis; they may be derived from grand nursing theories or non-nursing theories; or they may be derived from practice guidelines and standards.
- Before being used in a research study or applied in practice, middle range nursing theories should be analyzed or evaluated.

Learning Activities

1. Search current nursing journals for examples of the development, analysis, or use of middle range theories in the discipline of nursing. Can any trends be identified?
2. Select one of the middle range theories derived from a grand nursing theory and one derived from a non-nursing theory. Analyze both for ease of application to research and practice.
3. Annette, the nurse from the opening case study, determined that she wanted to develop a middle range theory of spiritual health. Consider a concept of interest or one relevant to your practice. How could you develop the concept into a preliminary middle range theory following one of the processes presented in this chapter?

REFERENCES

Ajzen, I., & Fishbein, M. (1980). *Understanding attitudes and predicting social behavior.* Englewood Cliffs, NJ: Prentice-Hall.

Alligood, M. R. (2014). State of the art and science of nursing theory. In M. R. Alligood (Ed.), *Nursing theorists and their work* (8th ed., pp. 712–720). St. Louis, MO: Mosby.

Bandura, A. (1977). *Social learning theory.* Englewood Cliffs, NJ: Prentice-Hall.

Bandura, A. (1986). *Social foundations of thought and action: A social cognitive theory.* Englewood Cliffs, NJ: Prentice-Hall.

Baumhover, N. C. (2015). The process of death imminence awareness by family members of patients in adult critical care. *Dimensions of Critical Care Nursing, 34*(3), 149–160.

Becker, M. H., & Maiman, L. A. (1975). Sociobehavioral determinates of compliance with health and medical care recommendations. *Medical Care, 13,* 10–24.

Benoit, R., & Mion, L. (2012). Risk factors for pressure ulcer development in critically ill patients: A conceptual model to guide research. *Research in Nursing & Health, 35*(4), 340–362.

Blegen, M. A., & Tripp-Reimer, T. (1997). Implications of nursing taxonomies for middle-range theory development. *ANS. Advances in Nursing Science, 19*(3), 37–49.

Brykczynski, K. A. (2014). Patricia Benner: Caring, clinical wisdom, and ethics in nursing practice. In M. R. Alligood (Ed.), *Nursing theorists and their work* (8th ed., pp. 120–146). St. Louis, MO: Mosby.

Burkhart, L., & Hogan, N. (2017). Spiritual care in nursing practice (SCiNP). In S. J. Peterson & T. S. Bredow (Eds.), *Middle range theories: Application to nursing research* (4th ed., pp. 106–115). Philadelphia, PA: Wolters Kluwer.

Carr, J. M. (2014). A middle range theory of family vigilance. *Medsurg Nursing, 23*(4), 251–255.

Cazzell, M. (2008). Linking theory, evidence, and practice in assessment of adolescent inhalant use. *Journal of Addictions Nursing, 19,* 17–25.

Chinn, P. L., & Kramer, M. K. (2015). *Theory and nursing: Integrated knowledge development* (9th ed.). St. Louis, MO: Mosby.

Cody, W. K. (1999). Middle-range theories: Do they foster the development of nursing science? *Nursing Science Quarterly, 12*(1), 9–14.

Covell, C. L. (2008). The middle-range theory of nursing intellectual capital. *Journal of Advanced Nursing, 63*(1), 94–103.

Davidson, J. E. (2010). Facilitated sensemaking: A strategy and new middle-range theory to support families of intensive care unit patients. *Critical Care Nurse, 30*(6), 28–39.

Dobratz, M. C. (2011). Toward development of a middle-range theory of psychological adaptation in death and dying. *Nursing Science Quarterly, 24*(4), 370–376.

Dobratz, M. C. (2016). Building a middle-range theory of adaptive spirituality. *Nursing Science Quarterly, 29*(2), 146–153.

Dowd, T. (2014). Katharine Kolcaba: Theory of comfort. In M. R. Alligood (Ed.), *Nursing theorists and their work* (8th ed., pp. 657–671). St. Louis, MO: Mosby.

Dunn, K. S. (2004). Toward a middle-range theory of adaptation to chronic pain. *Nursing Science Quarterly, 17*(1), 78–84.

Dyess, S. M., & Chase, S. K. (2012). Sustaining health in faith community nursing practice: Emerging processes that support the development of a middle-range theory. *Holistic Nursing Practice, 26*(4), 221–227.

Eakes, G. (2017). Chronic sorrow. In S. J. Peterson & T. S. Bredow (Eds.), *Middle range theories: Application to nursing research* (4th ed., pp. 93–105). Philadelphia, PA: Wolters Kluwer.

Fawcett, J., & DeSanto-Madeya, S. (2013). *Contemporary nursing knowledge: Analysis and evaluation of nursing models and theories* (3rd ed.). Philadelphia, PA: F.A. Davis.

Fitzpatrick, J. J. (2014). Foreword. In M. J. Smith & P. R. Liehr (Eds.), *Middle range theory for nursing* (3rd ed., pp. xi–xii). New York, NY: Springer Publishing.

Good, M. (1998). A middle-range theory of acute pain management: Use in research. *Nursing Outlook, 46*(3), 120–124.

Hamilton, R. J., & Bowers, B. J. (2007). The theory of genetic vulnerability: A Roy model exemplar. *Nursing Science Quarterly, 20*(3), 254–264.

Hastings-Tolsma, M. (2006). Toward a theory of diversity of human field pattern. *Visions: The Journal of Rogerian Nursing Science, 14*(2), 34–47.

Higgins, P. A., & Moore, S. M. (2000). Levels of theoretical thinking in nursing. *Nursing Outlook, 48*(4), 179–183.

Hodges, H. F., Troyan, P. J., & Keeley, A. C. (2010). Career persistence in baccalaureate-prepared acute care nurses. *Journal of Nursing Scholarship, 42*(1), 83–91.

Holland, B. E., Gray, J., & Pierce, T. B. (2011). The client experience model: Synthesis and application to African American with multiple sclerosis. *The Journal of Theory Construction & Testing, 15*(2), 36–40.

Huth, M. M., & Moore, S. M. (1998). Prescriptive theory of acute pain management in infants and children. *Journal of the Society of Pediatric Nurses, 3*(1), 23–32.

Johnson, M. J. (2002). The medication adherence model: A guide for assessing medication taking. *Research and Theory for Nursing Practice, 16*(3), 179–192.

Kelly, C. W. (2008). Commitment to health theory. *Research and Theory for Nursing Practice, 22*(2), 148–158.

Kim, H. S. (2010). *The nature of theoretical thinking in nursing* (3rd ed.). New York, NY: Springer Publishing.

Lauver, D. (1992). A theory of care-seeking behavior. *Image—The Journal of Nursing Scholarship, 24*(4), 281–287.

Lazarus, R. S., & Folkman, S. (1984). *Stress, appraisal, and coping.* New York, NY: Springer Publishing.

Lenz, E. R. (1996, May). *Middle range theory: Role in research and practice.* Paper presented at the Sixth Rosemary Ellis Scholar's Retreat, Cleveland, OH.

Lenz, E. R., Pugh, L. C., Milligan, R., & Gift, A. (2017). Unpleasant symptoms. In S. J. Peterson & T. S. Bredow (Eds.), *Middle range theories: Application to nursing research* (4th ed., pp. 67–78). Philadelphia, PA: Wolters Kluwer.

Lenz, E. R., & Shortridge-Baggett, L. (Eds.). (2002). *Self-efficacy and nursing.* New York, NY: Springer Publishing.

Liehr, P., & Smith, M. J. (1999). Middle range theory: Spinning research and practice to create knowledge for the new millennium. *ANS. Advances in Nursing Science, 21*(4), 81–91.

Martin, K. S. (2005). *The Omaha system: A key to practice, documentation, and information management.* St. Louis, MO: Elsevier Saunders.

Mefford, L. C. (2004). A theory of health promotion for preterm infants based on Levine's conservation model of nursing. *Nursing Science Quarterly, 17*(3), 260–266.

Meighan, M. (2014). Ramona T. Mercer: Maternal role attainment—becoming a mother. In M. R. Alligood (Ed.), *Nursing theorists and their work* (8th ed., pp. 538–554). St. Louis, MO: Mosby.

Meleis, A. I. (2012). *Theoretical nursing: Development and progress* (5th ed.). Philadelphia, PA: Lippincott Williams & Wilkins.

Meleis, A. I. (2015). Transitions theory. In M. C. Smith & M. E. Parker (Eds.), *Nursing theories & nursing practice* (4th ed., pp. 361–380). Philadelphia, PA: F.A. Davis.

Melzack, R., & Wall, P. D. (1992). Psychophysiology of pain. In D. C. Turk & R. Melzack (Eds.), *Handbook of pain and assessment* (pp. 3–25). New York, NY: Guilford Press.

Mishel, M. H. (2014). Theories of uncertainty in illness. In M. J. Smith & P. R. Liehr (Eds.), *Middle range theory for nursing* (3rd ed., pp. 53–86). New York, NY: Springer Publishing.

Murrock, C. J., & Higgins, P. A. (2009). The theory of music, mood and movement to improve health outcomes. *Journal of Advanced Nursing, 65*(10), 2249–2257.

Nivens, A. S., Herman, J., Pweinrich, S. P., & Weinrich, M. C. (2001). Cues to participation in prostate cancer screening: A theory for practice. *Oncology Nursing Forum, 28*(9), 1449–1456.

Pender, N. J., Murdaugh, C., & Parsons, M. A. (2015). *Health promotion in nursing practice* (7th ed.). Upper Saddle River, NJ: Prentice-Hall.

Peterson, S. J. (2017). Introduction to the nature of nursing knowledge. In S. J. Peterson & T. S. Bredow (Eds.), *Middle range theories: Application to nursing research* (4th ed., pp. 1–35). Philadelphia, PA: Wolters Kluwer.

Phillippi, J. C., & Roman, M. W. (2013). The motivation-facilitation theory of prenatal care access. *Journal of Midwifery & Women's Health, 58*(6), 509–515.

Pickering, C. E. Z., & Phillips, L. R. (2014). Development of a causal model for elder mistreatment. *Public Health Nursing, 31*(4), 363–372.

Pickett, S., Peters, R. M., & Jarosz, P. A. (2014). Toward a middle-range theory of weight management. *Nursing Science Quarterly, 27*(3), 242–247.

Polk, L. V. (1997). Toward a middle-range theory of resilience. *ANS. Advances in Nursing Science, 19*(3), 1–13.

Poss, J. E. (2001). Developing a new model for cross-cultural research: Synthesizing the health belief model and the theory of reasoned action. *ANS. Advances in Nursing Science, 23*(4), 1–15.

Reed, P. G. (2014). Theory of self-transcendence. In M. J. Smith & P. R. Liehr (Eds.), *Middle range theory for nursing* (3rd ed., pp. 109–140). New York, NY: Springer Publishing.

Riegel, B., Jaarsma, T., & Strömberg, A. (2012). A middle-range theory of self-care of chronic illness. *ANS. Advances in Nursing Science, 35*(3), 194–204.

Rosenstock, I. (1990). The health belief model: Explaining health behavior through expectancies. In K. Glanz, F. Lewis, & B. Rimer (Eds.), *Health behavior and health education* (pp. 39–62). San Francisco, CA: Jossey-Bass.

Roy, C. (2014). Synthesis of a middle range theory of coping. In C. Roy (Ed.), *Generating middle range theory: From evidence to practice* (pp. 211–232). New York, NY: Springer Publishing.

Ruland, C. M., & Moore, S. M. (1998). Theory construction based on standards of care: A proposed theory of the peaceful end of life. *Nursing Outlook, 46*(4), 169–175.

Shanley, E., & Jubb-Shanley, M. (2007). The recovery alliance theory of mental health nursing. *Journal of Psychiatric and Mental Health Nursing, 14*(8), 734–743.

Smith, K., & Bazini-Barakat, N. (2003). A public health nursing practice model: Melding public health principles with the nursing process. *Public Health Nursing, 20*(1), 42–48.

Smith, M. C. (2014). Evaluation of middle range theories for the discipline of nursing. In M. J. Smith & P. R. Liehr (Eds.), *Middle range theory for nursing* (3rd ed., pp. 35–50). New York, NY: Springer Publishing.

Smith, M. C., & Parker, M. E., (2015). *Nursing theories & nursing practice* (4th ed.). Philadelphia, PA: F.A. Davis.

Smith, M. J., & Liehr, P. R. (Eds.). (2014). *Middle range theory for nursing* (3rd ed.). New York, NY: Springer Publishing.

Sousa, V. D., & Zauszniewski, J. A. (2005). Toward a theory of diabetes self-care management. *Journal of Theory Construction and Testing, 9*(2), 61–67.

Suppe, F. (1996, May). *Middle range theory: Nursing theory and knowledge development.* Paper presented at the Sixth Rosemary Ellis Scholar's Retreat, Cleveland, OH.

Troutman-Jordan, M. (2015). Troutman-Jordan's theory of successful ageing. In M. C. Smith & M. E. Parker (Eds.), *Nursing theories & nursing practice* (4th ed., pp. 483–494). Philadelphia, PA: F.A. Davis.

Ulbrich, S. L. (1999). Nursing practice theory of exercise as self-care. *Image—The Journal of Nursing Scholarship, 31*(1), 65–70.

Wallace, R., Benson, H., & Wilson, A. F. (1971). A wakeful hypometabolic physiologic state. *The American Journal of Physiology, 221*(3), 795–799.

Watson, J. (2012). *Human caring science: A theory of nursing* (2nd ed.). Sudbury, MA: Jones & Bartlett Learning.

Whall, A. L. (2016). Philosophy of science positions and their importance in cross-national nursing. In J. J. Fitzpatrick & A. L. Whall (Eds.), *Conceptual models of nursing: Global perspectives* (5th ed., pp. 5–20). Upper Saddle River, NJ: Prentice-Hall.

Overview of Selected Middle Range Nursing Theories

Melanie McEwen

Elaine Chavez is employed as a nurse at a public health clinic in an urban area. She is also in her second semester of a graduate nursing program preparing to become a mental health nurse practitioner. In her practice, Elaine has worked with a number of women who have been abused by their partners, and she has observed a pattern of comorbidities in these women, including depression, alcoholism, substance abuse, and suicide attempts. Over the last few months, Elaine has reviewed the nursing literature and identified several intervention strategies that have been effective in working with women who have been victims of domestic violence. Using this information, she would like to implement a program to promote early identification of abuse and multiple-level interventions. This is a project that will work well with one of her master's portfolio assignments.

From her literature review, Elaine identified several theories related to her study. She was particularly interested in examining the set of circumstances that would cause the women to seek help. For this, she performed a more detailed literature review and identified Kolcaba's (2003, 2017) Theory of Comfort, which helped her conceptualize many of the issues faced by abused women. Indeed, the theory described individual characteristics that contributed to health-seeking behavior. These were stimulus situations, which can cause negative tension. By providing comfort measures, the nurse can help decrease negative tensions and promote positive tension. Elaine wanted to continue to identify comfort measures that would encourage the women to seek care for their problems.

For the next phase of her project, Elaine collected all of the information she could find on Kolcaba's theory. This included studies that had used the model as a conceptual framework and studies that had tested the model. From that information and the articles she had gathered previously about issues related to domestic violence, she was able to draft a set of interventions that she hoped to implement at the clinic following approval by her supervisor.

Previous chapters have described the growing emphasis on the development and testing of middle range theories in nursing. As a result, during the past two decades, a significant number of these theories have been presented in the nursing literature. The purpose of this chapter is to introduce some of the commonly used middle range nursing theories as well as some of the recently published ones to familiarize readers with these works and direct them to resources for more information. An attempt was made to include works from a variety of areas and from many scholars but by no means is the list presented here exhaustive. Nor does inclusion or exclusion relate to the quality or significance of the theory or its usefulness in research or practice.

To assist with organization of the chapter, the theories are divided into sections based on whether they appear to be "high," "middle," or "low" middle range theories. As explained in Chapter 10, the high/middle/low distinction relates to the level of abstraction as posed by Liehr and Smith (1999), with the "high" middle range theories being the most abstract and nearest to the grand theories. The "low" middle range theories, on the other hand, are the least abstract, and they are similar to practice or situation-specific theories. It is noted that these designations are arguably arbitrary and that one theory that is listed here as "high middle" may be considered by others to be a grand theory. Likewise, another theory listed here as "middle middle" might be considered by others to be a high middle range theory, and so forth.

Elements of theory description and theory analysis as explained in Chapter 5 serve as the basis for the more detailed discussions of selected theories. Each will include a brief overview, an outline of the purpose and major concepts of the theory, and context for use and nursing implications. Finally, evidence of empirical testing and application in practice are described (Box 11-1).

High Middle Range Theories

The high middle range theories presented here are some of the most well-known and widely used theories in nursing. Included are the works of Benner, Leininger, Pender, and Meleis. These theories may be considered grand theories or conceptual frameworks by other nursing scholars and possibly by the author of the theory. These theories, however, do not totally fit with the criteria for grand theories as outlined in this text and therefore are not covered in the chapters dealing with that content. In addition, the Synergy Model, a nursing model that is widely used in research and practice, particularly in critical care, will be discussed. Table 11-1 lists other high middle range theories or conceptual models, their purposes, and major concepts.

Benner's Model of Skill Acquisition in Nursing

Patricia Benner's theoretical model was first published in 1984. The model, which applies the Dreyfus model of skill acquisition to nursing, outlines five stages of skill

| Box 11-1 | American Association of Colleges of Nursing Essentials |

Middle range theory is vital for the ongoing development of the nursing profession. Indeed, according to the doctorate of nursing practice "essentials," "Nursing science frames the development of middle range theories and concepts to guide nursing practice" (American Association of Colleges of Nursing, 2006, p. 9).

Table 11-1 High Middle Range Nursing Theories

Theory/Model	Purpose	Major Concepts
Tidal model (psychiatric and mental health nursing) (Barker, 2001a, 2001b)	Describes psychiatric nursing practice focusing on three care processes; emphasizes the fluid nature of human experience characterized by change and unpredictability	Personhood (dimensions—world, self, others), discrete holistic (exploratory) assessment; focused (risk) assessment, empowerment, narrative as the medium of self
Spiritual Care in Nursing Practice Theory (Burkhart & Hogan, 2008)	Describes the process in which positive nurse–patient spiritual encounters can lead to positive spiritually growth-filled memories that will increase nurses' spiritual well-being	Patient cue, decision to engage/not engage, spiritual intervention, immediate emotional response (positive or negative), search for meaning, formation of a spiritual memory, spiritual well-being
Parish nursing (Bergquist & King, 1994)	Describes the integration of physical, emotional, and spiritual components in provision of holistic health care in a faith community	Client (spiritual, physical, emotional components), parish nurse (spiritual maturity, pastoral team member, autonomy, caring, effective communication), health (physical, emotional, and spiritual wellness and wholeness), environment (faith community)
Parish nursing (L. W. Miller, 1997)	Integrates the concepts of evangelical Christianity with application of parish nursing interventions	Person/parishioner, health, nurse/parish nurse, community/parish, the triune God
Neal Theory of Home Health Nursing (Neal, 1999a, 1999b)	Describes the practice of home health nurses as they use process of adaptation to attain autonomy	Autonomy, three stages (dependence, moderate dependence, and autonomy), logistics, client's home, client's resources, client's needs, and learning capacity
Occupational health nursing (Rogers, 1994)	Shows how the occupational health nurse works to improve, protect, maintain, and restore the health of the worker/workforce and depicts how practice is affected by both external and internal work setting influences	Work setting influences (corporate culture/mission, resources, work hazards, workforce characteristics), external factors (economics, population/health trends, legislation/politics, technology), occupational health nursing practice (health promotion, workplace hazard detection, case management/primary care, counseling, management, research, legal/ethical monitoring, community orientation)
Omaha System (Martin, 2005)	Comprehensive classification system that promotes documentation of client care, generally in community and home health nursing practice	Depicts the nursing process as circular rather than linear; steps are collect and assess data, state problems, identify admission problem rating, plan and intervene, identify interim/dismissal problem rating, and evaluate problem outcomes.
Schuler Nurse Practitioner Practice Model (Shuler & Davis, 1993)	Integrates essential nursing and medical orientations to provide a framework for holistic practice for nurse practitioners (NP)	Patient and NP inputs (noted as episodic and comprehensive with and without health problem); data gathering/role modeling; patient and NP throughputs include identification of problems and diagnosing, contracting, and planning and implementing of the plan of care. Outputs involve comprehensive evaluation of patient and NP outcomes.
Public health nursing practice (K. Smith & Bazini-Barakat, 2003)	Guides public health nurses to improve the health of communities and target populations	Interdisciplinary public health team, standards of public health nursing practice, essential public health services, health indicators, population-based practice (systems, community, individual, and family focus), healthy people in health communities
Rural nursing (Weinert & Long, 1991)	Guides rural nursing practice, research, and education by understanding and addressing the unique health care needs and preferences of rural persons	Health (health as ability to work), environment (distance and isolation), person (self-reliance and independence), nursing (lack of anonymity, outsider/insider, and old-timer/newcomer)

acquisition: novice, advanced beginner, competent, proficient, and expert. Although Benner's work is much more encompassing in regard to nursing domains and specific functions and interventions, it is the five stages of skill acquisition that has received the most attention with regard to application in administration, education, practice, and research.

Purpose and Major Concepts

Benner's model delineates the importance of retaining and rewarding nurse clinicians for their clinical expertise in practice settings because it describes the evolution of "excellent caring practices." She notes that research demonstrates that practice grows "through experiential learning and through transmitting that learning in practical settings" (Benner, 2001, p. vi). Expertise develops when the clinician tests and refines propositions, hypotheses, and principle-based expectations in actual practice situations. Finally, the model seeks to describe clinical expertise including six areas of practical knowledge (graded qualitative distinctions; common meanings; assumptions, expectations, and sets; paradigm cases and personal knowledge; maxims; and unplanned practices) (Benner, Tanner, & Chesla, 2009).

The central concepts of Benner's model are those of competence, skill acquisition, experience, clinical knowledge, and practical knowledge. She also identifies the following seven domains of nursing practice:

- Helping role
- Teaching or coaching function
- Diagnostic client-monitoring function
- Effective management of rapidly changing situations
- Administering and monitoring therapeutic interventions and regimens
- Monitoring and ensuring quality of health care practices
- Organizational and work-role competencies (Benner, 2001)

Context for Use and Nursing Implications

The Benner model has been used extensively as rationale for career development and continuing education in nursing. Areas specifically cited for utilization include nursing management, career enhancement, clinical specialization, staff development programs, staffing, evaluation, clinical internships, and precepting students and novice nurses (Benner, 2001; Benner et al., 2009).

Evidence of Empirical Testing and Application in Practice

Over the previous decade, dozens of articles have been written based on Benner's model, and a number of these were research-based studies. For example, Wilson, Harwood, and Oudshoorn (2015) examined the "perpetual novice phenomenon," and Cates and colleagues (2015) employed a Delphi method to develop a simulation-based competency assessment instrument for neonatal nurse practitioners, both based on Benner's model. In other research, Meretoja and Koponen (2012) used Benner's model to compare nurses' optimal and actual competencies in clinical settings, and Abraham (2011) reported on a study to evaluate a program based on Benner's model, which was designed to develop leadership skills and professionalism. Lastly, Homard (2013) reported on a correlational study which used Benner's novice-to-expert theory to compare exit examination scores and National Council Licensure Examination for Registered Nurses (NCLEX-RN) pass rates among students in a prelicensure nursing program following implementation of a program using standardized testing. Non–research-based articles included a report by Woody and Davis (2013) which described how to use Benner's model to develop and implement an educational module designed to improve nurse competence in peripheral intravenous therapy.

A fairly common theme was noted as several writers discussed Benner's applicability in development of procedures and protocols for orientation of new graduates or nurses into new specialty areas. For example, using Benner's model, Koharchik, Caputi, Robb, and Culleiton (2015) presented a process which can be used by clinical faculty and preceptors to develop clinical reasoning in nursing students; Coyle (2011) discussed an internship program in home health for new graduates; and Dumchin (2010) described a method for using online learning experiences to develop perioperative nurses. Finally, Benner's work was used in several articles (e.g., Bitanga & Austria, 2013; Haag-Heitman, 2012; Owens & Cleaves, 2012) to discuss the development or updating of career enhancement or clinical ladder programs.

Leininger's Cultural Care Diversity and Universality Theory

Madeleine Leininger was instrumental in demonstrating to nurses the importance of considering the impact of culture on health and healing (Leininger, 2002). Prior to her death in 2012, Leininger was a prolific nursing researcher and scholar, and she is credited with starting the specialty of transcultural nursing. In addition, she was a leading proponent of the idea that nursing is synonymous with caring.

Leininger reported that she conceptualized transcultural nursing as a distinct area of nursing practice in the late 1950s during her doctoral work in anthropology; she continued to study and develop a transcultural nursing conceptual framework throughout the 1960s. In the mid-1970s, she presented a "transcultural health model" that was expanded in 1978 and 1980. The Leininger Sunrise Model was first described as such in 1984 and depicts the transcultural dimensions of culturologic interviews, assessments, and therapies (McFarland, 2014; McFarland & Wehbe-Alamah, 2015).

Purpose and Major Concepts

The purpose of Leininger's theory is to generate knowledge related to the nursing care of people who value their cultural heritage and lifeways. Major concepts of the model are culture, culture care, and culture care differences (diversities) and similarities (universals) pertaining to transcultural human care. Other major concepts are care and caring, emic view (language expressions, perceptions, beliefs, and practice of individuals or groups of a particular culture in regard to certain phenomena), etic view (universal language expression beliefs and practices in regard to certain phenomena that pertain to several cultures or groups), lay system of health care, professional system of health care, and culturally congruent nursing care (Leininger, 2007; McFarland, 2014).

Context for Use and Nursing Implications

The goal for application of Leininger's theory is to provide culturally congruent nursing care to persons of diverse cultures. A central tenet of the theory is that it is important for the nurse to understand the individual's view of illness. Also, the focus is on recognizing and understanding cultural similarities and differences and using this information to positively influence nursing care and health (McFarland & Wehbe-Alamah, 2015). The theory has been widely used for research, and findings are appropriate for nurses in any setting who work with individuals, families, and groups from a cultural background different from the nurse's.

Evidence of Empirical Testing and Application in Practice

Leininger (2007) explained that her theory was derived and refined through a number of years of study. Over the past two decades, research on various groups was conducted, and she listed cultural values and culture care meanings and action modes for 23 cultural groups in her book. Many graduate students and nursing scholars have used Leininger's theory as a basis for research, and as a result, hundreds of examples of articles can be located in the literature. Many of these used Leininger's work as a conceptual framework to study cultural implications of a variety of health problems. For example, J. M. Long and colleagues (2012) examined health beliefs among four different Latino subgroups specifically related to type 2 diabetes; Gillum and colleagues (2011) researched cardiovascular disease in the Amish; Mixer, Fornehed, Varney, and Lindley (2014) examined end-of-life care for people in rural Appalachia; and López-Entrambasaguas, Granero-Molina, and Fernandez-Sola (2013) studied the incidence of HIV/AIDS among a group of sex workers in Bolivia.

Leininger's model has also been used by many authors to identify variables or characteristics of cultural groups or subcultures that might influence health. For example, Farren (2015) performed a comprehensive literature review of research that examined cultural differences in cancer survivors' perceptions and experiences to promote patient-centered, culturally congruent care for adult cancer patients, and Lee (2012) used Leininger-inspired "ethnonursing research methods" to discover care meanings and expression among Appalachian mothers living with their children in a homeless shelter. Other examples of research studies using Leininger's model are listed in Box 11-2.

Box 11-2	Research Studies Using Leininger's Theory of Cultural Care Diversity and Universality

Bhat, A. M., Wehbe-Alamah, H., McFarland, M., Filter, M., & Keiser, M. (2015). Advancing cultural assessments in palliative care using web-based education. *Journal of Hospice and Palliative Nursing, 17*(4), 348–354.

Doornbos, M. M., Zandee, G. L., & DeGroot, J. (2014). Attending to communication and patterns of interaction: Culturally sensitive mental health care for groups of urban, ethnically diverse, impoverished and underserved women. *Journal of the American Psychiatric Nurses Association, 29*(4), 239–249.

McCullagh, M. C., Sanon, M. A., & Foley, J. G. (2015). Cultural health practices of migrant seasonal farmworkers. *Journal of Cultural Diversity, 22*(2), 64–67.

Millender, E. (2012). Acculturation stress among Maya in the United States. *Journal of Cultural Diversity, 19*(2), 58–64.

Missal, B. (2013). Gulf Arab women's transition to motherhood. *Journal of Cultural Diversity, 20*(4), 170–176.

Morris, E. J. (2012). Respect, protection, faith, and love: Major care constructs identified within the subculture of selected urban African American adolescent gang members. *Journal of Transcultural Nursing, 23*(3), 262–269.

Street, D. J., & Lewallen, L. P. (2013). The influence of culture on breast-feeding decisions by African American and white women. *The Journal of Perinatal & Neonatal Nursing, 27*(1), 43–51.

Taşçi-Duran, E., & Sevil, U. (2013). A comparison of the prenatal health behaviors of women from four cultural groups in Turkey: An ethnonursing study. *Nursing Science Quarterly, 26*(3), 257–266.

Turk, M. T., Fapohunda, A., & Zoucha, R. (2015). Using photovoice to explore Nigerian immigrants' eating and physical activity in the United States. *Journal of Nursing Scholarship, 47*(1), 16–24.

A number of nonresearch articles describing aspects of transcultural nursing and focusing on Leininger's works have also been published in recent years. These include a review of a workshop to enhance cultural awareness for nurse practitioners (Elminowski, 2015); a report on how to provide culturally competent, patient-centered nursing care (Darnell & Hickson, 2015); and an article describing the impact of international service learning on nursing student's cultural competence (T. Long, 2016).

Pender's Health Promotion Model

Nola Pender began studying health-promoting behavior in the mid-1970s and first published the Health Promotion Model (HPM) in 1982. She reported that the model was constructed from expectancy-value theory and social cognitive theory using a nursing perspective. The model was modified slightly in the late 1980s and again in 1996 (Pender, Murdaugh, & Parsons, 2015).

Purpose and Major Concepts

The HPM was proposed as a framework for integrating nursing and behavioral science perspectives on factors that influence health behaviors. The model is to be used as a guide to explore the biopsychosocial processes that motivate individuals to engage in behaviors directed toward health enhancement (Pender et al., 2015). The model has been used extensively as a framework for research aimed at predicting health-promoting lifestyles as well as specific behaviors.

Major concepts of the HPM are individual characteristics and experiences (prior related behavior and personal factors), behavior-specific cognitions and affect (perceived benefits of action, perceived barriers to action, perceived self-efficacy, activity-related affect, interpersonal influences, and situational influences), and behavioral outcomes (commitment to a plan of action, immediate competing demands and preferences, and health-promoting behavior). Figure 11-1 shows the HPM.

Context for Use and Nursing Implications

Health promotion interventions are essential for improving the health of populations everywhere. It is noted that people of all ages can benefit from health promotion care, which should be delivered at sites where people spend much of their time (e.g., schools and workplaces). Nurses can develop and execute health-promoting interventions for individuals, groups, and families in schools, nursing centers, occupational health settings, and the community at large. Per the HPM, nurses should work toward empowerment for self-care and enhancing the client's capacity for self-care through education and personal development.

Evidence of Empirical Testing and Application in Practice

Pender and colleagues (2015) wrote that the model has been used by a very significant number of nursing scholars and researchers and has been useful in explaining and predicting specific health behaviors. Indeed, in the last decade, more than 250 English language articles that reported using or applying Pender's HPM have been published.

Most research studies used Pender's work as one component of a conceptual framework for study. For example, Park, Choi-Kwon, and Han (2015) used the HPM to study health behaviors of Korean nursing students related to obesity and osteoporosis, and Jackson and colleagues (2016) used the model to explain the relationship between several factors including physical functioning, personal factors, and behavioral influences on physical activity between prehypertensive and

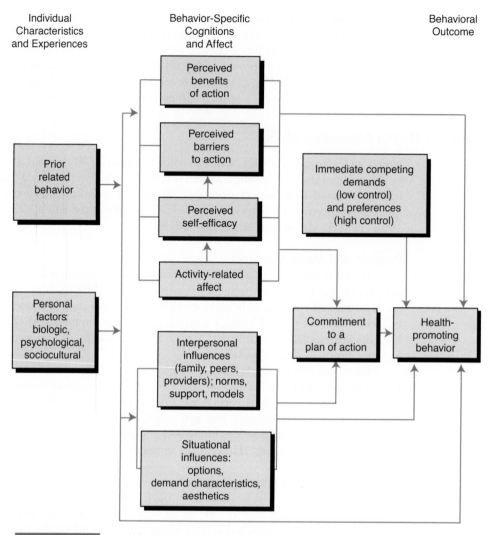

Individual
Characteristics
and Experiences

Behavior-Specific
Cognitions
and Affect

Behavioral
Outcome

Perceived
benefits
of action

Perceived
barriers
to action

Prior
related
behavior

Perceived
self-efficacy

Immediate competing
demands
(low control)
and preferences
(high control)

Activity-related
affect

Personal
factors:
biologic,
psychological,
sociocultural

Commitment
to a
plan of action

Health-
promoting
behavior

Interpersonal
influences
(family, peers,
providers); norms,
support, models

Situational
influences:
options,
demand characteristics,
aesthetics

Figure 11-1 Health Promotion Model.

(Adapted from Pender, N. J., Murdaugh, C. L., & Parsons, M. A. Health Promotion in Nursing Practice, 7th ed., © 2015. Reprinted by permission of Pearson Education, Inc., New York, New York.)

hypertensive African American women. Also focusing on physical activity, Hatzfeld, Nelson, Waters, and Jennings (2016) used the HPM to examine factors influencing health behaviors among active duty air force personnel.

Other studies use health promotion as an outcome or to predict behaviors. Burns, Murrock, and Graor (2012), for example, used the model to identify the relationship between body mass and injury severity among adolescents, concluding that overweight/obese adolescents may be at increased risk for serious injury. Additional examples of recent research studies using Pender's HPM are listed in Box 11-3.

Transitions Theory

Meleis (2010) wrote that the Transitions Theory evolved over the course of about four decades. She explained that it began in practice with her observations of the experiences that humans face as they deal with changes relating to health, well-being, and their

Box 11-3	Research Studies Using Pender's Health Promotion Model

Anderson, K. J., & Pullen, C. H. (2013). Physical activity with spiritual strategies intervention: A cluster randomized trial with older African American women. *Research in Gerontological Nursing, 6*(1), 11–21.

Bhandari, P., & Kim, M. Y. (2016). Predictors of the health-promoting behaviors of Nepalese migrant workers. *The Journal of Nursing Research, 24*(3), 232–239.

Bryer, J., Cherkis, F., & Raman, J. (2013). Health-promotion behaviors of undergraduate nursing students: A survey analysis. *Nursing Education Perspectives, 34*(6), 410–415.

Kim, H. J., Choi-Kwon, S., Kim, H., Park, Y. H., & Koh, C. K. (2015). Health-promoting lifestyle behaviors and psychological status among Arabs and Koreans in the United Arab Emirates. *Research in Nursing & Health, 38*(1), 133–141.

Lubinska-Welch, I., Pearson, T., Comer, L., & Metcalfe, S. E. (2016). Nurses as instruments of healing: Self-care practices of nursing in a rural hospital setting. *Journal of Holistic Nursing, 34*(3), 223–228.

McClune, A. J., & Conway, A. (2016). Farm safety: A tale of translational research and collaboration. *Pediatric Nursing, 42*(1), 31–35.

Valek, R. M., Greenwald, B. J., & Lewis, C. C. (2015). Psychological factors associated with weight loss maintenance: Theory-driven practice for nurse practitioners. *Nursing Science Quarterly, 28*(2), 129–135.

ability to care for themselves. Meleis's work moved through multiple steps, including concept analysis and several comprehensive literature reviews. The result was a conclusion that "transitions" is a central concept in nursing (Schumacher & Meleis, 1994). More focused attention through observation and research has contributed to formal development, testing, and application of the theory (Meleis, 2010).

Purpose and Major Concepts

Transitions Theory attempts to describe and attend to the interactions between nurses and patients, suggesting that nurses are concerned with the experiences of people as they undergo transitions whenever health and well-being are the desired outcome. The goal of "nursing therapeutics," then, is to conceptualize and address the potential problems that individuals encounter during transitional experiences and develop preventative and therapeutic interventions to support the patient during these occasions (George & Hickman, 2011; Im, 2014; Meleis, 2010).

Meleis (2010) defined transitions as "a passage from one fairly stable state to another fairly stable state, and it is a process triggered by a change" (p. 11). Furthermore, transitions are characterized by different stages, milestones, and turning points. These changes, or transitions, can be assisted or managed by nurses as they care for patients.

Numerous years of research and analysis into transitions led Meleis and her colleagues to the identification "of four major categories of transitions that nurses tend to be involved in" (Meleis, 2010, p. 3). These transitions and representative examples are:

- Developmental transitions—birth, adolescence, menopause, aging, death
- Situational transitions—changes in educational and professional roles, changes in family situations (e.g., divorce, widowhood), or changes in living arrangements (e.g., move to a nursing home, homelessness)
- Health–illness transitions—recovery process, hospital discharge, diagnosis of chronic illness
- Organizational transition—changing environmental conditions that affect the lives of clients; may be social, political, or economic (Im, 2014)

Other key concepts include "patterns" and "properties" of the transitions. Patterns denote whether the transitions are single, multiple, sequential, simultaneous, related, or unrelated. Properties of the transition experience are often interrelated in a complex way and refer to awareness, engagement, change/difference, time span, and critical points and events (Im, 2014).

In Transitions Theory, the nurse must consider the "facilitators" and "inhibitors" of the transition conditions. These include personal meanings, cultural beliefs and attitudes, socioeconomic status, preparation, and knowledge. Community conditions and societal conditions may also facilitate or inhibit transitions (Im, 2014).

"Nursing therapeutics" are those activities and actions that nurses may take during times of transitions (Schumacher & Meleis, 1994). These include assessment of readiness (assessment of each of the transition's conditions), preparation for transition (typically involves education to enhance optimal conditions to prepare for transition), and role supplementation (use of education and practice to facilitate the transitional process) (George & Hickman, 2011). The outcomes of transitions, and potential for nursing therapeutics, include the "patterns of response" of the patient. These are designated as process indicators (feeling connected, interacting, locating and being situated, developing confidence, and coping) and outcome indicators (mastery and "fluid integrative identities") (Im, 2014). Figure 11-2 shows the interaction of the major constructs of the theory.

Context for Use and Nursing Implications

According to Meleis (2010), most nursing care occurs during a transition that the patient is experiencing, and the goal of nursing care is to promote or encourage

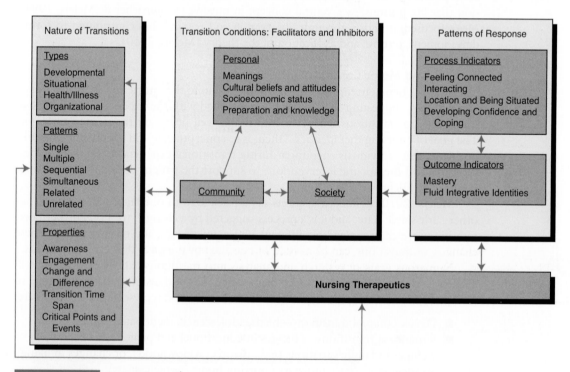

Figure 11-2 Transitions Theory.

(From Meleis, A. I., Sawyer, L. M., Im, E.-O., Messias, D. K. H., & Schumacher, K. [2000]. Experiencing transitions: An emerging middle range theory. *ANS. Advances in Nursing Science, 23*[10], 12–28. Used with permission.)

health outcomes during these occasions. Indeed, Meleis and Trangenstein (1994) defined nursing as the art and science of facilitation of the transitions of health and well-being and noted that nurses are concerned "with the processes and experiences of human beings undergoing transitions where health and perceived well-being is the outcome" (p. 257).

Transitions Theory is widely applicable and provides a comprehensive guide that considers cultural and social diversity. It was developed from multiple research studies among very diverse groups of people, during many types of transitions. Additionally, it has been shown repeatedly to be able to direct nursing practice, research, and education.

Evidence of Empirical Testing and Application in Practice

Transitions Theory has been based in both research and generated research (George & Hickman, 2011; Meleis, 2010). Meleis (2010) compiled and published a history of the development of the theory along with multiple examples of research and application in practice. Additional examples are becoming increasingly evident in the literature. Some of these focus on research examining patient transitions encountered by nurses in various specialty areas. For example, Joly (2016) addressed supportive care for young people with medically complex needs as they transition into adulthood; Rew, Tyler, Fredland, and Hannah (2012) examined adolescents' concerns as they transition through high school; Ekim and Ocakci (2016) looked at the transitions involved in discharge planning for children with asthma; and Häggström, Asplund, and Kristiansen (2012) researched patients' transition from the intensive care unit (ICU).

Several research studies using Transitions Theory focused on the experience of caregivers. One (Beaudet & Ducharme, 2013) such study identified transitions encountered by patients with Parkinson disease and their caregivers. The intent was to develop more focused interventions to assist the caregivers. In another example, Dossa, Bokhour, and Hoenig (2012) performed a grounded theory study that examined the transitions from hospital to home for patients with mobility impairments and their family caregivers; they concluded that health care providers need to improve systems to address patient concerns after discharge, focusing on improving communication and coordination to facilitate recovery and prevent complications.

Finally, Geary and Schumacher (2012) presented an interesting look at the integration of Transitions Theory with concepts from complexity science. They argued that the complexity of many of the transition situations encountered by nurses today is better described when the theories are integrated, concluding that the integration encourages recognition that transitions affect many, including the patients, their caregivers, health care providers, and the health care system. Integration of the theories should enhance dialogue and promote better understanding of the situations through changing outcomes for the better.

The Synergy Model

The Synergy Model for Patient Care was developed in the mid-1990s by a panel of nurses of the American Association of Critical-Care Nurses (AACN) Certification Corporation as a framework for certified practice. The initial model was revised somewhat, and the revised version was then used as the basis for the AACN's certification examination (Curley, 2007; Hardin, 2017).

Purpose and Major Concepts

The purpose of the Synergy Model is to articulate nurses' contributions, activities, and outcomes with regard to caring for critically ill patients. The model identifies eight

Box 11-4	The Synergy Model: Patient Characteristics and Nurse Competencies

Patient Characteristics	Nurse Competencies
Resiliency	Clinical judgment
Vulnerability	Clinical inquiry
Stability	Facilitation of learning
Complexity	Collaboration
Resource availability	Systems thinking
Participation in care	Advocacy and moral agency
Participation in decision making	Caring practices
Predictability	Response to diversity

Source: AACN (2016).

patient needs or characteristics and eight competencies of nurses in critical care situations (AACN, 2016; Pate, 2017). Of the many unique characteristics nurses assess, the eight most consistently observed are listed in Box 11-4. The nursing competencies denote how knowledge, skills, and experience are integrated within nursing care.

The Synergy Model also describes three levels of outcomes—those relating to the patient, the nurse, and the system. Patient outcomes include functional and behavioral change, trust, satisfaction, comfort, and quality of life. Nurse outcomes include physiologic changes, presence or absence of complications, and extent to which care objectives were attained. System outcomes include recidivism, costs, and resource utilization (Curley, 1998, 2007). For more information, see AACN (2017).

Context for Use and Nursing Implications

As mentioned, the Synergy Model was originally developed to structure the AACN's certification examination by identifying nursing competencies that are essential for those providing care to the critically ill. In 2002, assumptions of the model were expanded to establish it as a conceptual framework for designing practice and developing competencies required to care for critically ill patients. Use of the Synergy Model in practice is designed to optimize patient outcomes. When patient characteristics and nurse competencies match and synergize, outcomes for the patient are optimal (Curley, 2007; Hardin, 2017). In addition, the model can be used for developing nursing curricula and for conducting research (Curley, 2007; Hardin, 2017).

Evidence of Empirical Testing and Application in Practice

Although the Synergy Model is relatively new, a significant number of articles have been published describing its use in practice. Identified were two articles that tested application of the model in critical care situations. For example, Swickard, Swickard, Reimer, Lindell, and Winkelman (2014) described the process of development of a tool to determine the appropriate level of care needed for interfacility patient transport, using the Synergy Model as a guide. In another work, Stacy (2011) used the Synergy Model as a framework when reporting on "progressive care units," which are increasingly being used to bridge the gap between ICUs and medical-surgical units. A few works (Hardin, 2012; Hart, Hardin, Townsend, Ramsey, & Mahrle-Henson, 2013; Tejero, 2012) described research studies using the Synergy Model as a framework. Box 11-5 shows several examples of articles describing the model's use in leadership/administration, practice, and education.

| Box 11-5 | The Synergy Model in Practice and Education |

Goran, S. F. (2011). A new view: Tele-intensive care unit competencies. *Critical Care Nurse, 31*(5), 17–29.

Gralton, K. S., & Brett, S. A. (2012). Integrating the synergy model for patient care at Children's Hospital of Wisconsin. *Journal of Pediatric Nursing, 27*(1), 74–81.

Hardin, S. R. (2012). Engaging families to participate in care of older critical care patients. *Critical Care Nurse, 32*(3), 35–40.

Hardin, S. R. (2015). Vulnerability of older patients in critical care. *Critical Care Nurse, 35*(3), 55–61.

Helman, S., Lisanti, A. J., Adams, A., Field, C., & Davis, K. F. (2016). Just-in-time training for high-risk low-volume therapies: An approach to ensure patient safety. *Journal of Nursing Care Quality, 31*(1), 33–39.

Jeffery, A. D., Christen, M., & Moore, L. (2015). Beyond a piece of paper: Learning to hire with synergy. *Nursing Management, 46*(1), 52–54.

Kohr, L. M., Hickey, P. A., & Curley, M. A. Q. (2012). Building a nursing productivity measure based on the synergy model: First steps. *American Journal of Critical Care, 21*(6), 420–430.

Schleifer, S. J., Carroll, K., & Moseley, M. J. (2014). Developing criterion-based competencies for tele-intensive care unit. *Dimensions of Critical Care Nursing, 33*(3), 116–120.

Middle Middle Range Theories

A number of nursing theories may be categorized as "middle middle range." Four theories that have been cited in a considerable number of nursing studies are discussed in the following sections. They are Mishel's (1984) Uncertainty in Illness Theory, Kolcaba's (1994) Theory of Comfort, Lenz and colleagues' Theory of Unpleasant Symptoms (Lenz, Pugh, Milligan, Gift, & Suppe, 1997; Lenz, Suppe, Gift, Pugh, & Milligan, 1995), and Reed's (1991b) Self-Transcendence Theory. Table 11-2 lists other middle middle range theories that have been used in nursing practice and research.

Mishel's Uncertainty in Illness Theory

Merle Mishel began studying the concept of uncertainty in illness in the early 1980s when she desired to explain the stress that results from hospitalization (Mishel, 1981, 1984). In the late 1980s, she formally developed the theory, which she then revised in the early 1990s (Mishel, 2014). The Mishel Uncertainty in Illness Scale was created to better examine the concept, and since that time, her model and instruments have been used in numerous nursing studies (Bailey & Stewart, 2014; Mishel, 2014).

Purpose and Major Concepts

According to Mishel (1999, 2014), the Uncertainty in Illness Theory explains how clients cognitively process illness-related stimuli and construct meaning in these events. Uncertainty is seen as "the inability to structure meaning of illness-related events inclusive of inability to assign definite value and/or to accurately predict outcomes" (Mishel, 2014, p. 56).

The early iteration of the model (Mishel, 1988) described the concepts of "stimuli frame" (symptom pattern, event familiarity, event congruency), "cognitive capacities," and "structure providers" (credible authority, social support, education) that

Table 11-2 Middle Middle Range Nursing Theories

Theory/Model	Purpose	Major Concepts
Self-help (Braden, 1990)	Describes a process of factors that decrease self and life quality and factors that increase learning a self-help response and thus a greater quality of life	Disease characteristics, background inducements, monitoring (level of information about illness), severity of illness, dependency, uncertainty, enabling skill, self-help, life quality
Chronic Illness Trajectory Framework (Corbin & Strauss, 1991, 1992)	Describes a view of chronic illness with eight phases, from pretrajectory to dying, with each possessing the possibilities of reversals, plateaus, and upward or downward movement; allows for conceptualization of the course of illness to comprehensively direct care and conduct research	Trajectory, trajectory phases (pretrajectory, trajectory onset, crisis, acute, stable, unstable, downward, and dying), trajectory projection, trajectory scheme (shape illness course, control symptoms, and handle disability)
Motivation in health behavior (health behavior, self-determinism) (Cox, 1985)	Describes intrinsic motivation in health behavior	Individual's self-determined health judgments, self-determined health behavior, perceived competency in health matters, internal–external cue responsiveness
Theory of Care-Seeking Behavior (Lauver, 1992)	Explains the probability of engaging in health behavior as a function of psychosocial variables and facilitating conditions regarding the behavior	Clinical and sociodemographic variables, affect (feelings associated with care-seeking behavior), utility (expectations and values about outcomes), normative influences, habits, care-seeking behavior
Self-efficacy (Lenz & Shortridge-Baggett, 2002)	Applies Bandura's work in nursing to assist people to be as independent as possible in managing their health	Person (perception, self-referent), behavior (initiation, effort, persistence), efficacy–expectation (magnitude, strength, generality), information sources (performance, vicarious experiences, verbal persuasion, physiologic information), and outcome expectations
Model for social support (Norbeck, 1981)	Outlines the elements and relationships that must be studied to incorporate social support into nursing practice; emphasis placed on developing the environment	Properties of the person (age, demographic characteristics, needs), properties of the situation (role demands, resources, stressors), need for social support, available social support
Theory of Resilience (Polk, 1997)	Proposes interrelatedness of dispositional, relational, situational, and philosophical patterns to describe concept of resilience to guide generation of nursing interventions to assess and strengthen resilience	Dispositional pattern (pattern of physical and ego-related psychosocial attributes that contribute to manifestation of resilience), relational pattern (roles and relationships that influence resilience), situational pattern (characteristic approach to situations or stressors), philosophical pattern (personal beliefs)
Theory of Caring (Swanson, 1991)	Proposes a definition of caring and the five essential categories or processes that characterize caring	Knowing, being with, doing for, enabling, and maintaining belief
Theory of Successful Aging (Troutman-Jordan, 2015)	Describes the process in which individuals use various coping mechanism to progress toward desirable adaption to physiologic and functional changes over their lifetime	Successful aging (meaning, purpose in life), functional performance mechanisms (health promotion activities, physical health, physical activities), geotranscendence (decreased death anxiety, purpose in life), intrapsychic factors (creativity, personal control), spirituality (spiritual perspectives, religiosity)
Theory of Self-Care of Chronic Illness (Riegel, Jaarsma, & Strömberg, 2012)	Describes the process of maintaining health with health-promoting practices within the context of the management required of a chronic illness	Self-care maintenance, self-care monitoring, and self-care management, influencing factors (experience, skill, motivation, culture, confidence, habits, function, cognition, support, access to care)

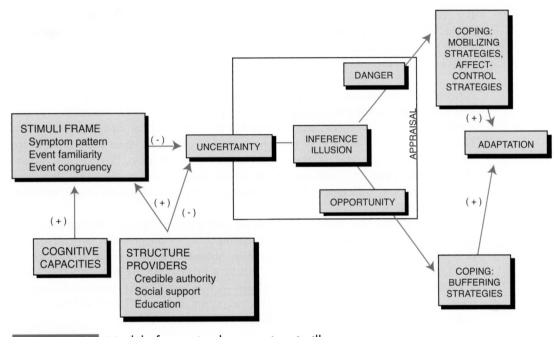

Figure 11-3   Model of perceived uncertainty in illness.

(From Mishel, M. H. [1990]. Reconceptualization of the uncertainty in illness theory. *Image—The Journal of Nursing Scholarship, 22*[4], 256–262. Used with permission of Wiley.)

may lead to uncertainty. Other concepts include appraisal, inference, illusion, and opportunity as well as coping mechanisms; these may lead to adaptation. In 1990, the process of theory derivation was used to update and revise the theory to address issues related to chronic uncertainty. Interestingly, chaos theory was used in this process (Mishel, 1990). Figure 11-3 shows the Uncertainty in Illness Theory.

Context for Use and Nursing Implications

The Uncertainty in Illness Theory explains how individuals cognitively process illness-related stimuli and how they structure meaning for those events. In the theory, adaptation is the desirable end-state achieved after coping with the uncertainty. Nurses may develop nursing interventions that attempt to influence the person's cognitive process to address the uncertainty. This, in turn, should produce positive coping and adaptation (Mishel, 1999, 2014).

Evidence of Empirical Testing and Application in Practice

During the process of theory development and refinement, Mishel developed and tested several research instruments. These are the Adult Uncertainty in Illness Scale and the Adult Uncertainty in Illness Scale—Community Form, the Parents' Perception of Uncertainty in Illness Scale, the Parents' Perception of Uncertainty in Illness Scale—Family Member (Mishel, 2014), and the Uncertainty Scale for Kids (Stewart, Lynn, & Mishel, 2010).

The Uncertainty in Illness Theory is becoming increasingly recognized in nursing literature as a resource for research and practice. A significant number of research studies were identified using Mishel's theory or instruments or both in addressing health issues among a wide variety of groups and covering many different health problems.

For example, in a longitudinal study, Bailey, Kazer, Polascik, and Robertson (2014) used Mishel's theory as part of the conceptual framework that examined uncertainty experienced by men who must have their prostate-specific antigen levels monitored following prostate cancer surgery. Other research employing Mishel's instruments included works by Kurita, Garon, Stanton, and Meyerowitz (2013), who studied uncertainty among patients with lung cancer and their psychological adjustment, and Cypress's (2016) examination of the uncertainty experienced by patients in the ICU. Interestingly, many studies using Mishel's theory were directed at patients and their families or caregivers. For example, White, Barrientos, and Dunn (2014) examined uncertainty experienced by stroke survivors and family caregivers; Unson, Flynn, Glendon, Haymes, and Sancho (2015) studied the stress and uncertainty of the caregivers of persons with dementia; and Germino and colleagues (2013) looked at uncertainty of breast cancer survivors and their families.

Mishel's work has achieved worldwide recognition, and her instruments have been translated into several languages including Italian (Giammanco, Gitto, Barberis, & Santoro, 2015), Persian (Saijadi, Rassouli, Abbaszadeh, Alavi Majd, & Zendehdel, 2014), and French (C. A. Miller, 2015). Finally, Christensen (2015) described development of the Health Change Trajectory Model—a new middle range theory—integrating concepts and relationships from Mishel's Uncertainty in Illness Theory and the Corbin and Strauss Chronic Illness Trajectory Framework (Corbin, 1998).

Kolcaba's Theory of Comfort

Katherine Kolcaba (2017) wrote that the first step in developing the Theory of Comfort was a concept analysis conducted in 1988 while she was a graduate student. Following a number of steps over several years, the Theory of Comfort was initially published in 1994 and later modified (Kolcaba, 1994, 2001).

Purpose and Major Concepts

Kolcaba (1994) defined comfort within nursing practice as "the satisfaction (actively, passively, or co-operatively) of the basic human needs for relief, ease, or transcendence arising from health care situations that are stressful" (p. 1178). She explained that a client's needs arise from a stimulus situation that can cause negative tension. Increasing comfort measures can result in having negative tensions reduced and positive tensions engaged. Comfort is viewed as an outcome of care that can promote or facilitate health-seeking behaviors. It is posited that increasing comfort can enhance health-seeking behaviors. One proposition notes that "if enhanced comfort is achieved, patients, family members and/or nurses are strengthened to engage in HSBs [health-seeking behaviors], which further enhance comfort" (Kolcaba, 2017, p. 200).

Major concepts described in the Theory of Comfort include comfort, comfort care, comfort measures, comfort needs, health-seeking behaviors, institutional integrity, and intervening variables. There are also eight defined propositions that link the defined concepts (Box 11-6) (Kolcaba, 2001, 2017). Figure 11-4 presents the Theory of Comfort.

Context for Use and Nursing Implications

Comfort Theory observes that patients experience needs for comfort in stressful health care situations. Some of these needs are identified by the nurse, who then implements interventions to meet the needs (Kolcaba, 1995). Kolcaba (2017) stated that "Comfort Theory can be adapted to any health care setting or age group . . . " (p. 200). Understanding of comfort can promote nursing care that is

Box 11-6	Propositions of Comfort Theory

1. Nurses and members of the health care team identify comfort needs of patients and family members.
2. Nurses design and coordinate interventions to address comfort needs.
3. Intervening variables are considered when designing interventions.
4. When interventions are delivered in a caring manner and are effective, the outcome of enhanced comfort is attained.
5. Patients, nurses, and other health care team members agree on desirable and realistic health-seeking behaviors.
6. If enhanced comfort is achieved, patients, family members, and/or nurses are more likely to engage in health-seeking behaviors; these further enhance comfort.
7. When patients and family members are given comfort care and engage in health-seeking behaviors, they are more satisfied with health care and have better health-related outcomes.
8. When patients, families, and nurses are satisfied with health care in an institution, public acknowledgment about that institution's contributions to health care will help the institution remain viable and flourish. Evidence-based practice or policy improvements may be guided by these propositions and the theoretical framework.

Sources: Kolcaba (2001, 2017).

holistic and inclusive of physical, psychospiritual, social, and environmental interventions. It is noted that any actually unhappy, unhealthy, or unwell patients can be made more comfortable (Kolcaba, 1994). Finally, outcomes of comfort can be measurable, holistic, positive, and nurse sensitive.

Evidence of Empirical Testing and Application in Practice

The General Comfort Questionnaire (GCQ) is a 48-item Likert-type scale that was developed to measure concepts and propositions described in the theory. The GCQ has been modified to be used for different populations in a number of studies, and a shortened GCQ (28 items) is also in use (Kolcaba, 2017).

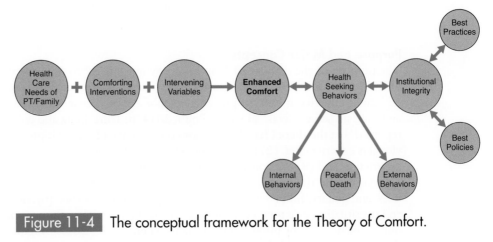

Figure 11-4	The conceptual framework for the Theory of Comfort.

(© Kolcaba [2007]. Used with permission. http://thecomfortline.com.)

Kolcaba (2017) described development of other tools to assist in research and practice application for the Theory of Comfort. These include the Verbal Rating Scale Questionnaire, the Radiation Therapy Comfort Questionnaire, the Hospice Comfort Questionnaire, the Urinary Incontinence and Frequency Comfort Questionnaire, and the Healing Touch Comfort Questionnaire. In addition, the Comfort Behaviors Checklist was developed to measure comfort in patient who can't use traditional questionnaires or other instruments.

A number of research studies have been conducted by Kolcaba and her colleagues using the instruments listed earlier. For example, Andersen, Jylli, and Ambuel (2014) used Kolcaba's Comfort Behaviors Checklist to evaluate the comfort care provided by a group of health providers and Seyedfatemi, Rafii, Rezaei, and Kolcaba (2014) used her instruments to study comfort and hope among preoperative patients. Whitehead, Anderson, Redican, and Stratton (2010) reported using Kolcaba's instruments to study the effects of an end-of-life nursing education program on nurses' death anxiety, knowledge of the dying process, and related concerns. Also examining nursing care at the end of life, Murray (2010) used Kolcaba's instruments to assess spiritual beliefs and practices of nurses caring for patients at the end of life, along with similarities and differences in spiritual beliefs and practices comparing hospice nurses and nurses working on oncology and other special care units.

In practice-specific examples, Marchuk (2016) described how Comfort Theory can be applied in end-of-life care in the neonatal intensive care unit (NICU), and Krinsky, Murillo, and Johnson (2014) explained how comfort measures can be used to improve nursing care for cardiac patients. Finally, Boudiab and Kolcaba (2015) presented a comprehensive look at the application of Comfort Theory in directing holistic, quality care for veterans and their families.

Lenz and Colleagues' Theory of Unpleasant Symptoms

The Theory of Unpleasant Symptoms was developed by a group of nurses interested in a variety of nursing issues, including symptom management, theory development, and nursing science (Lenz, Pugh, Milligan, & Gift, 2017). The theory was initially published in the nursing literature in the mid-1990s (Lenz et al., 1995) and then updated a few years later (Lenz et al., 1997). The theory was based on the premise that there are commonalities in experiencing different symptoms among different groups and in different situations. The theory was developed to integrate existing knowledge about a variety of symptoms to better prepare nurses in symptom management.

Purpose and Major Concepts

The purpose of the Theory of Unpleasant Symptoms is "to improve understanding of the symptom experience in various contexts and to provide information useful for designing effective means to prevent, ameliorate, or manage unpleasant symptoms and their negative effects" (Lenz & Pugh, 2014, p. 166). Lenz and colleagues (1997) reported that the theory has three major components: (1) the symptoms that the individual is experiencing, (2) the influencing factors that produce or affect the symptom experience, and (3) the consequences of the symptom experience.

Within the theory, symptoms are described in terms of duration, intensity, distress, and quality. Influencing factors can be physiologic factors, psychological factors, and/or situational factors. Performance is described in terms of functional status, cognitive functioning, or physical performance (Lenz et al., 2017). Figure 11-5 depicts the Theory of Unpleasant Symptoms.

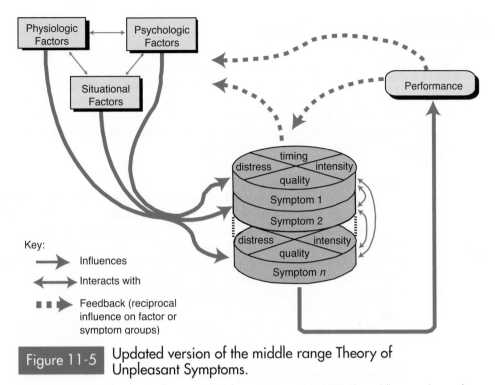

Figure 11-5   Updated version of the middle range Theory of Unpleasant Symptoms.

(From Lenz, E. R., Pugh, L. C., Milligan, R. A., Gift, A., & Suppe, F. [1997]. The middle range theory of unpleasant symptoms: An update. *ANS. Advances in Nursing Science, 19*[3], 14–27. Used with permission.)

Context for Use and Nursing Implications

The Theory of Unpleasant Symptoms helps nurses recognize the need to assess multiple aspects of symptoms, including characteristics of the symptom(s) itself; the underlying disease or other cause; as well as the frequency, intensity, duration, quality, and distress felt by the patient due to the symptom(s) (Lenz et al., 2017). The developers of the Theory of Unpleasant Symptoms note that it is clinically applicable to multiple client situations because it should stimulate nurses to consider factors that might influence more than one symptom and the ways in which symptoms interact with each other (Lenz et al., 1997). The theory's developers noted that it has been used in an emergency department (ED) to develop a symptom assessment scale for cardiac patients and has been useful in predicting the need for hospitalization among patients with chronic obstructive pulmonary disease (COPD).

Evidence of Empirical Testing and Application in Practice

A growing number of research studies using the Theory of Unpleasant Symptoms as a conceptual or organizing framework have been conducted. One study by Kim, Oh, Lee, Kim, and Kim (2015) used the theory in their investigation of predictors of symptoms and symptom experience among cancer patients undergoing chemotherapy. Also studying cancer patients, Hsu and Tu (2014) used the Theory of Unpleasant Symptoms to evaluate the effects of cancer treatments on functional status, depressive symptoms, fatigue, and quality of life. Other works applied the Theory of Unpleasant Symptoms in caring for patients undergoing bariatric surgery (Tyler & Pugh, 2009), patients with coronary heart disease (Eckhardt, Devon, Piano, Ryan, & Zerwic, 2014), and patients with inflammatory bowel disease (Farrell & Savage, 2010).

Reed's Self-Transcendence Theory

Pamela Reed first wrote about the concept of self-transcendence in 1983 and formally outlined her theory in 1991 (Reed, 1991b). She reported that she used "deductive reformulation" of theories of life span development in constructing the theory. These she integrated with Rogers's conceptual system, clinical experience, and empirical work (Reed, 1991b). Self-transcendence is developed by introspective activities and concerns about the welfare of others and by integrating perceptions of one's past and future to enhance the present (Reed, 1991a).

Purpose and Major Concepts

Self-transcendence is considered to be a "characteristic of developmental maturity whereby there is an expansion of self-boundaries and orientation toward broadened life perspectives and purposes" (Reed, 1991b, p. 64). Self-transcendence moves the individual beyond the immediate or constricted view of self and the world (Reed, 1996). Within self-transcendence, there is "an expansion of personal boundaries outwardly (toward others and the environment), inwardly (toward greater awareness of beliefs, values, and dreams), and temporally (toward integration of past and future in the present)" (Reed, 1996, p. 3). Other central concepts of the theory include well-being (a sense of wholeness and health) and vulnerability (awareness of personal mortality) (Coward, 2014; Reed, 2014).

Context for Use and Nursing Implications

Reed (1991b) reported that a theory of self-transcendence may be used by nurses to attend to spiritual and psychosocial expressions of self-transcendence in clients who are confronted with end-of-life issues. To promote self-transcendence, nurses may use interventions such as meditation, self-reflection, visualization, religious expression, counseling, and journaling to expand the individual's boundaries.

Evidence of Empirical Testing and Application in Practice

A number of nursing research studies have used the theory of self-transcendence. In an early work, Reed (1991a) found support for the theory in an examination of the mental health of older adults. In the study, she identified a relationship between self-transcendence and mental health and an inverse relationship between self-transcendence and depression. More recently, studies have been undertaken to examine self-transcendence and its effect on well-being or other variables. These studies are conducted among those with health issues such as spinal muscular atrophy (Ho, Tseng, Hsin, Chou, & Lin, 2016), Alzheimer disease (Walsh et al., 2011), hypertension (Thomas & Dunn, 2014), and at the end of life (Shockey-Stephenson & Berry, 2015).

Several projects have looked at self-transcendence among nurses and/or nursing students. For example, Hunnibell and colleagues (2008) studied differences in self-transcendence between hospice and oncology nurses, analyzing how it influenced burnout in those groups. In similar works, Palmer, Quinn Griffin, Reed, and Fitzpatrick (2010) studied self-transcendence and engagement in acute care registered nurses (RNs), and Haugan (2014) examined whether student nurses' self-transcendence could positively influence their attitudes toward caring for older adults. Finally, several works were identified that sought to enhance self-transcendence or to associate it with successful ageing. These included a study by McCarthy, Ling, and Carini (2013) and a second study by McCarthy, Ling, Bowland, Hall, and Connelly (2015).

Low Middle Range Theories

The number of low middle range theories appears to be growing as nursing researchers and nursing scholars describe phenomena directly related to practice. Three theories are examined in the following sections. They are Eakes, Burke, and Hainsworth's (1998) Theory of Chronic Sorrow; Beck's (1993) Postpartum Depression Theory; and Mercer's (1981) Conceptualization of Maternal Role Attainment/Becoming a Mother. Table 11-3 lists other low middle range theories.

Eakes, Burke, and Hainsworth's Theory of Chronic Sorrow

The concept of chronic sorrow was introduced in the early 1960s to describe grief observed in the parents of children with mental deficiencies. Subsequent research indicated similar patterns of chronic sorrow in parents of mentally or physically disabled children. The Nursing Consortium for Research on Chronic Sorrow expanded the concept to include individuals who experience a variety of loss situations and to their family caregivers (Eakes, 2017; Eakes et al., 1998).

The middle range Theory of Chronic Sorrow was formalized in 1998. The theory was inductively derived and validated through a series of studies and a critical review of the existing research. Chronic sorrow is defined as the "periodic recurrence of permanent, pervasive sadness or other grief related feelings associated with a significant loss" (Eakes et al., 1998, p. 179), which was described as a normal response to ongoing disparity associated with loss.

Purpose and Major Concepts

The Theory of Chronic Sorrow was developed to help analyze individual responses of people experiencing ongoing disparity due to chronic illness, caregiving responsibilities, loss of the "perfect" child, or bereavement. Chronic sorrow was characterized as pervasive, permanent, periodic, and potentially progressive in nature. The person has a perception of sadness or sorrow over time in a situation with no predictable end. The sadness or sorrow is cyclic or recurrent and brings to mind a person's losses, disappointments, or fears (Eakes, 2017).

The primary antecedent to chronic sorrow is involvement in an experience of significant loss. The loss is often ongoing with no predictable end. Disparity is a second antecedent and is created by loss experiences when the individual's current reality differs from the idealized. Trigger events (e.g., milestones, circumstances, situations, and conditions that create negative disparity resulting from the loss experience) focus or exacerbate the experience of disparity. The "lack of closure associated with ongoing disparity sets the stage for chronic sorrow, with the loss experienced in bits and pieces over time" (Eakes, 2017, p. 95).

Context for Use and Nursing Implications

Chronic sorrow is commonly experienced by individuals across the life span who have encountered significant loss or experience ongoing loss. The theory's developers suggest that nurses need to view chronic sorrow as a normal response to loss and provide support by fostering positive coping strategies and encouraging activities that increase comfort.

Interventions that demonstrate an empathic presence and a caring professional are helpful. These include taking time to listen, offering support and reassurance, recognizing and focusing on feelings, and appreciating the uniqueness of each individual. Other interventions include providing information in a manner that can be understood and offering practical tips for dealing with the challenges of caregiving.

Table 11-3 Low Middle Range Nursing Theories

Theory/Model	Purpose	Major Concepts
Theory of Adaptation to Chronic Pain (Dunn, 2004)	Describes the process and outcome of adaptation to chronic pain through use of religious and nonreligious coping to create human and environmental integration that promotes survival, growth, and integrity	Stimuli (background contextual variables, total pain intensity), compensatory life process (religious and nonreligious coping), adaptive modes (functional ability, psychological, and spiritual well-being)
Acute pain management (Good, 1998; Good & Moore, 1996)	Proposes prescriptions for nursing activities to reduce pain after surgery or trauma to ensure that clients have less intense pain with minimal side effects of medications	Potent pain medication, pharmacologic adjuvant, nonpharmacologic adjuvant, assessment of pain and side effects, goal setting, and balance between analgesia and side effects
Theory of Suffering (Morse, 2001)	Describes phases of suffering and relationship between states of enduring suffering and caregiver response	Enduring (emotional suppression) and emotional suffering, outcomes (recognition, acknowledgments, acceptance)
Theory of the Peaceful End of Life (Ruland & Moore, 1998)	Directs care necessary for terminally ill clients; enhances nursing care by combining the dimensions that are important to dying in a unifying whole	Not being in pain, experience of comfort, experience of dignity and respect, being at peace, closeness to significant others and people who care
Caregiving Effectiveness Model (C. E. Smith et al., 2002)	Explains and predicts outcomes of technology-based home caregiving provided by family members	Caregiving context (caregiving characteristics, caregiving/care-receiving interactions, patient education), adaptive context (family economic stability, caregiver health status, family adaptation, reactions to caregiving), caregiving effectiveness outcomes (patient quality of life, caregiver quality of life, patient condition, technologic side effects)
Theory of Caregiver Stress (Tsai, 2003)	Predicts caregiver stress and its outcomes from demographic characteristics, burden in care giving, stressful life events, social support, and social roles	Caregiver adaptation, input (objective burden, stressful life events, social support, social roles, demographic information), control process (perceived caregiver stress and depression), output (physical function, self-esteem, role enjoyment, marital satisfaction)
Theoretical model for the development of skin ulcers of nonsystemic origin and dependence-related lesions (García-Fernández, Agreda, Verdú, & Pancorbo-Hidalgo, 2013)	Explains the production mechanism of seven dependence-related lesions considered to lead to pressure ulcers	Moisture lesions (incontinence exposure), friction lesions (friction/grazing), pressure ulcers (pressure [decreased capacity for repositioning, decreased sensory perception], shear)
Theory of Family Vigilance (Carr, 2014)	Describes the meanings, patterns, and day-to-day experience of family members staying with hospitalized relatives	Commitment to care (advocacy, love, responsibility, solicitude, involvement), resilience (caring for self, perseverance, hope), emotional upheaval (anxiety, uncertainty, life and death decisions), dynamic nexus (relationships with family/friends, relationship with health care providers), transition (lifestyle, daily rhythm, comfort, space)

Evidence of Empirical Testing and Application in Practice

Eakes and colleagues (1998) reported that a number of research studies were used to develop and support the theory. Several recent research studies were identified using the Theory of Chronic Sorrow as a conceptual framework. These include Vitale and Falco's (2014) examination of parental chronic sorrow experienced with the premature birth of their infants; Nikfarid, Rassouli, Borimnejad, and Alavimajd's (2015) study of chronic sorrow in mothers of children with cancer; and Bowes, Lowes, Warner, and Gregory's (2009) study of chronic sorrow in parents of children with type 1 diabetes.

Other works focused on how to care for those experiencing chronic sorrow. Among them, Glenn (2015) described the use of online health communication technology to help mothers of children with rare diseases manage chronic sorrow. Also, Joseph (2012) described the importance of ED nurses recognizing chronic sorrow among family member of patients seen in the ED.

Beck's Postpartum Depression Theory

Building on a background of research on postpartum depression (Beck, Reynolds, & Rutowski, 1992), Cheryl Beck (1993) developed a theory regarding postpartum depression. A grounded theory approach was used to formulate the theory, which she described as a four-stage process of "teetering on the edge" into postpartum depression.

Purpose and Major Concepts

The purpose of the theory was to provide insight into the experience of postpartum depression. The concepts or stages in Beck's (1993) theory were defined as encountering terror (horrifying anxiety attacks, obsessive thinking, and enveloping fogginess), dying of self (alarming "unrealness," isolation of self, and contemplation of self-destruction), struggling to survive (battling the system, praying for relief, and seeking solace), and regaining control (making transitions, mounting lost time, and attaining a guarded recovery). A meta-synthesis of postpartum depression by Beck (2002a) produced a list of predictors or risk factors, including prenatal depression, child care stress, life stress, social support, prenatal anxiety, marital satisfaction, history of depression, infant temperament, maternity blues, self-esteem, socioeconomic status, marital status, and whether the pregnancy was planned. Distillation of predictors and risk factors of postpartum depression added these stressors/potential consequences: sleeping and eating disturbances, anxiety and insecurity, emotional lability, mental confusion, loss of self, guilt and shame, and suicidal thoughts (Maeve, 2014).

Context for Use and Nursing Implications

The model proposed nursing interventions to alert nurses to the incidence and impact of postpartum depression. Beck stressed the importance of identifying new mothers who might be suffering from postpartum depression and suggested interventions such as referral to postpartum depression support groups (Beck et al., 1992).

Evidence of Empirical Testing and Application in Practice

Beck's theory has been used in a significant number of nursing studies and in practice situations (Marsh, 2013). To further examine the concept of postpartum depression, Beck (1995, 1998) performed a meta-analysis to document its effects. Based on the information from a meta-analysis, Beck and Gable (2000) developed the Postpartum Depression Screening Scale (PDSS) to improve detection of the disorder. The tool was revised in 2002 (Beck, 2002b), translated into Spanish (Beck & Gable, 2003), and revised further in 2006 (Beck, Records, & Rice, 2006). These tools have been validated (Beck et al., 2006; Clemmens, Driscoll, & Beck, 2004) and used by nurses in a growing list of research studies in many countries and in additional languages (Maeve, 2014).

In one example, Le, Perry, and Sheng (2009) used the PDSS to examine the feasibility of using the Internet to screen for postpartum depressive symptoms, concluding that it is viable and feasible tool to screen for postpartum depression. In another work, Logsdon, Tomasulo, Eckert, Beck, and Dennis (2012) presented guidelines for hospital-based postpartum depression screening using the PDSS. A team lead by Thomason (Thomason et al., 2014) used the PDSS to examine parenting stress and depressive symptoms, and Lucero, Beckstrand, Callister, and Sanchez Birkhead (2012) used the Spanish version of the PDSS to examine the prevalence of postpartum depression among Hispanic immigrants in the United States.

Mercer's Conceptualization of Maternal Role Attainment/Becoming a Mother

Ramona Mercer first described a theoretical framework for the maternal role in the early 1980s; she expanded on the process in a subsequent publication in 1985. She reported that the theory was based on role theory, knowledge of the infant's traits, and a review of the literature to identify variables that influence or are influenced by maternal roles. She defined maternal role attainment as a process "in which the mother achieves competence in the role and integrates the mothering behaviors into her established role set so that she is comfortable with her identity as a mother" (Mercer, 1985, p. 198).

Following a review and synthesis of research related to the concept of "maternal role attainment," Mercer (2004) proposed changing the name of her theory to "Becoming a Mother." This change was later expanded on (Mercer, 2006), and a number of related nursing interventions were identified supporting the change (Mercer & Walker, 2006).

Purpose and Major Concepts

Mercer attempted to identify the "form and strength of the relationships between key maternal and infant variables and maternal role attainment" as well as "other factors that appear to influence maternal role attainment" (Mercer, 1981, p. 73). She proposed that the variables of age, perception of the birth experience, early maternal–infant separation, social stress, support system, self-concept and personality traits, maternal illness, childrearing attitudes, infant temperament, infant illness, culture, and socioeconomic level affect the maternal role.

In the more recent iteration of her theory, Mercer (2004) explains that the process of establishing maternal identity in becoming a mother is (1) commitment, attachment, and preparation (during pregnancy); (2) acquaintance, learning, and physical restoration (in the first 2 to 6 weeks following birth); (3) moving toward a new normal (2 weeks to 4 months); and (4) achievement of the maternal identity (around 4 months). She noted that these stages may overlap and may be highly variable due to maternal and infant variables as well as the social/environmental context. Additional key concepts and ideas identified in Mercer's works include infant temperament, infant health status, infant characteristics, and infant cues as well as family, family functioning, father or intimate partner, mother–father relationship, and social support (Meighan, 2014).

Context for Use and Nursing Implications

Nurses in postpartum situations should recognize that competency in the maternal role toward "becoming a mother" increases with age and experience. Also, the demands on first-time mothers challenge the nurse to be active in anticipatory socialization and guidance to prepare for the realities of the maternal role. Interventions suggested in Mercer's works include promoting parenting groups to highlight maternal needs during the first months (Noseff, 2014).

Evidence of Empirical Testing and Application in Practice

In early works, Mercer (1985) reported that mothering over the first year presents similar challenges for all groups, and a study by Fowles (1994) used Mercer's theory as part of her conceptual framework to examine the relationship between maternal attachment, postpartum depression, and maternal role attainment. More recently, a comprehensive study of maternal role attainment with medically fragile infants was undertaken to examine the quality of parenting (Holditch-Davis, Miles, Burchinal, & Goldman, 2011) and characteristics that influenced maternal role attachment longitudinally (Miles, Holditch-Davis, Burchinal, & Brunssen, 2011). In other works, Kinsey, Baptiste-Roberts, Zhu, and Kjerulff (2014) studied the effect of miscarriage history on maternal–infant bonding, and Sriyasak, Akerlind, and Akhavan (2013) examined childrearing among Thai teenage mothers using Mercer's theory as a framework. Lastly, Fouquier (2013) performed a comprehensive literature review to evaluate the applicability of Mercer's theory to African American women. She determined that the homogeneity of the samples for most of the research on Mercer's theory is not necessarily generalizable to African American women and concluded that more research is needed to identify attributes that influence maternal role attainment to that population.

Summary

This chapter presented a wide variety of middle range nursing theories. Because of space limitations, the descriptions are very brief and are intended to merely introduce the theories. The readers are directed to original and supporting sources for more information.

Elaine Chavez, the graduate student from the opening case study, saw how one of the numerous middle range nursing theories that have been published in recent years could be used to develop interventions in her practice. All nurses should likewise continue to review current nursing literature for new theories and ideas that are being presented to remain current and knowledgeable about nursing practice. To illustrate, Link to Practice 11-1 provides some thoughts on how nurses can apply middle range theories in their daily practice.

It must be mentioned again that the high, middle, and low range theories described here are by no means an exhaustive display of the growing number that have been presented in the nursing literature. Indeed, it was remarkable to observe the growth in middle range theory development over the last decade, and it is anticipated that this emphasis will continue well into the future.

Link to Practice 11-1

Applying Multiple Middle Range Theories in Practice

How might nurses apply multiple middle range theories in their practice? Consider these situations:

1. A nurse is providing care for a woman with ovarian cancer (Theory of Unpleasant Symptoms) who recently immigrated to the United States from Somalia (Leininger's Culture Care Diversity and Universality Theory) in an ICU (Synergy Model).
2. A nurse manager is charged with developing an orientation packet (Benner's Model of Skill Acquisition) for nurses new to a hospice practice (Kolcaba's Theory of Comfort) focusing on their awareness of beliefs, values, and well-being (Reed's Self-Transcendence Theory).
3. A family nurse practitioner is working with a new mother (Mercer's Theory of Becoming a Mother) who has just given birth to a child with a severe genetic disorder (Theory of Chronic Sorrow).
4. A public health nurse is charged with teaching a group of American Indian women (Leininger's Culture Care Diversity and Universality Theory) how to develop a healthy lifestyle (Pender's Health Promotion Model).

Key Points

- A growing number of widely used middle range theories have been proposed, applied, and tested and have been presented in the nursing literature.
- Among the "high" middle range nursing theories (theories that are relatively abstract and apply to a very broad aspect of nursing) frequently used by nurses for research and practice are the works of Benner, Pender, Leininger, and Meleis and the Synergy Model.
- "Middle" middle range nursing theories (theories that apply in a many aspects and situations) frequently used by nurses for research and practice include the Uncertainty in Illness Theory, the Theory of Comfort, the Theory of Unpleasant Symptoms, and Reed's Self-Transcendence Theory.
- "Low" middle range nursing theories (theories that are fairly concrete and apply to a narrow range of patients and situations) frequently used by nurses in research and practice include the Theory of Chronic Sorrow, Beck's Postpartum Depression Theory, and Mercer's Theory of Maternal Role Attainment.
- Many other middle range theories have been described in the nursing literature, and new ones are being developed by researchers and scholars to improve nursing care and patient outcomes.

Learning Activities

1. Select one of the middle range theories discussed in this chapter. Obtain a copy of the original work(s) and perform an analysis/evaluation using the criteria presented in Chapter 5.
2. Select one of the high middle range theories covered in this chapter and obtain a copy of the original work. Review three or four of the research studies cited for

that theory that either study relationships of the theory or use it as a conceptual framework. While reviewing these works, consider the following questions: Do the studies appear to use the theory appropriately? Are the works consistent in their use of the theory? Do the studies contribute to the knowledge base of the theory? How? Write a paper describing your findings.

3. Search current nursing journals for examples of the development, analysis, or use of middle range theories in the discipline of nursing. Debate trends with classmates or develop your analysis into a paper.

REFERENCES

Abraham, P. J. (2011). Developing nurse leaders: A program enhancing staff nurse leadership skills and professionalism. *Nursing Administration Quarterly, 35*(4), 306–312.

American Association of Colleges of Nursing. (2006). *The essentials of doctoral education for advanced nursing practice.* Retrieved from http://www.aacn.nche.edu/dnp/Essentials.pdf

American Association of Critical-Care Nurses. (2016). *The AACN synergy model for patient care.* Retrieved from https://www.aacn.org/nursing-excellence/aacn-standards/synergy-model

American Association of Critical-Care Nurses. (2017). *Standards: Synergy model.* Retrieved from https://www.aacn.org/nursing-excellence/aacn-standards/synergy-model

Andersen, R. D., Jylli, L., & Ambuel, B. (2014). Cultural adaptation of patient and observational outcome measures: A methodological example using the COMFORT behavioral rating scale. *International Journal of Nursing Studies, 51*(6), 934–942.

Bailey, D. E., Jr., Kazer, M. W., Polascik, T. J., & Robertson, C. (2014). Psychosocial trajectories of men monitoring prostate-specific antigen levels following surgery for prostate cancer. *Oncology Nursing Forum, 41*(4), 361–368.

Bailey, D. E., Jr., & Stewart, J. L. (2014). Merle H. Mishel: Uncertainty in illness theory. In M. R. Alligood (Ed.), *Nursing theorists and their work* (8th ed., pp. 555–573). St. Louis, MO: Mosby.

Barker, P. (2001a). The tidal model: Developing an empowering, person-centered approach to recovery within psychiatric and mental health nursing. *Journal of Psychiatric and Mental Health Nursing, 8,* 233–240.

Barker, P. (2001b). The tidal model: Developing a person-centered approach to psychiatric and mental health nursing. *Perspectives in Psychiatric Care, 37*(3), 79–87.

Beaudet, L., & Ducharme, F. (2013). Living with moderate-stage Parkinson disease: Intervention needs and preferences of elderly couples. *The Journal of Neuroscience Nursing, 45*(2), 88–95.

Beck, C. T. (1993). Teetering on the edge: A substantive theory of postpartum depression. *Nursing Research, 42*(1), 42–48.

Beck, C. T. (1995). The effects of postpartum depression on maternal–infant interaction: A meta-analysis. *Nursing Research, 44*(5), 298–304.

Beck, C. T. (1998). The effects of postpartum depression on child development: A meta-analysis. *Archives of Psychiatric Nursing, 12*(1), 12–20.

Beck, C. T. (2002a). Mothering multiples: A meta-synthesis of qualitative research. *MCN. The American Journal of Maternal Child Nursing, 27*(4), 214–221.

Beck, C. T. (2002b). Revision of the Postpartum Depression Predictors Inventory. *Journal of Obstetric, Gynecologic, and Neonatal Nursing, 31*(4), 394–402.

Beck, C. T., & Gable, R. K. (2000). Postpartum Depression Screening Scale: Development and psychometric testing. *Nursing Research, 49*(5), 272–282.

Beck, C. T., & Gable, R. K. (2003). Postpartum Depression Screening Scale: Spanish version. *Nursing Research, 52*(5), 296–306.

Beck, C. T., Records, K., & Rice, M. (2006). Further development of the Postpartum Depression Predictors Inventory-Revised. *Journal of Obstetric, Gynecologic, and Neonatal Nursing, 35*(6), 735–745.

Beck, C. T., Reynolds, M. A., & Rutowski, P. (1992). Maternity blues and postpartum depression. *Journal of Obstetric, Gynecologic, and Neonatal Nursing, 21*(4), 287–293.

Benner, P. (1984). *From novice to expert: Excellence and power in clinical nursing practice.* Menlo Park, CA: Addison-Wesley.

Benner, P. (2001). *From novice to expert: Excellence and power in clinical nursing practice* (Commemorative edition). Englewood Cliffs, NJ: Prentice Hall.

Benner, P., Tanner, C., & Chesla, C. (2009). *Expertise in nursing practice: Caring, clinical judgment, and ethics* (2nd ed.). New York, NY: Springer Publishing.

Bergquist, S., & King, J. (1994). Parish nursing—a conceptual framework. *Journal of Holistic Nursing, 12*(2), 155–170.

Bitanga, M. E., & Austria, M. (2013). Climbing the clinical ladder—one rung at a time. *Nursing Management, 44*(5), 23–4, 27.

Boudiab, L. D., & Kolcaba, K. (2015). Comfort theory: Unraveling the complexities of veteran's health care needs. *ANS. Advances in Nursing Science, 38*(4), 270–278.

Bowes, S., Lowes, L., Warner, J., & Gregory, J. W. (2009). Chronic sorrow in parent of children with type 1 diabetes. *Journal of Advanced Nursing, 65*(5), 992–1000.

Braden, C. J. (1990). A test of the self-help model: Learned response to chronic illness experience. *Nursing Research, 39*(1), 42–47.

Burkhart, L., & Hogan, N. S. (2008). An experiential theory of spiritual care in nursing practice. *Qualitative Health Research, 18*(7), 928–938.

Burns, K., Murrock, C. J., & Graor, C. H. (2012). Body mass index and injury severity in adolescent males. *Journal of Pediatric Nursing, 27*(5), 508–513.

Carr, J. M. (2014). A middle range theory of family vigilance. *Medsurg Nursing, 23*(4), 251–255.

Cates, L. A., Bishop, S., Armentrout, D., Verklan, T., Arnold, J., & Doughty, C. (2015). Initial development of C.A.T.E.S.: A simulation-based competency assessment instrument for neonatal nurse practitioners. *Neonatal Network, 34*(6), 329–336.

Christensen, D. (2015). The health change trajectory model: An integrated model of health change. *ANS. Advances in Nursing Science, 38*(1), 55–67.

Clemmens, D., Driscoll, J. W., & Beck, C. T. (2004). Postpartum depression as profiled through the depression screening scale. *MCN. The American Journal of Maternal Child Nursing, 29*(3), 180–185.

Corbin, J. M. (1998). The Corbin and Strauss chronic illness trajectory model: An update. *Scholarly Inquiry for Nursing Practice, 12*(1), 33–41.

Corbin, J. M., & Strauss, A. (1991). A nursing model for chronic illness management based upon the trajectory framework. *Scholarly Inquiry for Nursing Practice, 5*(3), 155–174.

Corbin, J. M., & Strauss, A. (1992). A nursing model for chronic illness management based upon the trajectory framework. In P. Woog (Ed.), *The chronic illness trajectory framework: The Corbin and Strauss nursing model* (pp. 9–28). New York, NY: Springer Publishing.

Coward, D. D. (2014). Pamela G. Reed: Self-transcendence theory. In M. R. Alligood (Ed.), *Nursing theorists and their work* (8th ed., pp. 574–592). St. Louis, MO: Mosby.

Cox, C. (1985). The Health Self-Determinism Index. *Nursing Research, 34*(3), 177–183.

Coyle, J. S. (2011). Development of a model home health nurse internship program for new graduates: Key lessons learned. *Journal of Continuing Education in Nursing, 42*(5), 201–214.

Curley, M. A. Q. (1998). Patient–nurse synergy: Optimizing patient's outcomes. *American Journal of Critical Care*, 7(1), 64–72.

Curley, M. A. Q. (2007). *Synergy: The unique relationship between nurses and patients*. Indianapolis, IN: Sigma Theta Tau International.

Cypress, B. S. (2016). Understanding uncertainty among critically ill patients in the intensive care units using Mishel's theory of uncertainty of illness. *Dimensions of Critical Care Nursing*, 35(1), 42–49.

Darnell, L. K., & Hickson, S. V. (2015). Cultural competent patient-centered nursing care. *The Nursing Clinics of North America*, 50(1), 99–108.

Dossa, A., Bokhour, B., & Hoenig, H. (2012). Care transitions from the hospital to home for patients with mobility impairments: Patient and family caregiver experiences. *Rehabilitation Nursing*, 37(6), 277–285.

Dumchin, M. (2010). Redefining the future of perioperative nursing education: A conceptual framework. *AORN Journal*, 92(1), 87–100.

Dunn, K. S. (2004). Toward a middle-range theory of adaptation to chronic pain. *Nursing Science Quarterly*, 17(1), 78–84.

Eakes, G. (2017). Chronic sorrow. In S. J. Peterson & T. S. Bredow (Eds.), *Middle range theories: Application to nursing research* (4th ed., pp. 93–105). Philadelphia, PA: Wolters Kluwer.

Eakes, G., Burke, M. L., & Hainsworth, M. A. (1998). Middle-range theory of chronic sorrow. *Image—The Journal of Nursing Scholarship*, 30(2), 179–184.

Eckhardt, A. L., DeVon, H. A., Piano, M., Ryan, C. J., & Zerwic, J. J. (2014). Fatigue in the presence of coronary heart disease. *Nursing Research*, 63(2), 83–93.

Ekim, A., & Ocakci, A. F. (2016). Efficacy of a transition theory-based discharge planning program for childhood asthma management. *International Journal of Nursing Knowledge*, 27(2), 70–78.

Elminowski, N. S. (2015). Developing and implementing a cultural awareness workshop for nurse practitioners. *Journal of Cultural Diversity*, 22(3), 105–113.

Farrell, D., & Savage, E. (2010). Symptom burden in inflammatory bowel disease: Rethinking conceptual and theoretical underpinnings. *International Journal of Nursing Practice*, 16(5), 437–442.

Farren, A. T. (2015). Leininger's ethnonursing research methodology and studies of cancer survivors: A review. *Journal of Transcultural Nursing*, 26(4), 418–427.

Fouquier, K. F. (2013). State of the science: Does the theory of maternal role attainment apply to African America motherhood? *Journal of Midwifery & Women's Health*, 58(2), 203–210.

Fowles, E. R. (1994). *The relationship between prenatal maternal attachment, postpartum depressive symptoms, and maternal role attainment*. Chicago, IL: Loyola University of Chicago.

García-Fernández, F. P., Agreda, J. J., Verdú, J., & Pancorbo-Hidalgo, P. L. (2014). A new theoretical model for development of pressure ulcers and other dependence-related lesions. *Journal of Nursing Scholarship*, 46(1), 28–38.

Geary, C. R., & Schumacher, K. L. (2012). Care transitions: Integrating transition theory and complexity science concepts. *ANS. Advances in Nursing Science*, 35(3), 236–248.

George, J. B., & Hickman, J. S. (2011). Other theories of the 1980s. In J. B. George (Ed.), *Nursing theories: The base for professional nursing practice* (6th ed., pp. 606–634). Upper Saddle River, NJ: Pearson Education.

Germino, B. B., Mishel, M. H., Crandell, J., Porter, L., Blyler, D., Jenerette, C., et al. (2013). Outcomes of an uncertainty management intervention in younger African American and Caucasian breast cancer survivors. *Oncology Nursing Forum*, 40(1), 82–92.

Giammanco, M. D., Gitto, L., Barberis, N., & Santoro, D. (2015). Adaption of the Mishel Uncertainty of Illness Scale (MUIS) for chronic patients in Italy. *Journal of Evaluation in Clinical Practice*, 21(4), 649–655.

Gillum, D. R., Staffileno, B. A., Schwartz, K. S., Coke, L., Fogg, L., & Reiling, D. (2011). Cardiovascular disease in the Amish: An exploratory study of knowledge, beliefs, and health care practices. *Holistic Nursing Practice*, 25(6), 289–297.

Glenn, A. D. (2015). Using online health communication to manage chronic sorrow: Mothers of children with rare diseases speak. *Journal of Pediatric Nursing*, 30(1), 17–24.

Good, M. (1998). A middle-range theory of acute pain management: Use in research. *Nursing Outlook*, 46(3), 120–124.

Good, M., & Moore, S. M. (1996). Clinical practice guidelines as a new source of middle-range theory: Focus on acute pain. *Nursing Outlook*, 44(2), 74–79.

Haag-Heitman, B. (2012). Supporting transitions in clinical practice development. *The Journal of Perinatal & Neonatal Nursing*, 26(1), 5–7.

Häggström, M., Asplund, K., & Kristiansen, L. (2012). How can nurses facilitate patient's transitions from intensive care? A grounded theory of nursing. *Intensive & Critical Care Nursing*, 28(4), 224–233.

Hardin, S. R. (2012). Hearing loss in older critical care patients: Participation in decision making. *Critical Care Nurse*, 32(6), 43–50.

Hardin, S. R. (2017). The AACN synergy model. In S. J. Peterson & T. S. Bredow (Eds.), *Middle range theories: Application to nursing research and practice* (4th ed., pp. 293–303). Philadelphia, PA: Wolters Kluwer.

Hart, A., Hardin, S. R., Townsend, A. P., Ramsey, S., & Mahrle-Henson, A. (2013). Critical care visitation: Nurse and family preference. *Dimensions of Critical Care Nursing*, 32(6), 289–299.

Hatzfeld, J. J., Nelson, M. S., Waters, C. M., & Jennings, B. M. (2016). Factors influencing health behaviors among active duty Air Force personnel. *Nursing Outlook*, 64(5), 440–449.

Haugan, G. (2014). Nurse-patient interaction is a resource for hope, meaning in life and self-transcendence in nursing home patients. *Scandinavian Journal of Caring Sciences*, 28(1), 74–88.

Ho, H. M., Tseng, Y. H., Hsin, Y. M., Chou, F. H., & Lin, W. T. (2016). Living with illness and self-transcendence: The lived experience of patients with spinal muscular atrophy. *Journal of Advanced Nursing*, 72(11), 2695–2705.

Holditch-Davis, D., Miles, M. S., Burchinal, M. R., & Goldman, B. D. (2011). Maternal role attainment with medically fragile infants: Part 2. Relationship to the quality of parenting. *Research in Nursing & Health*, 34(1), 35–48.

Homard, C. M. (2013). Impact of a standardized test package on exit examination scores and NCLEX-RN outcomes. *The Journal of Nursing Education*, 52(3), 175–178.

Hsu, M. C., & Tu, C. H. (2014). Improving quality-of-life outcomes for patients with cancer through mediating effects of depressive symptoms and functional status: A three-path mediation model. *Journal of Clinical Nursing*, 23(17–18), 2461–2472.

Hunnibell, L. S., Reed, P. G., Quinn-Griffin, M., & Fitzpatrick, J.J. (2008). Self-transcendence and burnout in hospice and oncology nurses. *Journal of Hospice and Palliative Nursing*, 10(3), 172–179.

Im, E.-O. (2014). Afaf Ibrahim Meleis: Transition theory. In M. R. Alligood (Ed.), *Nursing theorists and their work* (8th ed., pp. 378–395). St. Louis, MO: Mosby.

Jackson, H., Yates, B. C., Blanchard, S., Zimmerman, L. M., Hudson, D., & Pozehl, B. (2016). Behavior-specific influences for physical activity among African American women. *Western Journal of Nursing Research*, 38(8), 992–1011.

Joly, E. (2016). Integrating transition theory and bioecological theory: A theoretical perspective for nurses supporting the transition to adulthood for young people with medical complexity. *Journal of Advanced Nursing*, 72(6), 1251–1262.

Joseph, H. A. (2012). Recognizing chronic sorrow in the habitual ED patient. *Journal of Emergency Nursing*, 38(6), 539–540.

Kim, H. S., Oh, E. G., Lee, H., Kim, S. H., & Kim, H. K. (2015). Predictors of symptom experience in Korean patients with cancer undergoing chemotherapy. *European Journal of Oncology Nursing*, 19(6), 644–653.

Kinsey, C. B., Baptiste-Roberts, K., Zhu, J., & Kjerulff, K. H. (2014). Effect of miscarriage history on maternal–infant bonding during the first year postpartum in the First Baby Study: A longitudinal cohort study. *BMC Women's Health*, 14(1), 83–91.

Koharchik, L., Caputi, L., Robb, M., & Culleiton, A. L. (2015). Fostering clinical reasoning in nursing students. *The American Journal of Nursing*, 115(1), 58–61.

Kolcaba, K. Y. (1994). A theory of holistic comfort for nursing. *Journal of Advanced Nursing*, 19(6), 1178–1184.

Kolcaba, K. Y. (1995). The art of comfort care. *Image—The Journal of Nursing Scholarship*, 27(4), 287–289.

Kolcaba, K. Y. (2001). Evolution of the mid range theory of comfort for outcomes research. *Nursing Outlook, 49*(2), 86–92.

Kolcaba, K. Y. (2003). *Comfort theory and practice: A vision for holistic health care and research.* New York, NY: Springer Publishing.

Kolcaba, K. Y. (2017). Comfort. In S. J. Peterson & T. S. Bredow (Eds.), *Middle range theories: Application to nursing research and practice* (4th ed., pp. 196–211). Philadelphia, PA: Wolters Kluwer.

Krinsky, R., Murillo, I., & Johnson, J. (2014). A practical application of Katharine Kolcaba's comfort theory to cardiac patients. *Applied Nursing Research, 27*(2), 147–150.

Kurita, K., Garon, E. B., Stanton, A. L., & Meyerowitz, B. E. (2013). Uncertainty and psychological adjustment in patients with lung cancer. *Psycho-Oncology, 22*(6), 1396–1401.

Lauver, D. (1992). A theory of care-seeking behavior. *Image—The Journal of Nursing Scholarship, 24*(4), 281–287.

Le, H. N., Perry, D. F., & Sheng, X. (2009). Using the internet to screen for postpartum depression. *Maternal and Child Health Journal, 13*(2), 213–221.

Lee, R. C. (2012). Family homelessness viewed through the lens of health and human rights. *ANS. Advances in Nursing Science, 35*(2), E47–E59.

Leininger, M. M. (2002). Culture care theory: A major contribution to advance transcultural nursing knowledge and practices. *Journal of Transcultural Nursing, 13*(3), 189–192.

Leininger, M. M. (2007). Theoretical questions and concerns: Response from the theory of culture care diversity and universality perspective. *Nursing Science Quarterly, 20*(1), 9–13.

Lenz, E. R., & Pugh, L. C. (2014). The theory of unpleasant symptoms. In M. J. Smith & P. R. Liehr (Eds.), *Middle range theory for nursing* (3rd ed., pp. 165–196). New York, NY: Springer Publishing.

Lenz, E. R., Pugh, L. C., Milligan, R. A., & Gift, A. (2017). Unpleasant symptoms. In S. J. Peterson & T. S. Bredow (Eds.), *Middle range theories: Application to nursing research* (4th ed., pp. 67–78). Philadelphia, PA: Wolters Kluwer.

Lenz, E. R., Pugh, L. C., Milligan, R. A., Gift, A., & Suppe, F. (1997). The middle-range theory of unpleasant symptoms: An update. *ANS. Advances in Nursing Science, 19*(3), 14–27.

Lenz, E. R., & Shortridge-Baggett, L. M. (Eds.). (2002). *Self-efficacy in nursing: Research and measurement perspectives.* New York, NY: Springer Publishing.

Lenz, E. R., Suppe, F., Gift, A. G., Pugh, L. C., & Milligan, R. A. (1995). Collaborative development of middle-range nursing theories: Toward a theory of unpleasant symptoms. *ANS. Advances in Nursing Science, 17*(3), 1–13.

Liehr, P., & Smith, M. J. (1999). Middle range theory: Spinning research and practice to create knowledge for the new millennium. *ANS. Advances in Nursing Science, 21*(4), 81–91.

Logsdon, M. C., Tomasulo, R., Eckert, D., Beck, C., & Dennis, C. L. (2012). Identification of mothers at risk for postpartum depression by hospital-based perinatal nurses. *MCN. The American Journal of Maternal Child Nursing, 37*(4), 218–225.

Long, J. M., Sowell, R., Bairan, A., Holtz, C., Curtis, A. B., & Fogarty, K. J. (2012). Exploration of commonalities and variations in health related beliefs across four Latino subgroups using focus group methodology: Implications in care for Latinos with type 2 diabetes. *Journal of Cultural Diversity, 19*(4), 133–142.

Long, T. (2016). Influence of international service learning on nursing student's self efficacy towards cultural competence. *Journal of Cultural Diversity, 23*(1), 28–33.

López-Entrambasaguas, O. M., Granero-Molina, J., & Fernández-Sola, C. (2013). An ethnographic study of HIV/AIDS among Ayoreo sex workers: Cultural factors and risk perception. *Journal of Clinical Nursing, 22*(23–24), 3337–3348.

Lucero, N. B., Beckstrand, R. L., Callister, L. C., & Sanchez Birkhead, A. C. (2012). Prevalence of postpartum depression among Hispanic immigrant women. *Journal of the American Academy of Nurse Practitioners, 24*(12), 726–734.

Maeve, M. K. (2014). Cheryl Tatano Beck: Postpartum depression theory. In M. R. Alligood (Ed.), *Nursing theorists and their work* (8th ed., pp. 672–687). St. Louis, MO: Mosby.

Marchuk, A. (2016). End-of-life care in the neonatal intensive care unit: Applying comfort theory. *International Journal of Palliative Nursing, 22*(7), 317–323.

Marsh, J. R. (2013). A middle range theory of postpartum depression: Analysis and application. *International Journal of Childbirth Education, 28*(4), 50–54.

Martin, K. S. (2005). *The Omaha System: A key to practice, documentation, and information management* (2nd ed.). Philadelphia, PA: Elsevier Saunders.

McCarthy, V. L., Ling, J., Bowland, S., Hall, L. A., & Connelly, J. (2015). Promoting self-transcendence and well-being in community-dwelling older adults: A pilot study of a psychoeducational intervention. *Geriatric Nursing, 36*(6), 431–437.

McCarthy, V. L., Ling, J., & Carini, R. M. (2013). The role of self-transcendence: A missing variable in the pursuit of successful aging? *Research in Gerontological Nursing, 6*(3), 178–186.

McFarland, M. (2014). Madeleine M. Leininger: Culture care theory of diversity and universality. In M. R. Alligood (Ed.), *Nursing theorists and their work* (8th ed., pp. 417–441). St. Louis, MO: Mosby.

McFarland, M., & Wehbe-Alamah, H. B. (2015). *Leininger's culture care diversity and universality: A worldwide nursing theory* (3rd ed.). Burlington, MA: Jones & Bartlett.

Meighan, M. (2014). Ramona T. Mercer: Maternal role attainment—becoming a mother. In M. R. Alligood (Ed.), *Nursing theorists and their work* (8th ed., pp. 538–554). St. Louis, MO: Elsevier.

Meleis, A. I. (2010). *Transitions theory: Middle range and situation specific theories in nursing research and practice.* New York, NY: Springer Publishing.

Meleis, A. I., & Trangenstein, P. A. (1994). Facilitating transitions: Redefinition of the nursing mission. *Nursing Outlook, 42*(6), 255–259.

Mercer, R. T. (1981). A theoretical framework for studying factors that impact on the maternal role. *Nursing Research, 30*(2), 73–77.

Mercer, R. T. (1985). The process of maternal role attainment over the first year. *Nursing Research, 34*(4), 198–204.

Mercer, R. T. (2004). Becoming a mother versus maternal role attainment. *Journal of Nursing Scholarship, 36*(3), 226–232.

Mercer, R. T. (2006). Nursing support of the process of becoming a mother. *Journal of Obstetric, Gynecologic, and Neonatal Nursing, 35*(5), 649–651.

Mercer, R. T., & Walker, L. O. (2006). A review of nursing interventions to foster becoming a mother. *Journal of Obstetric, Gynecologic, and Neonatal Nursing, 35*(5), 568–582.

Meretoja, R., & Koponen, L. (2012). A systematic model to compare nurses' optimal and actual competencies in the clinical setting. *Journal of Advanced Nursing, 68*(2), 414–422.

Miles, M. S., Holditch-Davis, D., Burchinal, M. R., & Brunssen, S. (2011). Maternal role attainment with medically fragile infants: Part 1. Measurement and correlates during the first year of life. *Research in Nursing & Health, 34*(1), 20–34.

Miller, C. A. (2015). Pseudoprogression: Patient experience and nursing in uncertainty. *Canadian Journal of Neuroscience Nursing, 37*(2), 35–41.

Miller, L. W. (1997). Nursing through the lens of faith: A conceptual model. *Journal of Christian Nursing, 14*(1), 17–21.

Mishel, M. H. (1981). The measurement of uncertainty in illness. *Nursing Research, 30*(5), 258–263.

Mishel, M. H. (1984). Perceived uncertainty and stress in illness. *Research in Nursing & Health, 7*, 163–171.

Mishel, M. H. (1988). Uncertainty in illness. *Image—The Journal of Nursing Scholarship, 20*(4), 225–232.

Mishel, M. H. (1990). Reconceptualization of the uncertainty in illness theory. *Image—The Journal of Nursing Scholarship, 22*(4), 256–262.

Mishel, M. H. (1999). Uncertainty in chronic illness. *Annual Review of Nursing Research, 17*, 269–294.

Mishel, M. H. (2014). Theories of uncertainty in illness. In M. J. Smith & P. R. Liehr (Eds.), *Middle range theory for nursing* (3rd ed., pp. 53–86). New York, NY: Springer Publishing.

Mixer, S. J., Fornehed, M. L., Varney, J., & Lindley, L. C. (2014). Culturally congruent end-of-life care for rural Appalachian people and their families. *Journal of Hospice and Palliative Nursing, 16*(8), 526–535.

Morse, J. (2001). Toward a praxis theory of suffering. *ANS. Advances in Nursing Science, 24*(1), 47–59.

Murray, R. P. (2010). Spiritual care beliefs and practices of special care and oncology RNs at patients' end of life. *Journal of Hospice and Palliative Nursing, 12*(1), 51–58.

Neal, L. J. (1999a). Neal theory of home health nursing practice. *Image—The Journal of Nursing Scholarship, 31*(3), 251.

Neal, L. J. (1999b). The Neal theory: Implications for practice and administration. *Home Healthcare Nurse, 17*(3), 181–187.

Nikfarid, L., Rassouli, M., Borimnejad, L., & Alavimajd, H. (2015). Chronic sorrow in mothers of children with cancer. *Journal of Pediatric Oncology Nursing, 32*(5), 314–319.

Norbeck, J. S. (1981). Social support: A model for clinical research and application. *ANS. Advances in Nursing Science, 3*(4), 43–59.

Noseff, J. (2014). Theory usage and application paper: Maternal role attainment. *International Journal of Childbirth Education, 29*(3), 58–61.

Owens, A. L., & Cleaves, J. (2012). Then and now: Updating clinical nurse advancement programs. *Nursing, 42*(10), 15–17.

Palmer, B., Quinn Griffin, M. T., Reed, P., & Fitzpatrick, J. J. (2010). Self-transcendence and work engagement in acute care staff registered nurses. *Critical Care Nursing Quarterly, 33*(2), 138–147.

Park, D. I., Choi-Kwon, S., & Han, K. (2015). Health behaviors of Korean female nursing students in relation to obesity and osteoporosis. *Nursing Outlook, 63*(4), 504–511.

Pate, M. F. D. (2017). Introduction. In S. R. Hardin & R. Kaplow (Eds.), *Synergy for clinical excellence: The AACN synergy model for patient care* (2nd ed., pp. 3–10). Burlington, MA: Jones & Bartlett.

Pender, N. J., Murdaugh, C. L., & Parsons, M. A. (2015). *Health promotion in nursing practice* (7th ed.). Upper Saddle River, NJ: Prentice Hall.

Polk, L. V. (1997). Toward a middle-range theory of resilience. *ANS. Advances in Nursing Science, 19*(3), 1–13.

Reed, P. G. (1991a). Self-transcendence and mental health in oldest-old adults. *Nursing Research, 40*(1), 5–11.

Reed, P. G. (1991b). Toward a nursing theory of self-transcendence: Deductive reformulation using developmental theories. *ANS. Advances in Nursing Science, 13*(4), 64–77.

Reed, P. G. (1996). Transcendence: Formulating nursing perspectives. *Nursing Science Quarterly, 9*(1), 2–4.

Reed, P. G. (2014). Theory of self-transcendence. In M. J. Smith & P. R. Liehr (Eds.), *Middle range theory for nursing* (3rd ed., pp. 109–139). New York, NY: Springer Publishing.

Rew, L., Tyler, D., Fredland, N., & Hannah, D. (2012). Adolescents' concerns as they transition through high school. *ANS. Advances in Nursing Science, 35*(3), 205–221.

Riegel, B., Jaarsma, T., & Strömberg, A. (2012). A middle-range theory of self-care of chronic illness. *ANS. Advances in Nursing Science, 35*(3), 194–204.

Rogers, B. (1994). *Occupational health nursing: Concepts and practice.* Philadelphia, PA: Saunders.

Ruland, C. M., & Moore, S. M. (1998). Theory construction based on standards of care: A proposed theory of the peaceful end of life. *Nursing Outlook, 46*(4), 169–175.

Saijadi, N., Rassouli, M., Abbaszadeh, A., Alavi Majd, H., & Zendehdel, K. (2014). Psychometric properties of the Persian version of the Mishel's Uncertainty in Illness Scale in patients with cancer. *European Journal of Oncology Nursing, 18*(1), 52–57.

Schumacher, K. L., & Meleis, A. I. (1994). Transitions: A central concept in nursing. *Image—The Journal of Nursing Scholarship, 26*(2), 119–125.

Seyedfatemi, N., Rafii, F., Rezaei, M., & Kolcaba, K. (2014). Comfort and hope in the preanesthesia stage in patient undergoing surgery. *Journal of Perianesthesia Nursing, 29*(30), 213–220.

Shockey-Stephenson, P., & Berry, D. M. (2015). Describing spirituality at the end of life. *Western Journal of Nursing Research, 37*(9), 1229–1247.

Shuler, P. A., & Davis, J. E. (1993). The Shuler nurse practitioner model: A theoretical framework for nurse practitioner clinicians, educators and researcher. *Journal of the American Academy of Nurse Practitioners, 5*(1), 11–18.

Smith, C. E., Pace, K., Kochinda, C., Kleinbeck, S. V. M., Koehler, J., & Popkess-Vawter, S. (2002). Caregiving effectiveness model evolution to a midrange theory of home care: A process for critique and replication. *ANS. Advances in Nursing Science, 25*(1), 50–64.

Smith, K., & Bazini-Barakat, N. (2003). A public health nursing practice model: Melding public health principles with the nursing process. *Public Health Nursing, 20*(1), 42–48.

Sriyasak, A., Akerlind, I., & Akhavan, S. (2013). Childrearing among Thai first-time teenage mothers. *The Journal of Perinatal Education, 22*(4), 201–211.

Stacy, K. M. (2011). Progressive care units: Different but the same. *Critical Care Nurse, 31*(3), 77–83.

Stewart, J. L., Lynn, M. R., & Mishel, M. H. (2010). Psychometric evaluation of a new instrument to measure uncertainty in children and adolescents with cancer. *Nursing Research, 59*(2), 119–126.

Swanson, K. M. (1991). Empirical development of a middle range theory of caring. *Nursing Research, 40*(3), 161–166.

Swickard, S., Swickard, W., Reimer, A., Lindell, D., & Winkelman, C. (2014). Adaptation of the AACN synergy model for patient care to critical care transport. *Critical Care Nurse, 34*(1), 16–28.

Tejero, L. M. S. (2012). The mediating role of the nurse–patient dyad bonding in bringing about patient satisfaction. *Journal of Advanced Nursing, 68*(5), 994–1002.

Thomas, N. F., & Dunn, K. S. (2014). Self-transcendence and medication adherence in older adults with hypertension. *Journal of Holistic Nursing, 32*(4), 316–326.

Thomason, E., Volling, B. L., Flynn, H. A., McDonough, S. C., Marcus, S. M., Lopez, J. F., et al. (2014). Parenting stress and depressive symptoms in postpartum mothers: Bidirectional or unidirectional effects? *Infant Behavior & Development, 37*(3), 406–415.

Troutman-Jordan, M. (2015). Troutman-Jordan's theory of successful aging. In M. C. Smith & M. E. Parker (Eds.), *Nursing theories and nursing practice* (4th ed., pp. 483–508). Philadelphia, PA: F.A. Davis.

Tsai, P. F. (2003). A middle-range theory of caregiver stress. *Nursing Science Quarterly, 16*(2), 137–145.

Tyler, R., & Pugh, L. C. (2009). Application of the theory of unpleasant symptoms in bariatric surgery. *Bariatric Nursing and Surgical Patient Care, 4*(4), 270–276.

Unson, C., Flynn, D., Glendon, M. A., Haymes, E., & Sancho, D. (2015). Dementia and caregiver stress: An application of the reconceptualized uncertainty in illness theory. *Issues in Mental Health Nursing, 36*(6), 439–446.

Vitale, S. A., & Falco, C. (2014). Children born prematurely: Risk of parental chronic sorrow. *Journal of Pediatric Nursing, 29*(3), 248–251.

Walsh, S. M., Lamet, A. R., Lindgren, C. L., Rillstone, P., Little, D. J., Steffey, C. M., et al. (2011). Art in Alzheimer's care: Promoting well-being in people with late-stage Alzheimer's disease. *Rehabilitation Nursing, 36*(2), 66–72.

Weinert, C., & Long, K. A. (1991). The theory and research base for rural nursing practice. In A. Bush (Ed.), *Rural nursing* (pp. 21–38). Newbury Park, CA: Sage.

White, C. L., Barrientos, R., & Dunn, K. (2014). Dimensions of uncertainty after stroke: Perspectives of the stroke survivor and family caregiver. *The Journal of Neuroscience Nursing, 46*(4), 233–240.

Whitehead, P. B., Anderson, E. S., Redican, K. J., & Stratton, R. (2010). Studying the effects of the end-of-life nursing education consortium at the institutional level. *Journal of Hospice and Palliative Nursing, 12*(3), 184–193.

Wilson, B., Harwood, L., & Oudshoorn, A. (2015). Understanding skill acquisition among registered nurses: The "perpetual novice" phenomenon. *Journal of Clinical Nursing, 24*(23–24), 3564–3575.

Woody, G., & Davis, B. A. (2013). Increasing nurse competence in peripheral intravenous therapy. *Journal of Infusion Nursing, 36*(6), 413–419.

Evidence-Based Practice and Nursing Theory

Evelyn M. Wills and Melanie McEwen

Helen Soderstrom was stricken with changes in her vision, disturbances of gait, and occasional periods of severe fatigue during her senior year of nursing school. She experienced intermittent periods of normality as well as illness, and the periods when she had no symptoms lasted many months. During a time when her symptoms were unusually active, she sought medical help, and her physician determined that her symptoms were related to stress. Despite the periods of weakness and fatigue, she was able to complete the nursing program and graduated with honors.

During Helen's first year of practice, she experienced two periods of symptom exacerbation, but each was short-lived. With full insurance, she was able to see a neurologist who concluded that she was experiencing the beginning stages of a neuromuscular disease. Because there was no "cure," the neurologist worked with Helen to find interventions that helped her manage the symptoms when they became problematic.

After a few years in practice, Helen enrolled in a graduate program to work toward a career as a nurse educator. During her first year of graduate studies, she seldom experienced neurologic symptoms, but during her practice teaching course, they returned.

The recurrence of symptoms, along with a new understanding of evidence-based practice (EBP) from her graduate courses, led Helen to make her personal health experience the topic of her final, capstone paper. To learn more, she sought resources that would help her gain better control of the neuromuscular symptoms as well as assist her in her studies. To that end, she contacted her university hospital's neuroscience department and applied to join a clinical team to learn about the efficacy of treatments and evidence-based interventions currently being used for patients with neuromuscular diseases. As she gained more experience with EBP, she considered what system she would use to develop guidelines on symptom management and selected the Iowa Model of Evidence-Based Practice because of its basis in research applied to clinical problems.

Florence Nightingale, nursing's first investigator, devised a statistical means of deciphering her data from Scutari during the Crimean war (Cohen, 1984; McDonald, 2014). Despite her accomplishments as an epidemiologist and researcher, however, Nightingale failed to recognize this vital role for nurses as she described nursing as an "art" and medicine as a "science" (Nightingale, 1860/1957/1969). Focused on the "art" of nursing and the apprentice-style nature of early nursing education, Nightingale developed a systematic method for showing the results of nursing care in her own practice (see Chapter 2). In contrast, the idea of "science-based medicine" has been recognized since "mid-nineteenth century France and even earlier" (Sackett, Rosenberg, Gray, Haynes, & Richardson, 1996, p. 71). Furthermore, the ideal of science-based medicine was influenced by the great influenza epidemic of 1918 to 1919 when physicians learned that understanding factors leading to that health crisis were necessary to prevent similar occurrences (Barry, 2005).

In the 1960s, several physicians led by Dr. Archie Cochrane endeavored to begin teaching and practicing medicine based on data produced by scientific and epidemiologic research (Sur & Dahm, 2011). Cochrane questioned the efficacy of non–research-based practices in medicine (Sackett et al., 1996; Shah & Chung, 2009) and emphasized the critical review of research, focusing on randomized control trials (RCTs) to support medical practice. His influence led to development of the Cochrane Collaboration (now simply "Cochrane") in 1993, an endeavor supported by a group of 70 international physicians (Shah & Chung, 2009). That effort, originally termed "evidence-based medicine," and now "evidence-based practice," has grown exponentially. Today, the Cochrane initiative, and its attendant partners, is an organization charged with developing, maintaining, and updating systematic reviews of health care interventions (Cochrane, 2017). The intent of Cochrane is to help transform how health decisions are made by gathering and summarizing the best available evidence from health-related research to help patients and health providers make informed treatment choices.

Following efforts by Cochrane to collect and summarize research information, the requirement for scientific review of research and practice has become widespread in health disciplines. The Joanna Briggs Institute, for example, was named for an Australian nurse. Implemented in the 1990s, it now has worldwide influence in EBP (Joanna Briggs Institute, 2016; Polit & Beck, 2017). More recently, Sigma Theta Tau International, which has supported nursing research for decades, now sponsors a journal focused on publishing evidence-based nursing research (Polit & Beck, 2017). Although the notion of EBP was somewhat delayed in being recognized and implemented in nursing, over the past two decades, EBP has now essentially become the standard for research-based, informed decision making for nursing care.

In contrast to "research," which refers to the systematic, rigorous, critical investigation to answer question(s), EBP is an approach to problem solving that conscientiously collects, evaluates, and integrates the most current, or "best," evidence based on meta-analyses of the latest research for patient care (LoBiondo-Wood & Haber, 2018). Nurses have expanded the original EBP requirements (which largely espouse experimental research) by including qualitatively derived findings from phenomenologic, ethnographic, and grounded theory research and case studies (Polit & Beck, 2017). "Metasynthesis" is the term applied to the process of systematic review of qualitative studies on a topic and is a way to systematize such evidence for use in nursing situations (Butler, Hall, & Copnell, 2016; Melnyk & Fineout-Overholt, 2015).

Thus, EBP is a process that involves identifying a clinical problem, searching the literature, synthesizing the findings to critically evaluate the research evidence, and

Box 12-1	American Association of Colleges of Nursing Essentials and Evidence-Based Nursing Practice

Evidence-based practice (EBP) is one of the critical elements identified in the "Essentials of Master's Education" (American Association of Colleges of Nursing [AACN], 2011), and EBP is mentioned more than 50 times in the document. One statement helps summarize the relationship between EBP, theory, and professional nursing practice: "Master's-prepared nurses, when appropriate, lead the healthcare team in the implementation of evidence-based practice. . . . Integrate theory, evidence, clinical judgement, research and interprofessional perspectives using translational processes to improve practice and associated health outcomes for patient aggregates" (p. 16).

Similarly, according to the AACN (2006), doctor of nursing practice (DNP) programs are designed to prepare experts in specialized advanced nursing practice. It has been determined that DNP programs should " . . . focus heavily on practice that is innovative and evidence-based, reflecting the application of credible research findings" (p. 3). Indeed, Essential III explains the importance of "Analytical Models for Evidence-Based Practice" and includes a number of related competencies and objectives for DNP programs.

then determining appropriate interventions. Nursing scholars note that EBP relies on integrating research, theory, and practice and is equivalent to theory-based practice as the objective of both is the highest level of safety and efficacy for patients (Fawcett & Garity, 2009). Finally, EBP is an "essential" component of advanced nursing education and vital for both master's- and doctorate-prepared nurses (Box 12-1).

Overview of Evidence-Based Practice

The concept of EBP is widely accepted as a requisite in health care. EBP is based on the premise that health professionals should not center practice on tradition and belief but on sound information grounded in research findings and scientific development (Melnyk & Fineout-Overholt, 2015; Schmidt & Brown, 2015). Until the early part of the 21st century, the concept of EBP was more common in Canadian and British nursing literature than in U.S. nursing literature. Over the last decade, however, the term has become ubiquitous. This is attributed in part to the guideline initiatives of the Agency for Healthcare Research and Quality, the Institute of Medicine, and the U.S. Preventative Services Task Force, among others (Hudson, Duke, Haas, & Varnell, 2008; Melnyk & Fineout-Overholt, 2015).

Many nursing scholars (DiCenso, Guyatt, & Ciliska, 2005; Hall, 2014; Ingersoll, 2000; LoBiondo-Wood & Haber, 2018; Melnyk & Fineout-Overholt, 2015; Pugh, 2012; Rycroft-Malone, 2004) have pointed out that EBP and research are not synonymous. They are both scholarly processes but focus on different phases of knowledge development—application versus discovery. In general, EBP refers to the integration of individual clinical expertise with the best available external clinical evidence from systematic research. It is largely based on research studies, particularly studies using clinical trials, meta-analysis, and studies of client outcomes, and it is more likely to be applied in practice settings that value the use of new knowledge and in settings that provide resources to access that knowledge. However, nursing studies that employ qualitative methods or mixed method research are considered valuable to the discipline, as mentioned above (Hall, 2014).

Definition and Characteristics of Evidence-Based Practice

In medicine, EBP has been defined as the conscientious, explicit, and judicious use of the current best evidence in making decisions about the care of individual patients (Sackett, Straus, Richardson, Rosenberg, & Haynes, 2000). It is an approach to health care practice in which the clinician is aware of the evidence that relates to clinical practice and the strength of that evidence (Jennings & Loan, 2001; Tod, Palfreyman, & Burke, 2004).

To distinguish nursing from medicine in discussing EBP, a number of definitions have been presented in the literature. Sigma Theta Tau International (2005) defined "evidence-based nursing" as "an integration of the best evidence available, nursing expertise, and the values and preferences of the individuals, families, and communities who are served" (para. 4). Similarly, DiCenso and colleagues (2005) defined EBP as "the integration of best research evidence with clinical expertise and patient values to facilitate clinical decision making" (p. 4). Both of these definitions use similar terms (e.g., best evidence, expertise, patient values).

In nursing, EBP generally includes careful review of research findings according to guidelines that nurse scholars have used to measure the merit of a study or group of studies. Evidence-based nursing de-emphasizes ritual, isolated, and unsystematic clinical experiences; ungrounded opinions; and tradition as a basis for practice and stresses the use of research findings. Other measures or factors, including nursing expertise, health resources, patient/family preferences, quality improvement efforts, and the consensus of recognized experts, are also incorporated as appropriate (Melnyk & Fineout-Overholt, 2015; Schmidt & Brown, 2015).

In summary, EBP has several critical features. First, it is a problem-based approach and considers the context of the practitioner's current experience. In addition, EBP brings together the best available evidence and current practice by combining research results with tacit knowledge and theory. Third, it incorporates values, beliefs, and desires of the patients and their families. Finally, EBP facilitates the application of research findings by incorporating first- and secondhand knowledge into practice. Link to Practice 12-1 presents information on databases that nurses and others can access to find specific information on current guidelines and other collections of "evidence" that can be used to improve health care.

Concerns Related to Evidence-Based Practice in Nursing

Despite growing acceptance of application of EBP in nursing, some criticisms and concerns have been voiced in the nursing literature. For example, there is the concern that EBP is more focused on the science of nursing than on the art of nursing. Some authors have expressed concern that strict concentration on empirically based knowledge will lead to the failure to capture the uniqueness of nursing and the importance of holistic care in contemporary practice (Fawcett, Watson, Neuman, Walker, & Fitzpatrick, 2001; Hudson et al., 2008; Upton, 1999).

Another concern is that strict reliance on EBP will place nurses in the role of medical extender or medical technician, where nursing will be reduced to a technical practice. This concern was voiced as equating EBP with "cookbook care" and a disregard for individualized patient care (Finkelman & Kenner, 2016; Melnyk & Fineout-Overholt, 2015). Indeed, although evidence may provide direction for development of procedures, techniques, and protocols for nursing, it has been established that these are not

Link to Practice 12-1

Key Resources for Evidence-Based Practice

Several important databases have been set up over the last 20 years to promote integration of "evidence" in health care. Information on three of the most influential are presented here.

Cochrane Collaboration—http://www.cochrane.org/

The Cochrane Collaboration is an international network that helps health care practitioners, policy makers, patients, and their advocates make informed decisions about health care. The Cochrane Library prepares, updates, and promotes the accessibility of the *Cochrane Database of Systematic Reviews*.

Joanna Briggs Institute—http://www.joannabriggs.edu.au/

The Joanna Briggs Institute is an international research and development organization from the School of Translational Science at the University of Adelaide, South Australia. The Institute and its collaborating entities promote and support the synthesis, transfer, and utilization of evidence through identifying feasible, appropriate, meaningful, and effective health care practices to assist in the improvement of health care outcomes.

Agency for Healthcare Research and Quality (U.S. Preventative Services Task Force/National Guideline Clearinghouse)—http://www.guideline.gov/

The National Guideline Clearinghouse (NGC) is a database of evidence-based clinical practice guidelines. It is intended to be used by health professionals, practitioners, patients, and others to obtain objective, detailed information on clinical practice guidelines and to further their dissemination, implementation, and use.

the only knowledge that informs the nursing practice and that consideration of individual needs and values is essential (Hudson et al., 2008; Mitchell, 2013).

Third, because research involving humans is complex, findings may be open to interpretation and therefore should not be the sole basis for practice. Research must be considered within the context of the practice prescribed by theory, and it must integrate the values and beliefs of nursing philosophy (Chinn & Kramer, 2015; McKenna & Slevin, 2008; Walker & Avant, 2011).

A fourth concern relates to promoting a link with evidence-based medicine and its emphasis on positivist thinking and the dominance of randomized clinical trials as the major evidence. This concern is related to the absence of consideration of evidence gathered through qualitative research and theory development (Fawcett et al., 2001; Jennings & Loan, 2001; Stevens, 2002).

A fifth concern relates to the potential for linking health care reimbursement exclusively to interventions that can be substantiated by a documented body of evidence (Ingersoll, 2000). This leads to a number of ethical questions and issues that should be considered. For example, restricting "off-label" use of medications that may be helpful for certain patients or certain diagnoses, attempts to alter financial reimbursement to reduce emergency and specialty care, and adjusting payment to providers for over (or under) use of prescription pain medications.

Finally, it is argued that not all practice in the health professions can or should be based on science. In many cases, researchers have yet to accumulate a sufficient body of knowledge. In other cases, a different frame of reference provides a different rationale for action (McKenna & Slevin, 2008). In these instances, strict reliance on EBP may result in numerous voids when developing a plan of care.

Concerns such as these have been addressed by DiCenso and colleagues (2005), who assert that a fundamental principle of EBP is that research evidence alone is not sufficient to plan care. Other ethical and pragmatic factors, such as benefits and risks, associated costs, and patient's wishes, should be considered. Furthermore, they note that "best research evidence" can be quantitative or qualitative and does not necessarily rely on RCTs. These notions are also supported by Rycroft-Malone (2004), who maintains that well-conceived and well-conducted qualitative and quantitative research evidence, clinical experience, and patient experiences, combined with local or organizational influences, are necessary to facilitate EBP.

Evidence-Based Practice and Practice-Based Evidence

A new concept—"practice-based evidence" (PBE)—was introduced into the discussion of EBP a few years ago (Horn & Gassaway, 2007). The notion of PBE addresses many of the concerns noted previously and is grounded in the recognition that frequently interventions have limited formal research support, particularly in the number or quality of RCTs.

The premise of PBE is that large databases—not just clinical research—should be reviewed or "mined" to gather data to demonstrate quality and effectiveness. This type of review can provide comprehensive information about patient characteristics, care processes, and outcomes while controlling for patient differences (Walker & Avant, 2011). PBE acknowledges the importance of the environment in determining practice recommendations and recognizes that knowledge can be generated from practice as well as from research (Chinn & Kramer, 2015).

The intent behind PBE is to determine what works best for which patients, under what circumstances, and at what costs by providing a more comprehensive picture than RCTs, which typically examine one intervention with limited populations and under strictly controlled circumstances (Huston, 2017). Additional sources beyond formal research studies that are appropriate as PBE include benchmarking data, clinical expertise, cost-effective analyses, infection control data, medical record data, national standards of care, quality improvement data, and patient and family preferences (Huston, 2017).

Horn and Gassaway (2007) concluded that use of the PBE analyses can uncover better practices more rapidly leading to improved patient outcomes. Figure 12-1 illustrates one interpretation of the interrelationships among EBP, PBE, research, and theory in nursing.

Promotion of Evidence-Based Practice in Nursing

Implementation of EBP in nursing is still evolving, as often, nursing interventions are based on experience, tradition, intuition, common sense, and untested theories.

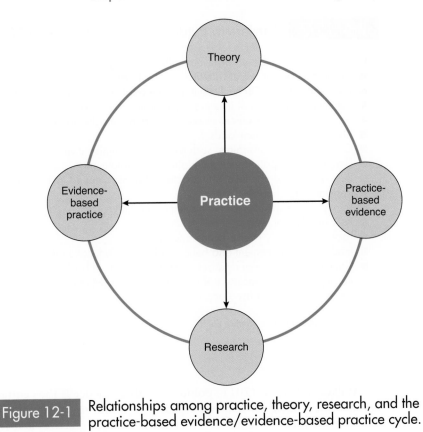

Figure 12-1   Relationships among practice, theory, research, and the practice-based evidence/evidence-based practice cycle.

(From Walker, L. O., & Avant, K. C. Strategies for Theory Construction in Nursing, 5th ed., © 2011. Reprinted by permission of Pearson Education, Inc., New York, New York.)

Although emphasis on EBP has grown rapidly, especially over the last decade, the actual incorporation of nursing research findings in practice has lagged. Melnyk and Fineout-Overholt (2015) have outlined barriers to implementation of research and EBP in nursing (Box 12-2).

There is significant support for increasing emphasis on EBP in nursing, and many organizations, such as the Institute of Medicine, Sigma Theta Tau International, and the Magnet Recognition Program of the American Nurses Credentialing Center, among others, have designed initiatives to advance EBP (Finkelman & Kenner, 2016; Huston, 2017; Melnyk & Fineout-Overholt, 2015). Indeed, practitioners, researchers, and scholars should welcome it because a systematic process of EBP may assist nurses in reducing the gap between theory and practice.

Theory and Evidence-Based Practice

The growing interest and appreciation of EBP in nursing, along with its considerable interconnectedness with research, has served in some ways to de-emphasize theory. As nurses become more aware of and attuned to EBP, however, they are renewing their appreciation of the linkages among research, theory, and practice. It has been observed that nursing focus on EBP has the potential to promote and draw new attention to this connection (Chinn & Kramer, 2015).

| Box 12-2 | Barriers to Evidence-Based Practice in Nursing |

■ Lack of evidence-based practice (EBP) knowledge and skills
■ Misperceptions or negative attitudes about research and evidence-based care
■ Lack of belief that EBP will result in more positive outcomes than traditional care
■ Voluminous amounts of information in professional journals
■ Lack of time and resources to search for and critically appraise evidence
■ Overwhelming patient loads
■ Organizational constraints, such as lack of administrative support or incentives
■ Demands from patients for a certain type of treatment
■ Peer pressure to continue with practices that are steeped in tradition
■ Resistance to change
■ Lack of consequences for not implementing EBP
■ Peer and leader/manager resistance
■ Lack of autonomy over practice and incentives
■ Inadequate EBP content and behavioral skills in educational programs
■ Continued teaching of rigorous research methods in bachelor of science in nursing (BSN) and master's of science in nursing (MSN) programs instead of teaching evidence-based approach to care

Source: Melnyk and Fineout-Overholt (2015).

Walker and Avant (2011) pointed out that practice is the central and core phenomenon and focus of nursing; arguably, it is the reason for nursing's existence. Thus, it is critical to remember that theory guides practice, and it also generates models of testing in research through both PBE and EBP. Furthermore, research and clinical data provide evidence for EBP or PBE and can generate practice guidelines and/or theories (e.g., situation-specific theories). This process is interactive and iterative (Walker & Avant, 2011). For nursing, therefore, practice must not only be evidence-based but also be theory-based, for when research validates a theory, it provides the evidence required for EBP. Finally, as more research is conduced about a specific theory, more evidence is provided to support practice (Chinn & Kramer, 2015; George, 2011).

Fawcett and colleagues (2001) wrote of a preference for the term "theory-guided, evidence-based practice," noting that theory is the reason for, and the value of, evidence. The "evidence," they stated, must extend beyond an emphasis on empirical research and RCTs to include evidence generated from theories. Indeed, the evidence itself refers to evidence about theories. Furthermore, they contend that theory determines what counts as evidence; thus, theory and evidence are inextricably linked.

Theoretical Models of Evidence-Based Practice

Numerous models of EBP have been developed by nurses to encourage translation of nursing research into practice. In many instances, the goal or intent is to create or establish EBP protocols, procedures, or guidelines. In some instances, universities and hospital groups have developed models to assist students or health care professionals in implementing EBP in their setting. In other instances, nurse researchers and scholars have interpreted the transfer of research evidence to nursing education and practice through processes that progressed from theory-based nursing, quality improvement, research utilization, and lately, evidence-based nursing practice. This section reviews five EBP models that are among the most frequently cited in the nursing literature. These have been widely studied and applied, many in multiple settings and for a variety of patient issues, situations, or nursing care processes. These models include:

- Academic Center for Evidence-Based Practice Star Model (ACE Star Model) (Stevens, 2005, 2012)
- Advancing Research and Clinical Practice Through Close Collaboration (ARCC Model) (Melnyk & Fineout-Overholt, 2015)
- Iowa Model (Titler et al., 2001)
- Johns Hopkins Nursing Evidence-Based Practice (JHNEBP) Model (Dearholt, 2012; Newhouse, Dearholt, Poe, Pugh, & White, 2007)
- Stetler Model of Evidence-Based Practice (Stetler, 2001)

These models can provide guidance for practicing nurses and advanced practice nurses to promote or enhance EBP and to develop practice guidelines, protocols, or interventions as appropriate. Each model will be described briefly and reviewed for its utility in nursing practice and education.

Academic Center for Evidence-Based Practice Star Model of Knowledge Transformation

The ACE Star Model was developed by faculty at the University of Texas Health Science Center at San Antonio (UTHSCSA) (Stevens, 2012). The Star Model is depicted by five points of knowledge transformation. The five forms of knowledge transformation occur in "relative sequence" when research evidence progresses through several cycles and is combined with other knowledge and then applied in practice.

Each point of the star represents a step in a process. The stepwise depiction allows for easy comprehension and is therefore useful even for novice nurses. In order, the points are:

1. Discovery research
2. Evidence summary
3. Translation to guidelines
4. Practice integration
5. Process, outcome evaluation (Stevens, 2012) (Figure 12-2)

This sequence allows the nurse to move research-based knowledge from one point to the next in sequence to provide a translation of evidence on which to base practice (Stevens, 2005, 2012). Knowledge transformation consists of eight premises that underlie and explain the position of the researchers who created the model. These are presented in Box 12-3. The rigor of the process the nurse or committee uses is part of the value of the knowledge transformation that occurs when using this model.

The model is used at UTHSCSA hospitals, and their nursing program maintains a very detailed and informative online educational site (http://www.acestar.uthscsa.edu/). The website provides an extensive online tutorial on the ACE Star Model complete with detailed information, resources, instructive videos, and slides. A quiz and a certificate of attendance are available for those completing instruction in the model (see Link to Practice 12-2). The ACE Star Model is useful in teaching nurses and nursing students the process of research evidence utilization in practice (Schaffer, Sandau, & Diedrick, 2013). One concern or criticism of the ACE Star Model has been noted by White (2016), who pointed out that it does not use evidence other than research per se.

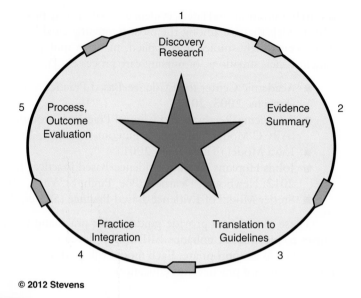

© 2012 Stevens

| Figure 12-2 | Diagram of the Academic Center for Evidence-Based Practice Star Model for evidence-based practice. |

(Used with permission from Stevens, K. R. [2012]. *Star model of EBP: Knowledge transformation.* San Antonio, TX: Academic Center for Evidence-Based Practice, University of Texas Health Science Center. Retrieved from http://nursing.uthscsa.edu/onrs/starmodel/star-model.asp.)

| Box 12-3 | Academic Center for Evidence-Based Practice Star Model: Knowledge Transformation—Underlying Premises |

1. Knowledge transformation (KT) is necessary prior to using research results in clinical decision making.
2. KT derives from multiple sources, including research, experience, authority, trial and error, and theoretical principles.
3. Systematic processes control bias; the research process is the most stable source of knowledge.
4. Evidence can be classified into a hierarchy of strength of evidence depending on the rigor of the science that produced the evidence.
5. Knowledge exists in a variety of forms. As research is converted through a system of steps, other knowledge is created.
6. The form in which knowledge exists can be referenced to its use.
7. The form of knowledge determines its usability.
8. Knowledge is transformed through steps, such as summarization, translation, application, integration, and evaluation.

Abstracted from Stevens, K. R. (2012). *Star model of EBP: Knowledge transformation.* San Antonio, TX: Academic Center for Evidence-Based Practice, University of Texas Health Science Center. Retrieved from http://nursing.uthscsa.edu/onrs/starmodel/star-model.asp

Link to Practice 12-2

Academic Center for Evidence-Based Practice Star Model of Knowledge Transformation

Access the website, take the tutorial, and complete the quiz to obtain a certificate of completion of the program at http://nursing.uthscsa.edu/onrs/starmodel/star-model.asp. This website may be useful for teaching the elements of evidence-based practice to nursing students.

Advancing Research and Clinical Practice Through Close Collaboration Model

Melnyk and Fineout-Overholt (2002) developed the ARCC Model through their work with many health care institutions seeking to advance and sustain EBP. This development was a process that involved many iterations and empirical testing of key relationships. The framework of the ARCC Model is taken from control theory and cognitive behavioral theories, which help guide nurses' behaviors as they gain acumen in EBP (Melnyk & Fineout-Overholt, 2015). Numerous studies and examples of how the ARCC Model has been implemented in clinical practice are available in the literature (Melnyk, 2002; Melnyk, 2017; Melnyk, Feinstein, & Fairbanks, 2002; Melnyk & Fineout-Overholt, 2011; Melnyk, Fineout-Overholt, Giggleman, & Choy, 2016; Melnyk, Rycroft-Malone, & Bucknall, 2004).

The AARC Model relates best to clinical practice, and much of the research supporting its development and implementation was conducted in acute care, pediatric settings. The central constructs are assessment of organizational culture and readiness for EBP, identification of strengths and major barriers to EBP, and development and use of EBP mentors. These constructs are done sequentially and followed by EBP implementation. Outcomes that should be evaluated include health care provider satisfaction, cohesion, intent to leave, turnover, improved patient outcomes, and hospital costs (Melnyk & Fineout-Overholt, 2015).

In employing the ARCC Model, the authors developed several scales to measure the ability to implement EBP. These are the Organizational Culture and Readiness Scale for System-Wide Integration of Evidence-Based Practice (OCRSIEP) and the EBP Beliefs (EBPB) scale (Melnyk & Fineout-Overholt, 2015). Organizational readiness is first assessed, and when feasible, mentors are identified and developed. The clinical nurses are then mentored through use of the ARCC system. Melnyk and Fineout-Overholt (2015) state that measuring the key constructs along with workshops and academic offerings assist organizations to adopt and sustain EBP. Finally, Melnyk and Fineout-Overholt (2015) developed a flow chart to assist in use of the model. Box 12-4 gives examples of research that has been conducted employing the ARCC Model of EBP.

The Iowa Model of Evidence-Based Practice to Promote Quality Care

The Iowa Model of EBP was developed in 1994 to promote quality care through research utilization. It is intended to provide guidance for nurses and others in making decisions about practice that affects patient outcomes. The Iowa Model incorporates starting points, which are nursing problems that are termed "triggers." It continues

Box 12-4   Research Based on the Advancing Research and Clinical Practice Through Close Collaboration Model of Evidence-Based Practice

Hanrahan, K., Wagner, M., Matthews, G., Stewart, S., Dawson, C., Greiner, J., et al. (2015). Sacred cow gone to pasture: A systematic evaluation and integration of evidence-based practice. *Worldviews on Evidence-Based Nursing, 12*(1), 3–11.

Kim, S. C., Stichler, J., Ecoff, L., Brown, C., Gallo, A.-M., & Davidson, J. (2016). Predictors of evidence-based practice implementation, job satisfaction, and group cohesion among regional fellowship program participants. *Worldviews on Evidence-Based Nursing, 13*(5), 340–348.

Thorsteinsson, H. S. (2013). Icelandic nurses' beliefs, skills, and resources associated with evidence-based practice and related factors: A national survey. *Worldviews on Evidence-Based Nursing, 10*(2), 116–126.

Underhill, M., Roper, K., Siefert, M. L., Boucher, J., & Berry, D. (2015). Evidence-based practice beliefs and implementation before and after an initiative to promote evidence-based nursing in an ambulatory oncology setting. *Worldviews on Evidence-Based Nursing, 12*(2), 70–78.

through multiple decision points and feedback loops to provide for evaluation of any changes (Titler et al., 2001).

The model has been refined over time to produce the current iteration (Titler, 2004, 2014). The diagram of the model shows the starting points, decision points, and feedback loops. When implemented, it will assist in providing quality care to clients of clinics, home health agencies, and hospitals (Titler et al., 2001) (Figure 12-3). The Iowa Model is very detailed and specific and has been applied to address a number of clinical topics. It is also one of the best researched EBP models. Box 12-5 shows some of the recent research studies that have used the Iowa model.

The Johns Hopkins Nursing Evidence-Based Practice Model

The JHNEBP Model was developed to accelerate the transfer of research to practice and to promote nurse autonomy, leadership, and engagement with interdisciplinary

Box 12-5   Research Based on the Iowa Model of Evidence-Based Practice to Promote Quality Care

Bankhead, S., Chong, K., & Kamai, S. (2014). Preventing extubation failures in a pediatric intensive care unit. *The Nursing Clinics of North America, 49*(2), 321–328.

Brown, C. G. (2014). The Iowa model of evidence-based practice to provide quality care: An illustrated example in oncology nursing. *Clinical Journal of Oncology Nursing, 18*(2), 157–159.

Estus, K. (2014). Cancer survivorship using IM & EBP to promote quality of care. *Clinical Nurse Specialist, 28*(3), 173–174.

Turenne, J. P., Héon, M., Aita, M., Faessler, J., & Doddridge, C. (2016). Educational intervention for an evidence-based nursing practice of skin to skin contact at birth. *The Journal of Perinatal Education, 25*(2), 116–128. doi:10.1891/1058-1243.25.2.116

White, S., & Spruce, L. (2015). Perioperative nursing leaders implement clinical practice guidelines using the Iowa model of evidence-based practice. *AORN Journal, 102*(1), 51–56. doi:10.1016/j.aorn.2015.04.001

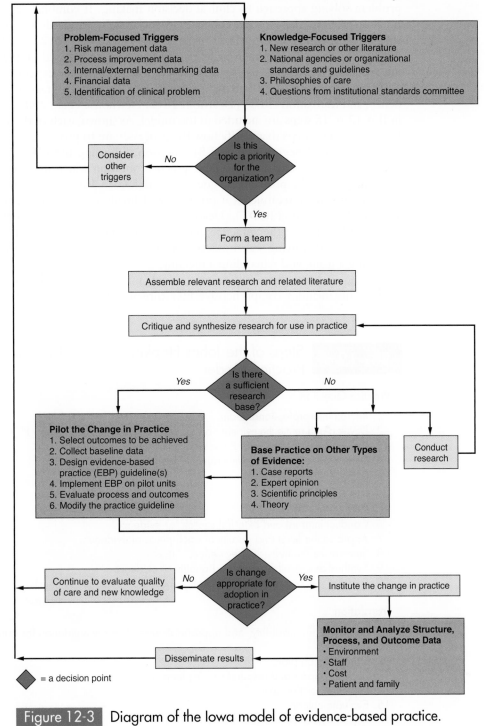

The Iowa Model of Evidence-Based Practice to Promote Quality Care

Problem-Focused Triggers
1. Risk management data
2. Process improvement data
3. Internal/external benchmarking data
4. Financial data
5. Identification of clinical problem

Knowledge-Focused Triggers
1. New research or other literature
2. National agencies or organizational standards and guidelines
3. Philosophies of care
4. Questions from institutional standards committee

Is this topic a priority for the organization?

Consider other triggers ← *No*

Yes

Form a team

Assemble relevant research and related literature

Critique and synthesize research for use in practice

Is there a sufficient research base?

Yes — *No*

Pilot the Change in Practice
1. Select outcomes to be achieved
2. Collect baseline data
3. Design evidence-based practice (EBP) guideline(s)
4. Implement EBP on pilot units
5. Evaluate process and outcomes
6. Modify the practice guideline

Base Practice on Other Types of Evidence:
1. Case reports
2. Expert opinion
3. Scientific principles
4. Theory

Conduct research

Is change appropriate for adoption in practice?

Continue to evaluate quality of care and new knowledge ← *No*

Yes → Institute the change in practice

Monitor and Analyze Structure, Process, and Outcome Data
• Environment
• Staff
• Cost
• Patient and family

Disseminate results

◆ = a decision point

Figure 12-3   Diagram of the Iowa model of evidence-based practice.

(Reprinted with permission from University of Iowa Hospitals and Clinics. © 1998. For permission to use or reproduce the model, please contact University of Iowa Hospitals and Clinics at 319-384-9098.)

colleagues (Dearholt & Dang, 2012). The JHNEBP Model was designed as a problem-solving approach to clinical decision making. It combines elements of the nursing process, the American Nurses Association's Standards of Practice, critical thinking, and research utilization processes (Dearholt, 2012; Newhouse et al., 2007). The model has numerous levels of activity, but it is based on practical teaching processes to promote use by novice nurses as well as more experienced nurses.

The JHNEBP process is based on three core elements: a practice question, evidence, and translation (PET) (Dearholt, 2012; Newhouse et al., 2007). As presented in Box 12-6, 18 steps are included in the model. As shown, each of the PET phases is based on several steps that clarify how the processes are to proceed.

This method begins with an EBP question, following the PICOT format. The first step is to generate an answerable practice question which includes the **P**atient, population, and the problem. It goes on to define an **I**ntervention, makes a **C**omparison with other treatments if possible, and finally defines the desired **O**utcome and the **T**ime table (PICOT) (Dearholt, 2012; Elias, Polancich, Jones, & Colvin, 2015). Other steps in the "practice question" phase include defining the scope of the question and identifying stakeholders, assigning responsibility for project leadership, recruiting a team, and scheduling a meeting.

In the evidence phase, the team conducts internal and external searches for evidence; this includes comprehensive literature searches. Appraisal of the level and

---

Box 12-6	Steps of the Johns Hopkins Nursing Evidence-Based Practice Model

Practice Question

1. Recruit interprofessional team.
2. Develop and refine the evidence-based practice (EBP) question. (Apply PICO elements.)
3. Define the scope of the EBP question and identify stakeholders.
4. Determine responsibility for project leadership.
5. Schedule team meetings.

Evidence

6. Conduct internal and external search for evidence.
7. Appraise the level and quality of each piece of evidence.
8. Summarize the individual evidence.
9. Synthesize overall strength and quality of evidence.
10. Develop recommendations for change based on evidence synthesis.

Translation

11. Determine fit, feasibility, and appropriateness of recommendation for translation pathway.
12. Create action plan.
13. Secure support and resources to implement action plan.
14. Implement action plan.
15. Evaluate outcomes.
16. Report outcomes to stakeholders.
17. Identify next steps.
18. Disseminate findings.

Source: Dearholt (2012, pp. 33–53).

quality of the evidence follows, and the evidence is summarized. This phase concludes with a synthesis of the overall strength and quality of the evidence leading to recommendations for change (Dearholt, 2012).

In the third phase, translation, the team decides whether or not and how to implement the changes. This involves determining the fit, feasibility, and appropriateness of the recommendations, before creating an action plan. Support and resources are secured, and the action plan is implemented and evaluated. The outcomes are reported to stakeholders and "next steps" are identified, and the findings are disseminated to appropriate individuals or groups (Dearholt, 2012). The JHNEBP Model is clearly explained and simple to apply. Related writings include the guidelines and definitions of the background, elements of the process, and the steps of the model (Dearholt & Dang, 2012; Newhouse et al., 2007). Lately, Elias et al. (2015) have added a "D" to the PICOT method to denote "digital data" components. This takes into account the factor of the current digital records and systems changes in the patient care industry.

Stetler Model of Evidence-Based Practice

The Stetler Model was initiated in the 1970s as a quality improvement (QI) effort employing the research utilization (RU) ideals then in widespread use (Melnyk & Fineout-Overholt, 2015). Over time and through several iterations, Stetler updated the approach and clarified the series of phases of the model such that it is readily implemented by practicing nurses and useful at the bedside (Stetler, Ritchie, Rycroft-Malone, Schultz, & Charns, 2007). Stetler and colleagues (1998) and Stetler and Caramanica (2007) argued that all research studies are not ready for use at the bedside. Furthermore, they explained that alternative sources of evidence are necessary to fill the gaps in nursing research evidence.

The current Stetler Model of EBP is similar to the nursing process; therefore, it is easily assimilated by practicing bedside nurses. The phases of the approach include preparation, validation, comparative evaluation/decision making, translation/application, and evaluation. It provides practitioners with stepwise directions for integrating research into practice. See Table 12-1 for description of the phases. The Stetler Model incorporates five steps to generate a process that takes into account the many other facets of nursing and the clinical situation prior to using research findings in the nurse's clinical practice. When implemented, the results should be systematically evaluated to track goal-oriented outcomes and proffer both formative and summative evaluation strategies. The major outcomes of RU or EBP should be improved patient results as well as enhanced professional practice (Stetler & Caramanica, 2007).

Theoretical Models: A Summary

The five EBP models described above are compared in Table 12-2 using the following criteria:

- Groups of health care professionals affected (groups affected)
- Environmental factors in which the model is useful (environment)
- Analysis of the model (analysis)
- Implementation: barriers/facilitators (implementation)
- Evaluation of effectiveness identified by the model (evaluation)

As shown, there are a number of similarities among the models. Schaffer and colleagues (2013) recently compiled a review of models for organizational change based on EBP. Similar to what has been presented here, their overview examined the

Table 12-1 Phases of the Stetler Model

Phase	Content	Actions
I	Preparation (purpose, control, and sources of research evidence)	■ Define potential issues ■ Seek sources of research evidence ■ Perceive problems ■ Focus on high-priority issues ■ Decide on need for a team ■ Consider other influential factors ■ Define desired outcomes ■ Seek systematic reviews ■ Determine need for explicit research evidence ■ Select research sources with conceptual fit
II	Validation (credibility of findings and potential for/detailed qualifiers of application)	■ Credibility of findings ■ Critique and synthesize resources ■ Critique systematic reviews ■ Reassess fit of individual sources ■ Rate the level and quality of evidence ■ Differentiate statistical and clinical significance ■ Eliminate noncredible sources ■ End the process if there is no evidence or clearly insufficient credible research evidence
III	Comparative evaluation/decision making (synthesis and decisions/ recommendations for criteria of applicability)	■ Synthesize the cumulative findings ■ Evaluate the degree and nature of other criteria ■ Make a decision whether/what to use ■ If decide to "not use," STOP use of the model ■ If decide to use, determine recommendations for a specific practice
IV	Translation/application (operational definition of use/actions for change)	■ Types ■ Methods ■ Levels ■ Direct instrumental use ■ Cognitive use ■ Symbolic use ■ Caution: Assess whether translation/product or use goes beyond actual findings/evidence ■ Formal dissemination and change strategies should be planned per relevant research ■ Consider need for appropriate reasoned variation
V	Evaluation (alternative types of evaluation)	■ Evaluation can be formal or informal, individual or institutional ■ Consider cost-benefit of evaluation efforts ■ Use RU as a process to enhance credibility of evaluation data ■ For both dynamic and pilot evaluations include two types of evaluative information

From Stetler, C. B. (2001). Updating the Stetler model of research utilization to facilitate evidence-based practice. *Nursing Outlook*, *49*(6), 272–279. From Figure 3B. Stetler Model Part II: Additional, per phase details.

key features of six models with the view to change practice in organizations. Most of the models incorporate the steps of the research process in some way, and all the models are focused on bringing the best in safe and effective nursing care to their major focus: the patient, or recipient of nursing care. Nurses who are actively engaged in promoting EBP are encouraged to review these as well as other published models and to select the one that best fits their needs and desired outcomes.

Table 12-2 Comparison of Selected Models of Evidence-Based Practice

Models of Evidence-Based Practice

Comparison Element	ACE Star Model	ARCC Model	Iowa Model	Johns Hopkins Model	Stetler Model
Groups of health care professionals (users)	Instructors, students, practicing nurses	Advanced practice nurses, practicing nurses	Instructors, students, practicing nurses	Practicing nurses	Practicing nurses or groups of nurses
Environmental factors in which the model is useful (environment)	Learning environments, hospitals	Patient care organizations	Nursing schools and patient care agencies	Learning environments, hospitals	Clinical situations
Analysis of the model (analysis)	Five major points similar to the nursing process	Five constructs with similarity to nursing process	Six steps of the model: Identify knowledge or problem-focused triggers (catalysts to critical thinking). Priority: organizational Form a team responsible for development, implementation, and evaluation of EBP	PET (see Figure 3-3, p. 42) steps are the basis for the model. Team approach to answer Practice questions, critique Evidence, and Translate it into usable form	Five phases: (I) Preparation (II) Validation (III) Comparative evaluation/ decision making (IV) Translation/ application (V) Evaluation
Implementation: barriers/ facilitators (implementation)	Implementation into practice is the fifth stage and involves bringing evidence to clinical decision making.	Implementation is based on the mentor's determination of organizational readiness.	Determine sufficiency of evidence. If yes: Pilot recommended change.	Team determines feasibility and creates an action plan to implement the change.	Translation and application is the fourth step.
Evaluation of the effectiveness of the model (evaluation)	Evaluation is the final stage and focuses on verification of the success EBP (Stevens, 2005).	Evaluation is the fifth of the constructs and has three levels that provide feedback (Melnyk & Fineout-Overholt, 2002).	Evaluate pilot success and disseminate results; implement into practice (Titler et al., 2001).	Evaluate outcomes. Report outcomes to stakeholders. Identify next steps (Dearholt, 2012, p. 51).	Evaluation is the last step (Stetler, 2001).

Helen, the nurse from the opening case study, conducted a systematic review of neuromuscular illnesses and management protocols using the Iowa Model of EBP. During this process and while working with the clinical team, she came to better understand her illness and the treatments that would most likely forestall deterioration of her condition. The complexity and high level of information she accumulated through her review of the research guided by theories of EBP brought Helen to a level of practice where she could not only help herself but also her patients and clients. Following graduation, she based her clinical practice on the expertise she had gained through her extensive study of the research and practice in neuromuscular diseases.

Summary

There is little doubt that EBP has become one of the key tenets of quality nursing care. As described, however, it is critical to remember that EBP must go beyond research per se and emphasis on RCT but must also be theory based. Many authors have written about the problems and barriers to EBP, and others have written on how to strengthen the process and make it relevant to practicing nurses.

Over the last decade, a number of models have been constructed to assist nurses to learn how to proceed in the development of evidence-based guidelines and promotion of EBP, as illustrated by the work of Helen in the case study. The five models described here, along with a number of others that have been mentioned in the nursing literature, give nurses information about the steps and processes necessary to elicit the evidence that is needed to provide safe interventions that are effective in nursing practice. Nurses who seek to use tested and published evidence in their clinical areas are advised to seek out a working model of EBP and follow it through to effect reasonable, safe, and effective changes for the benefit of their patients or clients.

Key Points

- Research, theory, and practice are integrated in nursing; EBP is a key element and outcome of that linkage.
- EBP is an approach to problem solving that uses the current best evidence in the care of patients.
- In nursing, EBP has been defined as "the conscientious, explicit, and judicious use of theory-derived, research-based information in making decisions about care delivery . . . in consideration of individual needs and preferences."
- Nursing as a profession has been relatively slow to incorporate EBP; this has changed in recent years.
- Some nurses are concerned that too much attention to EBP will draw attention away from the art of nursing care—that nursing will become lost in the science.
- Models of EBP have developed from early studies of research utilization and quality improvement. Many of these models have been developed with the impetus of hospitals or educational institutions' support.
- The major impetus for integration and implementation of research evidence—guided by EBP—should be reasonable, effective, and safe care for patients.

Learning Activities

1. Similar to the process used by Helen, the nurse in the opening case study, select one model of EBP presented. Using your current clinical setting and a practice problem you have noticed, determine what you would do to institute EBP into your current practice to address the problem.
2. Compare and contrast two EBP models and write a blog on which would most likely work in your agency or clinical unit. Explain why one model would work better than the other with your colleagues or your organizational culture.
3. Prepare a proposal for practice change in your agency or clinical unit using one of the models given in this chapter. Use as many of the steps of the model as possible and project the outcomes for the remaining steps.

REFERENCES

American Association of Colleges of Nursing. (2006). *The essentials of doctoral education for advanced nursing practice.* Retrieved from http://www.aacn.nche.edu/dnp/Essentials.pdf

American Association of Colleges of Nursing. (2011). *The essentials of masters education in nursing.* Washington, DC: Author. Retrieved from https://www.bc.edu/content/dam/files/schools/son/pdf2/MastersEssentials11.pdf

Barry, J. M. (2005). *The great influenza: The story of the deadliest pandemic in history.* New York, NY: Penguin Books.

Butler, A., Hall, H., & Copnell, B. (2016). A guide to writing a qualitative systematic review protocol to enhance evidence-based practice in nursing and health care. *Worldviews on Evidence-Based Nursing, 13*(3), 241–249. doi:10.1111/wvn.12134

Chinn, P. L., & Kramer, M. K. (2015). *Integrated theory and knowledge development in nursing* (9th ed.). St. Louis, MO: Elsevier.

Cochrane. (2017). *About us.* Retrieved from http://www.cochrane.org/about-us

Cohen, I. B. (1984). Florence Nightingale. *Scientific American, 250*(3), 128–137.

Dearholt, S. L. (2012). The Johns Hopkins nursing evidence-based practice model and process overview. In S. L. Dearholt & D. Dang (Eds.), *Johns Hopkins nursing evidence-based practice: Model and guidelines* (2nd ed., pp. 33–53). Indianapolis, IN: Sigma Theta Tau International.

Dearholt, S. L., & Dang, D. (2012). *Johns Hopkins nursing evidence-based practice: Model and guidelines* (2nd ed.) Indianapolis, IN: Sigma Theta Tau International.

DiCenso, A., Guyatt, G., & Ciliska, D. (2005). Introduction to evidence-based nursing. In A. DiCenso, D. Ciliska, & G. Guyatt (Eds.), *Evidence-based nursing: A guide to clinical practice* (pp. 3–19). St. Louis, MO: Elsevier.

Elias, B. L., Polancich, S., Jones, C., & Colvin, S. (2015). Evolving the PICOT method for the digital age: The PICOT-D. *The Journal of Nursing Education, 54*(10), 594–599. doi:10.3928/01484834-20150916-09

Fawcett, J., & Garity, J. (2009). *Evaluating research for evidence-based nursing practice.* Philadelphia, PA: F.A. Davis.

Fawcett, J., Watson, J., Neuman, B., Walker, P. H., & Fitzpatrick, J. J. (2001). On nursing theories and evidence. *Journal of Nursing Scholarship, 33*(2), 115–119.

Finkelman, A., & Kenner, C. (2016). *Professional nursing concepts: Competencies for quality leadership* (3rd ed.). Burlington, MA: Jones & Bartlett Learning.

George, J. B. (2011). Nursing theory and clinical practice. In J. B. George (Ed.), *Nursing theories: The base for professional nursing practice* (6th ed., pp. 35–58). Boston, MA: Pearson.

Hall, H. (2014). Qualitative research. In H. R. Hall & L. A. Roussel (Eds.), *Evidence-based practice: An integrative approach to research, administration and practice* (pp. 23–44). Burlington, MA: Jones & Bartlett Learning.

Horn, S. D., & Gassaway, J. (2007). Practice-based evidence study design for comparative effectiveness research. *Medical Care, 45*(10), S50–S57.

Hudson, K., Duke, G., Haas, B., & Varnell, G. (2008). Navigating the evidence-based practice maze. *Journal of Nursing Management, 16*(4), 409–416.

Huston, C. J. (2017). *Professional issues in nursing: Challenges & opportunities* (4th ed.). Philadelphia, PA: Wolters Kluwer.

Ingersoll, G. L. (2000). Evidence-based nursing: What it is and what it isn't. *Nursing Outlook, 48*(4), 151–152.

Jennings, B. M., & Loan, L. A. (2001). Misconceptions among nurses about evidence-based practice. *Journal of Nursing Scholarship, 33*(2), 121–127.

Joanna Briggs Institute. (2016). *About us.* Retrieved from http://joannabriggs.org/

LoBiondo-Wood, G., & Haber, J. (2018). Integrating research, evidence-based practice, and quality improvement processes. In G. LoBiondo-Wood & J. Haber (Eds.), *Nursing research: Methods and critical appraisal for evidence-based practice* (9th ed., pp. 5–24). St. Louis, MO: Elsevier.

McDonald, L. (2014). Florence Nightingale, statistics and the Crimean war. *Journal of the Royal Statistical Society, Series A (Statistics in Society), 177*(3), 569–586.

McKenna, H. P., & Slevin, O. D. (2008). *Nursing models, theories and practice.* Oxford, United Kingdom: Blackwell.

Melnyk, B. M. (2002). Strategies for overcoming barriers in implementing evidence-based practice. *Pediatric Nursing, 28*(2), 159–161.

Melnyk, B. M. (2017). Models to guide the implementation and sustainability of evidence-based practice: A call to action for further use and research. *Worldviews on Evidence-Based Nursing 14*(1), 255–256. doi:10.1111/wvn.12246

Melnyk, B. M., Feinstein, N. F., & Fairbanks, E. (2002). Effectiveness of informational/behavioral interventions with parents of low birth weight (LBW) premature infants: An evidence base to guide clinical practice. *Pediatric Nursing, 28*(5), 511–516.

Melnyk, B. M., & Fineout-Overholt, E. (2002). Key steps in implementing evidence-based practice: Asking compelling, searchable questions and searching for the best evidence. *Pediatric Nursing, 28*(3), 262–266.

Melnyk, B. M., & Fineout-Overholt, E. (2011). Making the case for evidence-based practice and cultivating a spirit of inquiry. In B. M. Melnyk & E. Fineout-Overhold (Eds.), *Evidence-based practice in nursing & healthcare: A guide to best practice* (2nd ed., pp. 3–24). Philadelphia, PA: Lippincott Williams & Wilkins.

Melnyk, B. M., & Fineout-Overholt, E. (2015). *Evidence-based practice in nursing & healthcare: A guide to best practice* (3rd ed.). Philadelphia, PA: Wolters Kluwer.

Melnyk, B. M., Fineout-Overholt, E., Giggleman, M., Choy, K. (2016). A test of the ARCC© model improves implementation of evidence-based practice, healthcare culture, and patient outcomes. *Worldviews on Evidence-Based Nursing, 14*(1), 5–9. doi:10.1111/wvn.12188

Melnyk, B. M., Rycroft-Malone, J., & Bucknall, T. (2004). Sparking a change to evidence-based practice in health care organizations. *Worldviews on Evidence-Based Nursing, 1*(2), 83–84.

Mitchell, G. J. (2013). Evidence-based practice: Critique and alternative view. In W. K. Cody (Ed.), *Philosophical and theoretical perspectives for advanced nursing practice* (5th ed., pp. 321–330). Burlington, MA: Jones & Bartlett Learning.

Newhouse, R. P., Dearholt, S., Poe, S., Pugh, L. C., & White, K. (2007). Organizational change strategies for evidence-based practice. *The Journal of Nursing Administration, 37*(12), 552–557.

Nightingale, F. (1860/1957/1969). *Notes on nursing: What it is and what it is not.* New York, NY: Dover.

Polit, D. F., & Beck, C. T. (2017). *Nursing research: Generating and assessing evidence for nursing practice* (10th ed.). Philadelphia, PA: Wolters Kluwer.

Pugh, L. C. (2012). Evidence-based practice: Context, concerns, and challenges. In .S. L. Dearholt & D. Dang (Eds.), *Johns Hopkins nursing evidence-based practice: Model and guidelines* (2nd ed., pp. 5–11). Indianapolis, IN: Sigma Theta Tau International.

Rycroft-Malone, J. (2004). The PARIHS framework—a framework for guiding the implementation of evidence-based practice. *Journal of Nursing Care Quality, 19*(4), 297–304.

Sackett, D. L., Rosenberg, W. M., Gray, J. A. M., Haynes, R. B., & Richardson, W. S. (1996). Evidence-based medicine: What it is and what it isn't. *BMJ, 312*, 71–72.

Sackett, D. L., Straus, S. E., Richardson, W. S., Rosenberg, W., & Haynes, R. B. (2000). *Evidence-based medicine: How to practice and teach EBM.* London, United Kingdom: Churchill Livingstone.

Schaffer, M. A., Sandau, K. E., & Diedrick, L. (2013). Evidence-based practice models for organizational change: Overview and practical applications. *Journal of Advanced Nursing, 69*(5), 1197–1209.

Schmidt, N. A., & Brown, J. M. (2015). *Evidence-based practice for nurses: Appraisal and application of research* (3rd ed.). Burlington, MA: Jones & Bartlett Learning.

Shah, H. M., & Chung, K. C. (2009). *Archie Cochrane and his vision for evidence-based medicine. Plastic and Reconstructive Surgery, 124*(3), 982–988. http://dx.doi.org/10.1097/PRS.0b013e3181b03928

Sigma Theta Tau International. (2005). *Position statement on evidence based nursing.* Retrieved from http://www.nursingsociety.org/why-stti/about-stti/position-statements-and-resource-papers/evidence-based-nursing-position-statement

Stetler, C. B. (2001). Updating the Stetler model of research utilization to facilitate evidence-based practice. *Nursing Outlook, 49*(6), 272–279.

Stetler, C. B., Brunell, M., Giuliano, K. K., Morsi, D., Prince, L., & Newell-Stokes, V. (1998). Evidence-based practice and the role of nursing leadership. *The Journal of Nursing Administration, 28*(7–8), 45–53.

Stetler, C. B., & Caramanica, L. (2007). Evaluation of an evidence-based practice initiative: Outcomes, strengths and limitations of a retrospective, conceptually-based approach. *Worldviews on Evidence-Based Nursing, 4*(4), 187–199.

Stetler, C. B., Ritchie, J., Rycroft-Malone, J., Schultz, A., & Charns, M. (2007). Improving quality of care through routine, successful implementation of evidenced-based practice at the bedside: An organizational case study protocol using the Pettigrew and Whipp model of strategic change. *Implementation Science, 2*, 3. doi:10.1186/1748-5908-2-3

Stevens, K. R. (2002). The truth about EBP and RCTs. *The Journal of Nursing Administration, 32*(5), 232–233.

Stevens, K. R. (2005). *Essential competencies for evidence-based practice in nursing.* San Antonio, TX: Academic Center for Evidence-Based Practice, University of Texas Health Science Center.

Stevens, K. R. (2012). *Star model of EBP: Knowledge transformation.* San Antonio, TX: Academic Center for Evidence-Based Practice, University of Texas Health Science Center. Retrieved from http://nursing.uthscsa.edu/onrs/starmodel/star-model.asp

Sur, R. L., & Dahm, P. (2011). History of evidence-based medicine. *Indian Journal of Urology, 27*(4), 487–489.

Titler, M. (2004). Methods in translation science. *Worldviews on Evidence-Based Nursing, 1*(1), 38–48.

Titler, M. (2014). Developing an evidence-based practice. In G. LoBiondo-Wood & J. Haber (Eds.), *Nursing research: Methods and critical appraisal for evidence-based practice* (8th ed., pp. 418–440). St. Louis, MO: Elsevier.

Titler, M. G., Kleiber, C., Steelman, V. J., Rakel, B. A., Budreau, G., Everett, L. Q., et al. (2001). The Iowa model of evidence-based practice to promote quality care. *Critical Care Nursing Clinics of North America, 13*(4), 497–509.

Tod, A., Palfreyman, S., & Burke, L. (2004). Evidence-based practice is a time of opportunity for nursing. *British Journal of Nursing, 13*(4), 211–216.

Upton, D. J. (1999). How can we achieve evidence-based practice if we have a theory–practice gap in nursing today? *Journal of Advanced Nursing, 29*(3), 549–555.

Walker, L. O., & Avant, K. C. (2011). *Strategies for theory construction in nursing* (5th ed.). Upper Saddle River, NJ: Prentice Hall.

White, K. M. (2016). Evidence-based practice. In K. M. White, S. Dudley-Brown, & M.F. Terhaar (Eds.), *Translation of evidence into nursing and health care practice* (2nd ed., pp. 3–24). New York, NY: Springer Publishing.

Shared Theories Used by Nurses

13

Theories From the Sociologic Sciences

Joan C. Engebretson

Simon Brown is a family nurse practitioner (FNP) who is currently working in a school-based clinic located within a high school in a disadvantaged, inner-city neighborhood. In his practice, Simon sees a number of students who are sexually active as well as some who are already parents. Although teen pregnancy and childbearing rates have dropped dramatically over the last few years elsewhere, they have remained disproportionately high at his school. Simon has conducted sex education classes, but he speculates that the key to a more effective intervention lies elsewhere.

A literature review reinforced what Simon suspected—that abstinence and contraception-focused programs for adolescents have had only modest results in reducing teen pregnancy rates and minimal impact on teens in disadvantaged inner-city communities. He confirmed that patterns of adolescent sexual risk behaviors are shaped by the social environment, social position, and gender. He also learned that in the United States, although very young motherhood is concentrated in disadvantaged groups, regardless of race and ethnicity, the very early adoption of the role of mother is not the typical first choice of young women who perceive themselves as having options.

From his review of the literature, Simon identified two sociologic perspectives, Role Theory and the Social-Ecological Model, which helped him conceptualize the major issues facing adolescents in his school. He understands the interrelatedness and complexity of the factors and roles which are deeply embedded in social structures and knows they are not easily changed. Furthermore, he recognizes that young people in inner-city neighborhoods typically have a scarcity of positive adult role models and often lack appropriate adult supervision and meaningful job networks.

Further study led Simon to realize that the reproductive role is one area over which poor, inner-city adolescents can exercise control. Young men can validate their masculine role by biologically fathering a child, and young women can demonstrate their capacity for love in the maternal role. It is sometimes perceived that postponing childbearing will not improve their circumstances and becoming a parent may elevate their personal status.

Armed with the information gathered from his literature searches, Simon is seeking to learn even more about cultural variations and social constructs of behavior. His goal is to use this knowledge to develop interventions that will promote adolescent health and facilitate developmentally appropriate and positive role behaviors among the students in his school.

Historically, nursing has been responsive to society's needs. Early nurse leaders such as Florence Nightingale, Clara Barton, Lillian Wald, Margaret Sanger, and Mabel Keaton Staupers were, to varying degrees, social activists. They observed and understood the historical and social forces that affected large aggregates of individuals. Their understanding was demonstrated through their population-focused nursing interventions. Mills (1959) coined the term *sociological imagination* to refer to this process of looking at social phenomena to discover the unseen and repetitive patterns that govern individuals' social existence.

Beginning in the early 1900s, as Americans became increasingly focused on the ideology of individualism, and as cures were discovered for dreaded infectious diseases, the emphasis of health care shifted from populations and social factors that affect health to the individual and personal lifestyles. Consideration of the influence of social forces on health became almost obsolete. An understanding of theories from sociology and related disciplines that focus on the interaction between human society and individuals is important for nurses, however, because sociologic factors have a dramatic impact on the health and well-being of individuals, families, groups, and society. Thus, advanced nursing practice and research must consider those social factors and issues that may promote, constrain, and/or shape health and health behaviors.

This chapter reviews selected sociologic concepts, theories, and frameworks for their relevance to nursing practice, research, administration, and education. Systems theories and the related Social-Ecological Model and social networks, which locate the individual within progressive spheres of influence, are discussed initially. This is followed by an overview of the classic social science theoretical perspectives of Social Constructionism and interaction theories, focusing on role theories and cultural diversity. A review of exchange theories and critical theories, which are focused on social economic and political perspectives follows. The chapter concludes with a look at Complexity Science, Complex Adaptive Systems, and Chaos Theory. Each section begins with a brief historical overview that is followed by a discussion of basic assumptions, central concepts, and related theoretical viewpoints. Examples of nursing practice or research application of the theories are included where available.

Systems Theories

Systems theories and systems thinking have been very important to the nursing profession. Indeed, several nursing theorists based their works on systems theory. Notable examples include Neuman, Rogers, Roy, and Johnson. These foundational theories generally depict the individual, their family, and their environment as holistic systems within a configuration of connected parts, continually influencing and being influenced by each other. In the late 20th century, however, following expansion of the reductionist approach of biomedicine, these theories and perspectives were somewhat eclipsed in nursing as the profession became more focused on clinical research and clinical practice.

Despite this change, it is vital to recognize that systems theories are extremely relevant in the human and social sciences. During the recent years, enhanced attention has been given to subsequent extensions of system theory. This section will describe the most basic systems model—General Systems Theory—as well as the more contemporary Social-Ecological Model and social networks. Complexity Science, an even more recent iteration of systems theory, will be described at the end of the chapter.

General Systems Theory

General Systems Theory (GST), or more specifically, *Open Systems Theory* (OST) (von Bertalanffy, 1968), is regarded as a universal grand theory because of its unique relevancy and applicability (B. M. Johnson & Webber, 2010).

Overview

The GST was initially introduced in the 1930s by biologist Ludwig von Bertalanffy. In GST, systems are composed of both structural and functional components that interact within a boundary that filters the type and rate of exchange with the environment. Living systems are open because there is an ongoing exchange of matter, energy, and information. Basic tenets of GST are that (1) a system is composed of subsystems, each with its own function; (2) systems contain energy and matter; (3) a system may be open or closed (open systems exchange energy and closed systems have clearly defined boundaries); and (4) open and closed systems reach stationary states (Mason & Attree, 1997).

The following elements are common to systems (Figure 13-1):

- Input—matter, energy, and information received from the environment
- Throughput—matter, energy, and information that is modified or transformed within the system
- Output—matter, energy, and information that is released from the system into the environment
- Feedback—information regarding environmental responses used by the system (may be positive, negative, or neutral) (Kenney, 1995)

For survival, a system must achieve a balance internally and externally (equilibrium). Equilibrium depends on the system's ability to regulate input and output to achieve a balanced relationship of the interactive parts. The system uses various adaptation mechanisms to maintain equilibrium. Adaptation may occur through accepting or rejecting the matter, energy, or information or by accommodating the input and modifying the systems responses (Kenney, 1995). Several GST principles that are purported to be applicable to all systems are shown in Box 13-1.

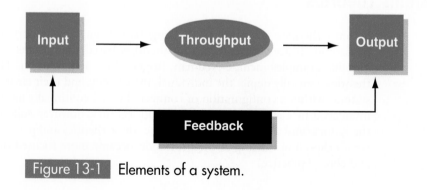

Figure 13-1   Elements of a system.

| Box 13-1 | Open Systems Theory Principles |

1. A system is a unit that is greater than the sum of its parts (wholeness is a major premise of both GST and OST).
2. A system comprises subsystems that are themselves part of suprasystems (hierarchically "nested").
3. A system has boundaries (i.e., abstract entities such as rules, norms, and values) that permit exchange of information and resources both into (inputs) and out of (outputs) the system (boundaries can also hinder or block exchange processes).
4. Communication and feedback mechanisms between system parts are essential for system function.
5. A change in one part leads to change in the whole system (*circular causality*).
6. A system goal or end point can be reached in different ways (*equifinality*).

Application to Nursing

In addition to widespread use of systems principles and perspectives in nursing theories as was mentioned, systems theory has been frequently applied to nursing practice. Meyer and O'Brien-Pallas (2010), for example, applied OST to large-scale organizations and from their data developed the "Nursing Services Delivery Theory." Reviewing the literature, Myny and colleagues (2011) identified five categories of nondirect patient care factors related to nurses' workload in acute care hospitals. Guided by systems theory, a conceptual model was built from the data. In educational situations, Zieber and Williams (2015) used systems theory to examine the experiences of nursing students who made errors in clinical practice, and Hamrin and colleagues (2016) described how nurse practitioner students could use systems thinking to develop effective and innovative quality improvement projects.

In direct-care clinical situations, major tenets of family systems theory, a derivative of systems theory, was applied to develop an intervention to assist families dealing with crisis (Tomlinson, Peden-McAlpine, & Sherman, 2012) and to help nurse practitioners work with family members of patients with mental illness (Haefner, 2014). Finally, Gerardi (2015) suggested that Complex Adaptive Systems Theory (described in more detail later in the chapter), another derivative of systems theory, should be applied by nurse managers and leaders to identify dysfunctional patterns and resolve conflicts in today's complex workplace environments.

Social Ecological Models

Scholars and researchers from sociology, anthropology, and social psychology applied tenets of systems theory to develop additional theories and perspectives to describe and explain behaviors. Social-Ecological Models (SEMs) are contemporary applications of the bio-psycho-social perspective to examine the patient/family experience of health or illness within the social ecological context.

Overview

The SEMs have been used in various forms for several decades to examine the complex interplay among individuals, social groups and other entities which influence health-related behaviors. As depicted in Figure 13-2, the SEM situates the individual within a series of concentric contextual systems: microsystems—the individual and immediate neighborhood; mesosystem—the larger local community;

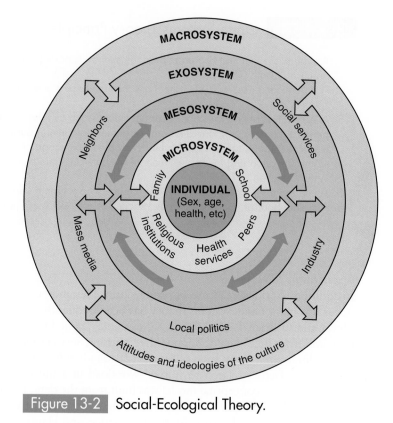

Figure 13-2 Social-Ecological Theory.

ecosystem—an even larger system (e.g., a country); and the macrosystem. This interdependent matrix allows for an examination of the more complex interactions of systems theory.

The SEM was expanded by Urie Bronfenbrenner (1979), a social psychologist. Bronfenbrenner's model is widely used by nurses and other health professionals to examine the reciprocal, causative relationships that ultimately influence human behavior from the perspective of humans in continuous interaction with their environment. Bronfenbrenner originally applied his conceptualization of the SEM to child development and then in later version included the trajectory of time to illustrate how social perspectives change or evolve.

Application to Nursing

Examples depicting use of SEMs in nursing research, education, and practice are easy to identify in the literature. In one work, Clary-Muronda (2016) reported on application of the SEM to evaluate facilitators and barriers to enhance success of culturally diverse nursing students. Through a systematic literature review, she was able to describe how the SEM provided a "multidimensional view" of potential problems and helped suggest possible solutions to improve workforce diversity. Similarly, Dwyer and Hunter-Revell (2016) explained how they used the SEM to organize the factors identified from a systematic literature review which influenced transition to practice in new graduate nurses.

Several recent examples of clinical practice application of the SEM were found. In community-based settings, the SEM was used as a guide to develop a school-based program to improve asthma symptoms among school children (Nuss et al., 2016), to discuss predictors of physical activity among adolescents (Spurr, Bally, Trinder, & Williamson, 2016), and to identify strategies to improve breastfeeding rates among African American women (Reeves & Woods-Giscombé, 2015). Finally, in acute care settings, the SEM was used as a framework to identify the multiple factors that influence the performance of the health team during neonatal resuscitation (Clary-Muronda & Pope, 2016) and to identify the factors that influence patient safety during the transfer of postoperative patients to the post anesthesia care unit (Rose & Newman, 2016).

Social Networks

The study of *social networks* can be a productive approach to understanding systems in nursing. In terms of the health and well-being of individuals, *social support networks*, as actual or potential resources, are especially relevant. This particularly relates to family networks (Logan & Spitze, 1996).

Overview

Social networks can also consider relationships, roles and positions of individuals, such as those found in health care organizations (e.g., nurses, physicians, pharmacists, and administrators). In *network analysis*, these units are referred to as *points*. Ties link points and represent the directional flow of resources. Figure 13-3 illustrates the exchange process in a simplistic diagram. In this figure, A, B, C, D, and E represent points, and arrows indicate ties. In the illustration, B has reciprocal ties to all other points, but A, C, D, and E have ties to only three other points. In the social world, resource exchanges can be instrumental, as in the exchange of information or materials, or *affective*, as shown by respect, approval, or an empathic ear.

Examples of techniques or tools for capturing and mapping network patterns include Moreno's (1953) *sociograms*, which plot the patterning of sentiments among group members; the echo map used in family assessments to diagram exchange relations between families and their external environment; and the exchange theory and network analysis program developed by Emerson (1981).

Application to Nursing

Variations in social networks are dependent on context and can be very influential in addressing health needs. Indeed, support from social networks is widely regarded as mediating the adverse effects of stressful events, as illustrated by a study examining grief reactions and posttraumatic growth among adolescents who had lost a parent (Hirooka, Fukahori, Ozawa, & Akita, 2017). In much the same way, Palmer, Saviet,

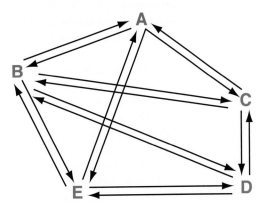

Figure 13-3 Example of resource flows in a noncomplex network.

and Tourish (2016) looked at social support networks, along with other variables, to help direct guidance to assist adolescents and young adults with grief over the loss of a loved one. Similarly, T. Y. Lee, Wang, Lin, and Kao (2013) found a significant moderating effect of perceived nurses' support on fathering ability and paternal stress for fathers of premature infants. In another work, lack of perceived social support was found to be significantly associated with antenatal depressive symptoms among Chinese women (Ngai & Chan, 2012). Thus, health care providers need to routinely assess the adequacy of individuals' perceived social support networks and target relevant interventions for those with inadequate support.

Social Construction and Interaction Theories

The philosophical base for much anthropologic and sociologic research is Interpretive Interactionism or Social Constructionism. "Social Constructionism" was first posited by Berger and Luckmann (1966) when they discussed how people share constructions or interpretations of reality. In this view, "taken for granted realities" arise from, and are maintained by, social interactions. A number of philosophers, sociologists, anthropologists, and influential thinkers have contributed to the understanding of Social Constructionism. Social Constructionism, then, refers to the collective ways of making sense of the world and giving meaning. It is based on the observation that knowledge and cognition are socially constructed and is considered to be accomplished through language acquisition and development of social processes (Denzin & Lincoln, 2003; Schwandt, 2007).

In the late 19th century, the focus of sociology moved to social interactional processes that link individuals to each other and to society. A diverse group of interactionist theories resulted from this shift. Three constructivist/interaction theories are discussed in this section. These are symbolic interactionism, cultural diversity, and Role Theory.

Symbolic Interactionism

George H. Mead (1934), the acknowledged father of symbolic interactionism, synthesized the concepts of self, mind, and society or social environment, which he perceived to be inseparable.

Overview

Central to Mead's work is the notion that humans adapt to, and survive in, their environment by sharing common symbols, both verbal and nonverbal. A distinctive feature of this symbolic interaction is that humans can imagine themselves in other social roles, a concept termed "role-taking," and internalize the attitudes, values, and norms of the "generalized other" or social group. Mead outlined stages of interactional learning by which he believed humans acquire social understanding. For Mead, the self is nonexistent at birth and emerges as the result of social experience. Mead's basic assumptions are listed in Box 13-2.

The focus for symbolic interactionism is on the connection between *symbols* (shared meanings) and *interactions*. Mead emphasized the process of role-taking as a basic mechanism by which interactions occur. Role-taking refers to the ability to not only put yourself in the role of another person but also anticipate how that person will think, feel, or respond (Mead, 1934). Although they are sometimes used interchangeably, role-taking and empathy are not synonymous. Role-taking is a cognitive

Box 13-2 Assumptions of Symbolic Interactionist Theories

1. Human beings have the capacity to create and use symbols.
2. Through the capacity to create and use symbols, humans have freed themselves from most of their instinctual and biologic programming.
3. Human beings adapt and survive in the social world.
4. Humans use words and language symbols to communicate, and they also use nonverbal gestures that have common meanings.
5. Humans can effectively communicate because of their ability to read symbols produced by others and to take on the position or point of view of another person.
6. Humans acquire a mind and self from interactions with others.
7. Human interactions form the basis of society.

Sources: Lindesmith and Strauss (1968); Turner (2013).

process, whereas empathy emphasizes the affective. The concept of role was extended to include the expectations attached to structural positions in society, and the concept of *self* became associated with the multiple roles played within these positions.

Application to Nursing

Social Constructionism and symbolic interactionism form the basic foundation for much of the qualitative research in nursing. Several qualitative research studies in nursing were found that used symbolic interaction as a conceptual framework. For example, Martsolf, Draucker, Bednarz, and Lea (2011) explored how adolescents make sense of their troubled dating relationships (i.e., verbal, emotional, sexual, or physical abuse). In another study, symbolic interactionism provided part of the theoretical framework in exploring young gay and bisexual men's definition of being healthy as well as describing their fears and concerns. Findings from this study can assist nurses in identifying culturally appropriate ways for interacting/intervening with this population (Guarnero, 2012). In another example rooted in symbolic interactionism, Horton and Dworkin (2013) explored the notion of gender-based power imbalances in HIV risk reduction and suggested moving beyond the interpersonal in HIV prevention policy solutions to include broader social inequalities and power imbalances that impact, for instance, condom negotiations.

Grounded theory methods were used to understand the social constructs in the decision-making processes that occur between persons with end-stage cancer and their family caregivers in a home setting. Implications for practice include palliative care education for nurses in all health care settings and health-promotion initiatives for advance directives education and end-stage illness management in home settings (Edwards, Olson, Koop, & Northcott, 2012). The perspective of the importance of social constructions has also been examined in dealing with several chronic conditions. To that end, Engebretson (2013) explored several individual studies of how patients experienced different chronic conditions and identified stigmas, concerns, and common issues.

Cultural Diversity

Culture refers to the shared beliefs and values that underlie and generate social behavior. It is how people make meaning of their experiences, operate in daily life, and develop social organization. The interest in and the study of culture within the

United States has been steadily pushing its way to the social forefront since the mid-1980s (Alexander & Smith, 2009). It was also during this time that a shift occurred in U.S. population demographics and the corresponding increase in diverse ethnic groups became more pronounced. Indeed, culture is very relevant to nursing practice because it is a significant determinant of health-related behaviors and a major factor in health care delivery.

Overview

Despite some variations, social scientists agree on the essential principles of culture. These principles are that (1) culture consists of tangible (material) and intangible (nonmaterial) components; (2) people inherit and learn a culture; (3) biologic, environmental, and historical forces shape and change culture; and (4) culture is a tool that people use to evaluate other societies and adapt to problems of living (Ferrante, 2015). Most people are so accustomed to these beliefs, perspectives, and practices they are often unaware of them until they encounter another culture. Equating ethnic perspectives or research only on ethnic or minority groups is a very limited view as everyone and every group has its own cultural beliefs and practices. The word *bias* refers to an inclination for or against some phenomenon that inhibits impartial and objective judgment and that can, in the extreme, constitute prejudice. *Cultural bias*, interpreting and judging phenomena in relation to one's own culture, is common among social and human societies and needs to be recognized. A multitude of historical and contemporary examples of cultural biases deal with the "isms": racism, sexism, classism, and ageism. An alternate perspective views cultural bias as a normative response to safeguard that which is known and familiar to the individual—*ethnocentrism*. Any normative belief about human beings can be reasonably isolated as a cultural belief and consequently lead to a biased perspective.

Cultural competence has become very important in clinical practice as ethnic diversity and awareness have challenged clinicians. Indeed, cultural competence has been linked to sensitivity to culture, race, ethnicity, gender, and sexual orientation in provision of patient-centered health care and improvement in health outcomes (Engebretson, 2011). Providing culturally sensitive health care is expected, or even mandated as Cultural and Linguistic Services (CLAS) standards were established by the Office on Minority Health (OMH) in 2001 and are incorporated into The Joint Commission's accreditation (The Joint Commission, 2010).

To be effective, health professionals should consider culturally embedded perspectives, but remember that one size does *not* fit all. Although promoting cultural competence and recognition of cultural differences or variations is welcome, some concerns with these emphases are essentializing this information into stereotyping individuals with group identities. To address such concerns and incorporate patient values and circumstances into care delivery, nursing theorists developed the Clinical Model of Cultural Competence (Engebretson, 2011; Engebretson, Mahoney, & Carlson, 2008). This model incorporated a cultural competency continuum. At one end of the continuum were cultural "destructiveness" and "incapacity"—where destructive behavior was directed at specific groups. Toward the middle of the continuum are "cultural blindness" and "precompetence"; here, clinicians seek to treat all groups with equality, and there are efforts to move toward understanding of the group. Cultural "competency" and "proficiency" are the highest levels of the model. Here, the clinician demonstrates an understanding of the cultural issues, and progresses toward provision of culturally competent, individual-based care.

Application to Nursing

In the social sciences, significant research is based on how members of a social group attend to their everyday lives (Holstein & Gubrium, 2008). Ethnography refers to both the product of an anthropologic study as well as a research approach and is often applied in nursing studies. In the literature, there are many examples of nursing studies that research cultural beliefs and practices, often using ethnographic techniques. For example, Higginbottom, Rivers, and Story (2014) conducted a focused ethnography look at the health and social needs of Somali refugees with visual impairment, concluding there is a significant need for social support and awareness of community outreach services for these individuals. Also researching refugees, Davenport (2017) performed a grounded theory study to examine issues faced by Iraqi refugees when they settle in the United States. In other examples, McCullagh, Sanon, and Foley (2015) used qualitative methods to examine health practices of migrant seasonal farmworkers and Opalinski, Dyess, and Grooper (2015) used ethnographic methods to research strategies that can be used by multicultural faith communities to address the problems of childhood obesity.

In several examples from the literature, "culture" did not necessarily refer to racial or ethnic groups. In one work, Christensen (2014) described how nurses who work in correctional facilities should consider the "culture of incarceration" in providing culturally sensitive care for incarcerated women. Then, Richardson (2014) discussed the importance of considering the specific needs of the "Deaf culture" to provide culturally competent care to those with hearing impairments.

Finally, information, strategies, and models to promote cultural competence are easily identified in the nursing literature. Elminowski (2015) reported on development of a workshop to promote cultural awareness for nurse practitioners, and Long (2016) described the implementation of international service learning experiences to promote cultural competence in nursing students. Finally, Shen (2015) performed a systematic literature review and reported on her analysis of the many cultural competence models and cultural competency assessment instruments that have been published over the past 35 years.

Current methods of research, practice, and training are challenged by multiculturalism. Results from these and other culturally based studies have implications for health care professionals to provide culture-specific and evidence-based care. Box 13-3 gives guidelines on how to avoid cultural bias in research and thereby improve health care for all.

Box 13-3 Recommendations for Avoidance of Cultural Biases in Research

- Acknowledge your own cultural beliefs and values through ongoing self-assessments.
- Question the value, purpose, cultural origins, and relevance of current practices wherever they are found.
- Critically examine any cross-cultural research in literature reviews for potential bias and pretension and be prepared for anti-intuitive findings and rejection of assumptions.
- Engage persons culturally similar to the study sample at each step of the research process.
- Promote cultural diversity in scientific nursing communities (local, state, national, and international) to provide checks and balances for individual biases.
- Create environments for egalitarian and pluralistic dialogue.
- Collaborate (or consult) with a multicultural interdisciplinary research group.
- Consider a qualitative ethnographic study for exploring differences.

Role Theory

The concept of "role" comes from the theater and conveys the notion that normative expectations and requirements, such as culturally defined behavioral rules, are attached to positions (status) in social organizations (e.g., family, corporation, society). Succinctly stated, an individual occupies a status but plays a role (Lindesmith & Strauss, 1968).

Overview

Through the enactment of roles, static social positions are brought to life. Roles can be assumed to carry not only certain rights and privileges but duties and obligations as well. For example, a registered nurse has the right to be paid on time and in turn has the obligation to report to work when scheduled and in a timely manner.

A status may include a number of roles, with each role appropriate to a specific social context. For instance, a woman who occupies the status of chief executive officer of a large company has multiple roles attached to that position. She may also have duties and obligations associated with other statuses, such as daughter, sister, wife, mother, Red Cross volunteer, and so on. Role behavior, in any given situation, depends on the statuses occupied by interacting individuals. Staff nurses, for example, behave one way toward their clients, another way toward their coworkers, and yet another way toward their supervisors.

Social positions are often *ascribed* based on such characteristics as class (e.g., poor, middle class, wealthy), gender, and racial or ethnic group membership or are *achieved* through education, training, and so forth. There are societal constraints on all statuses. For instance, an African American male nurse occupies several relevant statuses. He is a qualified professional, but there will undoubtedly be situations in which others will expect him to enact behaviors traditionally associated with his other ascribed status(es) (i.e., male, African American, son, brother, father).

Role strain, or role stress, is a subjective experience produced by such conditions as *role ambiguity, role incongruity, role overload,* and *role conflict.* Ill-defined, vague, or unclear role expectations can result in role ambiguity (e.g., the staff nurse assigned to temporarily act as head nurse with no preparation). Role incongruity can occur when role expectations run counter to the individual's values and self-perception; for example, a staff nurse who takes pride in her caring and supportive behaviors toward clients and coworkers is promoted to supervisor and must "trim the budget." The nurse faced with an imbalance in ratio of demands (excessive) and time (inadequate) on an understaffed acute intensive care unit may experience *role overload.* Occupying more than one status at a time increases the likelihood of an individual being unable to enact the roles associated with one status without violating those of another status (e.g., administrative/supervisor-professional nurse/client advocate). The individual faced with such mutually exclusive or contradictory role expectations will likely experience *role conflict.*

The roles an individual plays have a profound effect on attitude and behavior as well as on self-perceptions. As society in general, and health care systems in particular, become increasingly more complex and resources shrink, role stress can be expected to continue and expand. Various researchers have studied various roles. Link to Practice 13-1 focuses on role changes across generations.

Application to Nursing

In recent years, a significant amount of research on caregiver roles and related concepts has been performed. Friedemann and Buckwalter (2014), for example, conducted a

Link to Practice 13-1

Significant attention has recently focused on the notion of "generational differences" in nursing education and administration. The observations of the differences and subsequent implications are rooted in research and can be related to many of the theories and principles described in this chapter (e.g., culture, social exchange/social networks, Role Theory, conflict).

In one example, Hendricks and Cope (2013) explained that generational cohorts carry similar traits based on sharing of important life events at critical development stages. In their discussion of the commonly described "generations" (e.g., veterans or traditionals, baby boomers, generation Xers, and millennials), they explicitly discussed the "cultural" differences and distinctions of the different generations and focused on some of the variations in techniques of communication and potential sources of conflict. In another example, Sparks (2012) examined differences in "empowerment" and sentinel characteristics consistent with critical social theory in her study of job satisfaction in baby boomers and generation X nurses.

Hendricks, J. M., & Cope, V. C. (2013). Generational diversity: What nurse managers need to know. *Journal of Advanced Nursing, 69*(3), 717–725.
Sparks, A. M. (2012). Psychological empowerment and job satisfaction among Baby Boomer and Generation X nurses. *Journal of Nursing Management, 20,* 451–460.

study of gender and family relationship on caregiver role perception, focusing on workload, burden, and help among families receiving benefits from home health care agencies. They determined that roles, responsibilities, and responses varied considerably based on gender and ethnicity and urged community health nurses to recognize vulnerabilities of care providers. Similarly, Hansen and colleagues (2012) explored the concepts of role strain and satisfaction with family caregivers making life-sustaining treatment decisions within the context of ongoing care for elderly ill relatives in a variety of settings. In a final example, Frye (2016) studied issues experienced by fathers in their role as caregivers of children with autism spectrum disorder, noting that their need for support as they reported significant concerns related to responsibilities, finances, as well as their experiences of grief and loss.

Role Theory has also been used as one of the major components of some nursing theories. One example is Ramona Mercer's Theory of Maternal Role Attainment (Noseff, 2014) (described in Chapter 11). In another example, Déry, D'Amour, Blais, and Clarke (2015) reported using Role Theory as one of the "theoretical underpinnings" for development of the "Enacted Scope of Nursing Practice" model which promotes optimal use of nurses, operating within the full scope of nursing practice to improve health systems and ultimately patient care.

Exchange Theories, Conflict and Critical Theories

Many anthropologists and sociologists who study health issues recognize how the larger social system impacts health and health care. This has been labeled the "pol-econ" for the focus on political or economic issues and refers to a number of social science theories focused on how groups of people behave with respected to distribution of goods and services and development of power. These theories form the foundation for political and economic issues, applicable to small groups or aggregates at the local level, national level, and even international level. This section describes two major pol-econ perspectives: exchange theories and conflict or critical theories, with attention to critical social theory and feminist theories.

Exchange Theories

Theories that have become known as "exchange theories" have their basis in the philosophical perspective called *utilitarianism*.

Historical Overview

Utilitarianism developed between the late 18th century and the mid-19th century and is a legacy from both moral philosophy and classic economic theory. The moral philosophy component considers the satisfaction of an individual's desires or utility. Philosophically, maximization of each individual's satisfaction automatically leads to maximum satisfaction of the wants of all. Translated into more familiar terms, "the greatest good for the greatest number" is an underlying principle of utilitarianism (see Chapter 16 for a more detailed discussion of utilitarianism).

Three basic assumptions about individuals and exchange relations are added from classic economic theory. First, individuals are purposive and motivated to maximize material benefits from exchanges with others in a free and competitive marketplace. Second, as agents in a free market, individuals have access to all the information needed to weigh alternatives and calculate costs for each alternative. Third, based on their own calculations, individuals are able to rationally choose the activities that will maximize their profits (Turner, 2013).

Modern Social Exchange Theories

The influence of utilitarianism is evident in modern exchange theories to varying degrees. Utilitarian principles were reformulated for modern exchange theories in an attempt to explain human interactions in all social contexts and without the limitations imposed by a pure economic framework, hence the label "Social" Exchange Theory. Assumptions of Social Exchange Theories as outlined by Turner (2013) are listed in Box 13-4.

The *social exchange* perspective emerged in American sociology in the 1960s with the work of Homans (1961) and Blau (1964) and in social psychology with Thibaut and Kelley (1959). Modern exchange theories emphasize the social and psychological motivation of individuals. There are two major divisions of Social Exchange Theories: the individualistic or microlevel theories and the societal/collectivist or macrolevel theories.

Within the *individualistic social exchange* framework, the central focus is motivation; human beings are motivated by self-interest to act. Relationships are deemed successful and continue when each party feels that the nature of an exchange is fair and beneficial. Beneficial or rewarding relationships require commitment to sustain them. When *reciprocity* is absent or unrewarding within the relationship, or costs exceed rewards, individuals tend to withdraw from further exchanges. This premise applies to all social groups, including the family. Divorce is an example of withdrawing from an unsatisfactory exchange relationship.

In contrast to the individualistic or microlevel perspective are the macrolevel theories. This second broad division of Social Exchange Theories is derived from a *collectivist* tradition and gives greater weight to society. Collectivism has its roots in

Box 13-4   Assumptions of Social Exchange Theories

- Humans do not seek to maximize profits but attempt to make some profit in their social transactions with others.
- Humans are not perfectly rational, but they do engage in calculations of costs and benefits in social transactions.
- Humans do not have perfect information on all available alternatives, but they are usually aware of at least some alternatives, which form the basis for assessment of costs and benefits.
- Humans always act under constraints, but they still compete with one another in seeking to make a profit in their transactions.
- Humans always seek to make a profit in their transactions, but they are limited by the resources that they have when entering an exchange relation.
- Humans engage in economic transactions in clearly defined marketplaces in all societies, but these transactions are only special cases of more general exchange relations.
- Humans pursue material goals in exchanges, but they also mobilize and exchange nonmaterial resources, such as sentiments, services, and symbols.

Source: Turner (2013).

the perspective of French anthropologist Lévi-Strauss (1969), whose work emphasized the integration of exchanges from larger social structures. In this perspective, the focus is on reciprocity from an institutional level.

Three fundamental exchange principles relate to the concept of integration as proposed by Lévi-Strauss (1969). First, individuals incur costs in all exchange relations, but costs are attributed to the customs, rules, laws, and values of society, as opposed to the individual motives found in economic or psychological explanations of exchange. Second, social norms and values regulate the distribution of all scarce and valued resources. Third, the norm of reciprocity governs all exchange relations (Turner, 2013).

Rational Choice Theory (Coleman, 1990; Hechter, 1987) is the most recently proposed exchange theory. Rational Choice Theory attempts to explain the macrolevel behavioral processes of both small and large social systems. Rational Choice Theory has a systems focus, but the psychological needs and motives of individuals are removed.

Three major sociologic concepts, *agency*, *rationality*, and *structure*, are evident in the assumptions and propositions of contemporary Social Exchange Theories (Table 13-1). The individualistic perspective emphasizes agency and considers that individuals actively shape their social lives, rather than being passive recipients. Individuals affect their own lives by adapting to, negotiating with, and changing social structures.

Inherent in the concept of rationality is the assumption that every individual has control over a supply of socially valued resources, either material or psychological, that serve as bartering tools. Individuals barter these resources in the social "marketplace" to maximize rewards by enhancing the valuables they control. The last concept, *structure*, is highly abstract and not directly observable. Social structure generally refers to the enduring and recurring patterns of behavior in groups and society.

Subsumed in these concepts (agency, rationality, and structure) are related issues of *inequality*, *power*, and *conflict*. Prior to its appearance in exchange theorizing, Karl Marx (1977) noted that inequality exists in hierarchical class structures where

Table 13-1 Central Concepts in Social Exchange Theories

Concept	Meaning
Agency	Individuals actively create or construct their social world, and as thinking, feeling, and acting beings, they are motivated to control or to condition the situations that affect their social lives to maximize their advantage.
Rationality	Individuals are acquisitive and success oriented and motivated for immediate rewards. Therefore, to gain the most benefit, individuals calculate costs and the probabilities of receiving rewards or avoiding punishments in social interactions.
Structure	Social and cultural influences that constrain and shape an individual's behavior and conscious experiences are assumed to be located in the unconscious mind, in material relationships, in the symbolic relationships of myth or language, or in repetitive patterns of permanent interactions.

Source: Waters (1994).

those who have control of resources with high economic value also have the power to exploit those with fewer such resources. Conflict, according to Marx, is inevitable with oppression, and resolution of conflict requires emancipatory actions. Factors associated with positions of privilege and power include gender, age, ethnicity, and socioeconomic status.

Application to Nursing

Among recent nursing studies to use Social Exchange Theory as a conceptual framework is Shacklock, Brunetto, Teo, and Farr-Wharton (2014). They used Social Exchange Theory as a "lens" to study the relationships among nurses' "support antecedents" (supervisor relationship and perceived organizational support) and outcomes of job satisfaction, engagement, and organizational commitment. These findings suggested that support antecedents were positively associated with satisfaction and reduced intention to quit. Similarly, Brunetto and colleagues (2013) used Social Exchange Theory to examine the relationships between supervisors and teamwork activities and the outcomes of psychological well-being and turnover intention. They concluded that nursing managers must improve workplace relationships to help retain skilled nurses. In other works, focusing on caregivers, Picot, Youngblut, and Zeller (1997) combined Social Exchange Theory with equity theory to develop the *Picot Caregiver Rewards Scale* (PCRS) in order to obtain a more holistic view of the caregiver experience and to plan health promotion interventions for caregivers, and Carruth, Holland, and Larsen (2000) found that social exchange and equity theory provided a conceptual framework for studying reciprocal intergenerational exchanges of assistance and support and for developing a Caregiver Reciprocity Scale (CRS).

Conflict and Critical Theories

Conflict theories, also termed *critical theories*, share common ground in the elements analyzed in human societies: inequality, power/authority, domination/subjugation, interests, and conflict. Modern conflict theories have their roots in the writings of Karl Marx, the most famous conflict theorist, with later influences from Max Weber (1958) and Georg Simmel (1956). Marx argued that economic-based class conflict is the most basic and influential source of all social change. He viewed class conflict as inevitable because of the unequal allocation of goods and services in capitalist societies.

Marx's model of conflict was shaped by Europe's transition from a feudal to a capitalistic society, and to him, capitalism was an economic system that perpetuates inequality. Marx believed that the only means for emancipatory social change within a capitalist society was violent revolution, with the workers fighting against the capitalists. He argued that the ideology of any society is always the ideology of the ruling class or the powerful people, as those in power use ideology to ensure their value system reigns (Eitzen, Baca-Zinn, & Smith, 2017).

Modern critical/conflict theories have modified Marx's model. Dahrendorf (1958) regarded Marx's Theory of Class Conflict and Social Change as too simplistic because other social groups (e.g., political groups) also experience conflict. Implicit in his perspective is the notion that conflict meets systems' functional need for change. Society is characterized by struggles between social classes and between powerful and less powerful groups because of the inequality embedded in hierarchical social structures. The potential for conflict is inherent in the majority of human relationships because social organization means, among other things, the unequal distribution of power resulting in the "haves" and the "have-nots" (Eitzen et al., 2017). Two perspectives or types of conflict theory—Critical Social Theory and feminism are described here.

Critical Social Theory

The early foundation for Critical Social Theory (CST) can be found in Marx's argument that oppressive arrangements require revolutionary action. CST or critical theory is both theoretical and philosophical and has increasingly been used to address sociopolitical conditions that affect inequities in health and health care.

CST uses societal awareness to expose social inequalities that keep people from reaching their full potential. It is derived from the belief that social meanings structure life through social domination. Proponents of CST maintain that social exchanges that are not distorted by power imbalances will stimulate the evolution of a more just society. Furthermore, critical theory assumes that truth is socially determined (Martins, 2011).

Habermas (1991) is perhaps the best-known contemporary critical social theorist. In opposition to Marx's revolutionary action, Habermas argued that emancipation from domination is possible through "[rational] communicative [inter-]action." He supported employment of negotiation as integral to communicative action, realizing that negotiation must be conducted without the use of power or coercion by either of the interacting parties. With his emphasis on interaction through communication, Habermas discounted the importance of both material and structural constraints on changing social systems.

Freire (1970) applied critical theory to education and developed programs to liberate individuals and groups and make them economically independent. His work has greatly influenced pedagogy, focusing on the importance of education.

Critical Theory and Participatory Action Research. An important application of critical theories has been Action Research or Participatory Action Research (Wallerstein & Duran, 2010). Participatory Action Research (PAR) is sometimes employed in communities to stimulate community involvement and develop a solution to a community issue. A number of community-based PAR approaches have been used to support community action to improve community life. These projects are designed to reduce disparities in health and enlighten researchers.

In PAR, the researcher and the community or group members—often in underserved communities—work collaboratively to construct a particular activity or process to address health-related problems or needs. In PAR, the community members are encouraged to contribute important information about the realities of the current situation as well as to identify how it can be improved. This not only empowers the participants to create a better solution to an issue, it also allows for the participants to employ their unique perspectives to develop a more realistic, useful, and sustainable solutions (Wallerstein & Duran, 2006). In addition to empowering the community members in the process, many have developed projects that neither perspective could have generated independently.

Application to Nursing. Concepts from critical theory of CST have been examined in recent nursing literature, often within the context of working with disadvantaged groups. For example, in one work, Evans-Agnew, Boutain, and Rosemberg (2017) described the use of "photovoice" as a participatory tool in phenomenological research. Using critical theory and feminism as the framework, the authors detailed how photovoice can be employed to collect vital data from marginalized individuals. The authors explained how visual exposure of vulnerability through pictures can be used to address power relations and help seek transformative change.

In other examples, Stanley (2013) used CST as a framework for a project to expose nursing students to vulnerable populations—specifically homeless persons—to promote their awareness of health disparities and the complexity of social, cultural, and economic issues with this population. Similarly, K. E. Johnson, Guillet, Murphy, Horton, and Todd (2015) used aspects of CST to develop a simulation exercise for bachelor of science in nursing (BSN) students to illustrate for them some of the issues encountered by those in poverty. Finally, Bevan and colleagues (2012) used CST as a guide in their examination of the dilemmas faced by nurse researchers with respect to disclosure of incidental findings during genomic testing.

A number of examples of PAR were found in the nursing literature. One example was a project by Carlson and colleagues (2006) in which community resources were identified to address information needs about diabetes and its compactions among residents of low-income, African American communities. Another example of the action approach was an effort to reduce problems of MRSA infections in a rehabilitation hospital. Using action-based research strategies, a team found one unit that had much lower infection rates and discovered the cleaning staff for that unit had developed a unique manner of bagging the laundry and cleaning the unit (Webber, Macpherson, Meagher, Hutchinson, & Lewis, 2012). In a third example, Skene, Gerrish, Price, Pilling, and Bayliss (2016) use PAR methods to work with neonatal intensive care unit (NICU) staff and family members to promote more active involvement of parents in infant care and to promote family-centered care. Finally, Del Fabbro, Mitchell, and Shaw (2015) used PAR techniques to examine and enhance educational approaches for nursing faculty who teach international students.

Feminist Theory

Feminist theory is closely related to critical theories as often women have been less socially empowered than men. Gender differences and subordination have traditionally been viewed as both natural and inevitable, but some believe that gender is socially constructed and tends to justify the subordination and exploitation of women. A core assumption in feminist theories is that women are oppressed. This perspective has been determined to be too simplistic, however, and beginning in the 1960s, new views of feminism were presented (Eitzen et al., 2017; Waters, 1994).

A rather wide range of perspectives fall under the rubric of feminist theory. Feminist theory has been described as an analysis of women's subordination for the purpose of figuring out how to change it (Eitzen et al., 2017). There are many

Box 13-5   Themes in Feminist Theories

1. Women's experiences are central, normal, and valuable; experiences open new ways of knowing the world.
2. Gender is a basic organizing concept. The concept of *gender* involves two interrelated elements: (1) the social construction and exaggeration of differences between women and men (i.e., there is a fundamental basis of inequality, or social stratification, similar to social class and race) and (2) gender distinctions are used to legitimize and perpetuate power relations between women and men (i.e., compared with men, women are devalued and socially, economically, politically, and legally subordinated).
3. Gender distinctions occur in daily processes of constructing and reconstructing differences between women and men and devalues women. However, rather than passive victims, women participate in gendering processes as active agents, actors, and creators of culture.
4. Gender relations must be analyzed within specific sociocultural and historical contexts.
5. Monolithic, bounded notions (e.g., "the family") contribute to an ideology that contains class, cultural, and heterosexual biases and supports the oppression of women.

Source: Osmond and Thorne (1993).

issues, themes, and assumptions that are common in feminism. Osmond and Thorne (1993) discuss relevant themes in feminist theory; some of these are summarized in Box 13-5.

Variations of Feminist Theory. There is considerable variation among feminist perspectives. A few of the most commonly encountered are described in this section.

Liberal feminism is concerned with the political life and well-being of women and focuses on social justice and sexual equality. Friedan (1963) is probably the most well-known liberal feminist. She argued against the entrapment of women by the *feminine mystique*, an ideology that claims women are separate but special by extolling the virtues of women's traditional roles of wife and mother. Especially noteworthy is Freidan's examination of differences in women's pathologies (e.g., married women compared to unmarried women are more susceptible to diseases/disorders).

Socialist (Marxist) feminism focuses on the economic value of women's work (Marxist) and examines social structure in relation to women's roles and cultural practices (socialist). These approaches are exemplified by Millet's (1971) work describing the impact of patriarchy on the social structure, which she saw as a masculine system of political domination. She questioned the persistence of patriarchal beliefs and attitudes into an era where women are educated and free yet continue to be subordinate and devalued. She determined that because patriarchal domination is socially constructed, women can take emancipatory actions and reconstruct gender relations.

Firestone (1970) is perhaps the epitome of *radical feminism*. She refuted Marx's notion of economic class and argued instead that "sex class divisions" are at the root of women's oppression. "[T]o assure the elimination of sexual classes requires the revolt of the underclass (women) and the seizure of control of *reproduction*" (Waters, 1994, p. 267).

Application of Feminist Theory to Nursing. Feminist theory and philosophy have been frequently cited in the nursing literature. Beginning in the late 19th century, Florence Nightingale wrote on gender roles. Examples of Nightingale's feminist views included her efforts to obtain women's right to education, self-development, and occupations and her criticism of the double sexual standard of the times (Pfettscher, 2014). Nursing has a history of being a profession for females and one interpretation of nursing was "as handmaiden to the physician." This history illuminates the subordinate position of nurses in both profession and gender. Nursing has moved beyond this as more males enter the profession and the role of nurses as independent professionals has emerged. However, there are still vestiges of these nondominant positions in the profession. Thus, the feminist perspective has relevance for nurses to fully develop and exercise their professional role.

In more contemporary writings, feminist theory begins with the narratives of women from widely varied situations. For example, Cassidy, Goldberg, and Aston (2016) conducted a literature review of the feminist perspective on young women's sexual health and discovered "conflicting discourses" on sexuality and sexual health practices. They urged nurses to "challenge the status quo" and question sexual health norms for young women. Also addressing health needs of women, Burton (2016) described how using a feminist perspective can be effective for nurses to employ to improve care for adolescent girls and young adult women.

Considerable contemporary attention has been given in applying feminist concepts toward health needs of "transgendered" persons. For example, Rew, Thurman, and McDonald (2017) discussed sexual health and sexual rights and determined that additional work from theoretical development, research, and policy development must be undertaken to address unmet needs among "variant-gender" persons. Similarly, both MacDonnell (2014) and Fowler (2017) used a feminist perspective to describe the role of nurses with respect to promoting lesbian, gay, bisexual, and transgender (LGBT) health.

In more clinically focused examples, Antinuk (2013) used feminist theory to develop interventions for nurses who work with women who had experienced "forced genital cutting." In a final study, women's lived experiences with electroshock therapy (ECT) were explored and compared with nurses perceptions of ECT. Whereas nurses saw the treatment as beneficial, the women associated ECT with damage and devastating loss (van Daalen-Smith, 2011).

Complexity Science, Chaos Theory and Complex Adaptive Systems

The Newtonian-based theories of Western science that emerged from the Enlightenment period were "causal models," which focused on linearity, homeostasis, order, equilibrium, predictability, and control. These concepts formed a sort of invisible template that constrains many scientists from examining the "noise" or variation in their data (e.g., outliers). An emerging postmodern science of nonlinear dynamic systems—Complexity Science—takes science "outside that box." Simply stated, Complexity Science focuses on finding the underlying order in the apparent disorder of natural and social systems and understanding how change occurs in nonlinear dynamical systems over time (Walsh, 2000; Vicenzi, 1994).

Complexity Science (CS) is not a single theory but an evolving paradigm. Its focus is on the interconnection between individual units or agents that seek to explain relationships among variables and behaviors that are not fully predictable (Kauffman, 1995). Furthermore, CS examines the systems of diverse interacting agents to identify how they evolve and maintain order (Lindberg, Nash, & Lindberg, 2008).

Box 13-6   American Association of Colleges of Nursing Essentials

Chaos theory and Complexity Science are mentioned several times in *The Essentials of Master's Education in Nursing* (American Association of Colleges of Nursing [AACN], 2011). Specifically noted is that the master's degree program should prepare the graduate to " . . . demonstrate the ability to use Complexity Science and systems theory in the design, delivery, and evaluation of health care" (p. 12).

In addition, the DNP essentials (AACN, 2006) describes "complexity" with respect to practice and within the health care setting numerous times, suggesting the need for graduates of DNP programs to understand the concept and nature of complex systems.

Source: AACN (2006, 2011).

CS has been applied to various fields including weather forecasting, economics, neuroscience, and organizational behavior (Engebretson & Hickey, 2017). In health care, an understanding of complexity and nonlinear systems is important because "chaos" may be observed in the physical body in heart rhythms, electrical brain activity, and chemical reactions (e.g., neurotransmitters), as well as in other structures or organizations. The interdisciplinary application of CS has steadily gained momentum since the 1990s and is considered "essential" in advanced nursing education (Box 13-6). This section will introduce Chaos Theory, an early example or precursor of CS, and Complex Adaptive Systems, to be followed by a discussion of how CS is being applied in nursing and health care.

Chaos Theory

Chaos Theory has its origins in meteorology in the 1960s (B. M. Johnson & Webber, 2010). Chaos Theory is the study of unstable, aperiodic behavior in deterministic (nonrandom) nonlinear dynamical systems. *Dynamical* refers to the time-varying behavior of a system and *aperiodic* is the nonrepetitive but continuous behavior that results from the effects of any small disturbance. Based on Chaos Theory, natural and social systems change and ultimately survive because of alterations or disturbances and nonlinear behavior.

One of the key concepts of Chaos Theory is *sensitive dependence on initial conditions*—the notation that even a small difference can lead to dramatic, divergent paths. Because equilibrium is never reached in a dynamic system, trajectories that start from "arbitrarily close" points will ultimately diverge exponentially (Walsh, 2000). This sensitivity to initial conditions is commonly referred to as the "butterfly effect"—where hypothetically, a butterfly flapping its wings on one side of the world can cause a tornado the next month on the other side of the world.

In Chaos Theory, a *strange attractor* (strange because its appearance was unexpected) is similar to a magnet that exerts its pull on objects to return them to their original starting point. These patterns can be graphed in a way that illustrates the change behavior of the system (Haigh, 2008). Figure 13-4 is an example of a strange attractor showing chaotic motion from a simple three-dimensional model; note the butterfly resemblance.

A *bifurcation* is a sudden change or transition that will lead to a period of doubling, quadrupling and so forth at the onset of chaos (Walsh, 2000). This change occurs when a system is pushed so far from its steady state that it is unable to recover and a chaos or crisis state is reached. At this point, the system arrives at a "fork in

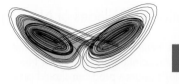

Figure 13-4 | Three-dimensional model of a strange attractor.

the road"—a choice of two or more alternative steady states, each different from the first (Prigogine & Stengers, 1984). The history of the system is influential as to which choice is made. When stressors again impact the system, the process is repeated. At each crisis point, the system reaches a bifurcation with choices. With successive bifurcations, choices become increasingly limited. A diagram of bifurcations would resemble a decision tree (Ward, 1995) or, with a more familiar analogy, the human vascular system.

Chaos is natural and universal and can be found in such diverse phenomena as the human heartbeat and the world economy (Vicenzi, 1994) and may be applied to brain wave patterns, as well as explaining complex lifestyle-choices or decisions (Coppa, 1993; Ray, 1998). Although chaos may cause uncertainty, it also offers opportunities that can create hope and bring about change; both are integral components of nursing practice (Haigh, 2008).

Complex Adaptive Systems

The term "Complex Adaptive System" (CAS) has been used to describe specific systems that have been applied to individual health, health threats, and health care organizations. Thus, when discussing CAS, the "system" can be one aspect of a patient (e.g., nervous or circulatory system), the individual, a family, a health care unit or clinic, or the entire health care apparatus (Engebretson & Hickey, 2017).

A CAS is an interconnected network of individual agents or components that interact within a system in ways that are not totally predictable (Holden, 2005). In a CAS, *agents* are units or components of the system, and *patterns* are formed by agents acting from a set of internalized rules (often labeled some simple rules). Some examples of CAS are a flock of birds or a hive of bees, where the birds or bees are the agents interacting in patterned ways. In this illustration, one can understand the functioning of the system (flock or hive) in ways that an examination of one of the components (birds or bees) does not. Furthermore, each agent or component may also be a CAS or part of a larger CAS.

There are other important characteristics of CAS. A CAS may develop new rules that shape the behavior of the CAS; this is a concept called *emergence*. Indeed, CAS are *dynamical and adaptive* to changes in both the internal and external environments (Smith, 2011). Complexity exists in the *dynamic balance between stability and instability*. An example from health care would be a patient who is stable but whose electrocardiogram (ECG) strip reveals variability in the form of heart block but in which the system is able to adapt to changes or demands. On the other extreme, fibrillation, in which the rhythm is irregular and unpatterned, which is not capable of adapting to the environment (Goldberger, 1996).

Self-organization describes how a CAS incorporates an aspect of *emergence* in which a CAS exhibits collective behaviors and possible new patterns and activates the nonlinearity within the system to adapt to new conditions. In CAS, *control is distributed, rather than centralized* and *simple rules* allow the system to adapt and function. The ability to adapt without a centralized control is another sign of a CAS. Finally, a CAS will utilize *coordination dynamics* within a part of a system, between different parts of the system, and between other systems (Kelso & Engstrom, 2006). Again, the flock of birds illustrates these characteristics as the self-organization, emergence, coordination, and so forth, combine to enable the birds to fly as a group with high velocity and not bumping into each other.

In CAS, *diversity* maximizes self-organization. This allows the system to provide for greater adaptation. These systems are also *deterministic*. In other words, the system can act on previous behavior, which contrasts with random systems. Finally, an additional characteristic of CAS is the idea of *coevolution* which allows these adaptive changes to be perpetuated and develop. Box 13-7 summarizes basic principles of CS.

Application to Nursing

The application of CS, CAS, and Chaos Theory has considerable relevance for nursing and nursing science. Understanding the human biologic organism as a CAS allows for application to all areas of clinical nursing. Application of the perspective of complexity in management/administration and education are also assistive. As nurses recognize and appreciate the complexity and adaptability of the person, group, or other entity, they can support and encourage this adaptability on both individual and organizational levels.

Box 13-7   Concepts and Principles from Complexity Science and Complex Adaptive Systems

- Complexity Science—application of principles of physics and mathematics to explain the relationship among variables that allow for variation and emergent behaviors that are not fully predictable; concepts can be applied to biomedicine, clinical issues, social science, and health care organizations.
- Dynamical system—a system whose state evolves over time according to a rule and initial conditions; the whole is not reducible to its parts.
- Nonlinear dynamics—application of mathematics (nonlinear algebra) to examine patterns of a system over time.
  - These time series patterns in a complex system (in contrast to a chaotic system) have a fractal pattern.
  - Self-similarity—the fractal patterns are similar at various times and levels or scales of resolution.
  - Attractor—a mathematical characteristic that describes the point to which a system tends to evolve.
- Complex Adaptive Systems (CAS)—a collection of individual agents (or components within the system) with freedom of behaviors that may not be predictable.
  - CAS are dynamical and adaptive and operates in response to initial conditions and to internal or external stimuli.
  - Internal rules—a system operates by internal rules which may not be explicit or shared. This is often referred to as operating by simple rules.
  - CAS are deterministic and not random; therefore, there is a pattern.
  - Systems are embedded within other systems; CAS have fuzzy boundaries—the environment or membership can change and adapt.
  - Self-organization—the system can spontaneously order itself without an external intervention.
  - Emergent properties—the behavior(s) emerging from interaction among agents may be new or novel; they are continually evolving.
  - Control is often distributed, rather than centralized.

Sources: Engebretson and Hickey (2017); Goldberger (1996); Kelso and Engstrom (2006); Lorenz (1993); Plsek and Greenhalgh (2001); Rickles, Hawe, and Shiell (2007).

The nursing literature contains multiple examples describing use of CS, CAS, and Chaos Theory in nursing. Aspects of CS, for example, were applied to critical care and critical care nursing in two works (Khan, Lasiter, & Boustani, 2015; Trinier, Liske, & Nenadovic, 2014). In another example, Hodges (2011) used principles of CS to develop a problem-based learning experience for community health nursing students. Then, in research, Oyeleye, Hanson, O'Connor, and Dunn (2013) used CS as the framework for a study examining the relationships among workplace incivility, stress, burnout, turnover, and psychological empowerment in acute care nurses, and Kneipp and Beeber (2015) used a CS perspective to study self-management behaviors and social withdrawal among disadvantaged women who suffer from migraines and depression.

The construct of CAS was used by Clancy (2014) to explain the importance of workflow management strategies in health systems. It was also used in another example to identify "best management practice" for new nurses who must learn to care for multiple patients with simultaneous complex needs (Kramer et al., 2013).

Several recent examples of clinical application of CAS focusing on various situations or settings were found. For example, CAS was used as a framework to discuss the care integration and networks of agents proving care in the NICU (D'Agata & McGrath, 2016). In a similar example, Glenn, Stocker-Schnieder, McCune, McClelland, and King (2014) used CAS as the framework for a qualitative study examining nursing care in the intrapartum setting. CS and the CAS were used to explain how sepsis is manifested within the human body, focusing on how nurses can conceptualize and recognize signs of sepsis to elicit more prompt intervention (Mann-Salinas, Engebretson, & Batchinsky, 2013). Finally, examples of application of CAS concepts in graduate nursing education was presented by Lis, Hanson, Burgermeister, and Banfield (2014), and Mulready-Shick and Flanagen (2014) used CAS concepts to discuss strategies for building and sustaining the "dedicated education unit" for academic partnerships.

Among the studies that apply Chaos Theory to nursing are Fisher and Wineman (2009), who presented the possibilities for conceptualizing and exploring complex physiologic patterns that occur in response to aging, disease, and treatment. Two indirect clinical applications were identified. Chaos Theory provided the framework for a study to predict nursing turnover in an acute care setting (Wagner, 2009), and Barker (1996) explored how chaos might contribute to a metaparadigm of nursing.

Summary

Theories from the sociologic sciences are integral to the discipline of nursing. Indeed, nurses in virtually all settings, caring for all types of clients, use concepts and principles from social theories daily. Simon, the nurse in the opening case study, recognized that in dealing with the problem of teenage pregnancy, it was essential to move beyond the logical intervention of providing more information on sexuality. Because he recognized that teen pregnancy is a social problem, he knew that it must be addressed using social science concepts, principles, and theories.

Sociologic theories are rich and substantively diverse. Because of this richness and diversity, it was impossible to include all theories and perspectives that are relevant to the discipline of nursing in this chapter. It is hoped, however, that the reader has gained an appreciation of the sociologic perspective and understands its significance to professional nursing.

Developing a sociologic perspective is not always comfortable because it calls for confronting and questioning existing ideologies and assumptions regarding social arrangements. It is important to do this, however, and the knowledge gained can benefit not only clients but also the health care system and professional nurses.

Key Points

- Theories from the sociologic sciences have greatly influenced nursing; indeed, many early nursing leaders (e.g., Nightingale, Barton, Wald, Sanger) were social activists.
- Systems theories, including GST, the Social-Ecological Model and social networks, provide a framework that allows nurses and other health care professionals to consider the patient(s) within the framework of their social environment and to recognize the interactions of the multitude of factors that can influence health decisions and ultimately health.
- Interactions frameworks, such as symbolic interactionism and Role Theory, describe how humans relate to each other (e.g., using language, gestures, and symbols to communicate) and in roles they take or are ascribed to them.
- Exchange theories are based on the philosophical perspective termed "utilitarianism," which supports the notion of "the greatest good for the greatest number." Exchange theories apply to human interactions in social context.
- Conflict/critical theories present the social processes of stability and change and explain how conflict is endemic to all social organizations because of unequal distribution of power. Critical social theory, feminist theory, and cultural diversity are examples of conflict theories and perspectives used by nurses.
- Complexity Science, Complex Adaptive Systems, and Chaos Theory seek to explain the interrelatedness and dependence of nonlinear dynamics, to find underlying order in apparent disorder of natural and social systems, and how changes occur in nonlinear systems over time.

Learning Activities

1. Consider a complex health problem or issue routinely encountered in your practice. Following the example of Simon, the nurse from the opening case study, apply a social-ecological perspective to consider how to better address the problem or issues from a more holistic perspective.
2. Select one of the theories presented in this chapter and obtain copies of the theorist's work(s). Read the work and consider ways to apply the concepts and principles in nursing. Are the concepts and principles more applicable in some settings than in others? Are the concepts and principles more applicable with some groups or aggregates than others?
3. Select a theory presented in this chapter. Review the nursing literature and identify nursing articles and studies describing how/when the theory is used in nursing. Present the findings in a paper or share them with colleagues.
4. Select one of the grand nursing theorists and review her work. Identify any concepts, principles, and theories drawn from the social sciences. Share findings with colleagues.

REFERENCES

Alexander, J. C., & Smith, P. (2009). The strong program in cultural sociology. In J. Turner (Ed.), *The handbook of sociological theory* (2nd ed., pp. 135–150). New York, NY: Springer Publishing.

American Association of Colleges of Nursing. (2006). *The essentials of doctoral education for advanced nursing practice*. Retrieved from http://www.aacn.nche.edu/dnp/Essentials.pdf

American Association of Colleges of Nursing. (2011). *The essentials of master's education in nursing*. Retrieved from http://www.aacn.nche.edu/education-resources/MastersEssentials11.pdf

Antinuk, K. (2013). Forced genital cutting in North America: Feminist theory and nursing considerations. *Nursing Ethics, 20*(6), 723–728.

Barker P. (1996). Chaos and the way of Zen: Psychiatric nursing and the 'uncertainty principle.' *Journal of Psychiatric and Mental Health Nursing, 3*(4), 235–43.

Berger, P. L., & Luckmann, T. (1966). *The social construction of reality: A treatise in the sociology of knowledge*. New York, NY: Anchor Books.

Bevan, J. L., Senn-Reeves, J. N., Inventor, B. R., Greiner, S. M., Mayer, K. M., Rivard, M. T., et al. (2012). Critical social theory approach to disclosure of genomic incidental findings. *Nursing Ethics, 19*(6), 819–828.

Blau, P. (1964). *Exchange and power in social life*. New York, NY: Wiley.

Bronfenbrenner, U. (1979). *The ecology of human development: Experiments by nature and design*. Cambridge, MA: Harvard University Press.

Brunetto, Y., Shriberg, A., Farr-Wharton, R., Shacklock, K., Newman, S., & Dienger, J. (2013). The importance of supervisor-nurse relationships, teamwork, wellbeing, affective commitment and retention of North American nurses. *Journal of Nursing Management, 21*(6), 827–837.

Burton, C. W. (2016). The health needs of young women: Applying a feminist philosophical lens to nursing science and practice. *ANS. Advances in Nursing Science, 39*(2), 108–118.

Carlson, B. A., Neal, D., Magwood, G., Jenkins, C., King, M. G., & Hossler, C. L. (2006). A community-based participatory health information needs assessment to help eliminate diabetes information disparities. *Health Promotion Practice, 7*(3), 213S–222S.

Carruth, A., Holland, C., & Larsen, L. (2000). Development and psychometric evaluation of the Caregiver Reciprocity Scale II. *Journal of Nursing Measurement, 8*(2), 179–191.

Cassidy, C., Goldberg, L., & Aston, M. (2016). The application of a feminist poststructural framework in nursing practice for addressing young women's sexual health. *Journal of Clinical Nursing, 25*(15–16), 2378–2386.

Christensen, S. (2014). Enhancing nurses' ability to care within the culture of incarceration. *Journal of Transcultural Nursing, 25*(3), 223–231.

Clancy, T. R. (2014). It's all about flow in a complex adaptive system. *The Journal of Nursing Administration, 44*(4), 190–193.

Clary-Muronda, V. (2016). The culturally diverse nursing student: A review of the literature. *Journal of Transcultural Nursing, 27*(4), 400–412.

Clary-Muronda, V., & Pope, C. (2016). Integrative review of instruments to measure team performance during neonatal resuscitation simulations in the birthing room. *Journal of Obstetric, Gynecologic, and Neonatal Nursing, 45*(5), 684–698.

Coleman, J. (1990). *Foundations of social theory*. Cambridge, MA: Belknap Press.

Coppa, D. F. (1993). Chaos theory suggests a new paradigm for nursing science. *Journal of Advance Nursing, 18*(6), 985–991.

D'Agata, A. L., & McGrath, J. M. (2016). A framework of complex adaptive systems: Parents as partners in the neonatal intensive care unit. *ANS. Advances in Nursing Science, 39*(3), 244–256.

Dahrendorf, R. (1958). Toward a theory of social conflict. *The Journal of Conflict Resolution, 2*, 170–183.

Davenport, L. A. (2017). Living with the choice: A grounded theory of Iraqi refugee resettlement to the U.S. *Issues in Mental Health Nursing, 38*(4), 352–360.

Del Fabbro, L., Mitchell, C., & Shaw, J. (2015). Learning among nursing faculty: Insights from a participatory action research project about teaching international students. *The Journal of Nursing Education, 54*(3), 153–158.

Denzin, N. K., & Lincoln, Y. S. (2003). *Strategies of qualitative inquiry*. Thousand Oaks, CA: Sage.

Déry, J., D'Amour, D., Blais, R., & Clarke, S. P. (2015). Influences on and outcomes of enacted scope of nursing practice: A new model. *ANS. Advances in Nursing Science, 38*(2), 136–143.

Dwyer, P., & Hunter-Revell, S. (2016). Influences on new graduate nurse transition: A literature review using a social ecological framework. *Nursing Research, 65*(2), E52.

Edwards, S. B., Olson, K., Koop, P. M., & Northcott, H. C. (2012). Patient and family caregiver decision making in the context of advanced cancer. *Cancer Nursing, 35*(3), 178–186.

Eitzen, D. S., Baca-Zinn, M., & Smith, K. E. (2017). *In conflict and order: Understanding society* (14th ed.). Boston, MA: Pearson.

Elminowski, N. S. (2015). Developing and implementing a cultural awareness worship for nurse practitioners. *Journal of Cultural Diversity, 22*(3), 105–113.

Emerson, R. (1981). Social exchange theory. In M. Rosenberg & R. Turner (Eds.), *Social psychology: Sociological perspectives* (pp. 30–65). New York, NY: Basic Books.

Engebretson, J. (2011). Clinically applied medical ethnography: Relevance to cultural competence in patient care. *The Nursing Clinics of North America, 46*(2), 145–154.

Engebretson, J. (2013). Understanding stigma in chronic health conditions: Implications for nursing. *Journal of the American Association of Nurse Practitioners, 25*(10), 545–550.

Engebretson, J. C., & Hickey, J. V. (2017). Complexity science and complex adaptive systems. In J. B. Butts & K. L. Rich (Eds.), *Philosophies and theories for advanced nursing practice* (3rd ed., pp. 115–141). Burlington, MA: Jones & Bartlett Learning.

Engebretson, J., Mahoney, J., & Carlson, E. (2008). Cultural competence in the era of evidence-based practice. *Journal of Professional Nursing, 24*(3), 172–178.

Evans-Agnew, R. A., Boutain, D. M., & Rosemberg, M. S. (2017). Advancing nursing research in the visual era: Reenvisioning the photovoice process across phenomenological, grounded theory, and critical theory methodologies. *Advances in Nursing Science, 40*(1), E1–E15.

Ferrante, J. (2015). *Sociology: A global perspective* (9th ed.). Stamford, CT: Cengage Learning.

Firestone, S. (1970). *The dialectic of sex: The case for feminist revolution*. London, United Kingdom: Paladin.

Fisher, E. M., & Wineman, N. M. (2009). Conceptualizing compensatory responses: Implications for treatment and research. *Biological Research for Nursing, 10*(4), 400–408.

Fowler, M. D. (2017). "Unladylike commotion": Early feminism and nursing's role in gender/trans dialogue. *Nursing Inquiry, 24*(1), e12179.

Freire, P. (1970). *Pedagogy of the oppressed*. New York, NY: Herder and Herder.

Friedan, B. (1963). *The feminine mystique*. London, United Kingdom: Penguin Books.

Friedemann, M. L., & Buckwalter, K. C. (2014). Family caregiver role and burden related to gender and family relationships. *Journal of Family Nursing, 20*(3), 313–336.

Frye, L. (2016). Fathers' experience with autism spectrum disorder: Nursing implications. *Journal of Pediatric Healthcare, 30*(5), 453–463.

Gerardi, D. (2015). Conflict engagement: Workplace dynamics. *The American Journal of Nursing, 115*(4), 62–65.

Glenn, L. A., Stocker-Schnieder, J., McCune, R., McClelland, M., & King, D. (2014). Caring nurse practice in the intrapartum setting: Nurses' perspectives on complexity, relationships and safety. *Journal of Advanced Nursing, 70*(9), 2019–2030.

Goldberger, A. (1996). Non-linear dynamics for clinicians: Chaos theory, fractals, and complexity at the bedside. *Lancet, 347*, 1312–1314.

Guarnero, P. (2012). Understanding health promotion behaviors among young men of color. *Communicating Nursing Research, 45*(6), 495.

Habermas, J. (1991). The critical theory of Jürgen Habermas. In J. Turner (Ed.), *The structure of sociological theory* (pp. 254–281). Belmont, CA: Wadsworth.

Haefner, J. (2014). An application of Bowen family systems theory. *Issues in Mental Health Nursing, 35*(11), 835–841.

Haigh, C. A. (2008). Using simplified chaos theory to manage nursing services. *Journal of Nursing Management, 16*(3), 298–304.

Hamrin, V., Vick, R., Brame, C., Simmons, M., Smith, L., & Vanderhoef, D. (2016). Teaching a systems approach: An innovative quality improvement project. *The Journal of Nursing Education, 55*(4), 209–214.

Hansen, L., Press, N., Rosenkranz, S. J., Baggs, J. G., Kendall, J., Kerber, A., et al. (2012). Life-sustaining treatment decisions in the ICU for patients with ESLD: A prospective investigation. *Research in Nursing & Health, 35*(5), 518–532.

Hechter, M. (1987). *Principles of group solidarity.* Berkeley, CA: University of California Press.

Higginbottom, G. M., Rivers, K., & Story, R. (2014). Health and social care needs of Somali refugees with visual impairment (VIP) living in the United Kingdom: A focused ethnography with Somali people with VIP, their caregivers, service providers, and members of the Horn of Africa Blind Society. *Journal of Transcultural Nursing, 25*(2), 192–201.

Hirooka, K., Fukahori, H., Ozawa, M., & Akita, Y. (2017). Differences in posttraumatic growth and grief reactions among adolescents by relationship with the deceased. *Journal of Advanced Nursing, 73*(4), 955–965.

Hodges, H. F. (2011). Preparing new nurses with complexity science and problem-based learning. *The Journal of Nursing Education, 50*(1), 7–13.

Holden, L. M. (2005). Complex adaptive systems: Concept analysis. *Journal of Advanced Nursing, 52*(6), 651–657.

Holstein, J. A., & Gubrium, J. F. (2008). *Handbook of constructionist research.* New York, NY: Guilford Press.

Homans, G. (1961). *Social behavior: Its elementary forms.* New York, NY: Harcourt Brace.

Horton, K. L., & Dworkin, S. L. (2013). Redefining gender-based power to move beyond interpersonal approaches to HIV prevention. *ANS. Advances in Nursing Science, 36*(1), 42–50.

Johnson, B. M., & Webber, P. B. (2010). *An introduction to theory and reasoning in nursing* (3rd ed.). Philadelphia, PA: Lippincott Williams & Wilkins.

Johnson, K. E., Guillet, N., Murphy, L., Horton, S. E., & Todd, A. T. (2015). "If only we could have them walk a mile in their shoes": A community-based poverty simulation exercise for baccalaureate nursing students. *The Journal of Nursing Education, 54*(9), S116–S119.

Kauffman, S. (1995). *At home in the universe: The search for laws of self-organization and complexity.* New York, NY: Oxford University Press.

Kelso, J. A. S., & Engstrom, D. A. (2006). *The complementary nature.* Cambridge, MA: MIT Press.

Kenney, J. W. (1995). Relevance of theory-based nursing practice. In P. J. Christensen & J. W. Kenney (Eds.), *Nursing process: Application of conceptual models* (4th ed., pp. 3–17). St. Louis, MO: Mosby.

Khan, B. A., Lasiter, S., & Boustani, M. A. (2015). CE: Critical care recovery center: An innovative collaborative care model for ICU survivors. *The American Journal of Nursing, 115*(3), 24–31, 46.

Kneipp, S. M., & Beeber, L. (2015). Social withdrawal as a self-management behavior for migraine: Implications for depression comorbidity among disadvantaged women. *ANS. Advances in Nursing Science, 38*(1), 34–44.

Kramer, M., Brewer, B. B., Halfer, D., Maguire, P., Beausoleil, S., Claman, K., et al. (2013). Changing our lens: Seeing the chaos of professional practice as complexity. *Journal of Nursing Management, 21*(4), 690–704.

Lee, T. Y., Wang, M. M., Lin, K. C., & Kao, C. H. (2013). The effectiveness of early intervention on paternal stress for fathers of premature infants admitted to a neonatal intensive care unit. *Journal of Advanced Nursing, 69*(5), 1085–1095.

Lévi-Strauss, C. (1969). *The elementary structures of kinship.* Boston, MA: Beacon Press.

Lindberg, C., Nash, S., & Lindberg, C. (2008). *On the edge: Nursing in the age of complexity.* Bordentown, NJ: Plexus Press.

Lindesmith, A., & Strauss, A. (1968). *Social psychology.* New York, NY: Holt, Rinehart & Winston.

Lis, G. A., Hanson, P., Burgermeister, D., & Banfield, B. (2014). Transforming graduate nursing education in the context of complex adaptive systems: Implications for master's and DNP curricula. *Journal of Professional Nursing, 30*(6), 456–462.

Logan, J. R., & Spitze, G. (1996). *Family ties: Enduring relations between parents and their grown children.* Philadelphia, PA: Temple University Press.

Long, T. (2016). Influence of international service learning on nursing students' self-efficacy towards cultural competence. *Journal of Cultural Diversity, 23*(1), 28–33.

Lorenz, E. N. (1993). *The essence of chaos.* Seattle, WA: University of Washington Press.

MacDonnell, J. A. (2014). Enhancing our understanding of emancipatory nursing: A reflection on the use of critical feminist methodologies. *ANS. Advances in Nursing Science, 37*(3), 271–280.

Mann-Salinas, E. A., Engebretson, J., & Batchinsky, A. I. (2013). A complex systems view of sepsis: Implications for nursing. *Dimensions of Critical Care Nursing, 32*(1), 12–17.

Martins, D. C. (2011). Thinking upstream: Nursing theories and population-focused nursing practice. In M. A. Nies & M. McEwen (Eds.), *Community/public health nursing: Promoting the health of populations* (4th ed., pp. 37–49). Philadelphia, PA: Elsevier/Saunders.

Martsolf, D. S., Draucker, C. B., Bednarz, L. C., & Lea, J. A. (2011). Listening to the voices of important others: How adolescents make sense of troubled dating relationships. *Archives in Psychiatric Nursing, 25*(6), 430–444.

Marx, K. (1977). *Capital: A critique of political economy* (Vol. 1, B. Folkes, Trans.). New York, NY: Vintage Books.

Mason, G., & Attree, M. (1997). The relationship between research and the nursing process in clinical practice. *Journal of Advanced Nursing, 26*(5), 1045–1049.

McCullagh, M. C., Sanon, M. A., & Foley, J. G. (2015). Cultural health practices of migrant seasonal farmworkers. *Journal of Cultural Diversity, 22*(2), 64–72.

Mead, G. H. (1934). *Mind, self, and society: From the standpoint of a social behaviorist* (C. W. Morris, Ed.). Chicago, IL: University of Chicago Press.

Meyer, R. M., & O'Brien-Pallas, L. L. (2010). Nursing services delivery theory: An open system approach. *Journal of Advanced Nursing, 66*(12), 2828–2838.

Millet, K. (1971). *Sexual politics.* New York, NY: Avon/Equinox.

Mills, C. W. (1959). *The sociological imagination.* New York, NY: Oxford University Press.

Moreno, J. (1953). *Who shall survive? Foundations of sociometry, group psychotherapy and sociodrama.* New York, NY: Beacon Press.

Mulready-Shick, J. A., & Flanagan, K. (2014). Building the evidence for dedicated education unit sustainability and partnership success. *Nursing Education Perspectives, 35*(5), 287–293.

Myny, D., Van Goubergen, D. V., Gobert, M., Vanderwee, K., Van Hecke, A., & Defloor, T. (2011). Non-direct patient care factors influencing nursing workload: A review of the literature. *Journal of Advanced Nursing, 67*(10), 2109–2129.

Ngai, F., & Chan, S. (2012). Stress, maternal role competence, and satisfaction among Chinese women in the perinatal period. *Research in Nursing & Health, 35*(1), 30–39.

Noseff, J. (2014). Theory usage and application paper: Maternal role attainment. *International Journal of Childbirth Education, 29*(3), 58–68.

Nuss, H. J., Hester, L. L., Perry, M. A., Stewart-Briley, C., Reagon, V. M., & Collins, P. (2016). Applying the social ecological model to creating asthma-friendly schools in Louisiana. *The Journal of School Health, 86*(3), 225–232.

Opalinski, A., Dyess, S., & Grooper, S. (2015). Do faith communities have a role in addressing childhood obesity? *Public Health Nursing, 32*(6), 721–730.

Osmond, M. W., & Thorne, B. (1993). Feminist theories: The social construction of gender in families and society. In P. G. Boss, W. J. Doherty, R. LaRossa, W. R. Schumm, & S. K. Steinmetz (Eds.), *Sourcebook of family theories and methods: A contextual approach* (pp. 591–623). New York, NY: Plenum Press.

Oyeleye, O., Hanson, P., O'Connor, N., & Dunn, D. (2013). Relationship of workplace incivility, stress, and burnout on nurses' turnover intentions and psychological empowerment. *The Journal of Nursing Administration, 43*(10), 536–542.

Palmer, M., Saviet, M., & Tourish, J. (2016). Understanding and supporting grieving adolescents and young adults. *Pediatric Nursing, 42*(6), 275–281.

Pfettscher, S. A. (2014). Florence Nightingale. In M. R. Alligood (Ed.), *Nursing theorists and their work* (8th ed., pp. 60–78). St. Louis, MO: Mosby.

Picot, S., Youngblut, J., & Zeller, R. (1997). Development and testing of a measure of perceived caregiver rewards in adults. *Journal of Nursing Measurement, 5*(1), 33–52.

Plsek, P., & Greenhalgh, T. (2001). The challenge of complexity in health care. *BMJ, 323*(7313), 625–628.

Prigogine, I., & Stengers, I. (1984). *Order out of chaos: Man's new dialogue with nature.* New York, NY: Bantam Books.

Ray, M. A. (1998). Complexity and nursing science. *Nursing Science Quarterly, 11*(3), 91–93.

Reeves, E. A., & Woods-Giscombé, C. L. (2015). Infant-feeding practices among African American women: Social-ecological analysis and implications for practice. *Journal of Transcultural Nursing, 26*(3), 219–226.

Rew, L., Thurman, W., & McDonald, K. (2017). A review and critique of Advances in Nursing Science articles that focus on sexual health and sexual rights: A call to leadership and policy development. *ANS. Advances in Nursing Science, 40*(1), 64–84.

Richardson, K. J. (2014). Deaf culture: Competencies and best practices. *The Nurse Practitioner, 39*(5), 20–28.

Rickles, D., Hawe, P., & Shiell, A. (2007). A simple guide to chaos and complexity. *Journal of Epidemiology and Community Health, 61,* 933–937.

Rose, M., & Newman, S. D. (2016). Factors influencing patient safety during postoperative handover. *AANA Journal, 84*(5), 329–335.

Schwandt, T. A. (2007). *The Sage dictionary of qualitative inquiry.* Thousand Oaks, CA: Sage.

Shacklock, K., Brunetto, Y., Teo, S., & Farr-Wharton, R. (2014). The role of support antecedents in nurses' intentions to quit: The case of Australia. *Journal of Advanced Nursing, 70*(4), 811–822.

Shen, Z. (2015). Cultural competence models and cultural competence assessment instruments in nursing: A literature review. *Journal of Transcultural Nursing, 26*(3), 308–321.

Simmel, G. (1956). *Conflict and the web of group affiliations* (K. H. Wolff, Trans.). Glencoe, IL: Free Press.

Skene, C., Gerrish, K., Price, F., Pilling, E., & Bayliss, P. (2016). Developing family-entered care in a neonatal intensive care unit: An action research study protocol. *Journal of Advanced Nursing, 72*(3), 658–668.

Smith, M. (2011). Philosophical and theoretical perspectives related to complexity science in nursing. In A. W. Davidson, M. A. Ray & M. C. Turkel (Eds.), *Nursing, caring, and complexity science: For human-environment well-being* (pp. 1–29). New York, NY: Springer Publishing.

Spurr, S., Bally, J., Trinder, K., & Williamson, L. (2016). A multidimensional investigation into the predictors of physical activity in Canadian adolescents. *Journal of Holistic Nursing, 34*(4), 390–401.

Stanley, M. J. (2013). Teaching about vulnerable populations: Nursing students' experience in a homeless center. *The Journal of Nursing Education, 52*(10), 585–588.

The Joint Commission. (2010). *Cultural and linguistic care in area hospitals—final report.* Retrieved from https://www.jointcommission.org/assets/1/18/FINAL_REPORT_MARCH_2010.pdf

Thibaut, J. W., & Kelley, H. M. (1959). *The social psychology of groups.* New York, NY: Wiley.

Tomlinson, P. S., Peden-McAlpine, C., & Sherman, S. (2012). A family systems nursing intervention model for paediatric health crisis. *Journal of Advanced Nursing, 68*(6), 705–714.

Trinier, R., Liske, L., & Nenadovic, V. (2014). Complexity science: Understanding the implications for crucial care nursing. *Canadian Association of Critical Care Nurses, 25*(2), 38–39.

Turner, J. H. (2013). *Contemporary sociological theory.* Los Angeles, CA: Sage.

van Daalen-Smith, C. (2011). Waiting for oblivion: Women's experiences with electroshock. *Issues in Mental Health Nursing, 32*(7), 457–472.

Vicenzi, A. E. (1994). Chaos theory and some nursing considerations. *Nursing Science Quarterly, 7*(1), 36–42.

von Bertalanffy, L. (1968). *General system theory: Foundations, development, applications.* New York, NY: Braziller.

Wagner, C. (2009). The value of a nonlinear model in predicting nursing turnover. *The Journal of Nursing Administration, 39*(5), 200–203.

Wallerstein, N. B., & Duran, B. (2006). Using community-based participatory research to address health disparities. *Health Promotion Practice, 7*(3), 312–323.

Wallerstein, N., & Duran, B. (2010). Community-based participatory research contributions to intervention research: The intersection of science and practice to improve health equity. *American Journal of Public Health, 100*(Suppl. 1), S40–S46.

Walsh, M. (2000). Chaos, complexity and nursing. *Nursing Standard, 14*(32), 39–42.

Ward, M. (1995). Butterflies and bifurcations: Can chaos theory contribute to our understanding of family systems? *Journal of Marriage and the Family, 57*(3), 629–638.

Waters, M. (1994). *Modern sociological theory.* London, United Kingdom: Sage.

Weber, M. (1958). *The Protestant ethic and the spirit of capitalism.* New York, NY: Charles Scribner.

Webber, K. L., Macpherson, S., Meagher, A., Hutchinson, S., & Lewis, B. (2012). The impact of strict isolation on MRSA positive patients: An action-based study undertaken in a rehabilitation center. *Rehabilitation Nursing, 37*(1), 43–50.

Zieber, M. P., & Williams, B. (2015). The experience of nursing students who make mistakes in clinical. *International Journal of Nursing Education Scholarship, 12*(1), 1–9.

Theories From the Behavioral Sciences

Melanie McEwen and Sattaria Smith Dilks

Tracy Simmons is in a master's degree program that will allow her to become an adult psychiatric/mental health advanced practice registered nurse (PMH-APRN). In a course on the application of theory in nursing, one of her assignments is to write a paper describing how she has applied a theory in providing care for a client. Although Tracy has been working as a nurse in a psychiatric hospital for the past 10 years, she is finding this assignment difficult because, thus far in the course, the instructor has focused primarily on grand nursing theories. Tracy knows little about these theories because in her practice, she uses a broad, eclectic approach, predominantly applying theories from the behavioral sciences.

Tracy discussed her dilemma with her professor and learned that she can use any theory or set of theories for the assignment; it is not necessary to rely strictly on nursing theories. The discussion with her professor enlightened Tracy about the necessity of applying non-nursing theories to nursing practice. With the realization of the importance of theories from other disciplines to nursing, Tracy's interest in the many psychologically based theories is piqued, and she conducted a literature review.

The person that Tracy chose for her assignment is Alan, a 41-year-old Caucasian male, who is married and the father of two adolescents. Alan was admitted to the hospital with diagnoses of major depression, substance dependence with physiologic dependency, and hepatitis C. Assessments revealed that he had problems with his primary support group, problems related to the social environment, occupational problems, and problems related to interaction with the legal system.

Although this is Alan's first hospitalization, he has had a long history of alcohol abuse. He also admits to using cocaine or marijuana occasionally on the weekends. His father was an alcoholic who died at the age of 44 years with cirrhosis of the liver. Although not actively suicidal, Alan expresses passive death wishes. Alan is a well-known member of the community and owns a large software business, which is on the verge of bankruptcy. His motivation for entering treatment is that his wife threatened to divorce him unless he stops using alcohol and drugs.

In reviewing Alan's care, Tracy planned to use a holistic approach, incorporating principles and concepts from various theories. The first theory that Tracy chooses is Freud's Psychoanalytic Theory because of Alan's denial. This theory is relevant because Freud discussed how an individual uses defense mechanisms to decrease anxiety, and Tracy knows that a major defense mechanism of alcoholism is denial. Tracy also thinks the cognitive-behavioral theories are appropriate because she believes that humans need to change cognition to change behavior. Because Tracy assumes that drinking and using drugs are means of coping, she plans to use Lazarus's Coping Theory to help Alan develop more effective coping strategies. Finally, Tracy plans to apply humanistic psychology because she believes that Alan, like all individuals, has the potential to change, and social psychology theories address health beliefs and intent to change.

As discussed in Chapter 1, nursing is a practice discipline, and practice disciplines are considered to be applied sciences rather than pure or basic sciences (Johnson, 1959). The object of both pure and applied sciences is the same (to achieve knowledge), but according to Folta (1968), the difference between the two is their emphasis. In pure science, the emphasis is on basic research, which focuses on the application of the scientific method to add abstract knowledge. In contrast, the emphasis in applied science is on research related to the application and testing of the abstract concepts. Thus, applied sciences use the scientific method to apply and test fundamental knowledge or principles in practice. Historically, nursing science has drawn much of its knowledge from the basic sciences and then applied that knowledge to the discipline of nursing.

In learning about theories used in nursing, it is important to remember that nursing has evolved over decades and that the knowledge base for the discipline is a compilation of phenomena from many different disciplines. In the case study, Tracy discovered the notion of "shared" or "borrowed" versus "unique" theory. Johnson (1968) has defined borrowed theories as knowledge that has been identified in other disciplines and is used in nursing. According to Johnson, knowledge does not belong to any discipline but is shared across many disciplines; thus, nursing science draws on the knowledge of other disciplines to enhance the knowledge required for nursing practice.

One of the areas from which nurses draw theoretical understanding are the psychological sciences, sometimes referred to as the behavioral sciences. The contribution of the behavioral sciences to knowledge in nursing science and nursing practice cannot be denied. Even though the basic theories, concepts, and frameworks are derived from another discipline, they are routinely applied in nursing practice. Additionally, they are frequently applied in nursing research as well as nursing education and administration.

There are many psychological theories, and it would be impossible to cover all of them in this chapter. Major theories were chosen to illustrate concepts that are used in nursing. For the purposes of this chapter, the psychological theories will be viewed in four categories: psychodynamic theories, behavioral and cognitive-behavioral theories, humanistic theories, and stress-adaptation theories. These theories look at an individual and how an individual responds to stimuli. In psychology, there is also a special field known as social psychology, which examines how society or groups of individuals respond to various stimuli. This chapter will examine three theories of social psychology commonly used in nursing: the Health Belief Model, the Theory of Reasoned Action, and the Transtheoretical Model (Stages of Change).

Psychodynamic Theories

The late 1800s saw the creation of a new discipline, psychology/psychiatry, with a new body of knowledge. Before Sigmund Freud presented his radical works describing human thoughts and behaviors, people were considered to be either "good" or "bad," "normal" or "crazy." Freud's work led to a major paradigm shift as scientists began to consider the thought processes of "man" and to speculate about human personality. From this paradigm shift came a number of psychological theories.

Freud's thinking was considered radical in the early 1900s. Even now in the early 21st century, many people still consider his work radical; yet, others believe it to be antiquated. Despite this, his basic ideas and concepts have been used and modified extensively in the development of numerous psychodynamic theories of human thought and behavior.

Psychodynamic theories attempt to explain the multidimensional nature of behavior and understand how an individual's personality and behavior interface. They also provide a systematic way of identifying and understanding behavior. This section describes three psychodynamic theories—the works of Freud, Erikson, and Sullivan. These three theories are also called "stage theories," meaning that they describe clearly defined stages at which new behaviors appear based on social and motivational influences. Table 14-1 compares the developmental stages of the three theories.

Psychoanalytic Theory: Freud

According to Freudian theory, behavior is nearly always the product of an interaction among the three major systems of the personality: the id, ego, and superego. Even though each of these systems has its own functions, properties, and components, they interact so closely that it is difficult to distinguish their effects on behavior.

Table 14-1 Stages of Development

Theorist	Developmental Emphasis	Stages
Sigmund Freud	Psychosexual	1. Oral 2. Anal 3. Phallic 4. Latency 5. Genital
Erik E. Erikson	Psychosocial	1. Trust versus mistrust 2. Autonomy versus shame and doubt 3. Initiative versus guilt 4. Industry versus inferiority 5. Identity versus identity confusion 6. Intimacy versus isolation 7. Generativity versus stagnation 8. Integrity versus despair
Harry S. Sullivan	Interpersonal	1. Infancy 2. Childhood 3. Juvenile 4. Preadolescence 5. Early adolescence 6. Late adolescence

Behavior is generally an interaction among these three systems; rarely does one system operate to the exclusion of the other two (Freud, 1923/1960).

Overview

According to Freud, the id is the original system of the personality, and it is the matrix in which the ego and superego differentiate. The id is unable to tolerate an increase in energy, which is experienced as an uncomfortable state of tension. This increased tension can be perceived either internally or externally. The id discharges the tension to return the body to a state of equilibrium. This tension release is known as the *pleasure principle* (Freud, 1923/1960).

The ego distinguishes between things in the mind and things in the external world. The ego is said to follow the reality principle with the aim of preventing tension until an appropriate object is found to satisfy the need. The ego has control over all cognitive and intellectual functions and is considered to be the executive of the personality because it controls behavior. It does this by mediating the conflicting demands of the id, superego, and external environment (Freud, 1923/1960).

The third system is the superego. The main functions of the superego are to (1) inhibit the impulses of the id, (2) encourage the ego to substitute moralistic goals for realistic goals, and (3) strive for perfection. The focus of the superego is on moral issues: "what is right" and "what is wrong" (Freud, 1923/1960).

Freud based his theory on the scientific view of the late 19th century, which regarded the human body as an energy system. He proposed that because the body derives its energy from the work of the body (e.g., respiration, digestion), then memory and thinking are also defined by the work they perform. He labeled this concept *psychic energy* and stated that an instinct is an inborn state of somatic excitement. Furthermore, an instinct is a quantum of psychic energy or, as Freud (1923/1960) said, "A measure of the demand made upon the mind for work" (p. 168). All the instincts together yield the sum total of psychic energy (Freud, 1905/1953).

The four characteristics of an instinct are source, aim, object, and impetus. Whereas source is the need, the aim is the removal of the tension. Object is what will satisfy the need and also includes all behaviors that occur to obtain the necessary object. The impetus of an instinct is the force or strength, which is determined by the intensity of the underlying need. Thus, psychic energy is displaced to the object to satisfy the instinctual need. Freud believed that instincts are the sole energy source for human behavior (Freud, 1905/1953).

The environment plays two roles with regard to instinct. It either satisfies or threatens the development of the person. The individual responds with increased tension; an increase in tension is known as *anxiety*. The function of anxiety is to warn the person of impending danger. Anxiety motivates the person to do something; thus, a behavior is seen. As a result of increased tension or anxiety, an individual is forced to learn new methods of reducing the tension. According to Freud (1926/1959), these new methods are called *ego defense mechanisms*. "All defense mechanisms have two characteristics in common: (1) They deny, falsify, or distort reality and (2) they operate unconsciously so that the person is not aware of what is taking place" (Hall & Lindzey, 1978, pp. 91–92).

Freud was one of the first theorists to emphasize the developmental aspect of personality. He believed that the personality was developed within the first 5 years of life. Each of his stages of development, excepting latency, during which focus lies outside of one's own body, is defined as a mode of reaction to a particular zone of the body. Freud's stages were related to psychosexual development and included oral, anal, phallic, latency, and genital stages (Freud, 1905/1953).

Application to Nursing

Although nursing theories are not based on Freud's theory, many of his ideas and concepts are relevant to nursing practice. These concepts include anxiety, developmental stages, defense mechanisms, and the identity of self.

Freud's theory helps to explain the complex nature of a person and how a person's past influences his or her personality. The complex processes of the past, which are found in the unconscious mind, suggest an explanation for the diversity in a person's behaviors. Even though the emphasis in much of nursing is on the "here and now," understanding the person's relevant past experiences can help the nurse identify underlying themes and improve care.

The id, ego, and superego are the components of the self. When there is an imbalance among these concepts, the self becomes lost and must be reconstructed. Nurses can help clients who have undergone a loss of self to discover a more active sense of self, put the self into action, and use the enhanced self as a refuge. Furthermore, an understanding of the concepts of id, ego, and superego helps the nurse understand the needs of the client and helps the nurse respond more appropriately to the behaviors.

In Alan's situation from the opening case study, the domination of the id would lead to increased substance use because of the pleasure principles. When Alan sobered, the superego would cause him to have feelings of shame and guilt. Tracy can now help Alan choose acceptable ways of behaving, thus causing an equilibrium among the id, ego, and superego. This equilibrium would help to relieve Alan's feelings of anxiety.

A behavior is the way an individual responds to increased tension or anxiety, and, in this case, Alan responded to increased tension by abusing substances (e.g., alcohol, cocaine, marijuana). Alan denied that he used substances inappropriately; he stated that he used alcohol "socially," and the drugs were only done on weekends and therefore "no big deal." Alan also stated that he had no marital problems when, in fact, his wife was going to divorce him. Alan was demonstrating Freud's concept of defense mechanisms, specifically denial. Defense mechanisms are used to help reduce anxiety and tension. Denial describes a client's behavior, and the main two definitions range from adaptive to maladaptive responses. In this case study, Alan uses denial as a maladaptive response. By using denial, Alan was able to decrease the feelings of rejection from his wife and the shame and guilt associated with abusing substances. Because Tracy recognized and understood the use of this maladaptive defense mechanism, she was able to develop a plan of care to help Alan develop more adaptive defense mechanisms to relieve anxiety.

Although denial is used in the case study to explain substance abuse, nurses encounter the use of denial with clients in almost all areas of nursing. Examples include those with obesity, cancer, hypertension, diabetes, and cardiac problems, just to mention a few. The use of denial is a way of protecting the self from a threat that could harm the person physically and decrease self-concept. When denial is used, the individual does not believe that he or she has a problem, and this can lead to noncompliant behavior.

Recent nursing literature that reports on application of Psychoanalytic Theory covers a variety of issues. For example, Steinberg and Cochrane (2013) examined the incorporation of psychodynamic theory in managing psychiatric mental health patients on an inpatient unit, and Walsh, Crisp, and Moss (2011) used a psychoanalytic perspective to describe how an intrapersonal mechanism influences organizational change. Other authors have used Psychoanalytic Theory to examine such concepts as denial in adolescent pregnancy (Platt, 2014), acceptance and denial-related chronic illness (Telford, Kralik, & Koch, 2006), and transference and countertransference in nursing care of patients with anorexia nervosa (Swatton, 2011).

Developmental (or Ego Developmental) Theory: Erikson

Erikson's Psychosocial Developmental Theory emerged as an expansion of Freud's concept of ego. In Erikson's theory, specific stages of a person's life from birth to death are formed by social influences that interact with the physical/psychological, maturing organism. Erikson described this as a "mutual fit of individual and environment" (Erikson, 1975, p. 102). Also, he is the only developmental theorist who extends development through adulthood; the other theorists stop with adolescence.

Overview

Erikson's theory lists eight stages of development: The first four stages occur in infancy and childhood, the fifth stage occurs in adolescence, and the last three stages occur during the adult years. In his work, Erikson emphasized the adolescent stage, that time in an individual's life when the person makes the transition from a child to an adult, and he determined that this transitional period has the greatest influence on the adult personality. Erikson believed that each stage of development builds on the next, thus contributing to the formation of the total person. Also, even though Erikson gave a chronologic timetable, it is not strict because he believed that each person has his or her own timetable for development (Erikson, 1963).

Erikson further developed the concept of ego to incorporate qualities that expanded the Freudian concept. He believed the ego is the most powerful of the three parts of the personality (id, ego, and superego) and described the ego as being robust and resilient. According to Erikson, the ego uses a combination of inner readiness and outer opportunities, with a sense of vigor and joy, to find creative solutions at each stage of development. This concentration of the potential strength of the ego empowers people to deal effectively with their problems (Erikson, 1968).

Application to Nursing

Developmental theory is a foundational element in some nursing theories, and it is important in nursing practice. For example, an essential part of the assessment process is to determine age appropriateness or development stage or status. Although developmental issues are generally thought to be associated only with pediatrics, this is not necessarily the case. By assessing the developmental stage of the adult and elderly person, data can be collected about interpersonal skills and behaviors because behavioral manifestations are clues to issues that need to be addressed in client care. Furthermore, individual responsibility and the capacity to improve one's functioning are issues to be addressed by nurses.

Erikson's theory identified the degree of mastery with regard to a person's chronologic age. This mastery is known as ego strength. Bjorklund (2000) believed that promoting assessment from the perspective of ego strengths, instead of ego deficits, is a valuable skill for nurses, who then can use the data for assessment and treatment outcomes. Besides using ego strengths for assessment and interventions, the nurse can also use them to empower the client to take control of his or her life and to deal effectively with problems.

Identifying and assessing Alan's ego strengths helped Tracy locate where Alan falls on the developmental continuum, thus providing data to develop therapeutic goals. When Tracy graduates and becomes a psychiatric/mental health advanced practice registered nurse (PMH-APRN), she can conduct family therapy, and Erikson's theory would be helpful in working with Alan's children, especially from the perspective of ego strength.

Developmental theory is used not only in psychiatric nursing but also in other specialty areas of nursing, and it is integral to holistic nursing practice (Reed, 1998). Nursing researchers and scholars commonly employ developmental theory in research studies or in describing practice guidelines for various groups. For example, Seal and Seal (2011) used developmental theory as the basis for interventions to promote self-competence in children to enhance their health behaviors while at a summer camp. Nurses have commonly used developmental theory to improve nursing care among older adults. For example, Giblin (2011) discussed the importance of nurses supporting older adults in "successful aging"; Jonsén, Norberg, and Lundman (2015) used developmental theory to study "meaning in life" among the "oldest old people"; and Ehlman and Ligon (2012) used a model based on Erikson's generative process to research the developmental issue of generativity versus stagnation in older adults who shared their life stories.

In other examples, Bailey (2012) wrote about vulnerability of adolescent girls, and Morgan and Stevens (2012) used developmental theory to examine issues of identity among transgender adults. These examples demonstrate that developmental theory is used throughout the life continuum (i.e., children, adolescents, adults, and older adults) and is used in pediatric, psychiatric, geriatric, and medical-surgical nursing. Further review of these research studies suggests that both ego strengths and ego deficits are being examined by nurses.

Interpersonal Theory: Sullivan

Harry Stack Sullivan based his developmental theory on the premise that an individual does not, and cannot, exist apart from his or her relations with other people.

Overview

Sullivan stated that from the first day of life, a baby is dependent on interpersonal situations and that this dependence continues throughout the person's life. Even if the person becomes a recluse and withdraws from society, the person carries the memories of interpersonal relationships, which continue to influence behavior and thinking. Sullivan stated that it is a "relatively enduring pattern of recurrent interpersonal relationships which characterize a human life" (Sullivan, 1953, p. 111).

To explain this phenomenon, the term *dynamism* must be understood. Dynamism, as defined by Sullivan, is "the relatively enduring pattern of energy transformation which recurrently characterizes the organism in its duration as a living organism" (Sullivan, 1953, p. 105). The individual's dynamisms characterize interpersonal relations. Although all people have the same dynamisms, the mode of expression varies with the situation and life experience of the individual. Although most dynamisms satisfy the basic needs of the individual, an important dynamism develops as a result of anxiety; this is known as the dynamism of self or the self-system (Sullivan, 1953). Anxiety is a product of interpersonal relationships. Anxiety may produce a threat to the security of the self, thus causing the person to use various types of protective and behavioral control measures. This, in turn, reduces anxiety but may interfere with being able to live constructively with others (Sullivan, 1953).

Sullivan also described the concept of personification, which is the image that a person has of himself or herself. Personification is a combination of feelings, attitudes, and conceptions that grow out of experiences with need satisfaction and anxiety. If interpersonal experiences are rewarding, it is known as the "good me" personification. On the other hand, if interpersonal experiences are anxiety arousing, it is known as the "bad me" personification. A synonym for personification is self-concept; thus, the "good me" personification is a high self-concept, and the "bad me" personification is a low self-concept (Sullivan, 1953).

Sullivan viewed the individual as an energy or tension system. The goal of the tension system is to reduce anxiety. According to Sullivan, the two main sources of anxiety are the tensions that arise from the needs of the organism and tensions that result from anxiety (Sullivan, 1953).

Sullivan (1953) believed that "tensions can be regarded as needs for particular energy transformations that will dissipate the tension of awareness with an accompanying change of 'mental' state, a change of awareness" (p. 85). Anxiety is the experience of tension that results from real or imagined threats to one's security. High levels of anxiety produce a reduction in the efficacy of satisfying needs, disturbance of interpersonal relationships, and confusion in thinking. Thus, Sullivan hypothesized that an individual learns to behave in a certain way related to the resolution or exacerbation of tension (Sullivan, 1953).

Sullivan took his theory further and described the sequence of interpersonal events to which a person is exposed from infancy to adulthood and ways in which these situations contribute to the development of that individual. Besides the six stages of interpersonal development, Sullivan also developed a threefold classification system of cognitions: prototaxic, parataxic, and syntaxic. Although Sullivan formally rejected the importance of instinct with regard to development, he acknowledged the importance of heredity. Furthermore, he did not believe that personality is set at an early age but that it may change at any given time because new interpersonal situations arise and the human organism is malleable (Sullivan, 1953).

From Sullivan's theory, a new paradigm developed; this was the conception of participant–observer. Prior to this conception, the therapist observed only what was occurring. Now, the therapist becomes an active part of the treatment. Another concept developed from Sullivan's interpersonal theory was that the environment plays an important role in treatment, thus creating the concept of a therapeutic milieu (Sullivan, 1953).

Application to Nursing

Peplau (1952, 1963) built her nursing theory, Interpersonal Relations in Nursing, on Sullivan's theory, Interpersonal Theory of Psychiatry. Similarly, Orlando (1961) based her nursing theory on Peplau's theory and Sullivan's theory. Thus, it is clear that Sullivan's theory has been important to nursing.

From Sullivan's concept of degree of anxiety, Peplau developed the four levels of anxiety (mild, moderate, severe, and panic levels) that are the standards nurses use in assessing anxiety. Peplau believed that nurses play an important role in helping clients reduce their anxiety and in converting it into constructive action. Peplau also believed that the nurse's role is to help the client decrease insecurity and improve functioning through interpersonal relationships. These interpersonal relationships can be seen as microcosms of the way the person functions in his or her relationships (Thompson, 1986). This is very similar to Sullivan's concepts of the development of interpersonal relationships.

To educate the client and assist the person in gaining personal insight, Peplau (1963) elaborated on Sullivan's concept of participant–observer. According to her, nurses cannot be isolated from the therapeutic milieu if they want to be effective. Peplau's belief was that the nurse must interact with the client as a human being, with respect, empathy, and acceptance.

A major focus of Orlando's theory is client participation, which correlates with both Sullivan's and Peplau's concept of participant–observer. The formation, development, use, and termination of the nurse–client relationship is a phenomenon that is studied in nursing because it is a vital component of care and helps to determine the efficacy of treatment outcomes (Abraham, 2011; Boylston & O'Rourke, 2013; Dmytryshyn, Jack, Ballantyne, Wahoush, & MacMillan, 2015; Rasheed, 2015; Senn, 2013).

Another important concept of Sullivan's theory is the therapeutic milieu (i.e., a therapeutic environment). Almost all facilities today support the concept of a therapeutic environment that aids in facilitating patient interactions. The therapeutic milieu is an important component of nursing practice, especially in the psychiatric setting as discussed by Espinosa and colleagues (2015). This concept was mentioned by Zugai, Stein-Parbury, and Roche (2013) in a discussion of caring for adolescents with anorexia nervosa, by Southard and colleagues (2012) in relation to renovation of nursing stations in adult care psychiatric units, and by Paterson, McIntosh, Wilkinson, McComish, and Smith (2013) when discussing use of restraints in mental health care.

Sullivan also acknowledged the importance of heredity in development. Even though the heredity concept is a biologic perspective, psychologists, such as Sullivan, acknowledge the importance of heredity in personality development. In the case study, Tracy thought consideration of hereditable influences was important in working with Alan because Alan's father was an alcoholic.

Behavioral and Cognitive-Behavioral Theories

The psychodynamic theories grew from the beliefs that (1) personality is based on how the person develops, (2) development stops at a certain age, and (3) behaviors associated with development cannot be changed. In other words, a person's destiny is set at an early age. Finding these theories problematic, the behavioral theorists postulated that personality consists of learned behaviors. More explicitly, personality is synonymous with behavior, and if the behavior is changed, the personality is changed.

Initially, behavioral studies focused on human actions without much attention to the internal thinking processes. When the complexity of behaviors could not be accounted for by strictly behavioral explanations, a new component was added: a component of cognitions or thought processes. The cognitive approach is an outgrowth of behavioral and psychodynamic theories and attempts to link thought processes with behaviors. Cognitive-behavioral theory, then, focuses on thinking and behaving rather than on feelings.

One of the best known behavioral theorists is B. F. Skinner. Additional cognitive-behavioral theories discussed in this section are those proposed by Beck and Ellis.

Operant Conditioning: Skinner

Like Freud, Skinner believed that all behavior is determined, but the two have different theories regarding the origin of the behavior. Although Skinner followed the ideologies of Pavlov and Watson (two early behaviorists), he expanded the notion of stimulus–response behavioral approaches of learning to include the concept of reinforcement. The Pavlovian theory, basically a biologic theory, states that a stimulus elicits a response. Skinner took this theoretical principle further and applied it to the psychological sciences. He held that it is possible to predict and control the behaviors of others through a contingency of human reinforcers, and he expanded on Pavlovian thinking by adding motivation and reinforcement to the principles of learning (B. F. Skinner, 1969).

Operant Conditioning was the term coined by Skinner to label his theory. Operant Conditioning refers to the manipulation of selected reinforcers to elicit and strengthen desired behavioral reinforcers. According to Skinner, an individual performs a behavior (discharges an operant) and receives a consequence (reinforcer) as a result of performing the behavior. The consequence is either positive or negative, and the consequence will most likely determine whether the behavior will be repeated. Thus, although negative consequences have a deterrent effect on the behavior, positive consequences generally result in repetition of the behavior. Absence of reinforcement generally decreases the behavior. Skinner's premise was that reinforcement ultimately determines the existence of behavior (B. F. Skinner, 1969).

Skinner defined a reinforcer as anything that increases the occurrence of a behavior. It is important to note that the value of the reinforcer depends on its meaning to a particular individual, and the same reinforcer may have different effects on different people. According to Skinner, there are two types of reinforcers: primary and secondary. Primary reinforcers are important to survival (e.g., food, water, and sex), and secondary reinforcers are conditioned reinforcers (e.g., money, material goods, and praise) (B. F. Skinner, 1969).

Behaviors are generally multidimensional, and complex behaviors need to be broken down into smaller steps. This allows for the shaping of behavior, which consists of progressively reinforcing the smaller steps needed to achieve a certain behavior (B. F. Skinner, 1987).

Cognitive Theory: Beck

Aaron Beck based his cognitive theory on the work he did with depressed persons. He posited that biased cognitions are faulty, and he labeled these thoughts as *cognitive distortions*. Cognitive distortions are habitual errors in thinking that Beck stated are verbal or pictorial events that are formed in the conscious mind. When cognitions are distorted, an individual incorrectly interprets life events, jumps to inaccurate conclusions, and judges himself or herself too harshly. These distorted cognitions create a false basis for beliefs, particularly regarding the self, and influence one's basic attitude about the self. Thought distortions are the catalysts for how an individual perceives events in his or her life; they may keep the individual from reaching a desired goal. The process of changing cognitive distortions is called *cognitive restructuring* (Beck, 1976).

Although cognitive distortions are in the conscious mind, Beck believed that they are influenced by an automatic thinking schema that originates in the unconscious mind. The automatic thinking schemata are themes that have developed in childhood and have been reinforced throughout life. The automatic thinking schemata influence cognitions and can cause them to be faulty. Beck stated that an individual expresses illness through thoughts and attitudes. In other words, thoughts influence emotions, and behavior is controlled by thoughts. If thoughts are distorted, then illness occurs. To treat the illness, the cognitive distortions must be changed (Beck, 1976).

Rational Emotive Theory: Ellis

Another cognitive theorist was Albert Ellis, who described Rational Emotive Theory, which focuses on an interconnectedness between thoughts, feelings, and actions.

An individual will think and act based on his or her perception of life events. The underlying premise is that an individual has the cognitive ability to think, decide, analyze, and do and that he or she thinks either rationally or irrationally. The repetition of irrational thoughts reinforces dysfunctional beliefs, which, in turn, produce dysfunctional behaviors. These dysfunctional beliefs lead to self-defeating behaviors, and the person experiences self-blame. Ellis stated that the individual learns these self-defeating behaviors and that the individual is capable of understanding his or her limitations. Ellis further posited that if behaviors are learned, they can be unlearned. A person can change beliefs by changing thoughts and thinking rationally. If this occurs, then the behavior is changed (Ellis & MacLaren, 2005).

Application of Behavioral and Cognitive-Behavioral Theories to Nursing

The behavioral approach is a concrete method of monitoring or managing behavior. Nurses often use it with children or adolescents and people with chronic illness because it is often successful in changing targeted behaviors.

By combining behavioral theory with cognitive theory, the nurse can help alter behaviors by encouraging the individual to change irrational beliefs through problem solving. An individual who is ill may express feelings of worthlessness, anger, and self-blame. The nurse using a cognitive-behavioral approach can point out specific positive qualities of the individual. This helps reduce self-blame, and the person gradually begins to feel better about himself or herself because the belief system is changing. In essence, the nurse has changed behavior by presenting positive (secondary) reinforcement to the person, thus helping to change self-cognitions. This, in turn, changes the individual's belief system.

A cognitive-behavioral approach also helps the nurse point out the use of maladaptive defense mechanisms (e.g., projection). Projection is an unconscious process in which the individual can ascribe undesirable thoughts, impulses, ideas, and/or feelings to another person in order to externalize what he or she feels are unacceptable attributes or traits. Through projection, the individual is able to decrease anxiety and deal with the situation as a detached entity (Sadock, 2009).

People sometimes blame others for their problems. This is particularly true for those who are addicted to drugs and alcohol (like Alan); addicts frequently do not take responsibility for their substance use, misuse, and abuse. Using a cognitive approach, specifically Ellis's, the nurse teaches the person to take responsibility for his or her own behaviors. Whereas Ellis's approach is used more with substance abuse because of the confrontational approach, Beck's is used more with depressed persons because it focuses on an empathic approach. In the case study, Alan has a dual diagnosis of depression and substance abuse, and Tracy would most likely use a cognitive-behavioral approach in planning his nursing care.

In nursing, cognitive-behavioral therapies have been used to help manage multiple sclerosis (Askey-Jones, Shaw, & Silber, 2012) and to treat women with postpartum depression (Scope, Booth, & Sutcliffe, 2012). Furthermore, a cognitive-behavioral approach has been shown to be successful in helping direct care for patients with schizophrenia in both inpatient settings (Carter, 2015) and community-based settings (Hartigan & Ranger, 2014). Additionally, cognitive-behavioral therapies have also been used to treat anxiety in children and adolescents with asthma (Marriage & Henderson, 2012) and caregivers of patients with depression (McCann, Songprakun, & Stephenson, 2015).

Humanistic Theories

Humanistic theories developed in response to the psychoanalytic thought that a person's destiny was determined early in life. Proponents of humanistic psychology believed that Psychoanalytic Theories explicitly exclude human potential. In other words, there was no hope for a person. Humanistic theories emphasize a person's capacity for self-actualization; thus, they present a relatively hopeful and optimistic perspective about humans. Humanists believe that the person contains within himself or herself the potential for healthy and creative growth. The theories of Maslow and Rogers are discussed in the following sections on humanistic theories.

Human Needs Theory: Maslow

Abraham Maslow, known as the father of humanistic psychology, believed that psychology takes a pessimistic, negative, and limited conception of humans. He charged the discipline to examine human strengths and to stress human virtue instead of human frailties, and he proposed that human science should explore individuals who realize their full potential. Furthermore, he believed that the inner core of the person is the self, which is a unique individual who possesses both characteristics similar to others and characteristics uniquely distinct to the person (Maslow, 1968).

Overview

Motivation is the key to Maslow's theory because he assumed that instead of being passive, an individual is an active participant who strives for self-actualization. Maslow's theory is basically a hierarchy of dynamic processes that are critical for development and growth of the total person. There are six incremental stages of Maslow's theory: physiologic needs, safety needs, love and belonging needs, self-esteem needs, self-actualizing needs, and self-transcendent needs. The goal of Maslow's theory is to attain the sixth level or stage: self-transcendent needs (Maslow, 1968).

In Maslow's scheme, needs are divided into "D" motives and "B" motives. "D" motives are deficiency needs. This means that these needs are basic and have the greatest strength because they are essential to human survival. "D" motive needs must be satisfied for a person to turn his or her attention to the satisfaction of the higher level needs. These higher level needs are called "B" motive needs and include self-esteem and self-actualization. Such needs are reflective of growth potential (Maslow, 1968).

Until basic deficiency needs are met, the individual does not pursue personal growth needs to develop his or her fullest potential as a human being. Maslow postulated an optimistic assessment by focusing on the individual's strengths instead of personal deficits. According to Maslow (1968), when a person strives for personal growth, it leads the person to his or her fullest potential. In other words, it is the person at his or her best. This means that the person develops a problem-solving approach to life, identifies with humankind, and transcends the environment. The person is able to look realistically at life and make rational decisions; this brings about inner peace. When a person accomplishes this, Maslow referred to the person as being self-actualized. Box 14-1 lists characteristics of a self-actualized person. This philosophical perspective helps a person get in touch with who he or she is and what he or she can become (Maslow, 1968).

Box 14-1   Characteristics of a Self-Actualized Person

- Realistic orientation
- Spontaneity
- Acceptance of self
- Acceptance of others
- Close relationships with others
- Autonomous thinking
- Appreciation of life
- Reactivity to others
- Consideration of others
- Respect for others

Application to Nursing

Maslow's theory can be applied to nursing practice in three ways:

1. It allows the nurse to emphasize the person's strengths instead of focusing on the individual's deficits.
2. It focuses on human potential, thus giving the person hope.
3. It provides a blueprint for prioritizing client care according to a hierarchy of needs.

By focusing on a person's strengths, the nurse empowers the individual. In the case study, when Tracy began planning Alan's care, she followed Maslow's hierarchy by giving priority to his "D" needs (i.e., physical and safety needs that help the individual feel safe and secure). She helped him withdraw safely from the addictive substances and treated active symptoms of hepatitis C. She knew that his physical needs must be met before she could address the "B" needs (i.e., his potential for personal growth, self-esteem, and self-actualization).

Considerable nursing research has been done in humanistic psychology, largely using Maslow's theory. One research study, for example, focused on identifying the needs of hemodialysis patients in order to improve quality of life (Bayoumi, 2012), another studied the development of a fall risk assessment for hospitalized patients (Abraham, 2011), and a third evaluated concepts to enhance retention rates of registered nurses in South Africa (Mokoka, Ehlers, & Oosthuizen, 2011). Additionally, Liu, Aungsuroch, and Yunibhand (2016) used Maslow's theory to help define the concept of job satisfaction in nursing, and Olson (2015) also used Maslow's hierarchy to describe the motivating factors for nurses returning to school to enhance their education.

Person-Centered Theory: Rogers

Carl Rogers developed a person-centered model of psychotherapy that emphasizes the uniqueness of the individual.

Overview

Rogers believed that every individual has the potential to develop his or her talents to the maximum potential; he called this the *actualizing tendency*. Furthermore, each individual possesses everything that is needed for self-understanding and for changing attitude and behavior (Rogers, 1959).

Two constructs are fundamental to Rogers' theory: organism and the self. Organism is the locus of all experience. Experience includes the awareness of everything potentially available that is going on within the organism at any given time. This totality of experience constitutes the phenomenal field, which has several components. The first component is that an individual's frame of reference can only be known by that person. The second component is that a person's behavior depends on the phenomenal field and is not dependent on stimulating conditions. The third component of a phenomenal field is that it is made up of conscious and unconscious experiences (Rogers, 1959).

A portion of the phenomenal field gradually differentiates; this is known as the self or self-concept. Self or self-concept denotes the "organized, consistent conceptual gestalt composed of perceptions of the characteristics of 'I' or 'me' and the perceptions of the relationship of the 'I' or 'me' to others and to various aspects of life with the values attached to these perceptions" (Rogers, 1959, p. 200). In addition to the self, there is an ideal self, which is what the person would like to be (Rogers, 1959).

The basic significance of the structural concepts organism and self is directly related to congruence and incongruence. These terms represent the acceptance or nonacceptance of the organism with the self. Congruence is when the self accepts the organismic experience without threat or anxiety; thus, the person is able to think realistically. Incongruence between self and organism makes an individual feel threatened and anxious, thus causing defensiveness and constricted and rigid thinking. This results in behavioral problems (Rogers, 1959).

According to Rogers (1951), "Behavior is basically the goal-oriented attempt of the organism to satisfy its needs as experienced" (p. 491). Behaviors occur for the organism to maintain and enhance itself. Rogers believed that an individual has two learned needs, positive regard and self-regard. Rogers (1959) stated, "If an individual should experience only unconditional positive regard, then no conditions of worth would develop, self-regard would be unconditional, the needs for positive regard and self-regard would never be at variance with organismic evaluation, and the individual would continue to be psychologically adjusted, and would be fully functioning" (p. 224). This is not the case when an individual receives both positive and negative evaluations by others, causing an individual to learn to differentiate between actions and feelings that are worthy or unworthy.

Organism and self are subject to strong influences from the environment, especially from the social environment. Rogers did not provide a timetable of significant changes through which an individual passes; instead, he focused on ways in which evaluation of an individual by others tends to influence the experience of the organism and the experience of the self (Rogers, 1951).

Application to Nursing

The major contribution that Rogers added to nursing practice is the understanding that each client is a unique individual who is basically good, with an inherent potential for self-actualization. He introduced the concept of a person-centered approach, which is easily adapted to nursing. Not only does this approach view the individual as unique, but there is also equal collaboration between the nurse and the client in the individual's care.

Tracy followed Rogers' philosophy that each individual is unique. Even though Alan had characteristics that were similar to others, he was an individual who had characteristics that were unique to him. Tracy collaborated with Alan to develop his plan of care. This is important in all areas of nursing because clients need to feel they are special and unique and that they have a say in their care. Their input into their treatment will motivate them to accomplish their goals; thus, treatment outcomes will be enhanced.

Rogers also identified the conditions that are needed for an effective nurse–client relationship: unconditional positive regard, empathic understanding, and genuineness. An effective nurse–client relationship will help to facilitate change in the person and produce a positive outcome of treatment.

Stress Theories

Although the previous theories have dealt with the development of personality and mental illness, the stress theories deal with normal human functioning. Stress, adaptation, and coping are all natural parts of life. Stress is inevitable in everyone's life, and people must deal with stress by adapting through coping. The stress theories provide nursing with a framework to understand the effects that stress has on the individual and how the individual responds to stressful situations or life events. Although the ability to successfully adapt to stress leads to the equilibrium of the individual, the inability to adapt successfully leads to disequilibrium. The disequilibrium may result in physiologic or psychological disorders. The important thing to remember with stress theories is that stress is different for everyone. The following sections discuss Selye's General Adaptation Syndrome in relation to Peplau's Levels of Anxiety and Lazarus' Stress Coping Adaptation Theory.

General Adaptation Syndrome: Selye

Hans Selye pioneered research into stress and proposed the General Adaptation Syndrome (GAS). Because Selye defined stress as wear and tear on the body, the GAS explains the physiologic responses to stress. An explanation of the GAS is presented in Chapter 15, but it will be discussed here briefly because Selye's GAS is also presented in psychological literature.

The GAS has three stages: alarm, resistance, and exhaustion. The first stage is the alarm reaction. This stage mobilizes the body's defense forces and activates the fight-or-flight syndrome, which puts the body in a state of disequilibrium. The second stage is resistance and focuses on the body's physiologic responses to regain homeostasis. The final stage is exhaustion. In this stage, the body has exhausted all its resources and a diseased state can occur (Selye, 1956).

Selye concentrated on the physiologic changes in the body and did not elaborate on the psychological changes. Kneisl and Ames (1986) correlated the three levels of the GAS with Peplau's Levels of Anxiety. Table 14-2 compares the stages of Selye's GAS with Peplau's Levels of Anxiety. In the alarm stage, there is an increased level of alertness, and anxiety is found at levels 1 (mild) and 2 (moderate). The individual focuses on the immediate task, which is to reduce the stressor. If the threat is eliminated, the person has adapted successfully. If the threat is not effectively resolved, the individual advances to the next stage (Kneisl & Ames, 1986).

In the resistance stage, the individual experiences level 2 (moderate) or 3 (severe) of anxiety. This is the stage when the individual increases the use of coping mechanisms to adapt to the stressor. Psychosomatic symptoms may appear in this stage. If the individual is unable to adapt to the stressor, the individual becomes overwhelmed with the stressor and advances to the next stage (Kneisl & Ames, 1986).

Table 14-2 Selye's and Peplau's Anxiety States

Selye's Stages of the General Adaptation Syndrome	Peplau's Levels of Anxiety	Characteristics of Levels of Anxiety
Alarm alert	Level 1 (mild) Level 2 (moderate)	Increased alertness Increased awareness Increased efforts to reduce anxiety Narrowing of perceptual field Problem solving is present. Coping is increased.
Resistance	Level 2 (moderate) Level 3 (severe)	Feels threatened Feels overloaded Problem-solving difficulties Selective inattention Depressed Irritable Psychosomatic symptoms
Exhaustion	Level 3 (severe) Level 4 (panic)	Feels helpless Feelings of awe, dread, and terror Loss of control Personality disorganization Loss of rational thoughts Decreased ability to relate rationally to others Out of touch with reality Dissociation Disease process (physical and emotional)

The stage of exhaustion results when the stressor is not or cannot be neutralized. This occurs because the stress may have lasted too long, the person is totally overwhelmed by the stressor, or the individual's normal coping mechanisms have been exhausted. At this stage, the individual experiences anxiety at level 3 (severe) or 4 (panic) of Peplau's Levels of Anxiety. The person becomes dysfunctional, and a multitude of psychopathologic symptoms can occur: disorganized thinking, disorganized personality, delusions, hallucinations, stupor, or violence (Kneisl & Ames, 1986).

Stress, Coping, and Adaptation Theory: Lazarus

Lazarus' theory deals with how a person copes with stressful situations. Whereas Selye's focus is on the body's physiologic responses, Lazarus focused on the person's psychological responses. He viewed these responses as a process and stated that a process-oriented approach is directed toward what an individual actually thinks and does within the context of a specific encounter and includes how these thoughts and actions change as the encounter unfolds. "Coping, when considered as a process, is characterized by dynamics and changes that are functions of continuous appraisals and reappraisals of the shifting person environmental relationship" (Folkman & Lazarus, 1988, p. 3).

The two major factors that are precedents to stress are the person–environment relationship and appraisals. The person–environment relationship includes such factors as personality, values, beliefs, commitments, social networks, social supports, demands and constraints, sociocultural factors, and life events. The three cognitive appraisals are primary, secondary, and reappraisal. Primary appraisal refers to the judgment that an individual makes about a particular event or stressor. Secondary appraisal is the evaluation of how an individual responds to an event. Reappraisal is simply appraisal after new or additional information has been received (Lazarus & Folkman, 1984).

Lazarus posited that stress is much more complicated than just stimulus and response. He focused on the idea that coping is not due to anxiety itself but how the person perceives the threat. Lazarus identified this perception as an appraisal and explained that a person's evaluation of a stressor or events is classified as a cognitive appraisal. He defined stress as "a particular relationship between the person and the environment that is appraised by the person as taxing or exceeding his/her resources" (Lazarus & Folkman, 1984, p. 18).

To manage the demands and emotions generated by the appraised stress, coping occurs. Coping is the process by which a person manages the appraisal. The two types are problem-focused and emotion-focused coping. Problem-focused coping actually changes the person–environment relationship, and emotion-focused coping changes the meaning of the situation. Once the person has successfully coped with a situation, reappraisal occurs. Reappraisal allows for feedback about the outcome and allows for adjustment to new information (Lazarus & Folkman, 1984).

Successful coping results in adaptation. Adaptation is "the capacity of a person to survive and flourish" (Lazarus & Folkman, 1984, p. 182). Adaptation affects three important areas: health, psychological well-being, and social functioning. These three areas are interdependent, and when one area is affected, all three areas are affected. For example, if a person develops an illness, it can cause problems in work performance, which in turn elicits a negative self-concept.

Application of Stress Theories to Nursing

Stress and adaptation are the basis of Roy's Adaptation Model (Roy, 2009) and Neuman's System Model (Neuman & Fawcett, 2011). Roy (2009) stated that the goal of nursing is the promotion of adaptive responses through the mode of coping. Neuman's theory deals with a person's responses to stress (Neuman & Fawcett, 2011).

The application of stress theories to nursing is important. Indeed, they provide a framework for nurses to assess the effects of stress, both physical and psychological, on the individual and the coping processes that the individual uses. When assessing a client's stressors, it is important for the nurse to also consider the meaning of the stressor to the individual and the resources and support that the person has in coping with the stressors. The nurse can help with problem solving or cognitive restructuring to facilitate effective coping and adaptation. This can also lead to the development of new coping strategies for the individual.

Stress theories are very important in nursing practice, and nurses using them as research frameworks have done considerable research. For example, McMeekin, Hickman, Douglas, and Kelley (2017) utilized Lazarus and Folkman's theory to research stress and coping behaviors reported by critical care nurses after they experience unsuccessful cardiopulmonary resuscitations. The relationship between community financial hardship and the perception of stress in African American adolescents was examined by Brenner, Zimmerman, Bauermeister, and Caldwell (2013), and Molina, Beresford, Espinoza, and Thompson (2014) examined and compared coping behaviors among women from different ethnic groups following receipt of an abnormal mammogram. Finally, an experimental study was conducted by Padden, Connors, and Agazio (2011) on perceived stress and coping by female spouses during their husband's active military deployment, using Lazarus and Folkman's theory.

Social Psychology

Health professionals use many different models for understanding behavior change because it is a complex process. Furthermore, behavior change is often difficult to achieve and sustain. When health professionals attempt to encourage healthy behaviors, they are competing against powerful influences. These powerful influences involve social, psychological, and environmental conditioning. In order for change to occur, the benefits of behavior must be desired and perceived to be beneficial to the person. Although education is an important factor in facilitating change, information is frequently not enough. The benefits of behavior change must be compelling. When implementing change, a multilevel, interactive perspective clearly shows the advantages of incorporating behavioral and environmental components. Social psychology helps to predict health behavior and is widely used in health-promoting activities.

Three models that address behavior change are the Health Belief Model (HBM), the Theory of Reasoned Action/Theory of Planned Behavior, and the Transtheoretical Model (and Stages of Change) (TTM). The HBM addresses a person's perceptions of the threat of a health problem and the accompanying appraisal of a recommended behavior for preventing or managing the problem, which is manifested as a behavior. The Theory of Reasoned Action assumes that people are rational and make decisions based on the information available to them. The important determinant of a person's behavior is intent. The TTM describes principals of change to explain the processes employed by people as they change their health-related behaviors. Each of these theories will be discussed in more detail in the following sections. For more information, see Link to Practice 14-1.

Link to Practice 14-1

Recently, a team headed by Plotnikoff (Plotnikoff, Costigan, Karunamuni, & Lubans, 2013) conducted a systematic literature review examining how several social cognitive theories—specifically the Health Belief Model, Theory of Planned Behavior, Protection Motivation Theory, Social Cognitive Theory/Self-Efficacy Theory, Transtheoretical Model, and Health Promotion Model—explained physical activity intention and behaviors in adolescents. Meta-analysis of the published research describing how these theories were supported (or not) revealed that the theories/models were more effective in explaining intention than behavior. The researchers concluded that very few studies have actually tested the predictive capacity of social cognitive theories for adolescent behavior related to physical activity and that more specific theoretical research is needed on these theories.

Based on these findings, what evidence-based interventions might nurses propose using the Health Belief Model to promote physical activity in this cohort? Using the Theory of Planned Behavior? Using the Transtheoretical Model? Social Cognitive Theory (see Chapter 13)? The Health Promotion Model (see Chapter 11)? Which theory might be best for explaining/researching/enhancing intention? Which might be best for explaining/researching/enhancing behavior?

Plotnikoff, R. C., Costigan, S. A., Karunamuni, N., & Lubans, D. R. (2013). Social cognitive theories used to explain physical activity behavior in adolescents: A systematic review and meta-analysis. *Preventive Medicine, 56*(5), 245–253.

Health Belief Model

The HBM was one of the first models that adapted theories from the behavioral sciences to predict health behaviors. This was done by focusing on the attitudes and beliefs of individuals. The HBM was originally developed in the 1950s by a group of social psychologists working for the U.S. Public Health Service who wanted to improve the public's use of preventive services (Rosenstock, 1974). Their assumption was that people fear disease and that health actions were motivated in relation to the degree of the fear and the benefits obtained. The HBM explained health behavior in terms of several constructs: perceived susceptibility of the health problem, perceived severity, perceived benefits, perceived barriers, and cues to action (Rosenstock, 1990).

Perceived susceptibility refers to one's opinion of chances of getting a condition, whereas perceived severity is one's opinion of how serious a condition and its sequelae are. One's opinion of the efficacy of the advised action to reduce risk or seriousness of impact is known as perceived benefits. Perceived barriers are one's opinion of the tangible and psychological cost of the advised action (Rosenstock, 1974). These four concepts were proposed as accounting for people's readiness to action. Thus, another concept was identified as "cues to action." These cues to action would activate the readiness to act and stimulate overt behaviors (Rosenstock, 1990; C. S. Skinner, Tiro, & Champion, 2015) (Figure 14-1).

In 1988, Rosenstock added another concept to the HBM, which he identified as self-efficacy. Self-efficacy is one's confidence in the ability to successfully perform an action. This concept was used to help the HBM better fit the challenges of changing habitual, unhealthy behaviors such as smoking, overeating, and being sedentary (C. S. Skinner et al., 2015). Table 14-3 summarizes the major concepts of the HBM.

Theory of Reasoned Action (Theory of Planned Behavior)

The Theory of Reasoned Action (TRA) was initially developed in the late 1960s by social psychologists Icek Ajzen and Martin Fishbein (Fishbein & Ajzen, 1975). The TRA explains the relationship among beliefs, attitudes, intentions, and behavior. It assumes that people are rational and make decisions based on the information available to them. The goal of the TRA, therefore, is to understand and predict behaviors that are largely under the individual's control (Poss, 2001). The TRA was later modified to the Theory of Planned Behavior (TPB) (Montano & Kasprzyk, 2015).

According to the TPB, the most important determinant of a person's behavior(s) is intention. Intention is the cognitive representation of the individual's readiness to perform a behavior and is determined by (1) attitude toward the behavior, (2) subjective norms, and (3) perceived behavioral control.

Attitude, or behavioral beliefs, refers to the individual's positive or negative evaluation of performing the behavior; it is concerned with his or her beliefs about the consequences of performing the behavior. Attitude has been viewed as a combination of feelings, beliefs, intentions, and perceptions. Combined with knowledge, these factors analyze the acceptability of performing a behavior in relation to a bipolar scale of positive/negative or yes/no. The determinant of attitude component is called "salient belief." A person's attitude toward a behavior can be predicted by multiplying the evaluation of each of the behavior's consequences by the strength of the belief. Beliefs are formed about an issue/object by associating it with all kinds of characteristics, qualities, and attributes. This leads to the development of an attitude (Ajzen & Fishbein, 1980).

Subjective norm, or normative beliefs, is seen as the social pressure upon a person to perform or not to perform a behavior. In deciding whether to perform an action

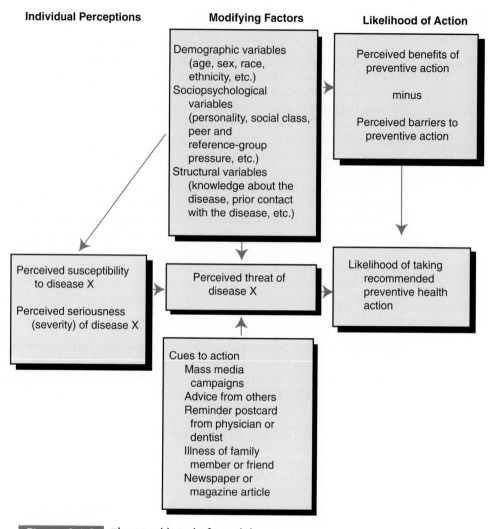

Figure 14-1   The Health Belief Model.

(From Becker, M. H., Haefner, D. P., Kasl, S. V., Kirscht, J. P., Maiman, L. A., & Rosenstock, I. M. [1977]. Selected psychosocial models and correlates of individual health-related behaviors. *Medical Care, 15,* 27–46, with permission.)

or behavior, an individual may consider what his or her parents, friends, or others will think about the behavior as well as how important it is to comply with the wishes of others. It involves both one's beliefs about the opinions of others and the person's motivation to conform to the wishes of those others. Thus, people often behave as they believe others expect them to behave.

Control beliefs, or perceived behavioral control, refer to the perceived power of factors that may facilitate or impede the behavior. In general, the more favorable the attitude and subjective norm, the greater the perceived control and the stronger would be the person's intention to perform the behavior. According to the TPB, behavioral intention is the most immediate determinant of any social behavior but only under conditions where the behavior in question is under volitional control.

The TPB proposes that an individual's intention is determined in turn by his or her attitude and subjective norm regarding the performance of the behavior.

Table 14-3 Health Belief Model Concepts

Concept	Definition	Examples
Perceived susceptibility	Subjective risk of contracting a condition; belief or opinion regarding chances of acquiring a health problem or threat	Does a teenage girl believe she will get pregnant during a single sexual encounter? Does an elderly man believe he will get the flu this winter? Does a middle-aged woman with a strong family history of breast cancer believe that she is vulnerable?
Perceived severity	Concern related to the seriousness of a health condition and understanding of potential difficulties the condition might cause; belief or perception of seriousness or consequences of a health threat or condition	A teenage girl believes that pregnancy would change her life dramatically. An elderly man understands that pneumonia is a potential complication of the flu. A middle-aged woman knows her grandmother died of breast cancer.
Perceived benefits	Beliefs related to the effectiveness of preventive actions; opinion that changing behavior(s) may reduce the treat	The teenage girl knows that using contraception will dramatically reduce the chances of a pregnancy. The elderly man believes that flu shots are effective in preventing illness. The middle-aged woman recognizes that yearly mammograms are effective in reducing deaths from breast cancer.
Perceived barriers	Perception of the obstacles to changing behavior; opinion related to tangible and/or psychological costs of action	The teenage girl may be embarrassed about going to a clinic to obtain contraceptives. The elderly man may not have transportation to take him to the clinic to receive a flu shot. The middle-aged woman's insurance does not cover the cost of mammograms.
Cues to action	A stimulus (external or internal) that triggers health-related behaviors; something that makes the individual aware of a health threat	The teenage girl attends a school-sponsored program on problems encountered by teenage mothers. The elderly man sees a posted flyer that a mobile van will be nearby the following week to provide free flu shots. The middle-aged woman learns from a public service radio ad that low-cost mammography is available at a nearby hospital.
Self-efficacy	Belief that one has the ability to change one's behaviors; recognition that personal health practices and choices can positively influence health	The teenage girl decides to postpone intercourse. The elderly man attends the shot clinic provided by the mobile van. The middle-aged woman makes an appointment for a mammogram.

Furthermore, attitude to the behavior is accounted for by beliefs about the outcomes of the behavior and evaluations of those outcomes. Subjective norm is determined by perceived pressure from specified significant others to carry out the behavior and motivation to comply with the wishes of significant others. Figure 14-2 depicts the components of the TPB.

Transtheoretical Model and Stages of Change

The TTM reportedly developed from an analysis of 25 theories of psychotherapy to describe the processes involved in how people make changes with regard to health-related behaviors (Prochaska, 1979). Initially building on the works of Freud, Skinner, and Rogers to focus on the processes of quitting smoking, DiClemente and Prochaska

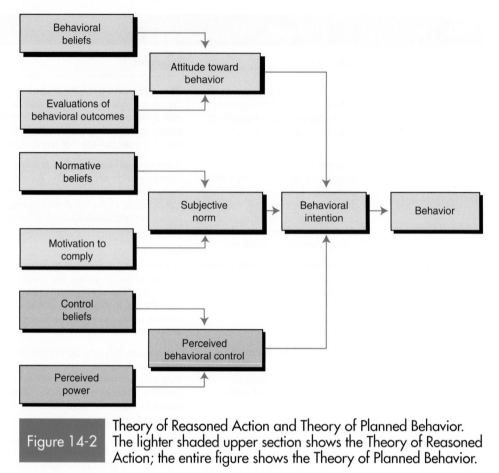

Figure 14-2   Theory of Reasoned Action and Theory of Planned Behavior. The lighter shaded upper section shows the Theory of Reasoned Action; the entire figure shows the Theory of Planned Behavior.

(From Ajzen, I., & Fishbein, M. [1980]. *Understanding attitudes and predicting social behavior* [p. 8]. Englewood Cliffs, NJ: Prentice Hall. Reproduced by permission of Pearson Education, Inc.)

(1982) determined that behavior change "unfolds through a series of stages," which involves different change processes at each stage. Their work quickly evolved from studies on smoking, and the TTM has been applied to many other health risks, behaviors, and problems such as substance abuse, depression, high-fat diets, mammography, pregnancy prevention, and sun exposure (Prochaska, Redding, & Evers, 2015).

At its core, the TTM focuses on the six "Stages of Change" (Box 14-2) (Prochaska et al., 2015). The stages are not necessarily linear; rather, change is seen as fluid or

Box 14-2   Transtheoretical Model's Stages of Change

- Precontemplation
- Contemplation
- Preparation
- Action
- Maintenance
- Termination

Source: Prochaska et al. (2015).

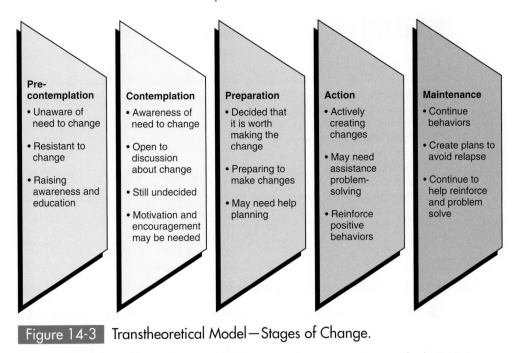

Pre-contemplation

- Unaware of need to change
- Resistant to change
- Raising awareness and education

Contemplation

- Awareness of need to change
- Open to discussion about change
- Still undecided
- Motivation and encouragement may be needed

Preparation

- Decided that it is worth making the change
- Preparing to make changes
- May need help planning

Action

- Actively creating changes
- May need assistance problem-solving
- Reinforce positive behaviors

Maintenance

- Continue behaviors
- Create plans to avoid relapse
- Continue to help reinforce and problem solve

Figure 14-3   Transtheoretical Model—Stages of Change.

(From American College of Sports Medicine. *ACSM's Resources for the Personal Trainer.* 4th ed., © 2013. Reprinted with permission from Lippincott Williams & Wilkins.)

dynamic and occurs through the unfolding of the processes over a period of time. Furthermore, "relapse" can occur at any stage, moving the individual back. Characteristics of each stage are depicted in Figure 14-3.

In the precontemplation stage, the individual does not anticipate immediate change; the person may not yet be motivated or they might not have enough information to determine a need to change. In the contemplation stage, individuals are aware of pros and cons of changing behaviors and will examine the balance between the costs and benefits of change. Sometimes, they will be stuck in chronic contemplation (behavioral procrastination) (Prochaska et al., 2015).

In the preparation stage, the individual is ready to make a change, and action is anticipated within in the next month (Prochaska et al., 2015). In the action stage, the individual has made lifestyle modifications and his or her actions are observable. In the maintenance stage, they have been able to sustain the action or changes, and the individual is working to prevent relapse. Maintenance lasts from 6 months to about 5 years, depending on the behavior being changed. Finally, in termination, individuals identify no temptation to relapse and report "self-efficacy" to maintain the behavior changes.

In addition to the Stages of Change, the TTM consists of 10 "Processes of Change" (Box 14-3). These are activities used to progress through the Stages of Change. Other key constructs are "decisional balance" and "self-efficacy." The integration of the "Processes" and "Stages" of change suggest that in the early stages (precontemplation/contemplation), individuals will experience the cognitive, affective, and evaluative processes of "consciousness raising," "dramatic relief," and "environmental reevaluation." In the action stages, individuals "draw more on commitments, conditioning, contingencies, environmental controls and support for progressing toward maintenance or termination" (Prochaska et al., 2015, p. 132). To enhance success in developing and implementing activities or interventions to promote positive change, Prochaska and colleagues (2015) recommend matching the stages and the processes and incorporating the elements of decisional balance and self-efficacy.

Box 14-3   Transtheoretical Model's Processes of Change

- Consciousness raising
- Dramatic relief
- Self-reevaluation
- Environmental reevaluation
- Self-liberation
- Helping relationships
- Social liberation
- Counterconditioning
- Stimulus control
- Reinforcement management

Source: Prochaska et al. (2015).

Application of Social Psychology Theories to Nursing

The application of social psychology theories in nursing typically relates to the area of health promotion. Nurses can propose strategies and develop programs to make people aware of health problems. They can then implement these programs using the social psychology theories to change unhealthy behaviors to healthy behaviors. That is the reason that nurses must advocate health promotion for patients using a multidimensional approach: organizational change efforts, policy development, economic supports, and environmental change. In today's society, disseminating the message is much easier. It can be delivered through printed educational material, electronic mass media, or directly in one-to-one counseling (Glanz, Rimer, & Viswanath, 2015). Social psychology theories are useful in promoting healthy behaviors, and nurses should be challenged to use them to make people aware of health problems and to propose positive behavioral change.

In the case study, Tracy might use a social psychology theory, such as the TPB, to examine factors that might influence Alan's intention to change his behavior. For example: What is Alan's attitude toward stopping drinking? What is his understanding of his family's attitudes and beliefs related to his alcohol use? What does he perceive as his level of control over his behavior? Examining each of these areas can help Tracy predict Alan's intention to change and, ultimately, his behavior relative to alcohol use and abuse.

As mentioned, the HBM was developed to help explain health-related behaviors. Besides being a guide to help identify leverage points for change, it can also be a useful framework for designing change strategies. Indeed, its use in nursing research and practice has been notable. During the last decade, more than 130 articles have been published in the nursing literature employing or testing the HBM.

For example, in classic application of the HBM, Dardis, Koharchik, and Dukes (2015) used the theory to develop an educational strategy to improve vaccination rates for pertussis among adults teaching in a preschool, and Adams, Hall, and Fulghum (2014) focused on cues to action and perceptions of severity and susceptibility to study vaccine acceptance among patients on hemodialysis. In other examples, Wu and Lin (2015) used the HBM to develop an intervention to improve adherence to mammography recommendations among Chinese American women, and Kvamme and Costanzo (2015) used the HBM as a guide to develop strategies to help prevent postthrombotic syndrome among inpatients with deep vein thrombosis. Numerous other works describing application of the HBM (e.g., Brown, Patrician, & Brosch, 2012; Davis, Buchanan, & Green, 2013; Klotzbaugh & Spencer, 2015) can be found in the nursing literature.

The TRA/TPB, likewise, has been used frequently in nursing studies. Review of the literature indicated scores of citations in recent nursing journals. Research examining the beliefs, attitudes, and intentions of health care providers was identified covering various topics. For example, Knowles and colleagues (2015) examined knowledge attitudes, beliefs, and intentions of intensive care unit (ICU) staff to implement bowel protocols; Youngcharoen and colleagues (2016) looked at nurses' beliefs attitudes, perceived norms, perceived control, and behavior intentions related to pain management among older adults with postoperative pain, and Bennett (2016) examined nurses' beliefs, behaviors, and perceived control in a study of behavior intentions for care of patients at the end of life.

Other researchers have used the TRA to look at health behaviors in diverse areas, including intention to care for patient with alcohol dependence (Talbot, Dorrian, & Chapman, 2015), intention to understand perceptions and beliefs of college students related to waterpipe smoking (Noonan, 2013), and intention to assess application of mobile technology in undergraduate nursing education (Mann, Medves, & Vanderkerkhof, 2015)

Similarly, the TTM has been widely used in nursing research studies and practice. In one example, a team led by Kamau-Small (Kamau-Small, Joyce, Bermingham, Roberts, & Robbins, 2015) used the Stages of Change as one element of an educational workshop to promote "cultural humility and care equity" (p. 169) among undergraduate nursing students; their intent was to promote behavior change related to cultural differences in clinical practice for public health nursing providers. Also targeting nursing students, Anderson and colleagues (2017) reported on a project using undergraduate students to help "super utilizers" of the emergency department (ED) access appropriate health care resources. The goal for the nursing students was to apply the TTM to promote behavior change among those clients using the ED for nonemergent health issues. Other examples using the TTM as a framework from the nursing literature were efforts to prevent cardiovascular disease using behavior modification (Farrell & Keeping-Burke, 2014), improving self-management for persons with chronic kidney disease (Vann et al., 2015), and interventions to improve exercise behavior among patients with coronary heart disease (Zhu, Ho, Sit, & He, 2014).

Finally, several examples were identified that used two or more of the social psychology theories or compared them. In one example, Barley and Lawson (2016) discussed the importance of using health psychology theories including the HBM, TTM, and TPB to help promote positive behavior changes and to develop and compare research. In other works, Othman, Kiviniemi, Wu, and Lally (2012) used both the HBM and the TRA as the conceptual framework for their study of how demographic factors, knowledge, and beliefs influence women's intention to undergo mammography screening, and Leach, Tonkin, Lancastle, and Kirk (2016) used both the TTM and the TPB as a framework of a strategy to enhance implementation of genomics into nursing practice. Lastly, Plotnikoff, Costigan, Karunamuni, and Lubans (2013) performed a systematic review of application of a number of social behavior theories including the TTM, HBM, and TRM to explain physical activity behaviors in adolescents (see Link to Practice 14-1).

Summary

This chapter has presented five families of theories that attempt to explain human behavior. Although each theory emphasizes a different concept or viewpoint, no one theory best explains the complexity of human behavior. The psychodynamic theories attempt to explain an individual's behavior in terms related to the development of the self that is formed by adulthood. The behavioral theorists believe that behavior is learned by reinforcement, whereas the cognitive theorists believe that the reinforcements are related to an individual's thought patterns.

Humanistic theories propose that individuals have within themselves the capacity to change. This potential for healthy and creative growth occurs throughout the individual's life span; thus, the behavior of an individual is a dynamic process. The stress-adaptation theories are associated with behaviors identified with the way a person adapts to stress through individual coping mechanisms. Finally, the social psychology theories look at how a person changes and explores ways to incorporate change through the promotion of health. Table 14-4 offers a brief comparison of these theories.

Tracy, in the opening case scenario, understands the complexity of humans and that using a single theory will not fully explain all of the variables that are associated with

Table 14-4 Comparison of Behavioral Theories

Theory	Theorist	Emphasis	Key Concepts
Psychodynamic	Freud	The study of unconscious mental processes of the psychodynamics of behavior	Personality structure: id, ego, superego; libido, pleasure principle, reality principle, instincts, stages of psychosexual development
	Erikson	Psychosocial factors that influence development	Id, ego, superego; conscious, preconscious, unconscious; developmental tasks; eight stages of biopsychosocial development
	Sullivan	Interpersonal experiences that influence development	Self-system, anxiety, security operations, personifications, modes of experience; stages of interpersonal growth and development
Cognitive-behavioral	Skinner	Analysis of human behavior observed in the current situation	Operant Conditioning; positive and negative reinforcement
	Beck	Cognitive distortions	Arbitrary inference, overgeneralization, selective abstraction, magnification and minimization, underlying assumptions, entitlement, perfection, automatic thoughts
	Ellis	The values and assumptions that govern much of people's lives	ABC theory of Rational Emotive Theory
Humanistic	Maslow	Fulfilling human potential	Hierarchy of needs; self-actualization
	Rogers	Person-centered	Organism and the self; congruence and incongruence; positive regard and self-regard
Stress-adaptation	Selye	Analysis of stress at the physiologic and biochemical levels of functioning	Stressor, General Adaptation Syndrome, alarm reaction, stages of resistance, stages of exhaustion
	Lazarus	Cognitive model of stress	Appraisal, coping, outcome
Social psychology	Rosenstock	Perceived threat and net benefits	Perceived susceptibility, perceived severity, perceived benefits, perceived barriers, cues of action, self-efficacy
	Ajzen and Fishbein	People make rational decisions based on the information they have.	Intent, attitude, subjective norms
	Prochaska	People go through several stages to make changes in health behaviors.	Stages of Change, processes of change, decisional balance; self-efficacy

behavior and its impact on health. Therefore, most nurses adopt an eclectic approach to theory utilization in providing care. This means that the nurse chooses concepts from various theories that best explain the behaviors of the person. Due to the interrelatedness of the concepts in the theories (e.g., the self, anxiety, hope, development, cognitions, reinforcements, empowerment, health promotion), concepts from multiple theories can be used. The concepts from the various theories chosen for the individual will depend on the patient's particular behavior, needs, or problems. By knowing how behavior is formed, the nurse can better plan effective care to change behaviors to improve health.

Key Points

- Theories from behavioral sciences are very widely used by nurses in practice and research.
- Psychodynamic theories and theories that focus on development stages that are studied and used by nurses include the works of Freud, Erikson, and Sullivan.
- Commonly used behavior and cognitive-behavioral theories include the works of Skinner, Beck, and Ellis.
- Human needs theories (e.g., Maslow and Rogers) and stress theories (e.g., Selye and Lazarus) are among the most commonly applied behavioral theories in nursing practice.
- The Health Belief Model, the Theory of Reasoned Action (Theory of Planned Behavior), and the Transtheoretical Model are social psychology theories widely used by nurse researchers.

Learning Activities

1. Consider the case of a school nurse who is working with a 14-year-old student suspected of being addicted to alcohol. Discuss with classmates what concepts from the various theories described could be used in planning nursing interventions. Using the theories from social psychology, how could the nurse set up a health-promotion campaign for a teenage drug and alcohol program?
2. Consider the following case: A 30-year-old woman arrives in the emergency department. She is diagnosed with a drug overdose. Assessment data reveal the following information: she has three children (18 months, 4 years old, and 14 years old); she is in the process of her second divorce; she took 25 diazepam (Valium) tablets (2 mg/tablet), which her doctor had given her for stress; she is unemployed; and she did not graduate from high school. Which theory (or theories) should be used to direct her care? What concepts from other theories could be used to enhance her care?
3. Consider the following case: A 65-year-old woman is being admitted for a mastectomy due to cancer. She expresses fear and depression during the nursing assessment. What concepts from the various theories could be used in planning her care? How might her care be changed if the woman were 25 years old or 45 years old? How have the social psychology theories been used in promoting breast cancer awareness?
4. Consider the following case: A 52-year-old man is admitted to the hospital for hypertension for the third time in the past year. Each time, he stopped taking his medications because he was "feeling good." What concepts from the various theories could be used to change his behavior? How could the nurse set up a health-promotion program for managing hypertension in the hospital? In the community?

REFERENCES

Abraham, S. (2011). Fall prevention conceptual framework. *The Health Care Manager, 30*(2), 179–184.

Adams, A., Hall, M., & Fulghum, J. (2014). Utilizing the health belief model to assess vaccine acceptance of patients on hemodialysis. *Nephrology Nursing Journal, 41*(4), 393–406.

Ajzen, I., & Fishbein, M. (1980). *Understanding attitudes and predicting social behavior.* Englewood Cliffs, NJ: Prentice Hall.

Anderson, D., Patch, E., Oxandale, B., Kincade, A., Gamber, A., & Ohm, R. (2017) Nursing student coaches for emergency department super utilizers. *The Journal of Nursing Education, 56*(1), 27–30.

Askey-Jones, S., Shaw, P., & Silber, E. (2012). Working together: Multiple sclerosis and mental health nurses. *British Journal of Neuroscience Nursing, 7*(6), 696–703.

Bailey, L. D. (2012). Adolescent girls: A vulnerable population. *Advances in Neonatal Care, 12*(2), 102–106.

Barley, E., & Lawson, V. (2016). Using health psychology to help patients: Theories of behaviour change. *British Journal of Nursing, 25*(16), 924–927.

Bayoumi, M. (2012). Identification of the needs of haemodialysis patients using the concept of Maslow's hierarchy of needs. *Journal of Renal Care, 38*(1), 43–49.

Beck, A. T. (1976). *Cognitive therapy and the emotional disorders.* New York, NY: International University Press.

Bennett, M. (2016). Nursing care at the end of life: 25 Years after the passage of the Patient Self-Determination Act. *Journal of Hospice & Palliative Nursing, 18*(6), 550–560.

Bjorklund, P. (2000). Assessing ego strength: Spinning straw into gold. *Perspectives in Psychiatric Care, 36*(1), 14–23.

Boylston, M. T., & O'Rourke, R. (2013). Second-degree bachelor of science in nursing students' preconceived attitudes toward the homeless and poor: A pilot study. *Journal of Professional Nursing, 29*(5), 309–317.

Brenner, A., Zimmerman, M., Bauermeister, J., & Caldwell, C. (2013). Neighborhood context and perceptions of stress over time: An ecological model of neighborhood stressors and intrapersonal and interpersonal resources. *American Journal of Community Psychology, 51*(3–4), 544–556. doi:10.1007/s10464-013-9571-9

Brown, C. G., Patrician, P. A., & Brosch, L. R. (2012). Increasing testicular self-examination in active duty soldiers: An intervention study. *Medsurg Nursing, 21*(2), 97–102.

Carter, R. (2015). Delivering cognitive behavior therapy in a secure setting. *Mental Health Practice, 19*(3), 23–30.

Dardis, M. R., Koharchik, L. S., & Dukes, D. (2015). Using the health belief model to develop educational strategies to improve pertussis vaccination rates among preschool staff. *NASN School Nurse, 30*(1), 20–25.

Davis, J., Buchanan, K., & Green, B. (2013). Racial/ethnic differences in cancer prevention beliefs: Applying the health belief model framework. *American Journal of Health Promotion, 27*(6), 384–389. doi:10.4278/ajhp.120113-QUAN-15

DiClemente, C. C., & Prochaska, J. O. (1982). Self-change and therapy change of smoking behavior: A comparison of processes of change in cessation and maintenance. *Addictive Behaviors, 7*(2), 133–142.

Dmytryshyn, A. L., Jack, S. M., Ballantyne, M., Wahoush, O., & MacMillan, H. L. (2015). Long-term home visiting with vulnerable young mothers: An interpretive description of the impact on public health nurses. *BMC Nursing, 14*(1), 12.

Ehlman, K., & Ligon, M. (2012). The application of a generativity model for older adults. *International Journal of Aging & Human Development, 74*(4), 331–344.

Ellis, A., & MacLaren, C. (2005). *Rational emotive behavior therapy: A therapist's guide* (2nd ed.). Atascadero, CA: Impact.

Erikson, E. H. (1963). *Childhood and society.* New York, NY: Norton.

Erikson, E. H. (1968). *Identity: Youth and crisis.* New York, NY: Norton.

Erikson, E. H. (1975). *Life history and the historical movement.* New York, NY: Norton.

Espinosa, L., Harris, B., Frank, J., Armstrong-Muth, J., Brous, E., Moran, J., et al. (2015). Milieu improvement in psychiatry using evidence-based practices: The long and winding road of culture change. *Archives of Psychiatric Nursing, 29*(4), 202–207.

Farrell, T. C., & Keeping-Burke, L. (2014). The primary prevention of cardiovascular disease: Nurse practitioners using behavior modification strategies. *Canadian Journal of Cardiovascular Nursing, 24*(1), 8–15.

Fishbein, M., & Ajzen, I. (1975). *Belief, attitude, intention and behavior: An introduction to theory and research.* Reading, MA: Addison-Wesley.

Folkman, S., & Lazarus, R. S. (1988). *Manual for the ways of coping questionnaire.* Palo Alto, CA: Consulting Psychologists Press.

Folta, J. R. (1968). Conference on the nature of science and nursing. Perspectives of an applied scientist. *Nursing Research, 17*(6), 502–507.

Freud, S. (1953). Three essays on the theory of sexuality. In J. Strachey (Ed. & Trans.), *The standard edition of the complete psychological works of Sigmund Freud* (Vol. 7, pp. 125–243). London, United Kingdom: Hogarth Press. (Original work published 1905)

Freud, S. (1959). Inhibitions, symptoms, and anxiety. In J. Strachey (Ed. & Trans.), *The standard edition of the complete psychological works of Sigmund Freud* (Vol. 20, pp. 75–175). London, United Kingdom: Hogarth Press. (Original work published 1926)

Freud, S. (1960). The ego and the id (J. Strachey, Ed. & Trans.), *The standard edition of the complete psychological works of Sigmund Freud* (Vol. 19, pp. 3–68). London, United Kingdom: Hogarth Press. (Original work published 1923)

Giblin, J. C. (2011). Successful aging: Choosing wisdom over despair. *Journal of Psychosocial Nursing and Mental Health Services, 49*(3), 23–26.

Glanz, K., Rimer, B. K., & Viswanath, K. (2015). *Health behavior: Theory, research, and practice* (5th ed.). San Francisco, CA: Jossey-Bass.

Hall, C. S., & Lindzey, G. (1978). *Theories of personality.* New York, NY: Wiley.

Hartigan, N., & Ranger, G. (2014). Cognitive behavior therapy for schizophrenia in a community mental health team. *Mental Health Practice, 18*(3), 22–28.

Johnson, D. E. (1959). The nature of a science in nursing. *Nursing Outlook, 7*(5), 291–294.

Johnson, D. E. (1968). Symposium on theory development in nursing. Theory in nursing: Borrowed and unique. *Nursing Research, 17*(3), 206–209.

Jonsén, E., Norberg, A., & Lundman, B. (2015). Sense of meaning in life among the oldest old people living in a rural area in norther Sweden. *International Journal of Older People Nursing, 10*(3), 221–229.

Kamau-Small, S., Joyce, B., Bermingham, N., Roberts, J., & Robbins, C. (2015). The impact of the care equity project with community/public health nursing students. *Public Health Nursing, 32*(2), 169–176.

Klotzbaugh, R., & Spencer, G. (2015). Cues-to-action in initiating lesbian, gay, bisexual, and transgender-related policies among Magnet hospital chief nursing officers: A demographic assessment. *ANS. Advances in Nursing Science, 38*(2), 110–120.

Kneisl, C. R., & Ames, S. W. (1986). *Adult health nursing: A biopsychosocial approach.* Menlo Park, CA: Addison-Wesley.

Knowles, S., Lam, L. T., McInnes, E., Elliott, D., Hardy, J. & Middleton, S. (2015). Knowledge, attitudes, beliefs and behaviour intentions for three bowel management practices in intensive care: Effects of a targeted protocol implementation for nursing and medical staff. *BMC Nursing, 14*, 6.

Kvamme, A. M., & Costanzo, C. (2015). Preventing progression of post-thrombotic syndrome for patients post-deep vein thrombosis. *Medsurg Nursing, 24*(1), 27–34.

Lazarus, R. S., & Folkman, S. (1984). *Stress, appraisal, and coping.* New York, NY: Springer Publishing.

Leach, V., Tonkin, E., Lancastle, D., & Kirk, M. (2016). A strategy for implementing genomics into nursing practice informed by three behaviour change theories. *International Journal of Nursing Practice, 22*(3), 307–315.

Liu, Y., Aungsuroch, Y., & Yunibhand, J. (2016). Job satisfaction in nursing: A concept analysis study. *International Nursing Review, 63*(1), 84–91.

Mann, E. G., Medves, J., & Vanderkerkhof, E. G. (2015). Accessing best practice resources using mobile technology in an undergraduate nursing program: A feasibility study. *CIN: Computers, Informatics, Nursing, 33*(3), 122–128.

Marriage, D., & Henderson, J. (2012). Cognitive behaviour therapy for anxiety in children with asthma. *Nursing Children and Young People, 24*(9), 30–34.

Maslow, A. H. (1968). *Toward a psychology of being* (2nd ed.). Princeton, NJ: Van Nostrand.

McCann, T. V., Songprakun, W., & Stephenson, J. (2015). A randomized controlled trial of guided self-help for improving the experience of caring for carers of clients with depression. *Journal of Advanced Nursing, 71*(7), 1600–1610.

McMeekin, D. E., Hickman, R. L., Jr., Douglas, S. L., & Kelley, C. G. (2017). Stress and coping of critical care nurses after unsuccessful cardiopulmonary resuscitation. *American Journal of Critical Care, 26*(2), 128–135.

Mokoka, K., Ehlers, V., & Oosthuizen, M. (2011). Factors influencing the retention of registered nurses in the Gauteng Province of South Africa. *Curationis, 34*(1), E1–E9.

Molina, Y., Beresford, S. A. A., Espinoza, N., & Thompson, B. (2014). Psychological distress, social withdrawal, and coping following receipt of an abnormal mammogram among different ethnicities: A mediation model. *Oncology Nursing Forum, 41*(5), 523–532.

Montano, D. E., & Kasprzyk, D. (2015). The theory of reasoned action, theory of planned behavior, and the integrated behavioral model. In K. Glanz, B. K. Rimer, & K. Viswanath (Eds.), *Health behavior: Theory, research and practice* (5th ed., pp. 95–124). San Francisco, CA: Jossey-Bass.

Morgan, S. W., & Stevens, P. E. (2012). Transgender identity development as represented by a group of transgendered adults. *Issues in Mental Health Nursing, 33*(5), 301–308.

Neuman, B., & Fawcett, J. (2011). *The Neuman systems model* (5th ed.). Upper Saddle River, NJ: Pearson.

Noonan, D. A. (2013). A descriptive study of waterpipe smoking among college students. *Journal of the American Association of Nurse Practitioners, 25*(1), 11–15.

Olson, S. E. (2015). Achieving success when returning to nursing education. *Nursing, 45*(2), 22–24.

Orlando, I. (1961). *The dynamic nurse–patient relationship.* New York, NY: Putnam.

Othman, A. K., Kiviniemi, M. T., Wu, Y. W., & Lally, R. M. (2012). Influence of demographic factors, knowledge, and beliefs on Jordanian women's intention to undergo mammography screening. *Journal of Nursing Scholarship, 44*(1), 19–26.

Padden, D. L., Connors, R., & Agazio, J. (2011). Stress, coping, and well-being in military spouses during deployment separation. *Western Journal of Nursing Research, 33*(2), 247–267.

Paterson, B., McIntosh, I., Wilkinson, D., McComish, S., & Smith, I. (2013). Corrupted cultures in mental health inpatient settings. Is restraint reduction the answer? *Journal of Psychiatric and Mental Health Nursing, 20*(3), 228–235.

Peplau, H. E. (1952). *Interpersonal relations in nursing.* New York, NY: Putnam.

Peplau, H. E. (1963). A working definition of anxiety. In S. F. Burd & M. A. Marshall (Eds.), *Some clinical approaches of psychiatric nursing* (pp. 323–327). New York, NY: Macmillan.

Platt, L. M. (2014). Preventing neonaticide by early detection and intervention in student pregnancy. *NASN School Nurse, 29*(6). 304–308.

Plotnikoff, R. C., Costigan, S. A., Karunamuni, N., & Lubans, D. R. (2013). Social cognitive theories used to explain physical activity behavior in adolescents: A systematic review and meta-analysis. *Preventive Medicine, 56*(5), 245–253.

Poss, J. E. (2001). Developing a new model for cross-cultural research: Synthesizing the health belief model and the theory of reasoned action. *ANS. Advances in Nursing Science, 23*(4), 1–15.

Prochaska, J. O. (1979). *Systems of psychotherapy: A transtheoretical analysis.* Homewood, IL: Dorsey Press.

Prochaska, J. O., Redding, A., & Evers, K. E. (2015). The transtheoretical model and stages of change. In K. Glanz, B. K. Rimer, & K. Viswanath (Eds.), *Health behavior and health education: Theory, research, and practice* (5th ed., pp. 125–148). San Francisco, CA: Jossey-Bass.

Rasheed, S. P. (2015). Self-awareness as a therapeutic tool for nurse/client relationship. *International Journal of Caring Sciences, 8*(1), 211–216.

Reed, P. G. (1998). A holistic view of nursing concepts and theories in practice. *Journal of Holistic Nursing, 16*(4), 415–419.

Rogers, C. R. (1951). *Client-centered therapy: Its current practice, implications, and theory.* Boston, MA: Houghton Mifflin.

Rogers, C. R. (1959). A theory of therapy, personality, and interpersonal relationships: As developed in the client-centered framework. In S. Koch (Ed.), *Psychology: A study of science* (Vol. 3, pp. 184–256). New York, NY: McGraw-Hill.

Rosenstock, I. M. (1974). The health belief model and preventive health behavior. *Health Education Monographs, 2*, 354–436.

Rosenstock, I. M. (1990). The health belief model: Explaining health behavior through expectancies. In K. Glanz, F. M. Lewis, & B. K. Rimer (Eds.), *Health behavior and health education: Theory, research and practice* (pp. 39–62). San Francisco, CA: Jossey-Bass.

Roy, C. (2009). *The Roy adaptation model* (3rd ed.). Upper Saddle River, NJ: Pearson.

Sadock, B. (2009). Signs and symptoms in psychiatry. In B. Sadock, V. Sadock, & P. Ruiz (Eds.), *Kaplan & Sadock's comprehensive textbook of psychiatry* (pp. 918–928). Philadelphia, PA: Lippincott Williams & Wilkins.

Scope, A., Booth, A., & Sutcliffe, P. (2012). Women's perceptions and experiences of group cognitive behaviour therapy and other group interventions for postnatal depression: A qualitative synthesis. *Journal of Advanced Nursing, 68*(9), 1909–1919.

Seal, N., & Seal, J. (2011). Developing healthy childhood behaviour: Outcomes of a summer camp experience. *International Journal of Nursing Practice, 17*(4), 428–434.

Selye, H. (1956). *The stress of life.* St. Louis, MO: McGraw-Hill.

Senn, J. F. (2013). Peplau's theory of interpersonal relations: Application in emergency and rural nursing. *Nursing Science Quarterly, 26*(1), 31–35.

Skinner, B. F. (1969). *Contingencies of reinforcement: A theoretical analysis.* New York, NY: Appleton-Century-Crofts.

Skinner, B. F. (1987). Whatever happened to psychology as the science of behavior? *American Psychologist, 42*, 780–786.

Skinner, C. S., Tiro, J., & Champion, V. L. (2015). The health belief model. In K. Glanz, B. K. Rimer, & K. Viswanath (Eds.), *Health behavior: Theory, research and practice* (5th ed., pp. 75–94). San Francisco, CA: Jossey-Bass.

Southard, K., Jarrell, A., Shattell, M. M., McCoy, T. P., Bartlett, R., & Judge, C. A. (2012). Enclosed versus open nursing stations in adult acute care psychiatric settings: Does the design affect the therapeutic milieu? *Journal of Psychosocial Nursing and Mental Health Services, 50*(5), 28–34.

Steinberg, P., & Cochrane, D. (2013). Integration of psychoanalytic concepts in the formulation and management of hospitalized psychiatric patients. *Bulletin of the Menninger Clinic, 77*(1), 23–40.

Sullivan, H. S. (1953). *The interpersonal theory of psychiatry.* New York, NY: Norton.

Swatton, A. (2011). Transference and countertransference in anorexia nervosa care. *Gastrointestinal Nursing, 9*(3), 38–43.

Talbot, A. L., Dorrian, J., & Chapman, J. (2015). Using the theory of planned behaviour to examine enrolled nursing students' intention to care for patient with alcohol dependence: A survey study. *Nurse Education Today, 35*(10), 1054–1061.

Telford, K., Kralik, D., & Koch, T. (2006). Acceptance and denial: Implications for people adapting to chronic illness: Literature review. *Journal of Advanced Nursing, 55*(4), 457–464.

Thompson, L. (1986). Peplau's theory. An application to short-term individual therapy. *Journal of Psychosocial Nursing and Mental Health Services, 24*(8), 26–31.

Vann, J. C., Hawley, J., Wegner, S., Falk, R. J., Harward, D. H., & Kshirsagar, A. V. (2015). Nursing intervention aimed at improving self-management for persons with chronic kidney disease in North Carolina Medicaid: A pilot project. *Nephrology Nursing Journal, 42*(3), 239–255.

Walsh, K. D., Crisp, J., & Moss, C. (2011). Psychodynamic perspectives on organizational change and their relevance to transformational practice development. *International Journal of Nursing Practice, 17*(2), 205–212.

Wu, T. Y., & Lin, C. (2015). Developing and evaluating an individual tailored intervention to increase mammography adherence among Chinese American women. *Cancer Nursing, 38*(1), 40–49.

Youngcharoen, P., Vincent, C., Park, C. G., Corte, C., Eisenstein, A. R., & Wilkie, D. J. (2016). Nurses' pain management for hospitalized elderly patients with postoperative pain. *Western Journal of Nursing Research, 38*(11), 1409–1432.

Zhu, L.-X., Ho, S.-C., Sit, J. W. H., & He, H.-G. (2014). Retraction: Effects of a transtheoretical model-based exercise stage-matched intervention on exercise behaviour and quality of life in patients with coronary heart disease: A randomized controlled trial. *Journal of Advanced Nursing, 70*(10), 2414.

Zugai, J., Stein-Parbury, J., & Roche, M. (2013). Effective nursing care of adolescents with anorexia nervosa: A consumer perspectives. *Journal of Clinical Nursing, 22*(13–14), 2020–2029.

Theories From the Biomedical Sciences

Melanie McEwen

Maria Leon is in her final year of a graduate program preparing to become a certified registered nurse anesthetist (CRNA). During the course of her graduate education, Maria observed that most people reported a burning sensation as propofol (a drug used to induce general anesthesia) was administered intravenously (IV). In conducting a review of the literature and discussing her observations with other CRNAs, Maria found several techniques used to minimize the injection pain. Based on this information, Maria decided that she would like to conduct a research study to examine the effectiveness of using lidocaine to reduce the injection pain of propofol. This project would fulfill the capstone requirement for her master's degree.

A literature review of pain management led Maria to the Gate Control Theory (GCT) (Melzak & Wall, 1982), which posits that there is a gating mechanism in the spinal cord. When pain impulses are transmitted from the periphery of the body by nerve fibers, the impulses travel to the dorsal horns of the spinal cord, specifically to the area of the cord called the *substantia gelatinosa*. According to the theory, when the gate is open, pain impulses ascend to the brain; when the gate is partially open, only some of the pain impulses can pass through. Pain medication has an effect on the gate, and if pain medication is administered before the onset of pain, it will help keep the gate closed, allowing fewer pain impulses to pass through.

In planning her research project, Maria used the GCT to guide the design and structure of the study. For the study, she decided to compare two techniques for pain prevention. One technique involved mixing 20 ml of a 1% propofol solution with 5 ml of a 2% lidocaine solution and injecting 1 ml of the mixture immediately before administration of the propofol. The second technique involved the placement of a tourniquet inflated to 50 mmHg on the arm in which the IV access device was placed. Then, 5 ml of 2% lidocaine would be injected, and the tourniquet would be removed 1 minute later; propofol would then be injected. A time frame of 20 seconds would allow the clients to report pain in the arm before the propofol took effect. Maria also planned to have a control group that did not have either of the pain prevention interventions.

If the theory was correct, Maria hypothesized that both experimental groups would have less pain from the injection because the gate that allowed pain sensations would not open or would only partially open. She did not know which of the two experimental procedures would be more effective in preventing pain but was enthusiastic about conducting the study and adding to the body of knowledge on pain prevention in anesthesia.

Theories from the biomedical sciences (e.g., biology, medicine, public health, physiology, pharmacology) have had a tremendous impact on nursing practice since Nightingale's time. Indeed, many of these theories are so integral to nursing practice that they are overlooked or taken for granted. For example, at the beginning of the 21st century, the Germ Theory seems almost too elemental to mention because even kindergarten children are taught the basic concept of germs and how to prevent infection. But nurses should recognize the relatively recent discovery of this revolutionary theory (late 1800s) and understand that a significant amount of nursing care is based on it. Other theories, concepts, and principles are similarly ingrained within nursing practice.

Biomedical theories have been the basis for research efforts of physiologists, physicians, and laboratory-based scientists for many years. Nurses have also been involved in research of this type and are increasingly directing studies that have a physiologic or biologic basis. As with any study, the underlying theories or conceptual frameworks may be broad (e.g., Germ Theory) or very narrow (e.g., Gate Control Theory [GCT]).

This chapter presents some of the most commonly used theories and principles from the biomedical sciences to illustrate how they are being used in studies conducted by nurses and applied in nursing practice. The number of these theories is staggering; thus, space allows for discussion of only a few. Although there is some overlap, the theories will be grouped into two large categories: theories of disease causation (e.g., Germ Theory, natural history of disease) and theories related to physiology (e.g., stress and adaptation, cancer causation, pain).

Theories and Models of Disease Causation

On a day-to-day, moment-to-moment basis, nurses in practice use any one of a number of concepts, principles, and theories from biology and public health. These theories are often related to disease causation and progression. This includes pathogenesis and infection as well as multiple epidemiologic concepts and principles (e.g., risk factor, exposure, prevention). This section provides a review of a few of these principles, theories, and models and shows how they are used in nursing practice and nursing research.

Evolution of Theories of Disease Causation

Disease refers to any condition that disturbs the normal functioning of an organism, whether it affects one organ or several systems. The term has also been defined as the failure of an organism to respond or adapt to its environment. The concept has changed dramatically over the course of time, however, and ideas about the cause of disease have been influenced by the prevailing culture and scientific thought.

In ancient times, disease was frequently viewed as a divine intervention or punishment. Early human beings attributed diseases to the influence of demons or spirits, and magic was a large part of treatment and prevention. As time passed, other interventions or treatments, such as the use of plant extracts, became more common.

As humans formed into societies and distinct cultural groups, two trends, or approaches, to medicine evolved. Sorcerers and priests embraced a magico-religious approach, whereas early physicians and scientists developed an empirico-rational approach. The empirico-rational approach was based on experience and observation and was practiced at first by priests but was adapted by nonclerical physicians. Modern medicine arose primarily from the empirico-rational approach as the human body and its functions became better known and as science led medical practice away from superstition and focus on the spiritual realm to include scientific processes and reasoning.

In the 17th century, William Harvey, an English physician and anatomist, demonstrated the dynamics of blood circulation (Donahue, 2011). Detailed studies of the organs, diseases, and processes, such as physiology and respiration, quickly followed, conducted by eminent physicians and scientists of the time. Medical debates focused on minute features of the body and how to treat particular diseases. Philosophies and theories developed that were largely reductionistic and deductive, focusing on cause and effect; the medical model quickly evolved.

In the latter part of the 19th century, scientists began to unravel the basic causes of infectious disease. Modern medicine began with the advent of Pasteur's Germ Theory, which posited that a specific microorganism was capable of causing an infectious disease (Black & Hawks, 2009). The focus on single-agent or single-organism cause for disease persisted for a number of decades and resulted in multiple successes in both treating and preventing communicable diseases. Today, however, the predominant general model of disease causation is multicausal, involving invasive agents, immune responses, genetics, environment, and behavior.

A number of theories and models describe disease causation and the properties that relate to disease processes and prevention. Some of the most frequently encountered models in nursing practice and research are discussed in the following sections.

Germ Theory and Principles of Infection

Louis Pasteur first proposed the Germ Theory in 1858. He theorized that a specific organism (i.e., a germ) was capable of causing an infectious disease (Kalisch & Kalisch, 2004). Today, this seems like a simple theory, but it is one that was critical to the development of modern medical care. Its impact has been phenomenal and has helped to radically reduce the number of deaths from infection.

Overview

At the beginning of the 21st century, theories of infection are most often applied to prevent infection (e.g., practicing strict handwashing, cleansing a scrape and applying antibiotic ointment, or prophylactically treating a surgery client with antibiotics) or to describe the process that seeks to identify, understand, and manage infectious diseases. This process initiates the search for the causative agent of an infection and method(s) of transmission. Once this has been accomplished, the focus can shift to the development of ways to prevent and treat the disease.

One of the most dramatic examples of this process was the outbreak of AIDS. The syndrome was first identified by the Centers for Disease Control and Prevention (CDC) in September of 1982, but months passed before it was determined that the causative agent was a retrovirus, later termed *HIV* (Shi & Singh, 2015). Early in the process, even before the virus was isolated, methods of transmission (e.g., sexual, transplacental, via blood products) were recognized and interventions for prevention proposed. Research on treatment has produced somewhat successful results in recent years and is ongoing.

Another example involves bovine spongiform encephalopathy (BSE), or mad cow disease, and its relationship with Creutzfeldt–Jakob disease (CJD). It has been hypothesized that the causative agent of BSE is a *prion*, which is not truly a germ, but a protein that is transmitted through ingestion of contaminated meat; the principles of infection, however, are similar (Secker, Hervé, & Keevil, 2011). Much additional work will be necessary to support this theory and to enhance preventive efforts. Ultimately, it is hoped that effective treatments for CJD will be found.

Lastly, a more recent example relates to Zika virus infection and severe birth defects—particularly microcephaly. In this example, an outbreak of Zika virus infection was initially recognized in Northeastern Brazil in early 2015 (Schuler-Faccini et al., 2016). By September of that year, 35 cases of microcephaly were reported in areas affected by the outbreak. This lead public health officials to determine a "possible association" between Zika virus and the birth defects. This designation was subsequently changed to a "causal" relationship following more detailed, in-depth review of the evidence (CDC, 2016).

Application to Nursing

Research studies use the Germ Theory to identify the causes or agents of infection. For an infection to occur, the host must be susceptible to the invasive organism. This susceptibility may be termed *risk*. For example, a person who has experienced severe burns is at higher risk of infection because one of the first lines of defense, the skin, is damaged. Many nursing articles that present practice guidelines and nursing research studies have focused on prevention and management of infection as well as identifying factors that place an individual at risk for developing infections. These studies and guidelines use principles from the Germ Theory, although this is rarely acknowledged.

Examples from recent literature that detail aspects of nursing practice related to prevention of infection include interventions to promote hand hygiene (Foote & El-Masri, 2016; Hohenberger, 2015; Kukanich, Kaur, Freeman, & Powell, 2013), guidelines for prevention of infections related to urinary catheters (P. Johnson, Gilman, Lintner, & Buckner, 2016; L. Williams, 2016b), and strategies to prevent ventilator-associated pneumonia in intensive care unit (ICU) patients (Klompas, 2015). Upshaw-Owens and Bailey (2012) and Chun, Kim, and Park (2015) described efforts nurses can use to prevent methicillin-resistant *Staphylococcus aureus* (MRSA) infection in hospitals and primary care settings, respectively. With respect to the previous discussion of Zika virus, strategies to prevent infection and manage complications were presented by Coyle (2016) and L. Williams (2016a).

The Epidemiologic Triangle

The classic epidemiologic model, particularly useful in the depiction of communicable disease, is the Epidemiologic Triangle (Figure 15-1). This model is often used to illustrate the interrelationships among the three essential components of host, agent, and environment with regard to disease causation. A change in any of the three components can result in the disease process. For example, exposure at school (environment) of a child who has not been immunized (host) to the measles virus (agent) will probably result in a case of measles.

Within the Epidemiologic Triangle, prevention of disease lies in averting exposure to the agent, enhancing the physical attributes of the host to resist the disease,

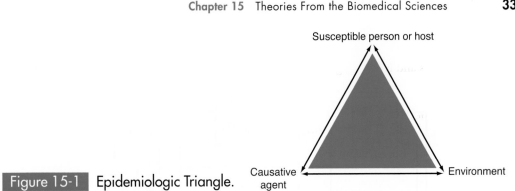

Figure 15-1 Epidemiologic Triangle.

and minimizing any environmental factors that might contribute to disease development. Host, agent, and environmental factors that affect health can also influence progression of the disease process. Host factors include age, gender, race/ethnicity, marital status, economic status, state of immunity, and lifestyle factors (e.g., diet, exercise patterns, hygiene, occupation, sexual health). Agent factors include presence or absence of biologic organisms (e.g., bacteria, fungi, viruses), exposure to physical factors (e.g., radiation, extremes of temperature, noise), and exposure to chemical agents (e.g., poisons, allergens, gases). Last, environmental factors include such things as physical elements or properties (e.g., climate, seasons, geology), biologic entities (e.g., animals, insects, food, drugs), or social/economic considerations (e.g., family, public policy, occupation, culture) (M. McEwen & Pullis, 2009).

The Web of Causation

To explain disease and disability caused by multiple factors, MacMahon and Pugh (1970) developed the concept of "Chain of Causation," later termed the "Web of Causation." Prior to that time, it had been observed that chronic diseases (i.e., coronary artery disease and most types of cancer) are not attributable to one or two factors or causative agents. Rather, they result from the interaction of multiple factors.

Overview

An example of the application of the Web of Causation to the development of coronary heart disease is presented in Figure 15-2. The Web of Causation can also be applied to many health-related threats and conditions. The problem of teenage pregnancy, for example, is attributable to a complex interaction among a number of causative and contributing factors, including lack of knowledge about sexuality and pregnancy prevention, lack of easily accessible contraception, peer pressure, low self-esteem, social patterns in which teen mothers are more likely to be children of teen mothers, use of alcohol or other drugs, and so on. Family violence, cocaine use, and gang membership are examples of other threats to health and well-being that can be more accurately explained through a model of multiple causations.

Recognition that many health problems have multiple causes leads to the recognition that there are rarely simple solutions to these health problems. When trying to manage teen pregnancy, for example, the solution is not as simple as addressing a knowledge deficit regarding sexuality and contraception. Many (if not most) teens are well informed about contraception and the mechanics of how one gets pregnant, and they still fail to take preventive measures. To prevent heart disease in an individual at risk, interventions include health education addressing a number of areas, including smoking cessation, weight loss, cholesterol reduction, and exercise. Likewise, to

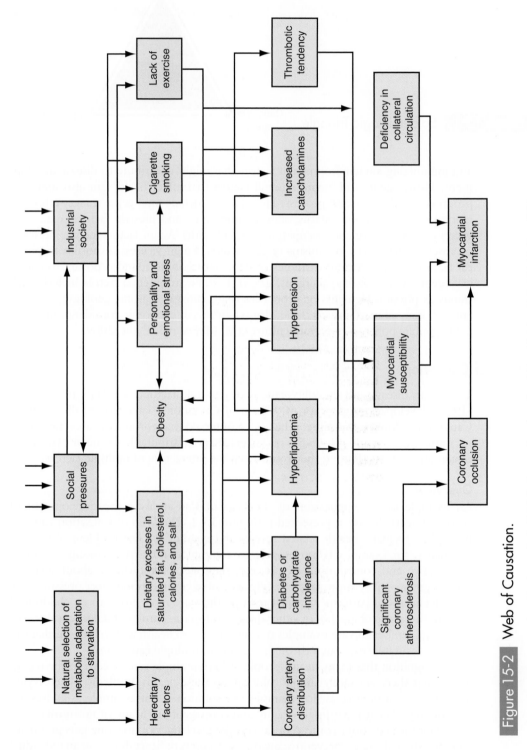

Figure 15-2 Web of Causation.

(Adapted with permission from Friedman, G. D. [1994]. *Primer of epidemiology* [4th ed.]. New York, NY: McGraw-Hill.)

prevent teen pregnancy, interventions should include health teaching on improving self-esteem, participating in role-playing exercises on how to say "no," encouraging orientation toward the future, enhancing parental supervision, and providing recreational alternatives (sports and other after-school activities), as well as giving information on sexuality, the mechanics of reproduction, and methods of contraception.

Application to Nursing

Nurses have developed interventions and proposed strategies to address complex health problems with multifactorial etiologies. For example, from a large-scale, literature synthesis, García-Fernández, Agreda, Verdú, and Pancorbo-Hidalgo (2014) organized risk factors for development of pressure ulcers among hospitalized individuals into a middle range theory. The risk factors included mobility, exposure to moisture/incontinence, mental state, nutrition, activity, predisposing disease, age, temperature and medications.

In another study, N. L. Johnson, Giarelli, Lewis, and Rice (2013) provided an overview of the correlational factors that are believed to contribute to development of autism spectrum disorder (ASD). These were broadly grouped into environmental factors (e.g., exposure to high levels of pollutants, viral infection during pregnancy, use of assisted reproductive therapies), and genetic factors (i.e., "genetic susceptibility" and "de novo mutations" [new, spontaneous mutations]). The researchers also described nursing implications including promotion of knowledge and skills to assess genetic risk, advocacy for families, and encouragement to assess for possible ASD in encounters with children.

In other works, Matthews and Moore (2013) examined the risk factors associated with sudden unexplained infant death (SUID)/sudden infant death syndrome (SIDS), and Phillippi and Roman (2013) reported on the factors that facilitated or hindered patient access to prenatal care. In theory-specific examples, Katerndahl, Burge, Ferrer, Becho, and Wood (2014) used the Web of Causation to describe the complex dynamics in violent familial relationships, and Siegel (2007) used the Web of Causation as the theoretical framework in her examination of the predictors of overweight in children in sixth, seventh, and eighth grades.

Natural History of Disease

The natural history of a disease refers to the progress of a disease process in an individual over time.

Overview

In their classic model, Leavell and Clark (1965) described two periods in the natural history of disease, prepathogenesis and pathogenesis. In this model, the prepathogenesis stage occurs prior to interaction of the disease agent and human host when the individual is susceptible. For example, an adult male smokes, a teenage girl considers becoming sexually active, or a preschooler attends a party also attended by a sick child. After exposure or interaction, the period of prepathogenesis proceeds to early pathogenesis (i.e., alterations in lung tissue, pregnancy, chicken pox) and on through the disease course to resolution—either death, disability, or recovery (i.e., lung cancer, teen motherhood, immunity to chicken pox).

In addition to the description of the natural history of disease progression, Leavell and Clark (1965) also outlined three levels of prevention—primary prevention, secondary prevention, and tertiary prevention—that correlate with the stages of disease progression (Box 15-1). Each of the three levels of prevention is applied at the appropriate

Box 15-1 Levels of Prevention

- *Primary prevention*: Activities that are directed at preventing a problem before it occurs. This includes altering susceptibility or reducing exposure for susceptible individuals in the period of prepathogenesis. Primary prevention consists of two categories: *general health promotion* (e.g., good nutrition, adequate shelter, rest, exercise) and *specific protection* (e.g., immunization, water purification).
- *Secondary prevention*: Early detection of and prompt intervention for a disease or health threat during the period of early pathogenesis. Screening for disease and prompt referral and treatment are secondary prevention.
- *Tertiary prevention*: Consists of limitation of disability and rehabilitation during the period of advanced disease and convalescence, where the disease has occurred and resulted in a degree of damage.

stage of pathogenesis in an attempt to halt progression (Figure 15-3). Thus, at the primary prevention stage, interventions focus on general health promotion activities (e.g., encouraging a healthful diet and promoting regular exercise) and efforts to prevent specific health problems (e.g., vaccination, encouraging use of seatbelts and car seats, promoting oral hygiene).

Secondary prevention is concerned with early detection and would include any screening activity (e.g., mammography, cholesterol screening) and subsequent efforts to limit disease progression for those identified with a health condition (e.g., taking statin medications, lumpectomy with radiation/chemotherapy). Last, tertiary prevention involves efforts to enhance rehabilitation and convalescence following advanced disease.

Application to Nursing

Much of nursing practice focuses on efforts to prevent the progression of disease at the earliest period or phase using the appropriate levels of prevention. There are many examples of applying primary prevention strategies in practice. These include efforts to prevent polypharmacy among community-dwelling older adults (Harvath, Lindauer, & Sexson, 2016); maternal morbidity and mortality (Logsdon, 2016); multidrug-resistant, gram-negative infection in surgical patients (Murphy, 2012); skin cancer in adults (Roebuck, Moran, MacDonald, Shumer, & McCune, 2015); falls among older adults (Morgan et al., 2017); and cardiovascular disease through use of statins (Sherrod, Sherrod, & Cheek, 2015).

Excellent examples of nursing interventions targeted to secondary prevention are also common in the nursing literature. Examples include a program to promote screening for perinatal depression among Special Supplemental Nutrition Program for Women, Infants, and Children (WIC) recipients (Fritz, 2015), discussion of the importance of screening for human papillomavirus (HPV)-related oral cancer (Katz, 2017), guidelines for depression screening among adolescents with diabetes (Dever, 2016), elder abuse screening (Stark, 2012), and community-based screening promotion to detect colorectal cancer (Weyl et al., 2015).

Tertiary prevention efforts include information to help nurses work to promote follow-up with recommendations among colorectal cancer survivors (Hawkins et al., 2015), prevent complications of hemodialysis through promotion of exercise (Hannan, 2016), and prevent tumor lysis syndrome among cancer patients (Kaplow & Iyere, 2016).

Finally, Jones-Parker (2012) presented a detailed overview examining all three levels of prevention intended to assist nurse practitioners in preventing cardiovascular disease in HIV-positive patients, and Klemp (2015) outlined multilevel preventive strategies for nurses to address breast cancer prevention across the cancer care continuum.

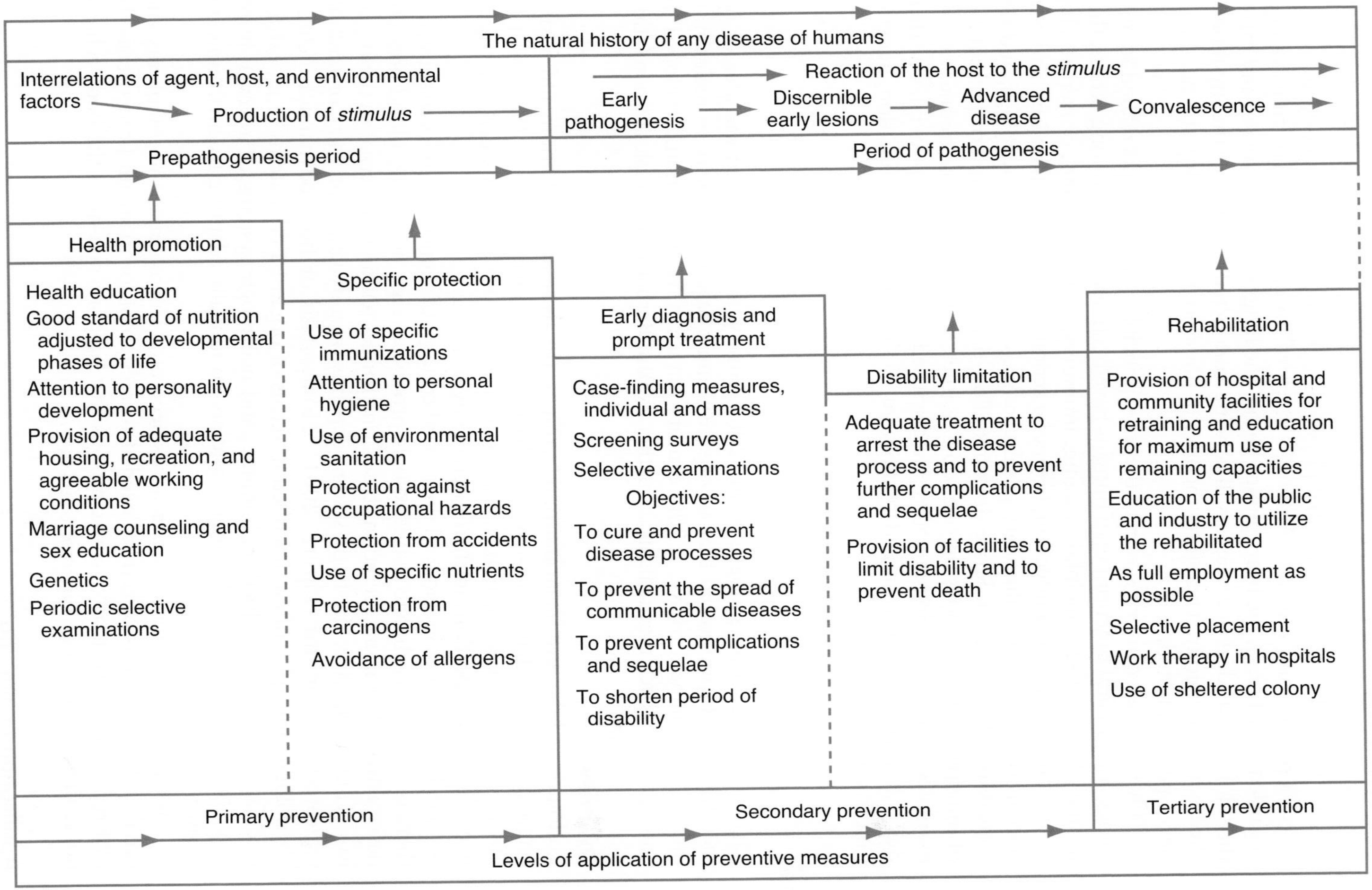

Figure 15-3 Natural history of disease.

(Adapted with permission from Leavell, H. R., & Clark, E. G. [1965]. *Preventive medicine for the doctor in his community: An epidemiologic approach* [p. 18]. New York, NY: McGraw-Hill.)

Theories and Principles Related to Physiology and Physical Functioning

Many theories based on the normal physiologic functioning of the body are used in nursing practice and research. Although much of normal physiologic functioning is regarded as fact (e.g., the heart pumps blood, the lungs exchange oxygen and carbon dioxide), a great deal of research still is being conducted to uncover the mysteries of the body's physiology. Therefore, theories of physiologic functioning still need to be developed and tested.

Over the past century, scores of theories, principles, and concepts related to physiology and physical functioning of humans have been developed. Among others, these include theories and principles of aging, immunity, wound healing, cancer development, inflammation and infection, hormone action, nutrition, metabolism, and body systems (renal system, pulmonary gas exchange, cardiovascular physiology, and nervous system functioning). Space does not allow detailed explanation or presentation of multiple, similar theories on one topic. Rather, some of the most frequently cited examples from the nursing literature are discussed. These include principles or theories of homeostasis, stress and adaptation, immunity and immune function, genetics, cancer, and pain.

Homeostasis

Claude Bernard, a physiologist in the 20th century, first conceived the idea of homeostasis. He hypothesized that an organism must have the capacity to maintain its internal environment to live. A 20th century physician, Walter Canon, developed the concept of feedback mechanisms to further explain Bernard's principles of regulation.

Overview

Canon coined the term *homeostasis*, referring to the dynamic equilibrium and flexible ongoing processes that maintain certain biologic factors within a range (S. Grossman, 2014b). The principles of homeostasis state that all healthy cells, tissues, and organs maintain static conditions in their internal environment.

Dr. Eugene Yates introduced the related concept of homeodynamics to show that there is continuous change in physiologic processes (e.g., heart rate, blood pressure, nerve activity, hormonal secretion) based on changes within or external to the organism. Thus, to survive, the body system depends on a dynamic interplay of multiple regulatory mechanisms (Lipsitz, 2001). Homeostasis or homeodynamics includes physiologic principles often described in terms of organ-based systems (e.g., cardiovascular, respiratory, endocrine, immune, and neurologic systems). However, in reality, the body systems are integrated and are continually adapting to environmental changes.

As a result, a new term, *allostasis*, has been used to recognize the complexity and variability of the levels of activity needed to reestablish or maintain homeostasis. In that regard, allostasis is a "dynamic process that supports and helps the body achieve homeostasis" (Jansen & Emerson, 2014, p. 13).

Application to Nursing

There are a number of illustrations of how principles of homeostasis are applied in nursing practice. For example, Walker (2016) reviewed the key assessment parameters for monitoring fluid and electrolyte imbalance, highlighting the need for maintenance of homeostasis. A team led by Chapa (Chapa et al., 2014) explained the complex pathophysiologic interactions of neurohormonal responses experienced by heart failure patients with comorbid diagnose of depression or anxiety. They concluded that understanding the role of neurohomones and the effect they have on the autonomic nervous system is key to developing and implementing appropriate interventions for complex heart failure patients. In an interesting article, Outland (2010) described homeostasis as "a cornerstone of holistic care" (p. 36) and presented the notion of "intuitive eating" to help restore and maintain "weight homeostasis" (a dynamic interaction between hormones, proteins, and neurotransmitters) to help control weight. Finally, Premji (2014) attempted to identify indicators of perinatal distress and protective factors and processes that promote resilience and allostasis—or ongoing adaptation—among pregnant women in low- and middle-income countries. Similarly, Ewen and Kinney (2014) focused on "allostasis" in their examination of adaptation of elderly women as they relocated to senior housing facilities.

Stress and Adaptation: General Adaptation Syndrome

In addition to the principles of homeostasis, Walter Canon also developed the concept of fight or flight to explain the body's reaction to emergencies.

Overview

The fight-or-flight response prepares the body for muscular activity (i.e., running, self-defense) when reacting to a perceived or actual threat. This process is a series of chemical reactions that are initiated by the adrenal medulla, which produces epinephrine (adrenaline) and norepinephrine. This reaction increases the heart rate, respiratory rate, blood pressure, and blood glucose levels. Blood is shunted to the muscles of the legs, heart, and lungs from the intestines; this prepares the body for quick response to danger (Jansen & Emerson, 2014).

In the 1960s and 1970s, Hans Selye built on Canon's work by developing a framework to describe how the body responds to stress. Selye derived his theories of stress from the observations he made while caring for people who were ill. The clinical manifestations he noted were loss of appetite, weight loss, feeling and looking ill, and generalized muscle aching and pains. Selye called this response the General Adaptation Syndrome (GAS) because it involved generalized changes that affect the body.

Selye believed that changes in organs occur in three stages. Stage 1, the alarm phase, begins with the fight-or-flight response. In this stage, the adrenal glands enlarge and release hormones including adrenocorticotropic hormone (ACTH). This increases blood glucose and depresses the immune system. If the stress continues, the body begins to experience detrimental changes (e.g., shrinkage of the thymus, spleen, lymph nodes, and other lymphatic structures). Other physical manifestations, such as gastric and duodenal ulcers, can also develop.

Stage 2 (resistance) occurs when the body starts to react and return to homeostasis. If the stressor ends, the body should be able to return to normal. Stage 3 (exhaustion) occurs when the stressor persists and the body cannot continue to produce hormones as in stage 1 or when damage has occurred to other organs (Table 15-1) (Selye, 1976).

Selye thought that the body's response to stress is nonspecific; that is, the body reacts as a whole organism. Also, it is not just bad things that cause stress but good things as well. Health conditions thought to be related to stress include cancer, hypertension, heart disease, cerebrovascular accident, peripheral vascular disease, asthma, tuberculosis, emphysema, irritable bowel syndrome, sexual dysfunction,

Table 15-1 Selye's Stages of Stress

Stage	Characteristics	Physical Responses
Alarm	Begins with alarm; body prepares for survival (fight or flight); physiologic changes are coordinated by the central nervous system (CNS) and the sympathetic nervous system (SNS), which stimulates the adrenal medulla to secrete norepinephrine and epinephrine; the adrenal cortex is stimulated by the pituitary gland's release of ACTH.	CNS involuntary responses include secretion of specific hormones and metabolism and fluid regulation. SNS responses include increased heart rate, contraction of the spleen, release of glucose, increase in respiratory rate, decrease in clotting time, dilation of pupils, increased perspiration, and piloerection (hairs standing on end).
Resistance	The body recognizes a continued threat and physiologic forces adapt to maintain increased resistance to stressors; begins with a decrease in adrenocorticotropic hormone (ACTH), and the body concentrates on organs that are most involved in the specific stress responses.	Adaptation implies return or improvement in physical health. Ineffective resistance leads to a state of maladaptation in which there is deterioration in the level of physical functioning. Chronic resistance eventually causes damage to the involved systems.
Exhaustion	The body enters exhaustion when all energy for adaptation has been used; ACTH secretion increases and the organ or organ systems show evidence of deterioration.	Symptoms include hypertrophy of the adrenal glands, ulceration in the gastrointestinal tract, and atrophy of the thymus gland.

obesity, anorexia, bulimia, connective tissue disease, ulcerative colitis, Crohn disease, infections, and allergic and hypersensitivity diseases.

Selye's syndrome theory has been the basis of many studies. Holmes and Rahe (1967) conducted one classic study. They proposed that a large number of life changes cause stress, which in turn may cause disease. The researchers asked individuals of various socioeconomic and cultural groups to rank a number of life changes according to the amount of energy needed to adapt to change. These events were ranked, and a certain number of life change units (LCUs) were assigned to each one. This scale was named the Social Readjustment Rating Scale (SRRS). The total number of LCUs experienced by a person accumulates over time and theoretically indicates the amount of stress a person has experienced. A significant accumulation of stress increases the likelihood of an incidence of major illness.

Application to Nursing

A number of nurses have used the SRRS in recent research studies. One study (Staniute, Brozaitiene, & Bunevicius, 2013) used the SRRS to examine the effects of social support and stressful life events on health-related quality of life among coronary artery disease patients. Another work (Ngai & Ngu, 2014) used the SRRS to study depressive symptoms in Chinese childbearing couples focusing on family sense of coherence, stress, and family and marital functioning, and a third study used the SRRS to examine whether self-esteem and self-efficacy were predictive of attrition among nursing students in associate degree programs (Peterson-Graziose, Bryer, & Nikolaidou, 2013). In a similar way, Ganz (2012) studied stress among ICU nurses, using the GAS as a framework.

In a discussion relative to nursing practice, Okonta (2012) conducted an integrative research review to examine whether yoga is effective in reducing high blood pressure using Selye's model as a framework. Finally, Kang, Rice, Park, Turner-Henson, and Downs (2010) described creation of an "integrated biobehavioral model" (p. 735) designed to be a framework for conducting research on stress and inflammation. This model was adapted from Selye (1976), Lazarus and Folkman (1984), and B. S. McEwen's (2003) Allostatic Load Theory.

Theories of Immunity and Immune Function

The immune system comprises a complex, coordinated group of systems that produces physiologic responses to injury or infection. The purpose of the immune system is to neutralize, eliminate, or destroy microorganisms that invade the body. Extensive interactions affect the manufacture of products that alter the structure and function of cells.

Overview

Immunity involves specific recognition of what is designated as an antigen, memory for particular antigens, and responsiveness on reexposure. The immune system is related to other systems involved in inflammation and healing. Each system is involved in the response of inflammation and has two characteristics: (1) recognition of a stimulating structure by specific receptors and (2) response by one or more effector elements that aims to alter or eliminate the stimulating structure.

The immune system contains a large variety of cells, called *leukocytes*, that protect the body against foreign invasion. The five classes of leukocytes are neutrophils, eosinophils, basophils, monocytes, and lymphocytes; each has a specific function in the immune response. The granulocytes (neutrophils, eosinophils, and basophils) are short-lived phagocytic cells. They search out bacteria or cell debris and destroy them through phagocytosis (Workman, 2016).

Monocytes mature into macrophages in tissues and defend against tumor cells. They secrete monokines (i.e., interleukin-1) that assist in immune and inflammatory responses. Lymphocytes originate from stem cells in the bone marrow and mature into either B or T cells. The T cells differentiate in the thymus gland, and the B cells mature in the bone marrow. Both T and B lymphocytes continually recirculate between blood, lymph, and lymph nodes. The surface of B lymphocytes is coated with immunoglobulin, and when the appropriately matched antigen is detected by a B cell, the surface immunoglobulin will bind with it. The T lymphocytes play a role in cell-mediated immunity. There are a variety of T cell subsets; some are regulatory T cells, which include helper T cells and suppressor T cells (Black & Hawks, 2009).

The complement system consists of around 20 plasma proteins found in serum and on cells. The complement system participates in inflammation by coordinating elements of the inflammatory response to microorganisms and tissue injury through generation of peptides that initiate effects such as leukocyte activation, chemotaxis, and mast cell degranulation. The system facilitates phagocytic function by coating the target particle with biologically active peptides and fragments of molecules activating the system. A series of proenzymes and other molecules initiate an attack on the cell membranes of microorganisms (Banasik, 2014b).

Antibody-mediated immunity involves antigen–antibody actions to neutralize, eliminate, or destroy foreign proteins. Antibodies for these actions are produced by B lymphocytes. The B lymphocytes become sensitized to a specific foreign protein (antigen) and synthesize an antibody directed specifically against that protein. The antibody (rather than the actual B lymphocyte) participates in action to neutralize, eliminate, or destroy that antigen. Cell-mediated immunity involves many leukocytic actions, reactions, and interactions. Lymphocyte stem cells and lymphoid tissues regulate activities and inflammation by producing and releasing cytokines. T lymphocytes can be natural killer cells or helper cells (T_4 or Th cells) (Workman, 2016).

Application to Nursing

Principles of immune function can be used as a theoretical framework for research. A number of recent nursing research studies can be identified that look at factors related to immune status. For example, a study by Hughes, Ladas, Rooney, and Kelly (2008) concluded that as an adjunct intervention, massage therapy helps reduce side effects of treatment and may boost immune function in children with cancer. In another example, Kang and colleagues (2011) concluded that persistent practice of relaxation techniques might positively influence immune responses in women diagnosed with breast cancer. Finally, in a correlational study, Starkweather (2013) examined the relationship among fatigue, pain, psychosocial factors, and immune activation in patients with persistent sciatica. She determined that immune activation associated with chronic pain affects fatigue severity and may also affect other behavioral responses.

The interrelatedness of the nervous, endocrine, and immune systems were described in two works on psychoimmunology. In one report, Yammine, Kang, Baun, and Meininger (2014) examined the literature and found that psychosocial risk factors for cardiovascular disease are associated with elevated plasma vasoconstrictive peptide endothelin-1. Another study led by Starkweather (Starkweather et al., 2017) examined "clusters of psychoneurological symptoms and inflammation" (p. 167) in a longitudinal study of women diagnosed with early-stage breast cancer.

Genetic Principles and Theories

Although genetic principles and theories date back to Gregor Mendel's work in the 1860s, advances in molecular biology have only recently begun to transform health care delivery. The Human Genome Project is an organized effort initiated in 1990 and completed in 2003 to create a biologically and medically useful database of the genome structure and sequence in humans. (The term *human genome* refers to the entire complement of genetic material contained on the 46 chromosomes.) It is anticipated that information gained from the Human Genome Project will increase understanding of inherited conditions, both single-gene and complex diseases, as well as responses to treatment (L. C. Grossman, 2014a; Quigley, 2015).

Overview

A gene is the fundamental and functional unit of heredity. It is composed of a double strand of DNA, and each of the strands has thousands to millions of bases. The order of the bases codes information that directs the manufacture of a specific protein (Banasik, 2014a). A gene mutation is an alteration in DNA coding that results in a change in the protein product. Mutations in some genes cause clinical disease because of the absence of the normal protein. Sickle cell anemia, for example, results when one base is substituted with another.

Gene discoveries have provided information on genetic disorders that cause symptoms in a large proportion of persons who have abnormal genotypes. Successes include the isolation of genes for cystic fibrosis, neurofibromatosis, muscular dystrophy, Huntington disease, and some types of breast cancer (Banasik, 2014a; L. C. Grossman, 2014b). Many other diseases have a genetic susceptibility component that results from the interaction of multiple genes with environmental factors. Because these diseases involve many genes and many possible mutations, an enormous number of combinations of genotypes are possible. Determining the molecular pathophysiology of human disease will provide opportunities for diagnosis, prevention, and treatment.

Box 15-2	American Association of Colleges of Nursing Essentials and Genetics

The American Association of Colleges of Nursing's master's of science in nursing (MSN) Essential 1 states, "The master's degree program prepares graduates to . . . Incorporate current and emerging genetic/genomic evidence in providing advanced nursing care to individuals, families, and communities while accounting for patient values and clinical judgment." (AACN, 2006, p. 8).

Application to Nursing

Genetics will greatly affect the way health care is practiced in the future, and nurses will need to incorporate genetic technology and discovery into practice and research at the individual, family, and community levels (see Box 15-2). Nurses familiar with genetics and who are able to "think genetically" can ask appropriate questions of patients to assess genetic risk factors, communicate with patients and their families about inherited risks, make referrals to genetic counselors, reinforce counseling, and administer gene therapy or genetically specific drugs (see Link to Practice 15-1) (Calzone et al., 2012; Quigley, 2015; T. Williams & Dale, 2016). Table 15-2 suggests a nursing model for application of genetics in health care illustrating how and where genetics education can be added to basic nursing science. The result is preparation of the nurses for "ecogenetic nursing."

Link to Practice 15-1

Calzone and colleagues (2013) discussed the expanding importance of genomics to nursing practice. They reviewed how genomics provides information that enhances understanding of the biology of disease and has resulted in new and more personalized therapies that can greatly influence health care decisions. They explained that nurses have a responsibility to be informed about the potential benefits and challenges of genomics and to use that knowledge to inform other health care professionals, individuals, families, and communities.

Several ways that nurses can integrate genomic information into clinical practice were presented. These are:

- Preconception and prenatal testing
- Newborn screening
- Disease susceptibility
- Screening and diagnosis
- Prognosis and therapeutic decisions
- Monitoring disease burden and recurrence

Calzone and Jenkins asserted that timely and effective translation of genomics into health care will require that currently practicing nurses be educated in genomics and future nurses must be taught essential genetic and genomic competencies.

From Calzone, K. A., Jenkins, J., Nicol, N., Skirton, H., Feero, W. G., & Green, E. D. (2013). Relevance of genomics to healthcare and nursing practice. *Journal of Nursing Scholarship, 45*(1), 1–2.

Table 15-2 A Nursing Model for Genetics in Health Care

	Nursing Science	Genetic Education	Ecogenetic Nursing
Individual	Caring behavior and support role	Predictive genetic testing	Educating patients on genetic testing
	Care across the life span	Gene discoveries for diseases	Assisting patients to determine need for testing
	Patient counseling	Genes in pedigrees	Genetic consulting
	Medication	Pharmacogenetics	Educating about individualized medication therapy
Family	Pedigrees	Genetic role in disease	Interpreting and sharing genetic risk and health promotion
	Health promotion	Molecular pathology	Individualizing genetic testing and health promotion
	Multidisciplinary practice	Genetic specialist on the health care team	Referring to and interfacing with genetic specialists
	Informed consent	Genetic research concerns	Explaining risks and benefits of genetic study
	Teaching and counseling families	Genetic risks	Assessing and counseling families—reproductive risks and prenatal diagnosis
Community	Community assessment	Population-based screening	Community readiness for genetic screening and intervention
	Design and implement screening programs and follow-up service	Genetic testing	Availability and voluntary access to genetic information, testing, and assurance of follow-up services
Population	Clinical trials	New technology	Coordinating genetically focused research
	Nursing research	Genetic research	Collaborative research: focusing on ecogenetics, ethics, and psychosocial issues
	Patient advocacy	Ethical issues surrounding genetic tests	Ensuring that patients remain the priority of clinical treatment and research

A practicing nurse must be sensitive to issues of ethics and confidentiality related to genetic testing and genetic information. Indeed, genetics is one area of health care where technology precedes the ethical framework for dealing with issues and creates problems previously unknown; nurses must be prepared to deal with these problems (Camak, 2016; Halloran, 2015; T. Williams & Dale, 2016). Nurses knowledgeable in genetics can ensure that patients and families make informed and voluntary decisions about genetic information. Nurses can also serve as patient advocates as they obtain informed consent to participate in genetic clinical trials or to undergo genetic tests.

Nurses knowledgeable in genetics can have an important role in counseling patients at risk for complex diseases. Because complex diseases occur much more frequently than single-gene disorders, and because the number of diseases found to have genetic determinates is increasing rapidly, there will not be enough genetic counselors to serve all who are at risk (Halloran, 2015; Quigley, 2015). Nurses must use their knowledge of genetics to identify and differentiate genetic risks in patients with complex disorders and refer these patients to a genetic counselor whenever appropriate (Prows, Hopkin, Barnoy, & Van Riper, 2013; Santos et al., 2013).

Nurses are becoming more involved with managing genetic information because it is often collected and recorded when the nurse takes a family history and obtains certain blood tests (e.g., screening for breast cancer, sickle cell trait). Genetic testing and counseling combines the provision of genetic information with psychosocial counseling. It is nondirective, voluntary, and personal and should precede testing to allow informed decision making. Counseling should include an explanation of risk factors, exploration of the person's perception of the condition, and discussion of childbearing options. Potential outcomes of decisions are examined to facilitate decision making, and follow-up counseling is recommended. Goals of genetic counseling are to help clients and family members comprehend the medical genetic information, appreciate the genetic contribution to health and illness, understand health options and alternatives, and make informed health choices (i.e., whether to pursue further testing, evaluation, and treatment). Genetic counseling frequently includes referral and follow-up for family members to gain more information and possible treatment.

Nurses have also studied specific genetically based illnesses. For example, Jacobson, Tedder, and Eggert (2016) reported on genetic implications for development and management of acute lymphoblastic leukemia in adults. In another example, Snow and Lu (2012) examined genetic "inheritability" of risk for addiction and described how understanding genetic predisposition to addiction to substances including nicotine, alcohol, or illicit drugs can help nurses develop better and more directed educational materials as well as treatment protocols. Finally, Plavskin (2016) reported on an interesting look at genetic and genomic-based approaches to examination of the mechanisms of resistance, infection, and transmission routes of pathogens.

Cancer Theories

The altered behavior of cancer cells is thought to result from several factors, including exposure to chronic irritants, chemicals, radiation, infectious agents, and genetic aberrations. Cancer cells are similar to normal cells in their basic biology and biochemistry, but regulation of their proliferation and differentiation is defective. Cells taken from malignant tumors typically differ from normal tissue cells in several ways. They are less sensitive to differentiation-inducing factors, and they can divide indefinitely. Also, key regulatory factors (i.e., oncogenes, tumor suppressor genes, and cyclins) are altered in cancer cells (S. Grossman, 2014a).

Overview

Cancer presents as a complex series of diseases involving multiple steps. In addition, there is often an interaction among multiple risk factors (e.g., genetics, hormonal factors, immunologic mechanisms, radiation, or cancer-causing viruses) or repeated exposure to a single carcinogenic agent (e.g., asbestos, nicotine). It is thought to begin with an event that leaves a cell premalignant; this is followed by a number of promotional steps that increase the potential for an initiated cell to become malignant. The strong age correlation (i.e., incidence increases with age) supports the concept that most cancers result from the cumulative impact of multiple exposures over the lifetime (S. Grossman, 2014a).

One theory of cancer development suggests that cancer arises as a series of genetic errors (Cavenee & White, 1995). In this theory, there are three stages of cancer development: (1) initiation (referred to as the original genetic error), (2) promotion (genetic changes that continue and favor uncontrolled growth and metastasis), and (3) progression or latency (uncontrolled growth and full-blown malignant activity) (Figure 15-4).

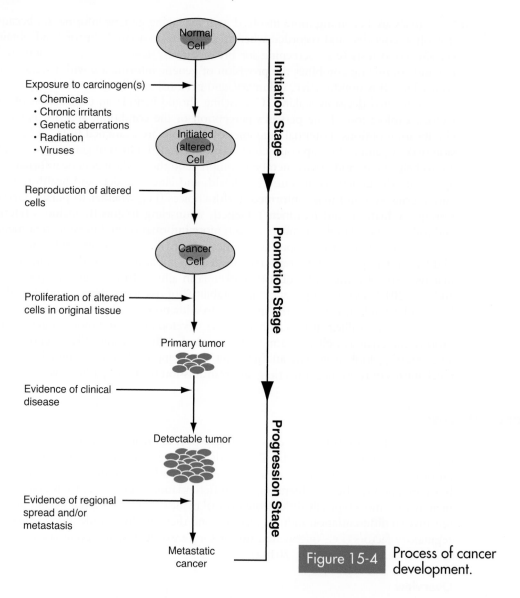

Figure 15-4   Process of cancer development.

This theory of cancer development states that cancer begins with one change in a normal cell. That change may alter cell production or cell function. This initiated cell may undergo additional malignant changes, especially if the environment supports the malignant activity. The cancer process can be stopped during the initiation stage, and even in the promotion stage, if the cellular environment is enabled to repair or control the carcinogenic genetic alteration (Banasik, 2014c).

Between 30% and 40% of all cancer deaths are preventable by modifying lifestyle factors, such as tobacco and alcohol use and diet. For example, it is thought that combined exposure to alcohol and smoking accounts for approximately 75% of all oral and pharyngeal cancers. Alcohol alone contributes to about 3% of all instances of colon, colorectal, esophageal, pancreatic, prostate, and breast cancers (Blattner, 2000). Table 15-3 lists some of the lifestyle, therapeutic, environmental, and host factors that appear to affect the development of cancer.

Table 15-3 Factors That Contribute to Cancer Development

Factor	Examples	Type of Cancer
Lifestyle factors	Use of tobacco and alcohol, diet	Lung, oral, and pharyngeal cancers (smoking and alcohol); colon and rectal cancer (alcohol, diet)
Therapeutic factors	Medically prescribed drugs (hormones, anticancer drugs, immunosuppressive agents)	Vaginal and cervical cancer (*in utero* exposure to diethylstilbestrol [DES]), endometrial cancer (synthetic estrogens), breast cancer (possible link to use of synthetic estrogens), leukemia (some anticancer drugs), non-Hodgkin lymphoma (drug-induced immunosuppression)
Environmental factors	Ionizing radiation, ultraviolet radiation, occupation, pollution, some infectious agents	Skin cancers (ultraviolet radiation), leukemia and thyroid cancer (ionizing radiation), lung cancer (some occupations and pollutants), cervical cancer (some subtypes of human papillomavirus), hepatocellular carcinoma (hepatitis B and C viruses)
Host factors	Inherent sensitivities to carcinogenesis	Colon and rectal cancers (familial adenomatous polyposis), site-specific breast cancers, cancer of the ovary, retinoblastoma

Source: Blattner (2000).

Theories dealing with cancer have been tested in a multitude of studies, with a goal of identifying the cause(s) of cancer, improving care, and ultimately finding cures. Studies that provided a basis for a relationship between lifestyle and cancer prevention have been conducted. For example, a growing body of evidence suggests that food choices, weight maintenance, and physical activity may have a protective effect on carcinogenesis (Bail, Meneses, & Demark-Wahnefried, 2016; Hoffman, 2016; Kushi et al., 2012).

Application to Nursing

Several works were found that addressed aspects of cancer prevention and how nurses can promote these activities. For example, a team lead by Mojica (Mojica et al., 2015) looked at factors that promote secondary prevention activities related to cancer (e.g., breast, cervical, and colorectal cancer screening) among Hispanics in the United States using community health workers. Weyl and colleagues (2015) also looked at interventions to promote colorectal screening in a community setting, and another work examined nursing interventions to increase women's intention to get pap smears (Guvenc, Akyuz, & Yenen, 2013). Lastly, Dickey, Cormier, Whyte, Graven, and Ralston (2016) reviewed protocols and recommendations to give nurses more information on how to promote prostate screening among African American men to reduce related health disparities.

An example of primary prevention for cancer was presented by Thomas (2016) who described strategies nurses can use to overcome barriers and promote vaccination against HPV. Another interesting look at primary prevention of cancer by nurses was presented by Rosenberg (2013) as she reviewed evidence of the relationship between cell phone use and brain cancer. Citing a number of recent studies, she summarized interventions to reduce exposure of children to radio frequency radiation and thereby potentially preventing associated brain cancer. Finally, Jablonski and Duke (2012) presented a tertiary prevention look at how to best manage pain in cancer patients living in rural areas.

Pain Management

Pain is a phenomenon that has received a great deal of attention in health care. Early pain theories emphasized the specific pathways of pain transmission. Later theories attempted to uncover the complexity of central processing of pain in specific areas of the brain. The specificity theory of pain, for example, was proposed in the early 1800s. The theory was based on the recognition that free nerve endings exist in the periphery of the body and suggested that there are highly specific structures and pathways responsible for pain transmission. These nerve endings act as pain receptors that are capable of accepting sensory input and transmitting this information along specific nerve fibers. This theory set the stage for further studies on pain and pain management (Keene, McMenamin, & Polomano, 2002).

A biochemical theory of pain perception was proposed in the 1970s following identification of endorphins and opioid receptors. This theory postulates that morphine-like substances attach to pain receptors to modulate or decrease pain. Endorphin, which is synthesized in the pituitary and basal hypothalamus, is released into the bloodstream from the pituitary gland and mediates pain at the spinal cord level through circulating spinal fluid. Opioid receptors modulate pain by binding endogenous opioid peptides. When acute pain is elicited, endogenous opioids are released and are associated with the stress response to modulate or decrease pain. If pain-relieving medications are administered, they will attach to specified sites and result in pain relief. Pain can be controlled with drugs that bind to receptors (Litwack, 2009).

Gate Control Theory

The GCT was proposed in 1965 to explain the relationship between pain and emotion. Melzack and Wall (1982) concluded that pain is not just a physiologic response but that psychological variables (i.e., behavioral and emotional responses) influence the perception of pain. According to the GCT, a gating mechanism occurs in the spinal cord. Pain impulses are transmitted from the periphery of the body by nerve fibers (A, delta, and C fibers). The impulses travel to the dorsal horns of the spinal cord, specifically to the area of the cord called the *substantia gelatinosa*. The cells of the *substantia gelatinosa* can inhibit or facilitate pain impulses that are conducted by the transmission cells. If the activity of the transmission cells is inhibited, the gate is closed and impulses are less likely to be conducted to the brain. When the gate is opened, pain impulses ascend to the brain. Similar gating mechanisms exist in the descending nerve fibers from the thalamus and cerebral cortex. A person's thoughts and emotions can influence whether pain impulses reach the level of conscious awareness (Bautista & Grossman, 2014; Helms & Barone, 2008).

The gate control model (Figure 15-5) differentiates the excitatory (white circle) and inhibitory (black circle) links from the *substantia gelatinosa* to the transmission cells as well as descending inhibitory control from brain stem systems. The round knob at the end of the inhibitor link implies that its action may be presynaptic, postsynaptic, or both. All connections are excitatory, except the inhibitory link from *substantia gelatinosa* to the transmission cell (Melzack & Wall, 1982).

As mentioned in the case study, it is believed that pain medication has an effect on the gating mechanism. If pain medication is administered before the onset of pain (i.e., before the gate is opened), it will help keep the gate closed longer and fewer pain impulses will be allowed to pass through. The greater the degree of pain, the greater the number of pain impulses passing through the gate. If fewer pain impulses are allowed through the gate, the person will experience less pain. If the gate is allowed to open completely, a higher dosage of pain medication is required to close the gate. Therefore, in theory, prevention and management of pain are linked to keeping the gate closed.

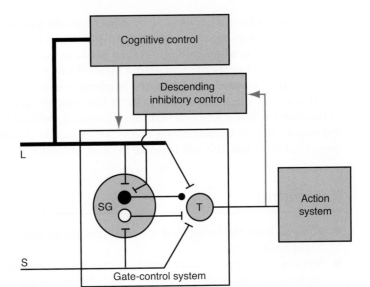

| Figure 15-5 | Gate Control Theory. L, large-diameter fibers; S, small-diameter fibers; SG, *substantia gelatinosa*; T, transmission. |

(Adapted with permission from Watt-Watson, J. H., & Donovan, M. I. [1992]. *Pain management* [p. 20]. St. Louis, MO: Mosby.)

Application to Nursing

The GCT has also been the model for several reports related to pain management. Lane and Latham (2009), for example, presented aspects of the GCT in use of heat and cold therapy as nonpharmacologic interventions to reduce pain in hospitalized children. Tansky and Lindberg (2010) performed a comprehensive literature review on the use of breastfeeding as an intervention to reduce pain caused by immunization using the GCT as a framework. They found that there is considerable evidence that it is an effective pain management technique.

In nursing research, one study (Ngamkham, Holden, & Wilkie, 2011) used the GCT to examine pain pattern responses in location, intensity, and quality among outpatients with cancer. Friesner, Curry, and Moddeman (2006) used GCT as the framework in a research study to compare two strategies for removal of chest tubes. They determined that encouraging slow, deep-breathing relaxation helps manage pain during chest tube removal. Finally, one experimental study, Hatfield (2008) showed that administration of an oral sucrose solution prior to immunization is effective in helping relieve pain in infants receiving routine vaccinations and a second experimental study (Jose, Sulochana, & Shetty, 2012) suggested that "skin tapping" prior to immunization reduced pain responses in infants receiving diphtheria-pertussis-tetanus (DPT) injection.

Summary

Nurses continually use concepts and principles from multiple biomedical theories in practice and in research. Indeed, these concepts, principles, and theories are so integral to nursing that they are difficult to differentiate and set aside for detailed inspection.

The biomedical theories used by nurses include theories of disease and disease causation as well as theories related to physiology and physical functioning. Nurses, particularly advanced practice nurses such as Maria from the case study, should study these theories. They should understand their relevance to nursing practice and recognize how they are used and supported in nursing research.

Because of length constraints, only a few concepts and theories were described in this chapter. But it is hoped that these discussions will lead the reader to recognize the importance of understanding theory and to apply theory to guide practice and research. Ultimately, this will improve the care of clients.

Key Points

- Theories from the biomedical sciences have greatly influenced nursing since Nightingale's time.
- Biomedical science theories used by nurses include theories from biology, medicine, public health, physiology, and pharmacology.
- Theories and models of disease causation commonly used by nurses include the "Germ Theory" (principles of infection) and public health theories, such as the Epidemiologic Triangle and the Web of Causation.
- The Natural History of Disease Model outlines the concepts of health promotion as well as primary, secondary, and tertiary prevention; these principles are used by nurses in all areas of practice and research.
- Theories and principles of physiology and physical functioning include homeostasis and theories of stress and adaptation; both are commonly used by nurses in practice and research.
- Theories and principles related to immunity and immune function are widely used in nursing practice and are increasingly being studied in nursing research.
- Nursing knowledge regarding genetics, genetic principles, and genetic counseling is growing, and nurses are recognizing the importance of genetic factors on health.
- Cancer theories, particularly related to prevention and early detection, are very important to nurses and a source for study for nursing research and review for nursing practice.
- Pain management is a vital part of nursing practice; nurses are continually researching how to improve pain management.

Learning Activities

1. Search current nursing journals for research studies that use epidemiologic, biologic, or physiologic theories as a framework. What theories are being tested?
2. Review the original work of one of the grand nursing theorists. Identify the epidemiologic, biologic, or physiologic concepts that are components of the theory.
3. Following the example of CRNA student Maria in the opening case study, outline a potential research study using one of the theories or models presented in this chapter as a framework as depicted in the opening case study. Show how the model or theory can be used to generate testable hypotheses.

REFERENCES

American Association of Colleges of Nursing. (2006). *The essentials of doctoral education for advanced nursing practice.* Retrieved from http://www.aacn.nche.edu/dnp/Essentials.pdf

Bail, J., Meneses, K., & Demark-Wahnefried, W. (2016). Nutritional status and diet in cancer prevention. *Seminars in Oncology Nursing, 32*(3), 206–214.

Banasik, J. L. (2014a). Genetic structure, regulation and tissue differentiation. In L. C. Copstead & J. L. Banasik (Eds.), *Pathophysiology* (5th ed., pp. 74–88). Philadelphia, PA: Elsevier.

Banasik, J. L. (2014b). Inflammation and immunity. In L. C. Copstead & J. L. Banasik (Eds.), *Pathophysiology* (5th ed., pp. 157–169). Philadelphia, PA: Elsevier.

Banasik, J. L. (2014c). Neoplasia. In L. C. Copstead & J. L. Banasik (Eds.), *Pathophysiology* (5th ed., pp. 113–137). Philadelphia, PA: Elsevier.

Bautista, C., & Grossman, S. (2014). Somatosensory function, pain, and headache. In S. C. Grossman & C. M. Porth (Eds.), *Porth's pathophysiology: Concepts of altered health states* (9th ed., pp. 422–451). Philadelphia, PA: Wolters Kluwer/Lippincott Williams & Wilkins.

Black, J. M., & Hawks, J. H. (2009). *Medical-surgical nursing: Clinical management for positive outcomes* (8th ed.). St. Louis, MO: Saunders.

Blattner, W. A. (2000). Etiology of malignant disease. In H. D. Humes (Ed.), *Kelley's textbook of internal medicine* (4th ed., pp. 141–147). Philadelphia, PA: Lippincott Williams & Wilkins.

Calzone, K. A., Jenkins, J., Yates, J., Cusack, G., Wallen, G. R., Liewehr, D. J., et al. (2012). Survey of nursing integration of genomics into nursing practice. *Journal of Nursing Scholarship, 44*(4), 428–436.

Camak, D. J. (2016). Increasing importance of genetics in nursing. *Nurse Education Today, 44,* 86–91.

Cavenee, W. K., & White, R. (1995). The genetic basis of cancer. *Scientific American, 272,* 72–79.

Centers for Disease Control and Prevention. (2016). *CDC concludes Zika causes microcephaly and other birth defects.* Retrieved from https://www.cdc.gov/media/releases/2016/s0413-zika-microcephaly.html

Chapa, D. W., Akintade, B., Son, H., Woltz, P., Hunt, D., Friedmann, E., et al. (2014). Pathophysiological relationships between heart failure and depression and anxiety. *Critical Care Nurse, 34*(2), 14–24.

Chun, H. K., Kim, K. M., & Park, H. R. (2015). Effects of hand hygiene education and individual feedback on hand hygiene behaviour, MRSA acquisition rate and MRSA colonization pressure among intensive care unit nurses. *International Journal of Nursing Practice, 21*(6), 709–715.

Coyle, A. L. (2016). Zika virus: What nurses need to know. *Nursing, 46*(5), 22–24.

Dever, M. (2016). Screening for depression in adolescents with diabetes. *Journal of Pediatric Nursing, 31*(1). 117–119.

Dickey, S. L., Cormier, E. M., Whyte, J., IV, Graven, L., & Ralston, P. A. (2016). Demographic, social support, and community differences in predictors of African-American and White men receiving prostate cancer screening in the United States. *Public Health Nursing, 33*(6), 483–492.

Donahue, M. P. (2011). *Nursing, the finest art: An illustrated history* (3rd ed.). Maryland Heights, MO: Mosby.

Ewen, H. H., & Kinney, J. (2014). Application of the model of allostasis to older women's relocation to senior housing. *Biological Research for Nursing, 16*(2), 197–208.

Foote, A., & El-Masri, M. (2016). Self-perceived hand hygiene practice among undergraduate nursing students. *Journal of Research in Nursing, 21*(1), 8–19.

Friesner, S. T., Curry, D. M., & Moddeman, G. R. (2006). Comparison of two pain-management strategies during chest tube removal: Relaxation exercise with opioids and opioids alone. *Heart & Lung, 35*(4), 269–276.

Fritz, B. J. (2015). Screening for perinatal depression at county WIC offices. *Journal of Obstetric, Gynecologic, and Neonatal Nursing, 44,* S13.

Ganz, F. D. (2012). Tend and befriend in the intensive care unit. *Critical Care Nurse, 32*(3), 25–33.

García-Fernández, F. P., Agreda, J. J., Verdú, J., & Pancorbo-Hidalgo, P. L. (2014). A new theoretical model for the development of pressure ulcers and other dependence-related lesions. *Journal of Nursing Scholarship, 46*(1), 28–38.

Grossman, L. C. (2014a). Genetic and congenital disorders. In S. C. Grossman & C. M. Porth (Eds.), *Porth's pathophysiology: Concepts of altered health states* (9th ed., pp. 138–159). Philadelphia, PA: Wolters Kluwer/Lippincott Williams & Wilkins.

Grossman, L. C. (2014b). Genetic control of cell function and inheritance. In S. C. Grossman & C. M. Porth (Eds.), *Porth's pathophysiology: Concepts of altered health states* (9th ed., pp. 118–137). Philadelphia, PA: Wolters Kluwer/Lippincott Williams & Wilkins.

Grossman, S. (2014a). Neoplasia. In S. C. Grossman & C. M. Porth (Eds.), *Porth's pathophysiology: Concepts of altered health states* (9th ed., pp. 160–199). Philadelphia, PA: Wolters Kluwer/Lippincott Williams & Wilkins.

Grossman, S. (2014b). Stress and adaptation. In S. C. Grossman & C. M. Porth (Eds.), *Porth's pathophysiology: Concepts of altered health states* (9th ed., pp. 202–215), Philadelphia, PA: Wolters Kluwer/Lippincott Williams & Wilkins.

Guvenc, G., Akyuz, A., & Yenen, M. C. (2013). Effectiveness of nursing interventions to increase pap smear test screening. *Research in Nursing & Health, 36*(2), 146–157.

Halloran, L. (2015). Genetics in practice: Ready or not. *The Journal for Nurse Practitioners, 11*(6), 654–655.

Hannan, M. (2016). Exercise and hemodialysis: The missing piece of tertiary prevention. *Nephrology Nursing Journal, 43*(4), 317–321.

Harvath, T. A., Lindauer, A., & Sexson, K. (2016). Managing complex medication regimens. *The American Journal of Nursing, 116*(11), 43–46.

Hatfield, L. A. (2008). Sucrose decreases infant biobehavioral pain response to immunizations: A randomized controlled trial. *Journal of Nursing Scholarship, 40*(3), 219–225.

Hawkins, N., Berkowitz, Z., Rodriguez, J. L., Miller, J. W., Sabatino, S. A., & Pollack, L. A. (2015). Examining adherence with recommendations for follow-up in the prevention among colorectal cancer survivors study. *Oncology Nursing Forum, 42*(3), 233–240.

Helms, J. E., & Barone, C. P. (2008). Physiology and treatment of pain. *Critical Care Nurse, 28*(6), 38–49.

Hoffman, A. J. (2016). The impact of physical activity for cancer prevention: Implications for nurses. *Seminars in Oncology Nursing, 32*(3), 255–272.

Hohenberger, H. (2015). The OR environment-hand hygiene, cleaning and clostridium difficile. *AORN Journal, 102*(6), 584–587.

Holmes, T., & Rahe, R. H. (1967). The Social Readjustment Rating Scale. *Journal of Psychosomatic Research, 11,* 213–218.

Hughes, D., Ladas, E. L., Rooney, D., & Kelly, K. (2008). Massage therapy as a supportive care intervention for children with cancer. *Oncology Nursing Forum, 35*(3), 431–442.

Jablonski, K., & Duke, G. (2012). Pain management in persons who are terminally ill in rural acute care: Barriers and facilitators. *Journal of Hospice & Palliative Nursing, 14*(8), 533–540.

Jacobson, S., Tedder, M., & Eggert, J. (2016). Adult acute lymphoblastic leukemia: A genetic overview and application to clinical practice. *Clinical Journal of Oncology Nursing, 20*(6), E147–E154.

Jansen, D. A., & Emerson, R. J. (2014). Homeostasis and adaptive responses to stressors. In L. C. Copstead & J. L. Banasik (Eds.), *Pathophysiology* (5th ed., pp. 12–24). Philadelphia, PA: Elsevier.

Johnson, N. L., Giarelli, E., Lewis, C., & Rice, C. E. (2013). Genomics and autism spectrum disorder. *Journal of Nursing Scholarship, 45*(1), 69–78.

Johnson, P., Gilman, A., Lintner, A., & Buckner, E. (2016). Nurse-driven catheter-associated urinary tract infection reduction process and protocol: Development through an academic-practice partnership. *Critical Care Nursing Quarterly, 39*(4), 352–362.

Jones-Parker, H. (2012). Primary, secondary, and tertiary prevention of cardiovascular disease in patients with HIV disease: A guide for nurse practitioners. *The Journal of the Association of Nurses in AIDS Care, 23*(2), 124–133.

Jose, R. M., Sulochana, B., & Shetty, S. (2012). Effectiveness of skin tap technique in reducing pain response. *International Journal of Nursing Education, 4*(1), 56–57.

Kalisch, P. A., & Kalisch, B. J. (2004). *American nursing: A history* (4th ed.). Philadelphia, PA: Lippincott Williams & Wilkins.

Kang, D. H., McArdle, T., Park, N. J., Weaver, M. T., Smith, B., & Carpenter, J. (2011). Dose effects of relaxation practice on immune responses in women newly diagnosed with breast cancer: An exploratory study. *Oncology Nursing Forum, 38*(3), E240–E252.

Kang, D. H., Rice, M., Park, N. J., Turner-Henson, A., & Downs, C. (2010). Stress and inflammation: A biobehavioral approach for nursing research. *Western Journal of Nursing Research, 32*(6), 730–760.

Kaplow, R., & Iyere, K. (2016). Recognizing and preventing tumor lysis syndrome. *Nursing, 46*(11), 26–32.

Katerndahl, D., Burge, S., Ferrer, R., Becho, J., & Wood, R. (2014). Webs of causation in violent relationships. *Journal of Evaluation in Clinical Practice, 20*(5), 703–710.

Katz, A. (2017). CE: Human papillomavirus-related oral cancers: The nurse's role in mitigating stigma and dispelling myths. *The American Journal of Nursing, 117*(1), 34–39.

Keene, A., McMenamin, E. M., & Polomano, R. C. (2002). Pain: The fifth vital sign. In D. D. Ignatavicius & M. L. Workman (Eds.), *Medical-surgical nursing: Critical thinking for collaborative care* (4th ed., pp. 61–94). Philadelphia, PA: Saunders.

Klemp, J. R. (2015). Breast cancer prevention across the cancer care continuum. *Seminars in Oncology Nursing, 31*(2), 89–99.

Klompas, M. (2015). Review: Does chlorhexidine prevent ventilator-associated pneumonia? *Evidence-Based Nursing, 18*(3), 90.

Kukanich, K. S., Kaur, R., Freeman, L. C., & Powell, D. A. (2013). Evaluation of a hand hygiene campaign in outpatient health care clinics. *The American Journal of Nursing, 113*(3), 36–42.

Kushi, L. H., Doyle, C., McCullough, M., Rock, C. L., Demark-Wahnefried, W., Bandera, E. V., et al. (2012). American Cancer Society guidelines on nutrition and physical activity for cancer prevention: Reducing the risk of cancer with healthy food choices and physical activity. *CA: A Cancer Journal for Clinicians, 62*(1), 30–67.

Lane, E., & Latham, T. (2009). Managing pain using heat and cold therapy. *Paediatric Nursing, 21*(6), 14–18.

Lazarus, R. S., & Folkman, S. (1984). *Stress, appraisal and coping.* New York, NY: Springer Publishing.

Leavell, H. R., & Clark, E. G. (1965). *Preventive medicine for the doctor in his community: An epidemiologic approach* (3rd ed.). New York, NY: McGraw-Hill.

Lipsitz, L. A. (2001). Clinical physiology of aging. In H. D. Humes (Ed.), *Kelley's textbook of internal medicine* (4th ed., pp. 118–127). Philadelphia, PA: Lippincott Williams & Wilkins.

Litwack, K. (2009). Somatosensory function, pain, and headache. In C. M. Porth & G. Matfin (Eds.), *Porth's pathophysiology: Concepts of altered health states* (8th ed., pp. 1225–1259). Philadelphia, PA: Lippincott Williams & Wilkins.

Logsdon, M. C. (2016). Nursing strategies to address maternal morbidity and mortality. *Journal of Obstetric, Gynecologic, and Neonatal Nursing, 45*(6), 857–860.

MacMahon, B., & Pugh, T. F. (1970). *Epidemiology: Principles and methods.* Boston, MA: Little, Brown.

Matthews, M., & Moore, A. (2013). Babies are still dying of SIDS: A safe sleep environment in child-care settings reduces risks. *The American Journal of Nursing, 113*(2), 59–65.

McEwen, B. S. (2003). Interacting mediators of allostasis and allostatic load: Towards an understanding of resilience in aging. *Metabolism, 52*(10 Suppl. 2), 10–16.

McEwen, M., & Pullis, B. (2009). *Community-based nursing: An introduction* (3rd ed.). St. Louis, MO: Saunders.

Melzack, R., & Wall, P. D. (1982). *The challenge of pain.* New York, NY: Penguin Books.

Mojica, C. M., Morales-Campos, D. Y., Carmona, C. M., Ouyang, Y., & Liang, Y. (2016). Breast, cervical, and colorectal cancer education and navigation: Results of a community health worker intervention. *Health Promotion Practice, 17*(3), 353–363.

Morgan, L., Flynn, L., Robertson, E., New, S., Forde-Johnston, C., & McCulloch, P. (2017). Intentional rounding: A staff-led quality improvement intervention in the prevention of patient falls. *Journal of Clinical Nursing, 26*(1–2), 115–124.

Murphy, R. J. (2012). Preventing multidrug-resistant gram-negative organisms in surgical patients. *AORN Journal, 96*(3), 315–329.

Ngai, F. W., & Ngu, S. F. (2014). Family sense of coherence and family adaptation among childbearing couples. *Journal of Nursing Scholarship, 46*(2), 82–90.

Ngamkham, S., Holden, J. E., & Wilkie, D. J. (2011). Differences in pain location, intensity, and quality by pain pattern in outpatients with cancer. *Cancer Nursing, 34*(3), 228–237.

Okonta, N. R. (2012). Does yoga therapy reduce blood pressure in patient with hypertension? *An integrative review. Holistic Nursing Practice, 26*(3), 137–141.

Outland, L. (2010). Intuitive eating: A holistic approach to weight control. *Holistic Nursing Practice, 24*(1), 35–43.

Peterson-Graziose, V., Bryer, J., & Nikolaidou, M. (2013). Self-esteem and self-efficacy as predictors of attrition in associate degree nursing students. *The Journal of Nursing Education, 52*(6), 351–354.

Phillippi, J. C., & Roman, M. W. (2013). The motivation-facilitation theory of prenatal care access. *Journal of Midwifery & Women's Health, 58*(5), 509–515.

Plavskin, A. (2016). Genetics and genomics of pathogens: Fighting infections with genome-sequencing technology. *Medsurg Nursing, 25*(2), 91–96.

Premji, S. (2014). Perinatal distress in women in low- and middle-income countries: Allostatic load as a framework to examine the effect of perinatal distress on preterm birth and infant health. *Maternal and Child Health Journal, 18*(10), 2393–2407.

Prows, C. A., Hopkin, R. J., Barnoy, S., & Van Riper, M. (2013). An update of childhood genetic disorders. *Journal of Nursing Scholarship, 45*(1), 34–42.

Quigley, P. (2015). Mapping the human genome: Implications for practice. *Nursing, 45*(9), 26–34.

Roebuck, H., Moran, K., MacDonald, D. A., Shumer, S., & McCune, R. L. (2015). Assessing skin cancer prevention and detection educational needs: An andragogical approach. *The Journal for Nurse Practitioners, 11*(4), 409–416.

Rosenberg, S. (2013). Cell phones and children: Follow the precautionary road. *Pediatric Nursing, 39*(2), 65–70.

Santos, E. M. M., Edwards, Q. I., Floria-Santos, M., Rogatto, S. R., Achatz, M. I. W., & MacDonald, D. J. (2013). Integration of genomics in cancer care. *Journal of Nursing Scholarship, 45*(1), 43–51.

Schuler-Faccini, L., Ribeiro, E. M., Feitosa, I. M., Horovitz, D. D., Cavalcanti, D. P., Pessoa, A., et al. (2016). Possible association between Zika virus infection and microcephaly—Brazil, 2015. *Morbidity and Mortality Weekly Report, 65*(3), 59–62.

Secker, T., Hervé, R., & Keevil, C. (2011). Adsorption of prion and tissue proteins to surgical stainless steel surfaces and the efficacy of decontamination following dry and wet storage conditions. *The Journal of Hospital Infection, 78*(4), 251–255.

Selye, H. (1976). *Stress in health and disease.* Boston, MA: Butterworths.

Sherrod, M. M., Sherrod, N. M., & Cheek, D. J. (2015). Follow the guideline for reducing cardiovascular risk with statins. *Nursing, 45*(6), 40–46.

Shi, L., & Singh, D. A. (2015). *Delivering health care in America: A systems approach* (6th ed.). Burlington, MA: Jones and Bartlett.

Siegel, J. H. (2007). *Predictors of overweight in children in grades six through eight* (Unpublished doctoral dissertation). University of Miami, FL.

Snow, D., & Lu, J. H. (2012). Genetics and genomics: Unraveling new opportunities for addiction treatment and education. *Journal of Addictions Nursing, 23*, 93–96.

Staniute, M., Brozaitiene, J., & Bunevicius, R. (2013). Effects of social support and stressful life events on health-related quality of life in coronary artery disease patients. *The Journal of Cardiovascular Nursing, 28*(1), 83–89.

Stark, S. (2012). Elder abuse: Screening, intervention, and prevention. *Nursing, 42*(10), 24–29.

Starkweather, A. (2013). Psychologic and biologic factors associated with fatigue in patients with persistent radiculopathy. *Pain Management Nursing, 14*(1), 41–49.

Starkweather, A., Kelly, D. L., Thacker, L., Wright, M. L., Jackson-Cook, C. K., & Lyon, D. E. (2017). Relationships among psychoneurological symptoms and levels of C-reactive protein over 2 years in women with early-stage breast cancer. *Supportive Care in Cancer, 25*(1), 167–176.

Tansky, C., & Lindberg, C. E. (2010). Breastfeeding as a pain intervention when immunizing infants. *The Journal for Nurse Practitioners, 6*(4), 287–295.

Thomas, T. L. (2016). Cancer prevention: HPV vaccination. *Seminars in Oncology Nursing, 32*(3), 273–280.

Upshaw-Owens, M., & Bailey, C. A. (2012). Preventing hospital-associated infection: MRSA. *Medsurg Nursing, 21*(2), 77–81.

Walker, M. D. (2016). Fluid and electrolyte imbalances: Interpretation and assessment. *Journal of Infusion Nursing, 39*(6), 382–386.

Weyl, H., Yackzan, S., Ross, K., Henson, A., Moe, K., & Lewis, C. P. (2015). Understanding colorectal screening behaviors and factors associated with screening in a community hospital setting. *Clinical Journal of Oncology Nursing, 19*(1), 89–93.

Williams, L. (2016a). What neonatal nurses need to know about the Zika virus. *Neonatal Network, 35*(3), 174–177.

Williams, L. (2016b). Zeroing in on safety: A pediatric approach to preventing catheter-associated urinary tract infections. *AACN Advanced Critical Care, 27*(4), 372–378.

Williams, T., & Dale, R. (2016). A partnership approach to genetic and genomic graduate nursing curriculum: Report of a new course's impact on student confidence. *Journal of Nursing Education, 55*(1), 574–578.

Workman, M. L. (2016). Inflammation and immunity. In D. D. Ignatavicius & M. L. Workman (Eds.), *Medical surgical nursing: Patient centered collaborative care* (8th ed., pp. 275–289). Philadelphia, PA: Elsevier.

Yammine, L., Kang, D. H., Baun, M. M., & Meininger, J. C. (2014). Endothelin-1 and psychosocial risk factors for cardiovascular disease: A systematic review. *Psychosomatic Medicine, 76*(2), 109–121.

Ethical Theories and Principles

Cathy L. Rozmus and Jeffrey P. Spike

Heather Benson is currently midway through a program to obtain her doctor of nursing practice (DNP). Heather is on faculty at a university-based nursing program where she has a group of eight undergraduate students on the medical-surgical floor of a community hospital. Early one morning, one of Heather's students approached her for advice. The student was assigned to a 55-year-old female, Ms. M., who has terminal liver cancer. Ms. M. has no immediate family and is jaundiced and cachectic with severe ascites. She is semiconscious and is moaning almost continuously. When Ms. M. is touched or moved, she screams in what appears to be pain. She is on a morphine drip for pain, and the student explained to Heather that the physician has just ordered an increase in the morphine drip dosage. The student is concerned because Ms. M.'s respiratory rate is 8 breaths per minute, and she is afraid that increasing the morphine dosage will reduce Ms. M.'s breathing even more or perhaps stop it completely.

Heather's educational program has included a course that presented various ethical theories and principles, and she and her classmates discussed and debated how the main principles can be applied in everyday situations encountered in their individual practices. In the course, she also completed an assignment applying the *Code of Ethics for Nurses With Interpretive Statements* (American Nurses Association [ANA], 2015a) in a case study. These activities helped her gain a much greater understanding of the ethical foundations for her roles and responsibilities.

In consideration of the various ethical theories and principles and nursing responsibilities, how should Heather advise her student?

Ethics is a branch of philosophy that involves the systematic study of how one should best live his or her life and treat others. Ethics should not be confused with personal opinions, the law, politics, or religion. Although all of these may influence how we make decisions, they are not "ethics." Socrates (469–399 BCE) first proposed the idea that ethics is a branch of philosophy. He posed the question, "Is something right because it is commanded by the gods, or is it commanded by the gods because it is right?" (Austin, n.d.).

An ethical perspective—to do what is right—is foundational to nursing. Indeed, as mentioned in Chapter 1, a code of ethics is one of the defining characteristics of a profession, and nursing has met this characteristic (ANA, 2015a). The nursing profession is widely respected, and nurses are perceived by the public as having the highest ethical standards of any profession (ANA, 2015b). In their role as patient care providers and advocates, nurses have defined responsibilities and expectations. These commitments involve basic duties to respect and care for patients that do not consider social or economic status, personal attributes, or the nature of their health problems (Winland-Brown, Lachman, & Swanson, 2015).

Bioethics is the systematic study of how to provide the best possible care in the health care delivery system by evaluating "the impact of biological and technological advances on humans and what is permissible" (Grace, 2009, p. 6). Ethical theories and principles present frameworks for how to examine patient health–related issues and make decisions on the best course of action in difficult circumstances where there is no single, obvious right or best decision or when there are two or more choices that are determined to be incompatible. It is vital for all practicing nurses to have a basic understanding of their responsibilities to society. For those who are in advanced practice or leadership roles, it is essential they are aware of the ethical foundations underlying the profession and how these ethical theories and principles are applied when making choices and decisions for patient care.

Ethics and Philosophy: An Overview

Before addressing theories of ethics in nursing, it is important to begin with some semantic clarifications.

Theory in the Humanities and Philosophy

Although confusing, what is often called "theory" in the humanities may be distinct from philosophical theories of ethics. "Theory" in the humanities usually refers to any one of a combination of ideas, hypotheses, or propositions derived from a range of the humanities fields such as literary theory, postmodern theory in sociology, and structuralism or poststructuralism in cultural anthropology. The word *theory* in these contexts means a general and abstract method of interpreting a text, but it does not suggest the "theory" is either rigorous or testable as is implied by the term *scientific theory.*

Philosophers generally regard something termed *theory* with indifference and consider that those inclined to examine "theory" will have little background in philosophy. With that distinction, this chapter provides an overview of "philosophical theories of ethics"—rather than "theory" per se.

Ethics Versus Morality

There is one more clarification that is important to the philosophical examination of ethics. One often sees the word *morality* used interchangeably with *ethics,* but there is a need to distinguish between these two terms. Although they have similar historical roots, they have diverged in meaning.

"Morality" is an accepted set of cultural beliefs about what is right and wrong behavior (Beauchamp & Childress, 2013). Morality can be used to recognize and enforce the traditional social customs and values that are widely shared by a cultural group. These customs or values, however, may be unsupported beliefs or biases of dominant groups but not applicable to all. Ethics, in contrast, is the careful, reflective, critical, and systematic study of morality with the objective of identifying rational and empirical justifications of how one ought to treat other people or, more generally, how one should lead one's life. Ethics, then, is the effort to overcome the biases created by cultural or historical context or circumstances in order to make decisions more fairly, objectively, or scientifically. The critical difference is the requirement of objective justifications (Adams, 2011).

The ANA (2015a) expanded on the distinctions by observing that morality refers to "personal values, character, or conduct of individuals or groups," whereas ethics is "the formal study of that morality from a wide range of perspectives including se-mantic, logical, analytics, epistemological and normative" (p. xi). One might describe ethics as evidence-based or critically assessed morality.

This chapter focuses on the accepted, foundational Western philosophical theo-ries of ethics. And after a brief review of the three most central ethical theories, the widely used, contemporary midlevel principles of bioethics will be presented.

Philosophical Theories of Ethics

In academia, ethics has been one of the main branches of philosophy since the time of Socrates in Ancient Greece. To focus on the most well-known and influential philosophical theories of ethics, three are presented here: one from the ancient world and two "modern" theories. To frame the introduction of these theories, it is important to recognize that although the two modern theories are in many ways the most powerful, the ancient theory, Virtue Ethics, has proven to be very conducive to generating different approaches to ethical reasoning.

Virtue Ethics

Virtue Ethics, or *Virtue Theory*, is the term used to describe Aristotle's views on ethics as well as newer approaches based on his writings.

Background

Aristotle's (384–322 BCE) *The Nicomachean Ethics*, the first book to explain ethics and ethical ideals, deeply influenced many medieval philosophers, including Jewish, Christian, and Muslim scholars. Thus, Virtue Ethics was widely accepted and revered through much of Europe prior to the Enlightenment (Butts & Rich, 2015).

Aristotle was concerned primarily with explaining human nature. Ethics, to Aristotle, was defined as fulfilling all of our potential as humans (Beauchamp & Childress, 2013). He explained that what makes humans different from other an-imals are our rational abilities; to flourish, humans need to excel at using these rational abilities. Aristotle provided an account of the character traits one needs in order to have good judgment. Subsequently, a good person is one who can control his or her emotions through practical knowledge or practical wisdom (*phronesis*) (Kraut, 2014).

One of Aristotle's best known insights was his "doctrine of the golden mean between two extremes." In short, he advocated for everything in moderation (Kraut, 2014). For example, courage is good but not the extremes of recklessness or cowardice. Similarly, he wrote about concern for one's looks (e.g., don't be slovenly, but don't be vain) and balance in exercise and diet and even drinking and joking. According to Aristotle, the right thing to do in any situation is whatever a wise, experienced, and perceptive person, with good practical judgment (*phronesis*), would do in the same situation (Beauchamp & Childress, 2013).

Another unique aspect of Aristotle's theory was the emphasis on not just knowing the right thing to do, a cognitive ability, but the importance of having the sort of confidant, action-oriented character that "gets it done." This is captured in the Greek word for virtue—*arête*—which applies to a person who sets lofty goals and achieves them. Virtue relates to "habit of character that predisposes one to do what is right; what we should be as moral agents" (ANA, 2015a, p. 46). Furthermore, virtue is viewed as excellence of character (Russell, 2014). Virtue Theory, then, is especially appealing to people who believe that good role models are the essence of good teaching (Paola, Walker, & Nixon, 2010). This sense of virtue is also concordant with the recent emphasis on the importance of leadership in nursing.

Aristotle was also the most important source of inspiration for the medieval approach to ethics known as *casuistry*. In casuistry, one analyzes a new case by comparing it to well-known and influential cases from the past, known as paradigm cases, by identifying the similarities and differences between the cases. In logic, this is known as analogical reasoning. Most legal reasoning, especially case law, is based on casuistry, and because legal cases are central to most discussions of clinical and research ethics, clearly, casuistry has a role in explaining the reasoning process of ethics (Butts & Rich, 2015; Grace, 2009).

Possibly, the one greatest weakness of Virtue Theory, including casuistry, is its foundational origin in established cultural norms. Many philosophers believe that because of its relationship with cultural norms, Virtue Theory does not provide a sufficiently objective approach to allow a critique of established traditions and instead tends too often to uncritically defend traditions (Beauchamp & Childress, 2013).

Application in Nursing

Despite its ancient origins, Virtue Theory is still relevant in contemporary health care. One recent example from the nursing literature involved application of Virtue Ethics as the philosophical framework for teaching undergraduate nursing students expectations for civility (Russell, 2014). Russell (2014) explained that virtue can be learned by practice through role modeling, critical reflection, and narrative exchange. Furthermore, commitment to virtue impacts conduct, and the virtues expressed in nursing should serve as a framework to promote ethical development of nursing students while simultaneously encouraging respect in relationships with clients, other health professionals, and other nurses.

Also focusing on nursing education, Crigger and Godfrey (2014) described the utilization of Virtue Ethics to enhance "professional identity formation" through character development. The authors stressed Aristotelian virtues such as courage, humility, and integrity, along with application of *phronesis* (e.g., deliberation, making good choices, and acting upon those choices in practice). They organized the constructs into the "Stair-Step Model" to illustrate to students the processes that lead to examination of the outcomes (*telos*) of actions, thereby aiding the formation of one's professional identity.

Finally, Newham (2015) presented a somewhat contrarian examination of the focus on Virtue Ethics in nursing. He suggested there is a need to move away from an overemphasis on character and examination of what sort of *person* one must be to be a "good" nurse. Noting that although Virtue Ethics (character) is important, there is also a need to recognize that "doing good" (or not) is not necessarily dependent on moral character. He concluded by suggesting that much of nursing practice involves complex situations that require objective judgment and decisions that are not dependent on the nurses' character but rather on knowledge and "praxis" that is independent of character.

Modern Ethical Theories

Before beginning to describe the two "modern" ethical theories—Deontology and Utilitarianism—it is important to point out that they are often viewed as mutually exclusive. The difference between them is fundamental, or, in philosophical terms, epistemologic. One—Utilitarianism—is a posteriori (knowledge dependent on experience or evidence) like the social sciences, whereas the other—Deontology—is a priori (knowledge independent of experience) like math and logic. As described in Chapter 1, the philosophical terms for these two contrasting types of epistemology are empiricist and rationalist. These perspectives often consider different viewpoints, seek different goals, and use different methods to explain and/or interpret truth and reality. Even in the many situations where the two theories agree about what is the right or best thing to do, the rationale for the conclusion would be different.

Deontology

The seminal theorist of Deontology is Immanuel Kant (1724–1804). Kant's ethics focused on rationality, and he formulated "the moral law" in the terms of universal maxims, or guiding principles every rational agent must agree to, precisely because they are rational.

Kant claimed to prove there was a single, ultimate rule for ethics, which he called the Categorical Imperative (Bandman & Bandman, 2002; Beauchamp & Childress, 2013). A paraphrase of his Categorical Imperative would be to "respect others' goals in life, and never treat them merely as a means to your own ends." But, even though he insisted there was only one rule, he added a second formulation of that rule, paraphrased as "only act according to rules which you would be willing to require everyone in the world to follow" (Link to Practice 16-1).

Link to Practice 16-1

Kant and the "Golden Rule"

Kant's formulations or rules sound very similar to Christianity's "Golden Rule"—"Do unto others as you would have them do unto you." Kant was aware of the similarities and hoped to defend Christian values by demonstrating that they were rational rather than revealed.

But the rule is also similar to other, even more ancient religious maxims found in the Hebrew Torah, Confucius's Analects, and the Mahabharata—all from around 600 to 900 BCE. Thus, it can be concluded that these early prephilosophical insights support the claim of Kant that this is the most fundamental rule of ethics. Furthermore, it is vital for philosophers to note that Kant did not claim his formulations were given to him by a divine source but that they were justified by reason—thus true for everyone.

Kant explained that the two formulations are isomorphic because of a necessary shared foundation in the concept of "autonomy." This implies that rational agents must dictate and follow their own laws (self-rule) as part of having a free will. Although autonomy is often considered a Kantian idea, for Kant, it is restricted to the choices of a purely rational agent (Kant, 1993).

Kant is often presented as the great synthesizing philosopher of the modern period, bringing together the truths of both the rationalists (Descartes, Spinoza, and Leibniz) and the empiricists (Locke, Berkeley, and Hume). He was the clear originator of the tradition known by philosophers as Deontology. *Deontology* is Greek for a system of duty-based laws, with duty implying absolute, non negotiable requirements. Kantian Deontology, then, posits that rational beings are obligated to act first and foremost from a sense of duty—irrespective of the consequences (Rich, 2015).

John Rawls (1971, 1993, 2001), the most influential academic philosopher in ethics over the last century, was a deontologist who was strongly influenced by Kant. Rawls was a proponent of egalitarianism, which is based on a notation of fairness where everyone should be treated equally (Paola et al., 2010). He proposed that fairness and equality be examined under a "Veil of Ignorance" where each person would shield themselves from their own biases and act neutrally when making decisions. Rawls promoted equal rights and basic liberty and suggested that social and economic inequalities be addressed impartially. He strongly advocated for those who are disadvantaged, writing that they should be given opportunities for improvement (Butts & Rich, 2015).

Rawls (1971) is known for a thought experiment he called The Veil of Ignorance. In this thought experiment, Rawls asks participants to imagine the souls in Heaven waiting to be born and looking down at the world and seeing all the different countries. He posed the question: Which country would they choose to be born in, assuming ignorance as to what family they will be born into? The goal was to make participants think objectively and remove implicit biases acquired through the social circumstances of birth and enculturation (Rawls, 1971).

The notion behind the thought experiment was to get people to agree on what is fair. For example, if one knows they would be born a girl, would they choose a country with powerful sexist traditions that deny women equal opportunity? If someone knows they will be born of African heritage, would they choose to be born into a country where "whites" live longer (and have better education and higher income) than "blacks"? In general, when assessing the ethics of a situation, a deontologist might start by asking questions such as these (Bandman & Bandman, 2002).

Utilitarianism

In the second more contemporary ethical theory, Utilitarianism, ethics is exemplified by choosing actions that maximize the pleasure and happiness and minimize the pain and suffering the choices may cause. Utilitarianism's most famous proponent was John Stuart Mill (1806–1873) who succinctly summarized its central principle as doing "the greatest good for the greatest number of people" (Bandman & Bandman, 2002). By making that the justification, Utilitarianism regards ethics as an empirical or scientific subject and ultimately a natural part of policy debates.

Utilitarianism is fundamentally practical and has succeeded in identifying many social ills that had become invisible to the ruling class in Europe following the Middle Ages and the Renaissance. For example, beginning over 150 years ago in England, utilitarians fought against child labor and slavery and in favor of free public schools, universal health care, women's right to vote, and animal welfare (the latter because all sentient beings are subject to pain and suffering; thus, animals are legitimate objects of ethical concern). In policy debates, when deciding on the most ethical course of action, the type of questions to be considered are: "How many people would be affected by a policy change?" "Who would a policy help?" and "What are the costs?"

The point of Utilitarianism is not so much the importance of setting pleasure or happiness as the goal, but the fact that everyone's pleasure or happiness counts as much as anyone else's. But in choosing happiness, it was also placing ethics into the realm of experience and potentially measurable outcomes. This made ethics appropriate for consideration into policy debates and politics. Mill, like his father (James Mill) and his godfather (Jeremy Bentham), was a member of the British Parliament. In that role, Mill introduced the first bill for women's suffrage into Parliament soon after he was elected in 1865. He coauthored a book with his wife Harriet Taylor (published in 1869) in which he argued for the "perfect equality" of women, noting that society was only harming itself by trying to preserve ancient traditions of marriage and family which limited the education and occupations of women. The utilitarian argument was very clear in his writings which pointed out that over half of the population was being denied the pleasures and happiness associated with freedom, education, fulfilling work, and income (Paola et al., 2010).

The persistent power of the utilitarian ethical theory can be seen in one of its most famous contemporary adherents, Peter Singer. Singer (2011) argued that being ethical in Utilitarianism means one should help everyone according to need, not just people in your city or country or in your family or religion. To give an idea of the degree of altruism Utilitarianism demands, the theory proposes that one must not take advantage of any benefits of position, such as gender, race/ethnicity, or inherited wealth or status. Just as Bentham's concern for animal suffering led him to propose and enact the first anti-vivesection laws in England 150 years ago, Singer has extended similar arguments to encourage vegan diets and other limits to the human use of animals (such as in research, and in zoos).

Deontology and Utilitarianism—A Summary

In most cases, Deontology and Utilitarianism perspectives agree on what is the right thing to do. The difference between them—the philosophically irreconcilable difference—is in the justification (i.e., what makes an action the right thing to do). In short, utilitarian theories of ethics are predicated on achieving good consequences for the most people, whereas Deontology leads us to make decisions based on duty rather than consequences (Butts & Rich, 2015) (Link to Practice 16-2). Despite their differences, or perhaps *because* of them, both Deontology and Utilitarianism provide rich but different approaches to ethics. Also, because of the fundamentally different nature of their arguments and justifications, it would be impossible to construct a single theory that combines them.

Both perspectives agree that ethics must be universal and result in an altruistic value system that does not allow one's self-interest to unfairly or unduly limit another's liberty. Thus, both theories can be of help when considering an ethics issue or question, but it is also important to consider *both* theories in case the perspectives lead to different conclusions. Practical ethics might best conclude that neither Utilitarianism nor Deontology can be considered complete and instead argue that they are each necessary and jointly sufficient.

Application to Nursing

Several examples comparing and contrasting the ethical theories of Utilitarianism and Deontology were identified in the recent nursing literature. In one example, Pieper (2008) presented an excellent review of the application of the two contrasting

Link to Practice 16-2

A Historical Example of Deontology and Utilitarianism

Dr. Gisella Perl was a Jewish Romanian gynecologist who was imprisoned in Auschwitz in 1944. She was chosen to work in the women's infirmary with few supplies or medications to treat the women prisoners in the camp. Soon after arrival in the camp, Dr. Perl learned that pregnant women were immediately sent to the gas chamber. Any women who avoided detection of their pregnancies and delivered their infants were also sent to gas chamber, along with their newborn infants. Furthermore, some pregnant women were the subjects of Dr. Mengele's horrendous research before they were killed. Despite her professional and religious beliefs, Dr. Perl began performing abortions on pregnant women with her bare hands (Brozan, 1982; Reamey, 2009).

Using deontologic theoretical approach, Dr. Perl's actions could be viewed as unethical. In this approach, the obligation of the health care provider is to maintain life in all circumstances—to do no harm. Aborting the pregnancies would be causing harm to the fetus and thus not following a major guiding principle. Using the utilitarian perspective, aborting the fetus would save the life of the mother; instead of the loss of two lives, only one life would be lost. Therefore, Dr. Perl's actions reflect the utilitarian perspective. She viewed herself as saving the mother's life and the lives of any future children the mother might have.

perspectives in the dilemma(s) encountered when obtaining the assent of children for research participation. She used historical examples to examine how the ethical theories can be applied to balance the determination of risks and benefits encountered when advising children of their autonomous choices while also considering the desires (and permission) of their parents. She explained that from a deontologic perspective, the only research with children that is ethically acceptable is that which has the potential to benefit the child or if the child is capable of assent. On the other hand, Utilitarianism suggests that research that is potentially beneficial to many children is justified and assent is not mandated, even if there is greater than minimal risk and the findings will not directly benefit the participants.

In another example, Hughes and Common (2015) discussed ethical decision making involved in treatment of patients with dementia. They described several issues and dilemmas frequently encountered from different perspectives (Deontology, Virtue Ethics, and "consequentialism" [Utilitarianism]). Several situations were presented in cases that questioned autonomy, use of restraints, and withholding treatment for this very vulnerable population. In a third example, Winters (2013) presented a case study examining the dilemma occasionally encountered in health care settings in which a nurse might be required to break patient confidentiality. She contrasted Utilitarianism and "Kantianism" in a situation in which a threat of violence was made by a patient against others. In this case, there was a duty for the nurse to consider the patient's "rights" versus the best outcome for all who are potentially involved. In short, she concluded that the nurse should consider all alternatives and consequences and choose that which will minimize potential harms and maximize benefits to all parties involved.

Bioethical Principles

For many people who study and apply ethics, the major ethical theories described earlier are too philosophical or too abstract to aid in making decisions—particularly in situations involving health and health care delivery. They desire guidance that is more concrete and reflective of the normative values that serve as ethical frameworks. A system of four bioethical principles has been proposed: autonomy, beneficence, nonmaleficence, and justice. Each of the four principles can be justified using either deontologic or utilitarian reasoning, and they have found much acceptance among health professionals, including nurses (ANA, 2015a).

Historical Perspective on the Bioethical Principles

A seminal event in the application of ethical theory and principles in health care can be traced to the mid-20th century. At the end of World War II, the United States directed a trial of the Nazi doctors accused of conducting "experiments" in the concentration camps that frequently resulted in the torture and murder of the research subjects (Shuster, 1997). Following the trials, in August 1947, the American judges developed a document known as the "Nuremberg Code" that outlined the basic principles of ethical human experimentation. The Nuremberg Code was widely praised and rapidly accepted as the guideline for research using human subjects; the main tenets are summarized in Box 16-1.

Building on the Nuremberg Code, in 1964, the World Medical Association developed a statement of "ethical principles for medical research involving human subjects" that became known as the Declaration of Helsinki (World Medical Association, 2013). The Declaration of Helsinki is more detailed than the Nuremberg Code and includes the need to obtain assent from those not able to consent themselves. Furthermore, it established the standard for submitting research protocols to an independent review board for approval of the research prior to initiation (Paola et al., 2010). The Declaration of Helsinki has been updated and modified several times since 1964 to address issues such as the requirement to publish negative benefits and to report sources of funding and declaring potential conflicts of interest (Paola et al., 2010; World Medical Association, 2013).

Box 16-1 Summary of the Basic Tents of the Nuremberg Code

- Consent of human subjects is voluntary and informed.
- Research should aim for positive results and seek to answer questions that cannot be procured any other way.
- Previous knowledge should justify the research.
- Unnecessary physical and mental suffering and injury should be avoided.
- Research should not be conducted if there is risk of death or disabling injury.
- Risks should be proportionate to expected benefits to humanity.
- Preparation and facilities should be provided to protect the subject against risk.
- Researchers should be scientifically qualified and fully trained.
- Subjects must be free to quit the research at any point.
- Researchers must stop the research when they observe that continuation would be unduly harmful.

Despite the widespread acceptance of the Nuremberg Code and the Declaration of Helsinki, unethical experimentation continued in many countries, including the United States. Indeed, the Tuskegee Study was one of the most infamous instances of unethical biomedical research in recent history. In this study, between 1932 and 1972, almost 400 low-income African American men with syphilis were not offered treatment; rather, they were monitored to evaluate the course of the disease. Left untreated, many of the men died and others were seriously harmed (Judkins-Cohn, Kielwasser-Withrow, Owen, & Ward, 2014).

Following the publication of the Tuskegee Study in 1972, the National Commission for the Protection of Human Subjects of Biomedical and Behavioral Research (NCPHSBBR) published *The Belmont Report: Ethical Principles and Guidelines for the Protection of Human Subjects of Research.* The Belmont Report outlined three basic ethical principles—respect for persons, beneficence, and justice—to serve as an "analytical framework that will guide the resolution of ethical problems arising from research involving human subjects" (NCPHSBBR, 1979, p. 2). The principle of nonmaleficence was later added (Beauchamp & Childress, 2013). Over time, these four principles moved beyond the narrowly focused concerns of biomedical research to become a framework used to analyze the multitude of ethical issues encountered in the provision of health care (Beauchamp & Childress, 2013; Farmer & Lundy, 2017).

Beauchamp and Childress (2013) describe these four principles as "midlevel principles" to make clear that each principle is less abstract than a philosophical theory and makes no claim to being self-sufficient. The four principles have been recognized as essential to ethical practice and adopted in hundreds of articles and textbooks, including all health care professions and allied health fields.

Part of the strength of application of these principles is that the principles of beneficence and nonmaleficence represent more traditional values of medicine (which some might want to differentiate as more patriarchal), whereas the other two principles, autonomy and justice, represent the two most important values in modern ethics. In short, the first two principles—beneficence and nonmaleficence—especially resonate with many older health care providers who are familiar with the traditional "paternalistic" values of the medical profession, as found in Hippocratic ethics, whereas the other two principles lay the groundwork for contemporary concepts such as "shared decision making" and "informed choice" which reflect the importance of the construct of patient-centered care. Each of the four principles will be discussed briefly, followed by additional examples illustrating how they have been applied in nursing.

Autonomy

The principle of autonomy, or respect for persons, focuses on the rights of individuals to make informed choices about their health care (Beauchamp & Childress, 2013; NCPHSBBR, 1979).

Overview
This principle is based on the conviction that the patient or subject is the ultimate authority on what is best for his or her well-being. With respect to the principle of autonomy, health care professionals should *always* provide *all* of the relevant information to the person about his or her health, illness, and treatment options in order to empower him or her to make an informed decision. This communication includes not only providing the information but also ensuring that the information is given in a way that can be understood by the person. Furthermore, there should be no bias

or undue influence or coercion to sway the person toward one action or another (Beauchamp & Childress, 2013; NCPHSBBR, 1979).

One consideration with this principle is the capacity of the person for "self-determination." Self-determination implies that the individual is capable of making reasoned decisions that reflect their own values and goals. Either developmental age, illness, or disability may leave the person unable to make an informed choice. In some cases, such as with minor children, there is a legal surrogate who makes the decisions. In other circumstances, however, it is less clear who has authority for a person with diminished decision-making capability (Beauchamp & Childress, 2013; NCPHSBBR, 1979).

The principle of autonomy refers to patient autonomy—not professional autonomy—and is the natural result of recognizing the patient's rights. This principle of autonomy changes the role of the clinician from being an authoritative expert and decision maker to being an educator and advocate. Currently, the preferred model of decision making is called shared decision making, which means clinicians have a responsibility to help patients understand their illness and all of the reasonable treatment options in order to help the patient make decisions that are best suited to the patient's goals and long-term life plans. Of note, autonomy protects pluralism because it acknowledges and allows different patients to make different choices, whether based on religious beliefs or other personal values (Spike & Lunstroth, 2016).

The concept of "informed consent" is derived from the principle of autonomy. Patients and potential research subjects should receive information on the risks and benefits of treatment or research. This information needs to include not only the risks and benefits of the potential treatments, interventions, or trials but also all available reasonable alternatives. Additionally, the person needs to be able to comprehend the information. Thus, the information should be presented in a format and with language that the receiver can understand. Finally, the choice needs to be voluntary. The person needs to make their decision free of coercion or undue influence (Beauchamp & Childress, 2013; NCPHSBBR, 1979). The context is also important for comprehension. A rushed presentation of facts in a noisy, busy room may preclude comprehension of the information. The consent process should not be seen as a trivial matter or formality but as part of patient education and requires active listening on the part of the health professional and thoughtful but honest answers to tough questions. For those individuals with limited ability for comprehension, a surrogate (i.e., parent or guardian) may be needed for making decisions on care. It is incumbent to note that surrogates are expected to represent the patient's wishes, not the surrogate's wishes (Beauchamp & Childress, 2013).

Application to Nursing

In nursing ethics, one might argue that the importance that is often given to being a patient advocate is best explained as a way to recognize and promote autonomy. As a patient advocate, it is the nurse's responsibility to ensure that the patient has not only been given all of the information but also understands the information. The accountability for advanced practice nurses is even higher (Farmer & Lundy, 2017). Both legal and accreditation standards for informed consent must be met; at a minimum, information should include "the patient's diagnosis or statement of his condition . . . the purpose and nature of the proposed procedure or treatment . . . risks, benefits, and potential outcomes, including anticipated course if treatment is refused . . . and alternatives to the proposed procedure/treatment" (Farmer & Lundy, 2017, p. 126).

This idea was explained succinctly in an essay by Rock and Hoebeke (2014) who discussed the ethical and legal basis for informed consent. The authors explained the duties of both the physician and the nurse in obtaining informed consent and concluded that as patient advocates, nurses must understand the legal and moral rights of patients for self-determination. Furthermore, the nurse must protect and preserve the patient's interests by ensuring that he or she understands the presented information and implications of treatment decisions.

In another example, Mitchell (2015) discussed the principles of autonomy and self-determination in a patient's decision to leave the emergency department (ED) "against medical advice" (AMA). She described the dilemma frequently faced by ED nurses who learn that a patient is planning on leaving AMA and noted the importance of recognizing the balance between respecting the patient's autonomy and promoting their safety. She explained that the nurse has an obligation to assess whether the patient has the capacity to make the decision to leave AMA and is fully appraised of possible risks, alternatives, and implications of leaving but concluded that if the patient has the mental capacity, his or her decision must be respected.

Finally, autonomy and self-determinism were the focus of a work by Olsen (2013). In this essay, the author discussed the challenge posed by patients who refuse to make lifestyle changes to positively benefit their health. Examples abound, including patients with lung disease who continue to smoke, those who have diabetes or are obese but who continue to eat poorly, and those who practice unsafe sex or use illicit drugs or abuse alcohol. Olsen explained that the nurse is to remember that the patient's "right" to make poor choices must be respected and that the nurse should avoid an adversarial relationship.

Beneficence

The principle of beneficence refers to doing what is in the patient's best interest and involves balancing benefits and burdens.

Overview

According to Beauchamp and Childress (2013), beneficence includes deeds of mercy, kindness, and charity. Health care providers have an obligation to act for the benefit of the patient and not in self-interest or in the interest of a third party. The risk/benefit analysis for the patient should consider quality of life issues, effectiveness of treatment, and cost of treatment as well as potential negative outcomes or side effects. The principle of beneficence identifies the clinician as a fiduciary, meaning that the clinician must *always* put the patient's best interest ahead of his or her own interests; the only benefits (or risks) that count are the patient's. Thus, beneficence is highly altruistic (Butts & Rich, 2015).

This principle, if not balanced by the principle of autonomy, is what helps justify paternalism—the practice of treating or making decisions for others in situations that rely on the expertise of the provider to decide what is in the patient's best interest without the input of the patient. In other words, there can be a conflict between the patient's autonomous choice and the provider's perceived benefits for the patient (Butts & Rich, 2015). Box 16-2 outlines five conditions that must be met to justify paternalism in health decision making.

Application to Nursing

One important question that is rarely addressed is the role of nurses in determining what is best for the patient. As the caregiver who spends the most time with the patient, nurses often find themselves questioning the judgments or actions of doctors.

Another issue with applying this principle in nursing revolves around the notion of who receives the benefit? In public/community health nursing where nurses are

> ### Box 16-2   Conditions That Justify Paternalism in Health Decisions
>
> - A patient is at risk for a significant, preventable harm.
> - The paternalistic action will probably prevent the harm.
> - The prevention of harm to the patient outweighs risks to the patient of the action taken.
> - There is no morally better alternative to the limitation of autonomy that occurs.
> - The least autonomy-restrictive alternative that will secure the benefit is adopted.
>
> Source: Beauchamp and Childress (2013, p. 222).

providing care to groups and populations, there are sometimes issues where the benefits to the group outweigh the benefit to the individual (ANA, 2015a). One example is the tension between parents who chose not to vaccinate their children and potentially risk exposing other children to an illness as a result. A similar tension occurs when public health nurses employ "direct observation therapy" to ensure that patients with tuberculosis take their medications, arguably negating their autonomy but benefiting society. A clear risk/benefit analysis must be done by first identifying the group that will be benefited and how those benefits compare to any risk for an individual within that group (Beauchamp & Childress, 2013; NCPHSBBR, 1979).

The principle of beneficence was examined in a work by Casarez and Engebretson (2012). They conducted an analysis of the propensity of health care providers to act in "omission" by failing to provide spiritual care—which would have potentially benefited a patient. They concluded that nurses should avoid both extreme secularization and imposition of one's own personal religious beliefs in the provision of spiritual care. Also focusing on the principle of beneficence, Denny and Guido (2012) discussed the nurse's ethical obligation to help relieve the pain of older adults.

Nonmaleficence

The principle of nonmaleficence relates to the Hippocratic principle of "first, do no harm." Health care professionals have an obligation to avoid causing bodily harm and death to patients and to minimize pain and suffering.

Overview

Beauchamp and Childress (2013) point out that nonmaleficence involves upholding professional standards of care, not being careless or negligent, judiciously withholding and withdrawing treatments, and careful consideration about providing extraordinary or "heroic" treatment. Of the four principles, nonmaleficence is the only one that is expressed in the negative, a prohibition; for that reason it is taken by many ethicists to be an inviolable minimum standard and thus to be more important clinically than the other principles.

Controversies surrounding this principle include end-of-life issues (prolonging death vs. quality of life) and withholding or withdrawing treatment at the end of life (Beauchamp & Childress, 2013; NCPHSBBR, 1979). Butts and Rich (2015) explained the "rule of double effect" which refers to performing an action that may have two potential outcomes—one is an intended or good outcome, but the other is a potentially detrimental outcome. In these situations, they explain, it is necessary to balance the positive effects with the potentially harmful effects.

This tension between beneficence and nonmaleficence was illustrated in the opening case study. Nonmaleficence may often counsel that hospice or palliative care is the best available treatment choice. Nonmaleficence in these situations is a conservative principle meant to *at least* avoid taking unnecessary risks or performing heroic interventions that may make things worse or protracting the patient's pain or suffering. It can also be interpreted to include a warning to know one's professional limits and to not attempt things that are beyond one's skills or training.

Application to Nursing

Nurses who find themselves in the position of trying to stop an aggressive treatment plan that is not working or achieving any reasonable goals can recognize the importance of the principle of nonmaleficence. Another issue with nonmaleficence for nurses can arise with military nurses. Military nurses have a dual loyalty—to country and to the patient. Sometimes, there may be conflict in those loyalties, and the perception of the military hierarchy may be that loyalty to country is higher priority than loyalty to the patient or enemy combatant. The role of nurses in torture is an extreme example of the ethical conflicts nurses may have with nonmaleficence (Holmes & Perron, 2007).

On a more routine level, many nurses report "moral distress" when told to provide care they think is causing unnecessary or undue suffering. For example, Choe, Kang, and Park (2015) reported on a study of "moral distress" among critical care nurses. This study noted themes or contributing factors to moral distress included unnecessary medical treatment, dilemmas from limited autonomy, and conflicts with physicians on treatment decisions. Similarly, Mason and colleagues (2014) studied moral distress among critical care unit nurses and identified themes of dealing with death and suffering, dealing with family, powerlessness, and medical values versus nursing values and contributory to moral distress. In a third example, Wagner and Dahnke (2015) stated that moral distress can affect nurses conducting disaster triage because it is very difficult to make life or death decisions for nurses who want to help and nurture all patients.

Justice

Justice is often described in terms of fairness in both treatment and research. Justice obligates health care professionals to provide necessary treatment for all members of society (Beauchamp & Childress, 2013; NCPHSBBR, 1979). Fair distribution of health care resources should include access to care but can also be applied to the notion of preventing waste and fraud.

Overview

In clinical care, justice requires providing health care to members of vulnerable populations, including the poor, the uninsured, and the undocumented, as well as the mentally and physically disabled. Perhaps, more controversially in the United States, the reality is that many people have access to health care based on ability to pay. There is a tension because given limited resources, the principle of justice also includes a duty to be careful stewards of those resources. To turn away an indigent patient for lack of ability to pay would be ethically condemned in any epoch, starting with Hippocrates. That duty has been built into the very definition of being a health care professional, as part of the "social contract" with society that authorizes exclusive privileges to practice (Butts & Rich, 2015; Grace, 2009). But there remains a tension when considering such issues as: Is everyone entitled to every available treatment without consideration of cost? Geographic location? Willingness or ability to follow up with care? Or age, as well as other potential issues?

Similarly in research, the principle of justice requires that one group not bear the risks of research to benefit another group. Research subjects should not be recruited simply because they are easily accessible, easily convinced, or easily coerced into participation. Vulnerable populations should not be exploited to the advantage of another group for research benefits or for profit. Research on prisoners is a good example of a practice that has become less common after ethical protections were put in place.

Issues in the principle of justice include allocation of resources at the unit, regional, or national level; setting priorities for and rationing of resources (Beauchamp & Childress, 2013; NCPHSBBR, 1979). This priority setting can often fall to public health and nursing in policy discussions.

Application to Nursing

Nursing leaders and managers must often address issues of justice involving allocation of resources. In extreme circumstances such as in disasters, pandemics, and war, the principle of justice may be a top priority. An example could be distribution of flu vaccine or antiviral medications during a flu pandemic. Allocation of intensive care unit (ICU) beds is another common allocation issue for nurses.

The most extreme example may have been the murder of disabled children and psychiatric patients by German nurses during the 1930s and 1940s. Nurses in Germany during the years of the Nazi government began to view the "volk," or people as a whole, as their patient instead of the individual. If resources were needed for wounded warriors, then killing children and psychiatric patients was seen as the better (more just) use of resources (Benedict & Rozmus, 2014; Benedict & Shields, 2014).

In a contemporary example, Douglas and Dahnke (2013) described the ethical issues health providers encounter in the case of "periviable" infants (neonates born between 22 and 24 weeks). The principle of justice was highlighted in this essay as the authors described the "burden" of health care to be "fair" to the population when only a small percentage of these infants will survive, and many of those who do will have major morbidities that will affect their life, their family's lives, and society as a whole. One notion posed by the authors is that what should be considered "is not looking at whether they can be treated, but whether they should be treated" (Douglas & Dahnke, 2013, p. 36). They concluded that it is "the moral obligation of the physicians and health professionals to provide the necessary information that will allow parents the ability to make an informed decision regarding their infants' care" (Douglas & Dahnke, 2013, p. 36).

Other Bioethical Principles

In addition to these ethical principles, ethical "rules" have also been widely described in the nursing and health care literature. These include veracity (or truth telling), privacy, confidentiality, and fidelity (Beauchamp & Childress, 2013). Other ethical principles found in the health care literature include fidelity to the profession, maintaining competence, and avoiding or managing conflicts of interest. All of these are important to providing quality, safe, patient-centered care, but none of them have the same level of generality as the four original principles.

Ethical Decision Making

The principles and philosophical theories of ethics can be used as an analytic framework to make decisions when encountering challenging issues or difficult choices—ethical dilemmas.

Overview

The first step in the process of ethical decision making is to recognize when an ethical issue or dilemma exists. Often, in the midst of a patient care situation or research project, the ethical issues and potential actions may not be obvious. Here, one might be advised to consider such questions as: What is the worst case scenario? What could possibly go wrong? Are we making any naïve assumptions? Or are we overlooking any stakeholders?

The second step in ethical decision making is to determine as many of the responses as possible to the issues or dilemma that might arise; this would be followed by an analysis of how the principles and philosophical theories relate to these possible responses. The four principles are mutually independent, and conflict among the principles is to be anticipated whenever there is an ethical dilemma. For example, as mentioned, autonomy may conflict with nonmaleficence in a situation in which a patient insists on a treatment plan that the nurse recognizes has a significant chance of causing harm.

Jonsen, Siegler, and Winslade (2010) proposed an approach to clinical decision making that superimposed the ethical principles within four "topics"—medical indication, patient preferences, quality of life, and contextual features. For each of the topics, they suggested questions that can be used to assist with the decision-making process. Table 16-1 summarizes these topics and questions. Butts and Rich (2015) explained that nurses as well as other health professionals should work to answer as many of the relevant questions as possible and to consider the patient's situation by involving the family and/or surrogates and members of an ethics team or committee when appropriate.

Understanding and applying the principles thus often explains the conflicts surrounding ethical issues but does not automatically resolve them. That still requires judgment of what is at stake, and for whom (the stakeholders), and then making a conscious, reasoned, and deliberate choice. Finally, there is personal action on the response that is chosen based on the analysis (Beauchamp & Childress, 2013; Carlin et al., 2011; NCPHSBBR, 1979).

Application to Nursing

A number of examples of nursing researchers and scholars comparing, studying, or applying the four major principles were identified in the recent nursing literature as examples of ethical decision making. In one example, Sundean and McGrath (2013) discussed each principle in their presentation of ethical considerations encountered by health care providers in the neonatal intensive care unit (NICU). Examining the heart-wrenching decisions made on a day-to-day basis as NICU providers treat critically ill infants, the authors described the many conflicts and dilemmas that arise because of the sometimes conflicting perspectives of the physicians, nurses, and parents, particularly in light of technologic advances. They concluded there is a need to consider all four principles to promote family-centered care that considers cultural differences.

Building on evolving guidelines and recommendations with respect to use of opioids for pain management, Bockhold and Hughes (2016) applied an ethical framework to examine how these highly addictive drugs can and should be used to manage chronic, noncancer pain. The authors noted the need to ensure that benefits outweigh potential harm in describing the challenges of helping to manage pain and the problems encountered when trying to taper patients off of opioid medications. In a similar work, Quinlan-Colwell (2014) applied the ethical principles to pain control,

Table 16-1 Four Topics Method for Analysis of Clinical Ethics Cases—Questions to Consider

Topic and Ethical Principle(s)	Questions to Consider
Medical indication (principles of beneficence and nonmaleficence)	What is the patient's diagnosis/health problem? What are goals of treatment? In what circumstances/situations is treatment not indicated? What is likelihood of success of different treatment options? How can the patient benefit from treatment? How can harm be avoided?
Patient preferences (autonomy)	Has the patient been informed of benefits and risks? Does the patient understand the information? Is the patient mentally capable and competent? What are the patient's preferences about treatment (if mentally competent)? Has consent been given? If the patient is *not* capable or competent— Have preferences been expressed in the past? Who is the appropriate surrogate? Is the patient willing and able to cooperate with treatment?
Quality of life (beneficence, nonmaleficence, and autonomy)	What are the prospects with and without treatment for return to normal life? Who would determine "quality of life" if the patient cannot make or express preferences? Are there biases that could prejudice the provider's evaluation of the patient's quality of life? Are there ethical issues related to improving or enhancing the patient's quality of life? What are plans or rationale to forgo life-sustaining treatment?
Contextual features (principles of justice and fairness)	Are there professional or business interests that might create conflicts of interest in the patient's treatment? Who are the stakeholders (i.e., clinicians, family members, insurers) that have an interest in the clinical decisions? What are the limits imposed on patient confidentiality by third parties (stakeholders)? What are the financial factors that could create conflicts of interest? Are there issues with allocation of scarce health resources? Are there religious or legal issues that might influence decisions? Are there public health or safety issues? Are there research and education considerations?

Source: Jonsen et al. (2010).

but their focus was on patients in the acute care setting, again pointing out the need to provide ethical, patient-centered care.

Several works were identified that described application of the four principles at the end of life. For example, Croft (2012) discussed issues related to attempting cardiopulmonary resuscitation, including the ethical, legal, and professional issues for "do not resuscitate" decisions. In other examples, Rising (2017) presented an ethical discussion of consideration of cultural differences with respect to veracity when talking with patients and family members at the end of life, and Hain, Diaz, and Paixao (2016) discussed ethical issues to consider when elders elect to stop dialysis. Several examples were found that applied the four principles in general contexts. These included public health nursing (Ivanov & Oden, 2013), hospice nursing (Cheon, Coyle, Wiegand, & Welsh, 2015), genetic research (Bevan et al., 2012), and nursing research (Doody & Noonan, 2016).

Summary

Three basic philosophical theories of Virtue Ethics, Deontology, and Utilitarianism provide a framework for making ethical decisions in nursing. Having an understanding of these theories can help nurses recognize their own and other people's viewpoints from an ethical perspective and to make decisions that are "right" or "good." The four principles of autonomy, beneficence, nonmaleficence, and justice provide an analytical framework for examining ethical issues and dilemmas encountered in nursing practice and research.

In the case presented at the beginning of this chapter, Heather's student is faced with the ethical dilemma of providing pain relief that might hasten the death of her patient, a frequent issue in health care—balancing length of life versus quality of life. Heather's student has two options: (1) increase the dose of the pain medication or (2) question the increase in the dosage or delay the increase in the pain medication. Increasing the pain medication may cause the patient to stop breathing and not increasing the dosage will mean the patient remains in what appears to be uncontrollable pain. In this case, the patient is semiconscious and cannot speak for herself so she cannot make her wishes known (autonomy) and she has no surrogate decision makers. The conflict in this case is between beneficence and nonmaleficence. Is pain control, even though it may hasten death, beneficence or maleficence? Pain control in general is usually viewed as an act of beneficence; however, hastening death is usually considered an act of maleficence.

As the ethical dilemma has been identified and different potential options for response (i.e., increase the morphine drip and risk respiratory depression or not increase the drip and leave the patient in pain) have been determined, the next step would be to consult with the stakeholders and review procedures and protocols to determine the best course forward.

Key Points

- Ethical theories are grounded in ancient and modern philosophy of what it means to do good.
- Although culture may be a major determinant of morality, ethics provides a more analytic approach to solving dilemmas in health care.
- Deontology is based on "duty" or obligation, whereas the utilitarian perspective focuses on what benefits the most; either perspective can lead to the same conclusion to an ethical dilemma, but the justification they offer will be different.
- The four principles of autonomy, beneficence, nonmaleficence, and justice are used by both clinicians and researchers in ethical decision making.

Learning Activities

1. Like Heather, the nurse from the opening case study, consider a situation or dilemma, an ethical issue you have encountered in clinical practice. What were all of the possible solutions to the issue? What ethical principles are involved in the possible solutions to the issue? What decision was ultimately made and why?
2. Think about an ethical dilemma you have encountered that caused you distress. Was the distress you felt because of a conflict in the philosophical theories or among those involved? Was the distress due to a conflict among the principles?
3. What ethical issues do you see in the news? What principles and philosophical theories might be involved, and how would they help resolve the issues?
4. Obtain a copy of the ANA's (2015a) Code of Ethics. With classmates, discuss how/when and to what extent it is applied in day-to-day practice.

REFERENCES

Adams, J. (2011). Nurse prescribing ethics and medical marketing. *Nursing Standard, 25*(29), 62–66.

American Nurses Association. (2015a). *Code of ethics for nurses with interpretive statements.* Silver Springs, MD: Author.

American Nurses Association. (2015b). *Nurses rank as most honest, ethical profession for 14th straight year.* Retrieved from http://nursingworld.org/FunctionalMenuCategories/MediaResources/PressReleases/2015-NR/Nurses-Rank-as-Most-Honest-Ethical-Profession-for-14th-Straight-Year.html

Austin, M. W. (n.d.). *Internet encyclopedia of philosophy.* Retrieved from http://www.iep.utm.edu/divine-c/

Bandman, E., & Bandman, B. (2002). *Nursing ethics through the life span* (4th ed.). Upper Saddle River, NJ: Prentice Hall.

Beauchamp, T. L., & Childress, J. F. (2013). *Principles of biomedical ethics* (7th ed.). New York, NY: Oxford University Press.

Benedict, S., & Rozmus, C. (2014). Nurses and human subjects research during the Third Reich and now. In S. Rubenfeld & S. Benedict (Eds.), *Human subjects research after the Holocaust* (pp. 87–98). Cham, Switzerland: Springer Publishing. doi:10.1007/978-3-319-05702-6_7

Benedict, S., & Shields, L. (2014). *Nurses and midwives in Nazi Germany: The "euthanasia programs."* New York, NY: Routledge.

Bevan, J. L., Senn-Reeves, J. N., Inventor, B. R., Greiner, S. M., Mayer, K. M., Rivard, M. T., et al. (2012). Critical social theory approach to disclosure of genomic incidental findings. *Nursing Ethics, 19*(6), 819–828.

Bockhold, C. R., & Hughes, A. K. (2016). The ethics of opioids for chronic noncancer pain. *Nursing, 46*(10), 63–67.

Brozan, N. (1982). *Out of death, a zest for life.* Retrieved from http://www.nytimes.com/1982/11/15/style/out-of-death-a-zest-for-life.html

Butts, J. B., & Rich, K. L. (2015). *Nursing ethics: Across the curriculum and into practice* (4th ed.). Burlington, MA: Jones & Bartlett.

Carlin, N., Rozmus, C. L., Spike, J., Wilcockson, I., Seifert, W., Chappell, C., et al. (2011). The health professional ethics rubric: Practical assessment in ethics education for health professional schools. *Journal of Academic Ethics, 9,* 277. doi:10.1007/s10805-011-9146-z

Casarez, R. L. P., & Engebretson, J. C. (2012). Ethical issues of incorporating spiritual care into clinical practice. *Journal of Clinical Nursing, 21,* 2099–2107.

Cheon, J., Coyle, N., Wiegand, D. L., & Welsh, S. (2015). Ethical issues experienced by hospice and palliative nurses. *Journal of Hospice & Palliative Nursing, 17*(1), 7–14.

Choe, K., Kang, Y., & Park, Y. (2015). Moral distress in critical care nurses: A phenomenological study. *Journal of Advanced Nursing, 71*(7), 1684–1693.

Crigger, N., & Godfrey, N. (2014). From the inside out: A new approach to teaching professional identity formation and professional ethics. *Journal of Professional Nursing, 30*(5), 376–382.

Croft, R. J. (2012). Cardiopulmonary resuscitation in end of life care. *Nursing Standard, 26*(51), 35–42.

Denny, D. L., & Guido, G. W. (2012). Undertreatment of pain in older adults: An application of beneficence. *Nursing Ethics, 19*(6), 800–809.

Doody, O., & Noonan, M. (2016). Nursing research ethics, guidance and application in practice. *British Journal of Nursing, 25*(14), 803–807.

Douglas, S. M., & Dahnke, M. D. (2013). Creating an ethical environment for parents and health providers dealing with the treatment dilemmas of neonates at the edge of viability. *Journal of Neonatal Nursing, 19*(1), 33–37.

Farmer, L., & Lundy, A. (2017). Informed consent: Ethical and legal considerations for advanced practice nurses. *The Journal for Nurse Practitioners, 13*(2), 124–130.

Grace, P. J. (2009). *Nursing ethics and professional responsibility in advanced practice.* Boston, MA: Jones & Bartlett Learning.

Hain, D. J., Diaz, D., & Paixao, R. (2016). What are ethical issues when honoring an older adult's decision to withdraw from dialysis? *Nephrology Nursing Journal, 43*(5), 429–434.

Holmes, D., & Perron, A. (2007). Violating ethics: Unlawful combatants, national security and health professionals. *Journal of Medical Ethics, 33,* 143–145. doi:10.1136/jme.2006.016550

Hughes, J., & Common, J. C. (2015). Ethical issues in caring for patients with dementia. *Nursing Standard, 29*(49), 42–47.

Ivanov, L. L., & Oden, T. L. (2013). Public health nursing, ethics and human rights. *Public Health Nursing, 30*(3), 231–238.

Jonsen, A. R., Siegler, M., & Winslade, W. J. (2010). *Clinical ethics: A practical approach to ethical decisions in clinical medicine* (7th ed.). New York, NY: McGraw-Hill.

Judkins-Cohn, T. M., Kielwasser-Withrow, K., Owen, M., & Ward, J. (2014). Ethical principles of informed consent: Exploring nurses' dual role of care provider and researcher. *Journal of Continuing Education in Nursing, 45*(1), 35–42.

Kant, I. (1993). *Grounding for the metaphysics of morals* (J. W. Ellington, Trans.) (3rd ed.). Indianapolis, IN: Hackett.

Kraut, R. (2014). *Aristotle's ethics. Stanford encyclopedia of philosophy.* Retrieved from https://plato.stanford.edu/entries/aristotle-ethics/

Mason, V. M., Leslie, G., Clark, K., Lyons, P., Walke, E., Butler, C., et al. (2014). Compassion fatigue, moral distress and work engagement in surgical intensive care unit trauma nurses: A pilot study. *Dimensions of Critical Care Nursing, 33*(4), 215–225.

Mitchell, M. A. (2015). Assessing patient decision-making capacity: It's about the through process. *Journal of Emergency Nursing, 41*(4), 307–313.

National Commission for the Protection of Human Subjects of Biomedical and Behavioral Research. (1979). *The Belmont report: Ethical principles and guidelines for the protection of human subjects of research* (DHEW Publication No. (OS) 78-0012). Retrieved from https://www.hhs.gov/ohrp/regulations-and-policy/belmont-report/

Newham, R. A. (2015). Virtue ethics and nursing: On what grounds? *Nursing Philosophy, 16*(1), 40–50.

Olsen, D. P. (2013). Helping patients who don't help themselves. *The American Journal of Nursing, 113*(7), 66–68.

Paola, F. A., Walker, R., & Nixon, L. L. (2010). *Medical ethics and humanities.* Sudbury, MA: Jones & Bartlett Learning.

Pieper, P. (2008). Ethical perspectives of children's assent for research participation: Deontology and utilitarianism. *Pediatric Nursing, 34*(4), 319–323.

Quinlan-Colwell, A. (2014). Making an ethical plan for treating patients in pain. *Dimensions of Critical Care Nursing, 33*(2), 91–95.

Rawls, J. (1971). *A theory of justice.* Cambridge, MA: Harvard University Press.

Rawls, J. (1993). *Political liberalism.* New York, NY: Columbia University Press.

Rawls, J. (2001). *Justice as fairness.* Cambridge, MA: Harvard University Press.

Reamey, A. S. (2009). *Gisella Perl: Angel and abortionist in the Auschwitz Death Camp.* Retrieved from http://www.phdn.org/archives/holocaust-history.org/auschwitz/gisella-perl/

Rich, K. L. (2015). Theories and methods in ethics. In J. B. Butts & K. L. Rich (Eds.), *Philosophies and theories for advance nursing practice* (2nd ed., pp. 177–194). Burlington, MA: Jones & Bartlett Learning.

Rising, M. L. (2017). Truth telling as an element of culturally competent care at end of life. *Journal of Transcultural Nursing, 28*(1), 48–55.

Rock, M. J., & Hoebeke, R. (2014). Informed consent: Whose duty to inform? *Medsurg Nursing, 23*(3), 189–191.

Russell, M. J. (2014). Teaching civility to undergraduate nursing students using a virtue ethics-based curriculum. *The Journal of Nursing Education, 53*(6), 313–319.

Shuster, E. (1997). Fifty years later: The significance of the Nuremberg Code. *The New England Journal of Medicine, 337*(20), 1436–1440.

Singer, P. (2011). *The expanding circle: Ethics, evolution, and moral progress.* Princeton, NJ: Princeton University Press.

Spike, J. P., & Lunstroth, R. B. (2016). *A casebook in interprofessional ethics: A succinct introduction to ethics for the health professions.* New York, NY: Springer Publishing.

Sundean, L. J., & McGrath, J. M. (2013). Ethical considerations in the neonatal intensive care unit. *Newborn & Infant Nursing Reviews, 13*, 117–120.

Wagner, J. M., & Dahnke, M. D. (2015). Nursing ethics and disaster triage: Applying utilitarian ethical theory. *Journal of Emergency Nursing, 41*(4), 300–306.

Winland-Brown, J., Lachman, V. D., & Swanson, E. O. (2015). The new "Code of Ethics for Nurses With Interpretive Statements" (2015): Practical clinical application, part 1. *Medsurg Nursing, 24*(4), 268–271.

Winters, N. (2013). Whether to break confidentiality: An ethical dilemma. *Journal of Emergency Nursing, 39*(3), 233–235.

World Medical Association. (2013). *WMA Declaration of Helsinki— ethical principles for medical research involving human subjects.* Retrieved from https://www.wma.net/policies-post/wma-declaration-of-helsinki-ethical-principles-for-medical-research-involving-human-subjects/

17

Theories, Models, and Frameworks From Leadership and Management

Melinda Granger Oberleitner

Marci Noble, an acute care nurse practitioner (NP), has been hired by a local integrated health system to work with a multidisciplinary team implementing practices across entities affiliated with the system. One goal for the team is to reduce the hospital readmission rates of patients diagnosed with congestive heart failure. Although she is an experienced NP, Marci is not yet familiar with the expectations of her new position. She envisions her role as that of clinical leader in performance improvement and in implementing best practices related to the care of heart failure patients and based on the latest clinical evidence.

Although Marci does not consider her role to be that of an administrator or manager, she recognizes that as a clinical leader, the information she learned about leadership styles and management practices in graduate school (e.g., motivating people, implementing change, and leading performance improvement) will be especially helpful to her as she transitions into her new position. Considerations for her new role include: How does she work within the management team? How can she be an effective agent for change? How can she support the team's performance improvement activities to positively affect patient care?

Nurses in management or leadership positions, regardless of role or practice setting, should have a working knowledge of theories, models, and frameworks of administration and management, which can help to guide practice. Furthermore, even though advanced practice nurses (APNs) (i.e., clinical nurse specialists [CNS], nurse practitioners, nurse anesthetists, and nurse midwives) are viewed primarily as clinicians, each role often has an administrative or management component. For example, APNs, who are being increasingly employed in traditional acute care facilities, are often responsible for performance improvement activities related to a specific product or service line. Similarly, an NP in a rural clinic may have administrative responsibilities for ancillary and secretarial staff assigned to the clinic in addition to the responsibilities of a client care provider.

This chapter provides a foundation in administration for nurses in any setting. Topics presented are historical and contemporary theories and models of leadership and management, organizational theories, motivational theories, and theories related to power, change, decision-making processes, conflict management, quality control, and quality improvement (QI).

Overview of Concepts of Leadership and Management

Leadership and management are closely related and sometimes intertwined concepts. Leadership is the ability to influence followers, to inspire confidence, and to generate support among followers for the leader's direction and vision. Leadership is viewed as a component of management; however, it is not the same thing. Leaders empower others and lead others willingly; in simplistic terms, leadership usually involves one individual trying to change the behavior of others. Furthermore, leaders challenge the current or prevailing wisdom and, by doing so, create new meaning for members of an organization (Peters, 1987).

Leaders in an organization can be formal or informal. Formal leaders are appointed by official or legislative authority. Informal leaders derive power through influence and, in reality, may be more important to staff or groups than the formal, appointed, or designated leaders. Influencing followers is perhaps the most essential aspect of leadership. Leaders can influence others by utilization of their expertise, by charisma, by coercion, or by virtue of the formal position they hold in organizations. Leaders who use expertise and charisma to influence others are the most effective in creating a sense of commitment in followers (Hellriegel, Jackson, & Slocum, 2008).

Management can be defined as the process of accomplishing work through and with other people. Effective management is often expected of a leader. In contrast to leaders, managers always have an official or appointed position within an organization through which they derive a legitimate source of power. Because of this official status, managers may direct willing and unwilling subordinates and are expected to perform specific, delineated functions, duties, and responsibilities. Effective leaders and managers are both required in today's workplace (DuBrin, 2007).

Early Leadership Theories

If one considers great historical leaders, names such as Alexander the Great, Julius Caesar, Napoleon Bonaparte, Thomas Jefferson, and Winston Churchill might come to mind. The Great Man Theory holds that leaders are born, not created. That is, certain individuals are born with the ability to lead, whereas most others are born to be led.

Trait Theories of Leadership

The Great Man Theory approach to defining leadership evolved into trait theories in the 1930s and 1940s. The trait theories assert that leaders possess certain characteristics (i.e., physical or personality traits and talents) that nonleaders do not.

Attributes, such as shyness, laziness, and timidity, are considered the antithesis of characteristics a leader should possess. An example of a physical attribute associated with leadership is height (i.e., a tall person may be able to look down on others and, therefore, may cut an imposing figure of authority). The converse may be true as well. Some individuals believe if someone is born shorter than most people, the individual may have to be more assertive or aggressive, and those behaviors may result in the development of a strong leader.

Personality traits or characteristics associated with leaders include intelligence, self-confidence, charisma, initiative, self-awareness, self-control, the ability to communicate effectively with individuals and in groups, goal orientation, self-directedness, the ability to assume consequences for actions and decisions, and the ability to tolerate stress. In lesser leadership positions, technical competence is important because it would be difficult to establish rapport with group members if the leader did not understand the technical details of the work (DuBrin, 2007). For example, Marci, as an acute care NP whose clinical area of expertise is focused on adults with acute illnesses, would have a difficult time assuming the position of director of perioperative services because of the level of technical expertise required in managing a perioperative nursing area.

Research studies designed to test trait theories of leadership have been inconsistent. The trait theories are limited by focusing only on leadership characteristics to the exclusion of the environment, the situation, and other possible confounding variables. Additionally, they focus on the attributes the leader brings to a particular situation rather than focusing on what specific actions the leader takes to address the situation.

Research attempts to identify traits consistently associated with leadership over time have been successful. Six traits have been identified that seem to best delineate the differences between leaders and nonleaders. These leader traits are the desire to lead, honesty and integrity, self-confidence, drive, intelligence, and job-relevant knowledge (Drafke, 2009). Another framework, the Big Five personality framework, advances the premise that five major personality traits or factors—extroversion, agreeableness, conscientiousness, emotional stability, and openness to experience—are predictors of leadership (Robbins & Judge, 2015). Research in this area concluded that relationships between personality traits and leadership style do indeed vary depending on the context (De Hoog, Den Hartog, & Koopman, 2005).

Emotional Intelligence

An interest in the inner or personal qualities of leaders has recently reemerged, particularly with respect to ethical qualities and charisma. This interest has been fueled by the demand for leaders with vision and charisma. Personality traits and characteristics have an important influence on leader effectiveness. The traits and characteristics that are most relevant tend to vary with the situation at hand. A foundational trait for leadership effectiveness that does not vary from situation to situation is self-awareness (DuBrin, 2007).

Self-awareness is one of the four key factors in emotional intelligence (EI). According to Goleman, Boyatzis, and McKee (2001), EI is a major contributor to leader effectiveness. The concept of EI refers to managing one's self and one's relationships effectively. EI includes the abilities of self-confidence, empathy, and visionary leadership. Passion for the work and for the people who do the work is particularly important to a leader with a high degree of EI. It is difficult, if not impossible, to inspire or motivate others if the leader is not passionate about the major work activities. The leader with high EI is able to sense and articulate a group's shared, yet possibly unexpressed, feelings and is able to develop a mission that inspires others to achieve a common goal (DuBrin, 2007). EI includes understanding one's own feelings, sensitivity, and empathy for others and the regulation of emotions.

Goleman and colleagues (2001) define four key competencies of EI:

- Self-awareness—the ability to understand and modulate one's own emotions. Goleman and colleagues (2001) contend this is the most essential of the four major competencies. A self-aware individual knows his or her own strengths and weaknesses and has a high level of self-esteem. The self-aware leader seeks feedback continually to determine how well his or her actions and decisions are received by others.
- Self-management/self-control—the ability to control one's emotions; control over mood and temper. The leader who is self-controlled acts with honesty and integrity in a consistent and dependable manner.
- Social awareness—the leader has empathy for others, including subordinates, and is intuitive about organizational "political" forces. The socially aware leader shows genuine care for others in the organization.
- Social skills/relationship skills—the ability to communicate clearly and convincingly. The leader who has social and relationship skills disarms conflicts, builds strong personal and professional bonds, uses social skills to spread enthusiasm and to solve disagreements and problems, uses kindness and humor often, and constantly expands network of contacts and supporters within and outside of the organization (DuBrin, 2007; Hellriegel et al., 2008).

Goleman and colleagues (2001) discovered that the most effective leaders are alike in one essential way—they all possess a high degree of EI. Without a high degree of EI, some experts contend a leader will never become a great leader (DuBrin, 2007).

Behavioral Theories of Leadership

Movement away from trait theories to explain and define leadership began as early as the 1940s. Leadership research from the 1940s through the mid-1960s focused instead on behavioral styles that leaders demonstrated (i.e., specific behaviors of leaders that make some more effective than others) (Hitt, Black, & Porter, 2011). This set of theories is referred to as the behavioral or functional theory of leadership. The major difference between trait theories and behavioral theories is that trait theories are concerned with the leader's individual characteristics, whereas behavioral theories seek to explain specific actions taken by the leader (Wagner & Hollenbeck, 2014).

Lewin and Lippitt conducted some of the first studies of leadership behavior at the University of Iowa in the late 1930s. The researchers, using an afterschool study group of 20 boys, aged 11 years, explored autocratic, democratic, and laissez-faire leadership behaviors or styles. The results of this study revealed that when the boys had a democratic leader, groups were more cohesive, the boys were more motivated, and originality of work was higher. With a democratic leader, the boys produced less work, but the work was of a higher quality than the work produced when the group leader used an authoritarian or laissez-faire leadership style. Nineteen of the 20 boys preferred the democratic style of group leadership over the other two styles (Lewin & Lippitt, 1938).

Other studies of autocratic versus democratic leadership styles concluded that democratic leadership styles produced higher performance results in some studies, whereas in other studies, performance was higher in groups with an authoritarian leader. However, what was consistent among study groups was that the level of satisfaction of group members was higher with the democratic style of leadership than with other styles.

Tannenbaum and Schmidt (1973) further explored satisfaction with leadership style and developed a model known as the continuum of leader behavior. This model provides for a range of leadership behaviors from leader centered (autocratic) to employee centered (laissez-faire). In determining which leader behavior the manager should implement, the authors proposed that the manager evaluate the following three variables: characteristics of the manager (i.e., experience with a certain leadership style), characteristics of the employees (i.e., level of experience with the process/job), and characteristics of the situation (i.e., offering a new product or service for the first time). Tannenbaum and Schmidt recommended an employee-centered approach or style because this approach most often led to increased employee satisfaction, motivation, and high performance and quality of the work product.

Leader–Member Exchange Theory

Leader–Member Exchange (LMX) Theory was developed by George Graen and James Cashman. The central focus of LMX Theory is the relationship and interaction between the supervisor (leader) and the subordinate (group member). The exchange between the superior and the subordinate is the unique, underlying premise of LMX. Interest in LMX has increased in recent years, leading to many field studies to test the propositions of the theory.

The theory recognizes that superiors develop unique working relationships with each subordinate or group member. According to LMX Theory, leaders categorize subordinates into one of two groups: the in-group (high-quality relationship with the leader) or the out-group (low-quality relationship). Often, the leader's first impression of the subordinate's competence heavily influences the leader's assignment of the subordinate to the in- or the out-group. The theory proposes that leaders do not interact with subordinates equally because supervisors have limited time and resources (Graen & Cashman, 1975).

Members of the in-group often have attitudes and values similar to the leader and interact frequently with the leader. They have a special exchange or relationship with the leader. In-group members perform their jobs in accordance with the expectations of their employment contracts. In addition, they can be counted on by the leader to volunteer for extra work and to take on additional tasks and responsibilities. As a result, in-group members are given additional rewards (increased job latitude, extra attention from the leader, and inside information that is not available to all employees), responsibility, and trust by the supervisor in exchange for their loyalty and performance. Research on LMX in field studies reveals that members of the in-group enjoy higher degrees of autonomy, job satisfaction, and trust from the supervisor as compared to members of the out-group.

Out-group members have less in common with the leader and are detached from the leader. There is limited reciprocal trust and support in the leader–subordinate relationship. Members of the out-group receive few rewards from supervisors and are more likely to quit because of job dissatisfaction.

Supervisors who aspire to be the most effective leaders create a special exchange relationship with all of their subordinates (Graen & Uhl-Bien, 1995; Wang, Law, Hackett, Wang, & Chen, 2005). The intent is not necessarily to treat all employees the same. Those subordinates who by virtue of their position in the organization have greater responsibility or administrative authority will have a deeper level of exchange with the superior. However, it is possible and highly desirable that the leader engender relationships of mutual trust, respect, and support with all followers.

LMX Theory postulates that the quality of the subordinate's relationship with the supervisor has a large impact on job behavior and performance and that the quality of that relationship has important job consequences (Bolino, 2007). Therefore, it is imperative that subordinates be evaluated based on their competencies rather than on the leader's favoritism (Graen & Uhl-Bien, 1995).

Motivational Theories of Leadership

The motivational theories expanded on the behavioral theories of leadership by focusing on factors that enhance worker/employee satisfaction and motivation and identifying factors that have a negative impact on those factors. Many of the motivational theories were based on the work of Maslow's (1968) Hierarchy of Needs Theory. Maslow's work included the concepts of five basic needs (i.e., physiologic, safety, love, esteem, and self-actualization), which he described as being the driving forces or motivators of human behavior. Lower level physiologic needs, including food and rest, must be satisfied before an individual can work on accomplishing higher level needs such as self-esteem and self-actualization. Even though his theory was derived as a motivational theory, Maslow's early works were not originally applied to motivation in the workplace.

Theory X and Theory Y
Douglas McGregor first published his work on Theory X and Theory Y in an article in 1957. McGregor was influenced by the works of Maslow, Herzberg, Argyris, and Likert. McGregor believed the structure of bureaucratic organizations, as well as prevailing management philosophy and policies, resulted in a situation in which power resided exclusively with management. In this structure, the role of management was to direct workers under the assumption that all workers were unmotivated, unambitious, lazy, and preferred to be led. These assumptions were labeled by McGregor as Theory X. McGregor's theory was that workers who had no input in the performance of the job lacked interest in the job and satisfaction with the work, resulting in resistance to change.

McGregor proposed a different set of assumptions and practices for meeting organizational goals in a more effective, humanistic manner; he designated this Theory Y. Management's priorities in Theory Y are to develop worker potential, remove obstacles, create opportunities for worker growth, and provide guidance, rather than control direction, for the worker. Theory Y encourages worker responsibility and participation in decision making. McGregor believed this style of participatory management would result in greater productivity, creativity, and worker satisfaction.

Because McGregor failed to operationalize concepts in his theories, there have been few direct tests of his theories. When the theories were tested, conflicting results were obtained (Caplan, 1971; Gray, 1978; Green, 1981; Kay, 1973; Malone, 1975; Morse & Lorsch, 1970). Most recently, Kopelman, Prottas, and Davis (2008) attempted to test the substantive validity of McGregor's theory by measuring the focal construct of the central concept utilizing an investigator-developed Theory X/Y attitude measure. The researchers viewed this as a critical first step in testing the many assumptions of the theory. The new measure is content valid and has adequate reliability. Finally, although a few contemporary companies are using Theory X management, many companies subscribe to the tenets of Theory Y (Daft & Marcic, 2015).

Motivation–Hygiene Theory (Herzberg's Two-Factor Theory)
Motivation–Hygiene Theory, or Two-Factor Theory, was established by psychologist Frederick Herzberg in 1959. Herzberg sought to describe the differences between factors that are true motivators for individuals (i.e., recognition for a job well done,

opportunities for promotion or advancement, challenging and rewarding work) and hygiene or maintenance factors. Examples of hygiene or maintenance factors include salary, quality of supervision, interpersonal relationships with coworkers, and good working conditions (Herzberg, 1966).

According to Herzberg (1966), hygiene factors, although they keep workers from becoming dissatisfied, do not act as real motivators. Hygiene factors are most often extrinsic and usually cannot be changed by employee behaviors; hygiene factors do not motivate employees. Motivators are most often intrinsic factors and are correlated with increased job satisfaction. Thus, when managers want to motivate employees, motivators should be emphasized.

Cerasoli, Nicklin, and Ford (2014) conducted a meta-analysis, the 10th such analysis, of more than 40 years of research to discern whether providing extrinsic incentives overcomes intrinsic motivation and the resultant effects on performance. In answer to the question, which matters most for performance, incentives or intrinsic motivation, the researchers determined that application of extrinsic motivators impacts the *quantity* of performance more so than the *quality* of the performance. Other findings of the analysis included intrinsic motivation alone (without incentives) is also a strong predictor of quantity of performance, incentives alone have little impact on intrinsic motivation, and intrinsic motivation appears to increase as age increases.

Contingency Theories of Leadership: Leadership and Management by Situation

As research into leadership became increasingly complex, it was recognized that leader characteristics, traits, and behaviors were not sufficient to explain the concept. The focus of research then shifted to include components of the situation or the environment into the equation as well. In other words, various external factors, such as conditions in the situation and the nature of the task to be accomplished, help to determine the leadership style that would be most effective in a particular situation.

The Fiedler Contingency Theory of Leadership

One of the earlier efforts to address contingencies in leadership situations was the Fiedler (1967) Contingency Theory of Leadership. Fiedler, Chemers, and Mahar (1976) state,

> This theory holds that the effectiveness of a group or organization depends on two interacting or "contingent" factors. The first is the personality of the leaders to determine their leadership style. The second factor is the amount of control and influence which the situation provides leaders over the group's behavior, the task, and the outcome. This factor is called situational control. (p. 3)

Fiedler (1967) developed the Least Preferred Coworker (LPC) Scale to determine and classify leadership styles. The instrument, an 18-item semantic differential scale, uses contrasting adjectives (e.g., friendly/unfriendly, open/guarded, and insincere/sincere) to direct the leader to describe an LPC. From the leader's responses on the scale, an LPC score is obtained. A leader with a high LPC score describes an LPC in a generally favorable manner. Fiedler believed this leader tends to be relationship-oriented and considerate about the feelings of coworkers. Conversely, a leader with a low LPC score would be described by Fiedler as task oriented. Leaders who fall in the midrange of scores are a mix of the two types of leaders and should determine for themselves to which group they ultimately belong. Fiedler's assumption is that a leader's style is innately either relationship or task oriented and that style cannot be changed as the situation changes (Fiedler et al., 1976).

Box 17-1 Group Classifications

- *Leader–member relations*: Confidence in the leader and support of the group is effective in influencing the group's performance. (This is the most important factor in determining the leader's control and influence over the group.)
- *Task structure*: Structure of the task is on a continuum from a well-defined, step-by-step procedure to a vague and undefined one.
- *Position power*: Authority is vested in the leader's position by the organization.

Once the leader's style has been determined by the LPC score, the next step is to match or fit the leader with the situation. Fiedler used the term *situational control* to describe three major group classifications or variables that may be used to evaluate an individual situation (Box 17-1).

Leader–member relations can be classified as good or poor, task structure as high or low, and position power as strong or weak. According to Fiedler, the better the leader–member relations, the higher the task structure; the stronger the position power, the more control or influence the leader has. For example, a nurse who is in an autonomous position as the vice president of patient care services (strong position power) is highly respected (good leader–member relations) by a group of nurse practitioners (high task structure) and is employed by the hospital is influential to the nurse practitioner group.

In Fiedler's studies of more than 1,200 groups since the 1950s, the low LPC leader (task oriented) has been found to be most effective in very favorable situations (position power is strong and leader–member relations are strong) and in very unfavorable situations (position power is weak and leader–member relations are weak). Also, the low LPC leader is most effective when tasks are clear and highly structured. The high LPC leader (relationship oriented) is most effective in moderately favorable situations when position power is weak, task structure is low, and leader–member relations are good (Hitt et al., 2011).

Numerous studies have been undertaken to test the validity of the contingency model's assumptions (Chemers, Harp, Rhodewalt, & Wysocki, 1985; Fiedler, 1969; Minor, 1980). These comprehensive studies, including a meta-analysis of 125 tests of the contingency model, provide strong support for the model's validity.

Path–Goal Theory

Robert House (1971, 1996) developed the Path–Goal Theory as an extension of the earlier work of Georgopoulos, Mahoney, and Jones (1957) and from research related to the expectancy theories of motivation (Vroom, 1964). Situational factors that are examined in this theory include the nature and scope of the task to be accomplished, the employee's perceptions and expectations of the task, and the role of the leader in the work process. Expectations of the leader in this theory are to assist followers in determining and attaining goals and to provide the necessary direction and support to ensure that employee goals are compatible with those of the organization. The role of the leader is also to provide motivation and some type of reward (i.e., recognition for the employee once the task has been completed or the goal has been reached) (Podsakoff, Bommer, Podsakoff, & Mackenzie, 2006). The leader is responsible for helping the employee determine and clarify the path the worker is to take to reach the goal. An important aspect of the leader's role is to identify and remove obstacles from the path of the worker to enable him or her to successfully attain the goal.

House (1971) identified four leadership behaviors to test the assumptions of his theory. The *directive* leader provides specific guidance and direction to workers on how the task is to be accomplished; the *supportive* leader is concerned with the accomplishment of the task as well as the needs of the worker; the *participative* leader involves workers in making decisions about how the task or goal should be accomplished; and the *achievement-oriented* leader sets challenging goals and has high expectations that employees will perform at the highest level. House assumes leaders are flexible and are able to use any of these leadership behaviors as the situation warrants.

The Path–Goal Theory also proposes two sets or classes of situational or contingency variables that influence the relationship between the leadership behavior and the outcomes. These two variables are environmental variables (those outside of the control of the employee) and variables that are part of the personal attributes of the employee. Examples of environmental variables include the nature and structure of the task or the goal to be accomplished and the composition of the work group to which the employee has been assigned. Employee contingency factors include ability, locus of control, and experience. House (1971) proposed that employee performance and satisfaction are enhanced when the leader is able to compensate in some way for any shortcomings with either the employee or the work setting.

Path–Goal Theory remains one of the most respected approaches to understanding leadership. Research related to the path–goal model is generally supportive of the major assumptions of the model (Robbins & Coulter, 2013; Schriesheim, Castro, Zhou, & DeChurch, 2006; Vecchio, Justin, & Pearce, 2008).

Situational Leadership Theory

Situational Leadership Theory, developed by Paul Hersey and Kenneth Blanchard in the 1970s, is a contingency theory that examines the relationship among three concepts of management: task behavior, relationship behavior, and maturity level of the follower or worker. *Task behavior* is the amount of direction given by the leader to ensure that the task is accomplished. *Relationship behavior* is the amount of emotional support and energy the leader provides to the follower or worker. According to Hersey and Blanchard (1977), task behavior and relationship behavior are directly related to the *maturity level* exhibited by the employee toward the job or task.

Leaders must adjust leadership style depending on the maturity level of the employee. That is, a more directive leadership style is required with an immature worker, and a less directive style is adequate for a mature worker. In this theory, a mature employee or worker is described as one who has the willingness, capacity, and initiative to set goals for himself or herself and to accomplish tasks with minimal direction. The immature employee requires more direction from the leader to accomplish the task or objective.

A worker's maturity level is not fixed or constant. Maturity levels may change when the task or objective changes; therefore, a worker's maturity level may be placed on a continuum from immature to mature. Frequent assessments of the follower or worker by the leader are necessary for the appropriate leadership style to be used.

In this theory, the leader must be able to adapt leadership styles to meet individual and situational demands. If workers in a situation are immature, the leader should provide a high level of task direction and a low level of support or relationship behavior. As the worker matures, the reverse may be true (i.e., with a mature worker, the leader's task direction decreases and relationship behavior increases). Eventually, the mature worker may need minimal task direction and relationship support from the leader (DuBrin, 2012).

Contemporary Leadership Theories

Since the late 1970s, theories of leadership have expanded the number of variables that affect effective leadership. These variables include increasing complexities of the work environment, the culture of the organization, values of the organization, leaders and followers within the organization, and the influence of the leader/manager (Vroom & Jago, 2007). Transactional and transformational leadership, authentic leadership, charismatic leadership, and servant leadership are considered some of the leading, emerging contemporary leadership theories.

Transactional and Transformational Leadership

Burns (1978), a scholar in the area of leader–follower interactions, maintained that there are two types of leaders in management, the transactional leader and the transformational leader. The transactional leader is viewed as the traditional manager, a manager who is concerned with day-to-day operations. The transformational leader is a long-term visionary who can inspire and empower others with his or her vision (Avolio, Zhu, Koh, & Puja, 2004; Bass, Avolio, Jung, & Berson, 2003; Bono & Judge, 2003; Schaubroeck, Lam, & Cha, 2007; Walumbwa, Avolio, & Zhu, 2008). In health care organizations, the transactional leadership model appears to be the most prevalent (Schwartz & Tumblin, 2002), although transformational leadership is ideally suited for environments, such as health care, which are continually changing and transforming (Borkowski, 2016).

Characteristics of transformational leaders include strong commitment to the profession and to the organization, the ability to help their followers look at old problems in new ways, as well as the ability to excite and motivate followers to produce extra effort to achieve group goals. The hallmark of the transformational leader is vision and the ability to communicate that vision to others so that it becomes a shared vision. This shared vision between leader and follower is translated as inspiring movement to achieve a common cause or a common goal for the organization. Research studies conducted in various settings such as in the military and business sectors support the effectiveness of transformational leadership as compared to transactional leadership in regard to employee performance and satisfaction (Robbins & Coulter, 2013).

Transformational leadership is built on transactional leadership (Judge & Piccolo, 2004). Transformational and transactional leadership should not be viewed as opposing forces (Robbins & Coulter, 2013). Contemporary management theorists caution that characteristics of both transactional and transformational leadership must be in the repertoire of the effective leader to accomplish the goals of the organization (Washington, 2007).

The concept of transformational leadership is one of the most widely researched concepts in the field of leadership (Harms & Crede, 2010). Research has validated the positive relationship between transformational leadership style and the performance and effectiveness of the leader. In addition, the impact of transformational leadership on follower satisfaction and motivation has also been extensively studied and positively validated (Judge & Piccolo, 2004).

Some contend that EI is an antecedent of transformational leadership. The concept of EI as it relates to leadership ability, especially transformational leadership, has been researched extensively in the past few years with mixed results. For example, Harms and Crede (2010) reported the results of a meta-analysis conducted to determine whether EI is related to transformational leadership and, if so, to what extent.

Results indicated a moderate relationship between EI and transformational leadership and suggested that EI may contribute to successful leadership. The authors caution, however, that the results of this study also seem to suggest that commonly marketed EI assessment tools, which are often used by organizations for management screening or training, should not be overemphasized and should be used only for self-awareness and self-reflection until better screening tools are available and have been psychometrically validated and empirically tested (Harms & Crede, 2010).

The results of Lindebaum and Cartwright's (2010) research revealed that when using a strong methodologic design to evaluate the relationship between EI and transformational leadership, no relationship between EI and transformational leadership is found. Conversely, the results of another meta-analysis conducted by O'Boyle, Humphrey, Pollack, Hawver, and Story (2011) validated the relationship between EI and job performance and supported the overall validity of EI.

Authentic Leadership

Authentic leadership is a construct derived from the works of the humanistic psychologists, particularly Carl Rogers and Abraham Maslow, who focused on the human potential for achieving self-actualization. Maslow (1971) viewed the self-actualized person as someone who has full personal awareness, holds an accurate self-picture of his or her capabilities, upholds the highest ethical standards, and is not easily swayed or influenced by others. Early application of the concept of authentic leadership occurred in the disciplines of sociology and education (Avolio & Gardner, 2005).

Shamir and Eilam (2005) advance four characteristics of authentic leaders. This type of leader:

1. Does not change to meet the expectations of others; he or she remains constant in his or her convictions.
2. Is not preoccupied with attempting to achieve higher personal status or honors.
3. Makes leadership decisions based on his or her personal point of view and not based on what he or she thinks others would want him or her to do.
4. Bases actions on personal values and belief systems.

Banks, McCauley, Garner, and Guler (2016) conducted a meta-analysis to compare authentic leadership and transformational leadership theories to address concerns by some regarding the contribution of authentic leadership to the leadership literature. The results of the analysis indicated a strong correlation between authentic and transformational leadership. However, there is significant construct redundancy between the two theories which elicits concerns that the two are not stand-alone constructs.

Charismatic Leadership

Charismatic leadership is an extension of attribution theory; that is, followers attribute heroic or extraordinary leadership abilities when they observe certain behaviors in their leaders (Conger & Kanungo, 1988). Several researchers, including House (1977), Bennis (1984), Conger and Kanungo (1988), and Rowold and Heinitz (2007), have attempted to describe and define attributes and characteristics of the charismatic leader. These characteristics include complete and compelling self-confidence in themselves and in their abilities, strong convictions and vision, and the ability to clearly and forcefully articulate that vision to others (Jung & Sosik, 2006).

Charismatic leaders are viewed as strong agents for change rather than as caretakers or managers of the current situation or environment. They are perceived as having behavioral characteristics that are unconventional and out of the ordinary. Charismatic leaders are risk takers and often arise from areas in society or business in which there is a common or shared ideology, such as the military, religious, political, or business sectors. These leaders often emerge when the organization has undergone a crisis.

Servant Leadership

A term first used in the late 1960s, *servant leadership* refers to a leadership style which is focused on listening, awareness, and stewardship by the leader. The servant leader is viewed as a moral leader who is driven to help followers meet their goals in order for organizational initiatives to be achieved. Servant leaders exhibit a commitment to helping others meet their potential by performance coaching which consists of performance planning, identification of professional development needs, frequent coaching, and consistent performance evaluation (Blanchard & Hodges, 2003). Although characteristics of servant leaders and transformational leaders are similar, the focus of the leader is different. The transformational leader's focus is on the organization, whereas the servant leader's focus is on followers (Stone, Russell, & Patterson, 2003).

Followership Theory

The literature on leadership abounds with theories and research related to the outcomes of application of the theories. Recently, focus has also shifted to followership theory and how it relates to leadership, as presumably, one cannot lead without followers. Following is a behavior which another person (a leader) is allowed to influence (DeRue & Ashford, 2010). Uhl-Bien, Riggio, Lowe, and Carsten (2014) assert that although most research on leadership acknowledges followers in some way, examining the behaviors of followers is crucial to fully understand the leadership process.

Organizational/Management Theories

Frederick Taylor, a mechanical engineer in steel plants in Pennsylvania, is recognized as the father of scientific management (Williams, 2013). In 1911, Taylor published *The Principles of Scientific Management*, which revolutionized the way work was accomplished in organizations in the United States. This change led to the use of the scientific method to help determine the "one best way" for a job to be done. Taylor's work is credited with beginning modern management theory.

Scientific Management

Taylor's work evolved because of what he perceived as inefficiencies on the job by workers and management, which he believed led to only one-third of the possible output. These inefficiencies included workers applying differing techniques to get the same job done, employees working at a deliberately slow pace, management not matching worker expertise and talents to the job, and management making decisions based on hunches and intuition. Taylor (1911) devised four principles of management (Box 17-2).

As a result of implementation of Taylor's principles and ideas, profits and productivity in American organizations rose dramatically. His methods gave U.S. companies a competitive advantage over foreign companies—an advantage that lasted for approximately 50 years.

> ### Box 17-2   Taylor's Principles of Management
>
> - Using scientific methods (i.e., time and motion studies), work can be organized to produce maximum efficiency and productivity while capitalizing on the expertise of the individual worker.
> - Workers with specific attributes and qualifications should be hired and then trained and matched to the job that would make the best use of their capabilities.
> - Workers should be rewarded monetarily if production exceeds established goals rather than being paid an hourly wage; workers should know where and how they fit into the organization and should be informed of the organization's mission and how they can help to accomplish the mission.
> - Managers and workers should work cooperatively; however, the role of management is to plan and supervise, and the role of the worker is to get the work done.

Theory of Bureaucracy/Organizational Theory

Max Weber, a political theorist and sociologist in prewar Germany, was attempting to address social and political concerns when he developed his definition of bureaucracy (Williams, 2013). Weber considered a bureaucracy to be an ideal form for an organization in which there is a clearly defined hierarchy and division of labor operating in a system of detailed rules and regulations. Weber's theory emphasized the concepts of authority, command, power, domination, and discipline. For example, in a bureaucracy, the authority for decision making depends on the individual's position in the organization (i.e., the higher the individual is ranked in the organization, the greater the level of authority of that individual) (Weber, 1970). Many of Weber's principles are still used in large health care organizations today.

Classic Management Theory

Henri Fayol, a French mining engineer and industrialist, successfully brought the Commentry-Fourchambault Mining Company from the brink of bankruptcy in 1888 and made it into a thriving, successful company. He accomplished this by using 14 principles of administration and management (DuBrin, 2012). These principles address areas such as division or specialization of work, authority, employee discipline, unity of direction or supervision, remuneration of workers, chain of command, equity, initiative, and esprit de corps (Fayol, 1949). Examples of Fayol's principles of management are included in Box 17-3. Many, if not most, of Fayol's principles are used in organizations today.

> ### Box 17-3   Fayol's Principles of Management
>
> - To ensure maximum efficiency and effectiveness, there should be specialization of work regardless of whether the work is technical or administrative.
> - Managers must have the right and the power to give orders; however, with authority comes responsibility. Responsibility and authority must be commensurate.
> - Good discipline is essential to the organization; however, management has the responsibility to inform workers of expectations and to provide good supervision.
> - When sanctions must be applied, they should be applied fairly and appropriately.
> - Every employee should have only one supervisor from whom he or she receives orders and directions. Compensation for work should be judged as fair by both management and the worker.

Motivational Theories

The ability to motivate others is a characteristic shared by leaders. Motivational theories are derived predominantly from the work of psychologist Abraham Maslow and his theory. McGregor's and Herzberg's theories were presented as evolving from Maslow's theory. The following sections discuss contemporary theories of motivation, including Achievement–Motivation or Three Needs Theory, Expectancy Theory, and Equity Theory.

Achievement–Motivation Theory

The Achievement–Motivation Theory was developed by Atkinson, McClelland, and Veroff. It focuses on aspects of personality characteristics and proposes three forms of motivation or needs in work situations (Drafke, 2009; Robbins & Judge, 2015). These three factors or motives are labeled social motives and are presented in Table 17-1.

Individuals with a high need for achievement (n-Ach) are not as concerned with the rewards of achievement as they are with the actual achievement. These individuals seek out characteristic situations in which the probability of success is neither too high nor too low, in which success can be achieved through one's own efforts, and in which personal credit can be received for a good or successful outcome. For example, if the probability of success is too high, an individual with n-Ach will find motive satisfaction low—he or she perceives that there is not a sufficient challenge. Individuals with high n-Ach are often attracted to entrepreneurial activities, such as developing their own businesses (Rue & Byars, 1977).

Research indicates that a high need to achieve is not necessarily synonymous with being a good manager. Other research has revealed that the needs for affiliation and power are closely related to managerial success. That is, the best managers appear to be those individuals who have a high need for power and a low need for affiliation (Robbins & Judge, 2015).

Expectancy Theory

Victor Vroom developed Expectancy Theory in the 1960s. Major concepts of this theory include the effects of ability and motivation on performance; they can be expressed as a mathematical statement:

$$\text{Performance} = \text{Ability} \times \text{Motivation}$$

Vroom (1960) concluded that managers should attempt to develop and motivate employees simultaneously. However, he recognized that the successful motivation of employees depends on the employee's aptitude and ability as well.

Table 17-1 Motivation Needs in Work Situations

Need	Characteristics
Achievement (n-Ach)	Need to strive for success and excellence in the work situation to accomplish what has not been accomplished before
Power (n-Pow)	Need to be influential and to control others; to be in charge or in authority
Affiliation (n-Aff)	Need to be liked, accepted, and respected by others

n-Ach, need for achievement; n-Pow, need for power; n-Aff, need for affiliation.

In a later work, Vroom (1964) added the concepts of expectancy, instrumentality, and valence to motivation. This premise can also be expressed as a mathematical statement:

$$\text{Motivation} = \text{Expectancy} \times \text{Instrumentality} \times \text{Valence}$$

Expectancy is defined as the association between the action and the outcome of the action. Action will lead to the achievement of a goal. *Instrumentality* describes the type of outcome derived because of an action; it is the perception that achievement of a goal will lead to a reward. *Valence* is the value placed on the desirability of the outcome by the employee (Vroom, 1964).

In short, the Expectancy Theory states that an individual will act (performance) in a certain manner because there is an expectation (motivation) that the act will result in an outcome. Employee performance is also based on the attractiveness of that outcome (reward) to the individual. Note that the attractiveness of the outcome or reward is what the *employee* perceives it to be, not what the manager perceives. An individual's own perceptions of performance and reward will determine the employee's level of effort. Therefore, it behooves managers to make certain employees understand and see the connection between performance and rewards and to determine what rewards are valued (and expected) by workers.

Equity Theory

J. Stacy Adams, a research psychologist, developed Equity Theory in 1963. This theory is based on the concepts of cognitive dissonance and distributive justice. It attempts to describe the relationship in which an individual gives something (input) and in exchange receives something (outcome) (Adams, 1965).

In a work situation, an individual expects that if he or she works hard at a job (input), he or she will receive compensation or recognition (outcome) based on what he or she has put in. The individual then compares this input–outcome ratio with relevant others in the same job situation (inside or outside of the organization). If the worker perceives the input–outcome ratio of the relevant others is equal to his or her own, then a state of equity exists. If the ratios are not equal (i.e., if the workers perceive themselves to be over- or underrewarded), a state of inequity exists, and the employee will attempt to correct the inequity (Robbins & Judge, 2015). The corrections may take several forms and include lower or higher inputs or outputs and increased absenteeism. The presence of inequity results in employee dissatisfaction.

Concepts of Power, Empowerment, and Change

In society and in organizations, the words *power* and *authority* are often used synonymously and sometimes interchangeably. However, the two concepts are not synonymous.

Power

Power is the larger concept from which authority is derived. Power can be defined as influence wielded by an individual or group of individuals to change behaviors and attitudes and to sway decisions. Power implies a dependency relationship. In other words, the more dependent an individual is on another, the more power is generated by the individual in possession of the desired attribute (e.g., wealth, information, prestige). Power can have positive or negative connotations. For example, among disenfranchised groups, power may have a negative connotation, as in abusing power or by engendering feelings of powerlessness.

Authority, on the other hand, is a formal right based on the manager's position in the organization. Authority is a source of legitimate power; however, some individuals (and organizations) are more proficient than others in using and delegating authority. Authority can be under- and overused. Usually, the higher one is (by virtue of vertical position) in an organization, the greater one's authority.

French and Raven (1959) conducted early research related to the concept of power. They classified five bases or sources of power: *reward, coercive, legitimate, referent,* and *expert power* (Table 17-2). Coercive, reward, and legitimate power are considered formal bases of power; referent and expert power are personal bases of power. Hersey and Blanchard (1982) described two other power sources: *informational power*—access to information that others do not have—and *connection power*. Connection power relates to networks and contacts within, especially vertical contacts, and outside of organizations—in other words, who you know. Another base of power, *charismatic power*, was subsequently identified in the literature (Heineken & McCloskey, 1985). Charismatic power can be distinguished from referent power as a type of personal power rather than reflected power. Charismatic power is the power that attracts one individual to another.

Power bases can be used individually or in combination. The effect of the power bases is additive; that is, the more power bases an individual uses, the greater or broader the power that individual will exert or exercise. Research indicates that personal sources of power are most effective (Carson, Carson, & Roe, 1993).

In organizations, *subordinate employees* can also achieve power by having superiors become dependent on them which is recognized as the most effective method of achieving power by lower level personnel (Borkowski, 2016). The most common ways lower level employees exercise personal power is by limiting or withholding access to people, resources, and information which is critical to doing business within the organization. Ways that *managers* can develop a successful power base include (1) creating a sense of obligation among employees to return favors done on their

Table 17-2 Sources of Power

Type of Power	Characteristics	Examples
Reward	The transfer of positive reinforcers from the leader to the follower	Praise, compensation, and other rewards the follower values
Coercive	The use of negative sanctions to achieve results desired by the leader	Unfavorable work assignments; unappealing work schedules
Legitimate	Power derived by virtue of the position or title held within the organization	Vice president of patient care services; chief nursing officer; charge nurse; team leader
Referent	Power that some individuals possess by virtue of their association with a more powerful individual or entity	Being on the faculty of a well-known university; working for a renowned nurse
Expert	Power derived through an individual's knowledge, experience, and expertise or skill in a certain discipline or area of specialization	A clinical nurse specialist consulting in the case of a pregnant oncology patient; a nursing professor chairing a curriculum change committee

behalf by the manager, (2) establishing a reputation or track record as an expert in a particular discipline or area, and (3) fostering dependence on the manager by employees especially as relates to the allocation or withholding of resources (Kotter, 1977).

Researchers such as McClelland (1975), Winter (1973), and Raven (2008) have determined that there are three major motivators that influence leader behavior when selecting a power strategy: need for power, need for affiliation, and n-Ach. For example, a manager with a high need for power may be more likely to operate from a base of impersonal coercive power and legitimate position power, whereas a supervisor with a high n-Ach may make more use of informational and expert power (Raven, 2008). Self-esteem, high or low, may also play a role in which power strategy is ultimately selected. It is theorized that individuals with low self-esteem may be more likely to utilize harsh or hard power bases such as coercion power (Kipnis, 1976).

An emerging area of research explored the use of body language to increase one's power position and influence which is also referred to as the power pose (Carney, Cuddy, & Yap, 2010). Positioning oneself in a high power pose results in positive psychological, physiologic, and behavioral changes which dictate how ultimately a person thinks and feels about himself or herself.

Empowerment

In many organizations, including some health care organizations, power has shifted from residing exclusively with management to the worker or a group of workers, often in a team configuration. *Empowerment*, in organizational terminology, is the transfer or delegation of responsibility and authority from managers to employees; empowerment is the sharing of power. Empowerment also involves the sharing of vision, mission, knowledge, expertise, decision making, and resources necessary for employees to reach organizational goals. The concept of empowerment can be operationalized as a continuum with employees in some organizations having virtually no say in how the work is to be accomplished and employers on the other end of the continuum having complete control over work processes (Daft & Marcic, 2015).

Empowerment is consistent with the contemporary views of leadership (e.g., transformational, visionary). In today's competitive economic environment, organizations that have been successful from an economic and quality standpoint are those that have empowered employees to "get the job done." This usually involves removing bureaucratic barriers to success, such as forcing workers to wait days or weeks for management approval of new work methods or for allocation of necessary resources to accomplish a task or goal. To exploit competitive marketplace advantages, decisions and changes are made rapidly and at a lower level in the organizational structure than in traditional companies. Empowered employees are often more creative and responsive to the needs of the customer or consumer.

Change

Today, nursing and, in a broader view, health care are arenas that seem to be in a constant state of flux or change. For most individuals, change elicits feelings of uncertainty, anxiety, and upheaval. Kurt Lewin, a German psychologist, proposed a method of planned change, which is controlled change or change by design. Theorists who have expanded the work of Lewin include Havelock, whose theories on change include six phases; Kilmann, who postulated five stages of organizational planned change; Kotter, who describes a process that includes eight stages for leading change; and Smith, who identified seven levels of change (Tomey, 2009).

Planned Change Theory

Lewin (1951) described a method in his field theory that provides a basis for considering the process of *planned* change. Planned change occurs by design, as opposed to change that is spontaneous or that occurs by happenstance or by accident. When Lewin's process is used correctly and in its entirety by a group or a system, effective change is implemented.

Central to Lewin's theories on planned change are the concepts of field and force. A *field* can be viewed as a system; therefore, when change occurs in one part or aspect of the system, the whole system must be examined to determine the effect of that change. *Force* is defined as a directed entity that has the characteristics of direction, focus, and strength. Lewin (1951) states that change is a move from the status quo that results in a disruption in the balance of forces or disequilibrium between opposing forces.

According to Lewin (1951), there are two forces involved in change, *driving forces* and *restraining forces*. As the name implies, a driving force encourages or facilitates movement to a new direction, goal, or outcome. A restraining force has the opposite effect; restraining forces block or impede progress toward the goal. In planned change, driving forces should be identified and accentuated. If possible, restraining forces should also be identified and minimized to achieve the desired outcome or change. Lewin describes effective change as the return to equilibrium as a result of balancing opposing forces. If driving forces and restraining forces can be identified, it may be possible to predict if and when change would be successful. Lewin identifies three phases that must occur if planned change is to be successful: unfreezing the status quo, moving to a new state, and refreezing the change to make it permanent. In the unfreezing stage, individuals involved must be informed of the need for change and should agree that change is needed. Change, particularly in the work environment, often leads to feelings of uneasiness, uncertainty, and loss of control. Change, just for the sake of change, is viewed by most individuals as stressful and unnecessary.

Driving forces should exceed restraining forces during movement, the second phase of the planned change process. The initiator of the change, the change agent, should recognize that change takes time, should be accomplished gradually, and should be thoughtfully and comprehensively planned before implementation.

During the refreezing phase, stabilization occurs. If stabilization is successful, the change is assimilated into the system. Change disrupts the comfort of the status quo; it leads to disequilibrium. Therefore, resistance to change should always be anticipated and expected.

Kotter (1995) expanded Lewin's theory by devising a more detailed eight-step approach for implementing change that correlates to the unfreezing, movement, and refreezing phases in Lewin's model. Kotter analyzed common mistakes made when managers attempt to initiate a change. Based on these mistakes, Kotter's Eight-Step Plan for Implementing Change was devised. The eight steps include:

1. Create a sense of urgency for the change.
2. Form coalitions to have enough power to lead the change.
3. Create a new vision to direct the change; strategies must be developed to achieve the new vision.
4. Communicate the new vision purposefully and effectively throughout the organization.
5. Remove barriers to change, empower others to act on the new vision, encourage an atmosphere of creativity and risk taking.
6. Plan rewards for short-term "wins" when the organization begins to move toward the new vision.

7. Continually assess the effects of the change and make adjustments as necessary in new programs.
8. Reinforce the changes by linking new behaviors to organizational success (Robbins & Judge, 2015).

Link to Practice 17-1 illustrates an example of one workplace's successful use of Kotter's Eight-Step Plan for Implementing Change.

Uncertain and dynamic environments often characterize the environments of organizations today. In this environment, stability and predictability rarely exist. Disruptions in the status quo are the norm. Organizations today face constant change, often bordering on chaos. Leaders in today's environments of continual change must be prepared to efficiently and effectively adapt to change and must be able to manage all aspects of change—from both external and internal forces.

Most of the time, drivers or the impetus for change originate because of pressure or factors external to organizations. The organization attempts to adjust or redesign the internal environment in attempt to respond to outside factors driving the change. Examples of external factors driving change in health care organizations today include evolving

Link to Practice 17-1

It has been estimated that over 70% of patient care errors occur because of lack of adequate communication during transitions in care between one provider and another, that is, during handoffs. Benefits of nursing bedside handoffs have been widely reported in the literature. This article reports on the efforts of one surgical orthopedic trauma unit in adopting a successful change of shift report process after attempting to make the change unsuccessfully several times before.

Kotter's Eight-Step Change Model was utilized to guide the process change. In the first step, a sense of urgency was created by illustrating risk for harm to patients as a result of miscommunication during poor handoff. During the second step, a diverse coalition of nurses committed to making the change was formed. Steps 3 and 4 involved creating the vision for the new process and communicating the change to all stakeholders. In this example, staff meetings and educational sessions were scheduled to communicate the vision. During step 5, empowering others to actualize the vision, staff members were instrumental in developing a new process for handoffs which created a sense of ownership. In the new process, it was determined it was safer for patients who were sleeping during handoffs to be awakened so that they could be involved. Identifying quick wins, step 6, reinforced the impetus for the change. A quick win in this example is staff were more likely to be able to leave on time at the end of shift times as a result of efficiencies generated with the new handoff process. Steps 7, build on the change, and 8, institutionalize the change, involved integrating and sustaining the change on the unit. Nurse satisfaction was measured postimplementation; almost 90% of the unit nurses agreed that conferencing with their patients prior to the start of the shift left them with a greater sense of satisfaction. The nurses also strongly agreed that incorporating bedside handoff improved the overall efficiency of the unit and, most importantly, played a significant role in reducing potential and actual errors in patient care.

Small, A., Gist, D., Souza, D., Dalton, J., Magny-Normilus, C., & David, D. (2016). Using Kotter's change model for implementing beside handoff: A quality improvement project. *Journal of Nursing Care Quality,* 31(4), 304–309.

health care policy, fluctuating government and private insurer payment practices, integration of data analytics, and the expanding role and power of consumers in the selection and evaluation of health services providers and organizations (Borkowski, 2016).

Resilience

Resilience is a concept or attribute which can be ascribed to individuals and to organizations. The word *resilience* is derived from a Latin term and refers to the ability to adapt to adversity and/or to change. Today's health care organizations, and the individuals who work in those organizations, are experiencing unprecedented periods of rapid change. Pressures placed on health care organizations from external forces such as the government, insurers, physicians, and customers, as well as from internal sources, demand organizational resilience, adaptability, and the ability to respond and react rapidly to change if the organization is to succeed and flourish.

Individuals with high levels of personal resilience are highly valued, especially in turbulent times, as they seem to be able to better manage their reactions to stressful situations and circumstances. In addition, resilient individuals tend to make more effective team members and leaders (Shirey, 2012).

Problem-Solving and Decision-Making Processes

Decision making is typically viewed as but one component of problem solving. Decision making can occur without taking the time to complete a comprehensive analysis, a step that is usually required in problem solving. Also, a decision can be made without identifying the real problem. Factors that play a role in an individual's process or method of decision making include the individual's values, life experiences, preferences, and inherent ways of thinking.

Early attempts to arrive at a scientific or rational method of decision making were described in the Rational Decision-Making Model. Research conducted by Vroom and Yetton (1973) and Vroom and Jago (1988) related to decision making has resulted in quantitative decision technology. This method can help managers select a decision-making style based on input and mathematical computation of effects of leader and situational variables.

The Rational Decision-Making Model

The primary assumption of the Rational Decision-Making Model, which has ties to the classic theories of economic behavior, is that of economic rationality. Economic rationality contends that people always attempt to maximize their individual economic outcomes when weighing decisions. Individuals or managers evaluate potential outcomes of their decisions based on current or prospective monetary worth. In a business decision-making situation, a manager weighs the alternative outcomes of a decision based in terms of profit-and-loss potential. The alternative selected as part of the decision-making process is the alternative that reaps the highest expected worth. *Expected worth* equals the sum of the expected values of the associated costs and benefits of the outcomes resulting from that alternative (Wagner & Hollenbeck, 2014).

Other assumptions of the model include the following:

- The problem is easy to discern and is without ambiguity.
- There is one well-defined goal to be achieved.
- All possible alternatives and consequences to action are known to the decision maker.

■ There are no time or cost constraints.
■ The final choice that is made will have the maximum economic payoff.

However, the assumptions of rationality often do not hold true. For example, in today's health care environment, how often does the manager have the luxury of no time or cost constraints?

Simon (1965), an economist and psychologist, concluded that most managers did not make decisions based on objective rationality. Simon proposed that there are bounds or limits to the ability of humans to make rational decisions at all times. *Bounded rationality*, a term devised by Simon, means that humans are unable to make entirely rational decisions because of the limits of human mental abilities and because of the influence of external factors on decision making. As a result, most people who make decisions do not have the time or capability to wait for the best possible solution to every problem. Decisions are made using incomplete knowledge and without attempting to determine all possible consequences. The final decision is good enough or "satisficing." Most people stop the search for alternatives when they find a satisficing alternative.

There are several influences on the decision-making process, which contribute to bounded rationality. These include intuition, personality and cognitive intelligence, EI, quality and accessibility of information, political considerations, degree of certainty, crisis and conflict, the values of the decision maker, procrastination, and decision-making styles (DuBrin, 2012).

Group Decision Making

In organizations, groups or teams of people typically make decisions rather than individuals. Group decision making is often used when the decision is complex, such as when a new process or product is being developed. Advantages of group decision making include the following: The decision made may be of higher quality because of the collective wisdom of the group members, major errors may be avoided because of the ability of the group members to evaluate each member's thinking, and commitment or "buy-in" of the group may be increased because of members' role in the outcome of the decision (DuBrin, 2012).

There are several disadvantages to group decision making. It often takes a group longer to reach a decision. In addition, decision making in groups may lead to compromises that really do not solve the problem. Because of the increased time involved for group decision making, group decision making should be reserved for problems that are multifaceted, complex, and important enough to warrant the efforts of the group (DuBrin, 2012).

An example of a group decision-making process is the Nominal Group Technique (NGT). Use of this technique allows a manager to explore potential alternatives to a problem and the reaction to implementation of specific alternatives. NGT follows a very structured format that begins by identifying the problem and ends with developing an action plan to implement a chosen solution. Once the plan is implemented, the group reconvenes to discuss progress and to evaluate outcomes (DuBrin, 2012).

Organizational Quantitative Decision-Making Techniques

Many organizations today, particularly health care organizations, rely on data-based decision making. That is, leaders and managers in those organizations rely on results of facts and quantitative measures to make decisions, although intuition and judgment still influence the decision-making process.

Examples of quantitative approaches used in decision making include the utilization of the following: Pareto diagrams for problem identification, Gantt charts and milestone charts to monitor the progress of scheduled projects, time-flow analyses, break even analyses (a method to determine profitability of new ventures or programs), decision trees, graphic illustrations of all possible alternatives to solve a particular problem, and sophisticated inventory-control techniques (DuBrin, 2012). Interactive performance management tools such as data visualization dashboards and scorecards are frequently used by managers and clinicians to determine the level of performance on quality metrics important to the organization. Data on key performance indicators retrieved from performance dashboards are integral to decision making and inform strategic and performance planning (Ross, 2014).

Conflict Management

Conflict can be positive or negative and functional or dysfunctional, although most people tend to shy away from situations in which there may be conflict. Negative conflict can be detrimental if allowed to continue for long periods without intervention from management. In general, a conflict situation has the following characteristics:

- At least two parties are involved.
- Strong emotions and behavior, directed toward defeating or suppressing the opponent, are apparent.
- Mutually exclusive needs or values exist or are perceived to exist.
- Opposing parties attempt to gain power over each other (Katz & Lawyer, 1985).

Thomas and Kilmann (1974) defined five conflict-handling modes or strategies: competing, accommodating, avoiding, collaborating, and compromising. *Competing* or *forcing* is used when the issue is important, needs speedy resolution, and "buy-in" from individuals other than the manager is unnecessary. When the issue in conflict is of relative unimportance to the manager or when the manager "gives in" to the other party involved in the conflict, *accommodation* is used. *Avoidance* should be used when emotions are still high and when the conflict is trivial; confrontation should be postponed until a more opportune time arrives. *Collaboration* is the opposite of avoidance and is used when the issue is too important to each side to be compromised; all parties want a win–win solution. *Compromise* is used for complex issues when conflicting parties are similar in power. Compromise can also be used to craft a temporary solution (Daft & Marcic, 2015).

Integrating the five conflict-handling modes with the two dimensions of cooperativeness and assertiveness results in the following conflict resolution options for managers: competing (assertive but uncooperative), collaborating (assertive and cooperative), avoiding (unassertive and uncooperative), accommodating (unassertive but cooperative), and compromising (midrange on both assertiveness and cooperation). Each option has its inherent strengths and weaknesses, and no one option is ideal for every situation.

Quality Improvement

"In God we trust. All others bring data."—W. Edwards Deming

One of the integral values of American society that has evolved in the last several decades is access to health care at reasonable cost in terms of resources. With increasing demands on health service organizations for improved quality and lower costs, the entire health care system has been forced to evaluate modes of operation. As a result, many health care organizations have incorporated concepts of QI.

QI is the commitment and approach used to scrupulously examine and continuously improve every process in every part of an organization. The ultimate intent of this methodology is meeting and exceeding customer expectations. QI empowers individuals and teams within systems to look at the way service is delivered to customers, to identify root causes of problems in the system, and then to creatively adopt solutions to the problems. Many health care organizations can accurately claim substantial improvements in both service effectiveness and efficiency as a result of this commitment and approach to quality.

In the field of QI, there exists a complex, ever-changing vocabulary. Even the term QI is not consistently used as the primary label for quality-related concepts. Other labels (and their abbreviations) frequently noted in the literature include continuous quality improvement (CQI), total quality management (TQM), total quality systems (TQS), quality systems improvement (QSI), and total quality (TQ), among others. Other related terms include performance improvement and process improvement.

The Case for Quality Improvement in Health Care

Early pioneers of QI in health care included the 19th century physician, Semmelweis, who introduced the importance of handwashing, and Florence Nightingale, whose work led to decreasing mortality rates among English soldiers in army hospitals by imposing strict sanitary conditions in the hospitals. Other momentous steps in QI, especially in the United States, was the formation of the Hospital Standardization Program by the American College of Surgeons, which eventually transformed into today's The Joint Commission, the organization which accredits health care organizations.

In 1966, 1 year after the implementation of Medicare, Donebedian first proposed quality could be measured by examining the structures, processes, and outcomes of care, which became the first conceptual approach widely used to measure the quality of health care (Chassin & Loeb, 2011). In 1996, The Joint Commission implemented its Agenda for Change, a quality-focused methodology to improve the systems, processes, and outcomes of care (Andel, Davidow, Hollander, & Moreno, 2012) (Table 17-3).

Despite the focus on QI and on cost reduction in the health care system, the industry in the United States remains plagued with inefficiencies and with all too common instances of poor quality. This results in alarming and unsustainable increase in costs and negatively impacts the ability of U.S. companies to remain competitive in a global economy. Aside from the staggering economic costs of an inefficient health care system, poor quality often leads to well-publicized errors, mistakes, premature deaths, and diminished quality of life for health care consumers.

Prior to the successful passage of national health care reform legislation, the Patient Protection and Affordable Care Act (PPACA), it was projected that approximately 32 to 45 million Americans who were uninsured or underinsured at that time would be entering the health care system. According to statistics posted on the U.S. Department of Health and Human Services website as of March 3, 2016, it is estimated that approximately 20 million additional Americans were afforded the opportunity to access health insurance coverage from the time the law was passed in 2010 through early 2016 (U.S. Department of Health and Human Services, 2016). PPACA makes heavy use of accountable care organizations and value-based purchasing. Another provision of the

Table 17-3 Health Care Quality Timeline

Date	Quality Innovation
19th century	Ignaz Semmelweis, an obstetrician, introduces handwashing to the care of patients.
	Florence Nightingale, an English nurse, recognizes the impact of unsanitary living conditions in English Army hospitals on the morbidity and mortality of patients.
1918	The American College of Surgeons forms the Hospital Standardization Program, the predecessor of The Joint Commission, and begins on-site hospital inspections using the Minimum Standards for Hospitals, a one-page document.
1948	The modern randomized clinical trial is instituted and used in a report from the United Kingdom Research Council on the treatment of pulmonary tuberculosis.
1951	The Joint Commission on Accreditation of Hospitals (JCAH) is created.
1953	JCAH publishes Standards for Hospital Accreditation.
1965	Legislation creating Medicare is enacted. Mandatory utilization review committees are established by the law that created Medicare.
1966	Donebedian proposes the first conceptual framework for measuring health care quality.
1970	The Joint Commission modifies its traditional accreditation process, which is based on standards, to comply with Donebedian's framework.
1971	Congress creates experimental review organizations to review inpatient and ambulatory services for quality and appropriateness of care.
1972	Medicare's Professional Standards Review Organizations established by the Social Security Administration Amendment.
1979	National Committee for Quality Assurance (NCQA) established.
1983	Professional Standards Review Organizations is replaced by Medicare Utilization and Quality Control Peer Review Organizations program; later became the Quality Improvement Organization Program.
1983	Forces of Magnetism are identified as a result of the work environment study conducted by the American Academy of Nursing Task Force on Nursing Practice in Hospitals. Hospitals that were able to recruit and retain nurses at higher levels were described as "Magnet" hospitals.
1989	Agency for Healthcare Policy and Research is created to replace the National Center for Health Services Research; later renamed the Agency for Healthcare Research and Quality (AHRQ). Initially, this agency was charged by Congress with developing practice guidelines and conducting health care research.
1994	University of Washington Medical Center, Seattle, becomes the first American Nurses Credentialing Center (ANCC) Magnet-designated organization.
1999	National Quality Forum is created; mission is to improve health care delivery by promoting the use of standardized quality measures and public reporting of resulting data and outcomes.
1999	Institute of Medicine releases the report, *To Err Is Human: Building a Safer Health System*.
2000	AHRQ receives a modified mandate from Congress; no longer directly responsible for developing new clinical practice guidelines.
2001	Institute of Medicine releases the report, *Crossing the Quality Chasm: A New Health System for the 21st Century*.
2010	The Patient Protection and Affordable Care Act (ACA) legislation is approved by the United States Congress; a stated aim of the ACA is to improve quality and efficiency of health care. A value-based purchasing program for hospitals is introduced with Medicare reimbursement payments to hospitals linked to performance on key quality indicators associated with high-volume, high-cost conditions.

(continued)

Table 17-3 Health Care Quality Timeline (Continued)

Date	Quality Innovation
2011	The U.S. Department of Health and Human Services submits the National Strategy for Quality Improvement in Health Care report to Congress; six priority areas are identified: patient safety, person-centered care, care coordination, effective treatment, healthy living, and care affordability.
2012	"Health care quality and safety are best characterized as showing pockets of excellence in specific measures or in particular services at individual health care facilities. Excellence across the board is emerging on some important quality measures. What has eluded us so far, however, is maintaining consistently high levels of safety and quality over time across all health care services and settings" (Chassin & Loeb, 2011, p. 562).
2017	The Centers for Medicare & Medicaid Services (CMS) continue to move Medicare provider payments to alternative payment models which emphasize value and quality outcomes.
	Growing reliance on "big data" to guide health care systems' decision-making capabilities in quality and cost-effectiveness initiatives.

Sources: American Nurses Credentialing Center, 2013; Chassin & Loeb, 2011; Institute of Medicine, 2013; The Joint Commission, 2013.

PPACA is the Centers for Medicare & Medicaid Services (CMS) no longer reimburse health care agencies for preventable readmissions and for health care facility–acquired conditions (Andel et al., 2012). Health care organizations not currently functioning at optimal levels in terms of efficiency and with the highest levels of quality outcomes are not likely to survive in today's pay-for-performance environment.

Quality Improvement Frameworks

For more than four decades, two Americans, W. Edwards Deming and J. M. Juran, were the primary champions of the quality movement throughout the world (Port, 1991). Deming was the developer of statistical quality control, whereas Juran was the innovator of total quality control. Both are credited with playing major roles as statistical and managerial consultants to Japanese industry in Japan's successful revitalization after the devastation of World War II (Port, 1991).

Since the 1970s, the literature on QI has grown, and many experts have contributed their ideas on QI. In the United States, the quality theories of Shewhart, Deming, Juran, and Crosby predominate. Walter Shewhart, a physicist at Bell Laboratories in the 1920s, was asked to investigate production processes at Western Electric's facilities to determine the source of variations in the quality of products produced. Shewhart coined the terms *common-cause* and *special-cause* variation and introduced the Plan-Do-Check-Act (PDCA) Model for improving work flow processes which are still used in many organizations today as part of their QI initiatives (Buchbinder & Shanks, 2017).

Deming's (1986) major thesis is that the cause of inefficiency and low quality can generally be traced back to system inadequacies rather than individual worker inadequacy. It is management's responsibility to improve the system with the involvement of all employees. This management theory focuses on improving quality, productivity, and competitive position in the marketplace and is referred to in the literature as Deming's 14 points (Box 17-4).

Deming's goal was to gear an organization's workforce to pursue specific organization-wide goals that were aimed at satisfying customer requirements for

---

Box 17-4   Deming's 14 Points

1. Create constancy of purpose for improvement.
2. Adopt the new philosophy.
3. Cease dependence on mass inspections.
4. End the practice of awarding business on the basis of price tags alone.
5. Institute on-the-job training and research.
6. Adopt and institute leadership.
7. Drive out fear among the organization's employees.
8. Improve constantly and forever every process for planning, production, and service.
9. Dismantle barriers between departments.
10. Eliminate slogans, exhortations, and production targets for employees.
11. Eliminate numerical quotas for employees and numerical goals for managers.
12. Remove barriers to pride of workmanship.
13. Institute a vigorous program of education and self-improvement.
14. Put everyone in the organization to work to accomplish the transformation.

Sources: Aguayo (1990); Deming (1986); Gillem (1988); Masters and Masters (1993).

---

quality, price, and service. Juran (1988) defined quality as "fitness for use." To satisfy customers, a product or service must have two components—features that a customer wants and as free from deficiencies as possible. According to Juran, one or the other of these two components alone does not constitute high quality. Juran offered three processes whereby managers can maintain and improve quality. These are commonly referred to as Juran's Trilogy (Table 17-4) (Juran, 1988).

Crosby (1979) emphasized the importance of systems knowledge and improvement, the disadvantages of reliance on inspections, and the need for statistical quality control. Crosby termed his major concepts the *four absolutes*:

1. The definition of quality is conformance requirements.
2. The system of quality is prevention and on not relying solely on "after-the-fact" methods to improve quality.
3. The performance standard is zero defects.
4. The measurement of quality is the price of nonconformance, which involves all costs in doing things wrong. In service companies, the cost of nonconformance is 35% of operating costs, whereas the cost of conformance is a far lower figure (Crosby, 1979).

Table 17-4 Juran's Trilogy: Processes Used to Maintain and Improve Quality

Process	Activities
Quality planning	Building quality into the processes and the product
Quality control	Evaluating actual performance, comparing that performance to predetermined goals, and taking action on the differences
Quality improvement (breakthrough)	Encouraging attainment of previously unprecedented levels of performance by the organization

Although experts on QI differ somewhat on their approaches, their theories share several characteristics (Daft & Marcic, 2015). These include the following:

- QI is driven by the leaders of the organization.
- Customer-mindedness permeates the organization.
- A transition is made from inspection-based management to process improvement.
- Formal process-improvement methods and statistical tools are used.
- All employees are involved in the exploration and refinement of work processes.

Quality Improvement Processes and Tools

Common terms utilized in QI are measurement and metrics (Buchbinder & Shanks, 2017). Measurement is a numerical expression of observable events or occurrences. Metrics refers to how those events or occurrences are tracked, recorded, or measured. Time is often an important unit of measurement in health care. For example, the wait time for patients to be seen in emergency departments (EDs) is frequently calculated as a quality measure and may even be advertised to gain competitive advantage. The metric for calculating or measuring wait times can be derived from the electronic health record (EHR). However, for the ED wait time to be calculated reliably and consistently over time by different people, the definition of wait time must first be determined. Is the wait time calculated beginning from the time the patient first registers in the ED, or is the time calculated from the time the patient is seen by the triage nurse, or is it the time which has elapsed before the patient is evaluated by the ED physician or NP? Once the metric is determined, the wait time can be evaluated and trended over time and can be benchmarked or compared against published local, regional, and/or national ED wait time statistics.

Contemporary approaches to the measurement of quality in health care organizations today rely heavily on statistical process control, which emphasizes the use of data analytics. QI tools used in data analytics include scorecards, data visualization dashboards, sophisticated statistical analyses, Pareto charts, cause-and-effect diagrams, run charts, and control charts, in addition to other similar methods.

Determining and measuring variation in a product or service is a key component of QI. Statistical process control is used to determine sources of variation in a process or outcome that impacts service quality. For example, large variation in the quality of a product or service is indicative of an aspect that is out of control. To use a health care–related example, a health system may monitor the readmission rates of patients with sternal wound infection after open-heart surgery. Extracting data from the EHR, representatives of the health system will calculate the average readmission rate for all cardiac surgery patients and compare the rates to preestablished national benchmarks for open-heart surgery. Data related to readmission rates postsurgery will then be calculated by cardiac surgery practice, usually composed of a team or group of physicians, and then may be calculated relative to each specific surgeon in the practice. A cardiac surgery practice and/or a cardiac surgeon whose patients are readmitted with sternal wound infections at statistically higher rates than the average rate when compared to local and national benchmarks would most likely be asked by the health system to address the problem as more frequent infections and readmission rates would indicate a quality variance.

Approaches to QI, which started in other industries and which have been adapted for use in health care, include Lean process management and Six Sigma. Lean

Thinking, also referred to as Lean, originated in the 1920s in the Ford Motor Company (Ford & Crowther, 1926), whereas Six Sigma was introduced by the Motorola company. Six Sigma is an extension of Juran's Trilogy as well as other QI approaches. Today, both approaches are used extensively in administration and service areas, although their roots are in manufacturing (Snee & Hoerl, 2004).

Lean represented a fundamental shift from traditional Western manufacturing approaches and beliefs, which included:

1. Separation of thinking from doing for workers is essential.
2. Deficiencies in products or services cannot be eliminated or avoided.
3. Organizations are most efficient when structured in a chain of command that is based on a hierarchy.
4. Inventories are essential to meet fluctuating production demands (de Koning, Verver, van den Heuvel, Bisgaard, & Does, 2006).

Japanese companies, such as Toyota, revolutionized automobile manufacturing implementing Lean Thinking processes as an alternative to the Western model of manufacturing. Lean focuses on producing what the customer wants and expects from a product—everything else is considered to be non–value-added activity. Another focus of Lean is reduction of waste and variability in production and in outcomes during the manufacturing process by synchronizing the flow of work. The strengths of Lean Thinking are the focus on the needs and wants of the customer and on its set of standardized solutions to frequently occurring problems in the process (de Koning et al., 2006).

Six Sigma was introduced as a company-wide QI initiative by Motorola in the late 1980s and then adapted and developed more extensively by General Electric (GE) in the following decade. Hallmarks of the Six Sigma approach are focus on customer satisfaction with the product or service, decision making that is driven by quantitative data analysis, and an emphasis on reducing costs. Six Sigma is a project-based QI strategy. Projects are selected and prioritized based on the importance of the project to the organization's mission and strategic goals. Project leaders are called Black Belts (BBs) and Green Belts (GBs), a reference to skill acquisition in the martial arts. Members of upper management to whom the BB and GB report are viewed as project owners and are referred to as "champions" (de Koning et al., 2006).

The steps used in Six Sigma are somewhat analogous to the scientific method, the nursing process, and similar problem-solving methods and include five steps or phases—define, measure, analyze, improve, and control—also referred to by the acronym DMAIC. The steps of DMAIC can be used to investigate any problem in an organization regardless of the scope or scale of the problem. A cost-benefit analysis is conducted in the define stage; if the analysis is favorable to the organization, the project is accepted and then proceeds to all stages or phases of DMAIC. Once the project is accepted, it is assigned to a project team headed by a GB or BB. Strengths associated with Six Sigma include its structured, analytic, and logical progression to problem solving. Organizational buy-in at all levels to the processes used by Six Sigma is also viewed as a strength. Weaknesses of the Six Sigma approach include its complexity when used to solve smaller scale or simpler problems (de Koning et al., 2006).

Some institutions use principles from different QI methodologies on the same QI project. An example is the use of the "Lean-Sigma" approach, which is a combination of the Lean and Six Sigma approaches (Varkey, Reller, & Resar, 2007). Link to Practice 17-2 shows how one QI project was used.

Link to Practice 17-2

Increasingly, QI tools and processes, such as Six Sigma, are being utilized in health care organizations. For example, staff affiliated with a 714-bed hospital in New York designed and implemented a QI project using Six Sigma methodology to correct issues associated with delayed transfer of patients to the intensive care units (ICUs) in the facility. An interdisciplinary team of clinicians and nonclinicians, led by a hospital administrator project Black Belt, analyzed components associated with inpatient transfers into the ICUs and identified eight steps which significantly impacted the transfer process.

Initially, it was determined by the team that the average time associated with a transfer from a floor bed to an ICU bed was 214 minutes; however, the time could extend to as long as 420 minutes. After conducting an initial capability analysis, the master Black Belt recommended a goal of an average of 90 minutes for average transfer time. During the improvement phase of the process, critical elements which impeded the transfer process were identified and a solution plan integrating new processes was developed. For example, the process for writing transfer orders to move patients out of the ICU was changed to ensure that transfer orders were completed by residents immediately following completion of morning rounds so that ICU beds could become available in a shorter time frame.

Following implementation of the new processes associated with transfer, data were collected and analyzed over a 1-year period (462 consecutive transfers to the ICU). The target performance goal was attained by the fourth month. The mean time for patient transfer from a floor bed to the ICU improved to 84 minutes.

Silich, S. J., Wetz, R. V., Riebling, N., Coleman, C., Khoueiry, G., Rafeh, N. A., et al. (2012). Using Six Sigma methodology to reduce patient transfer times from floor to critical-care beds. *Journal for Healthcare Quality, 34*(1), 44–54.

Evidence-Based Practice

In recent years, terms, such as *evidence-based medicine* (EBM), *evidence-based practice* (EBP), *evidence-based nursing*, *evidence-based health care*, and *best practices guidelines* (BPGs), have emerged and assumed a significant position in health care literature. These terms are probably best understood as decision-making frameworks that assist health care providers with making complex decisions utilizing research and other forms of evidence on a routine basis when formulating those decisions (Melnyk & Fineout-Overholt, 2015). Evidence-based decision frameworks are used to describe methods adopted by practitioners and others in an effort to increase the quality of health care, to decrease variability of care, and to decrease the costs related to providing health care.

Utilization of EBP and BPGs increases the quality of care by attempting to bridge the gap between the discovery of knowledge in health care and the time that knowledge is applied in practice. The Institute of Medicine (IOM) suggests that time lag may be as long as 20 years (IOM, 2001). The use of EBP and BPGs should decrease inappropriate variability in practice patterns, which often leads to increased costs. For example, a woman diagnosed with stage II breast cancer in Provo, Utah, should receive the same level of care as a woman who is diagnosed with the same stage of breast cancer in Tampa, Florida, if health care practitioners subscribe to and utilize the latest evidence-based or practice guidelines for the treatment and management of stage II breast cancer.

EBM utilizes a defined method in four major steps:

1. Eliciting, describing, defining, and refining a structured question about a target population, outcome, and, typically, an intervention
2. Systematic and comprehensive review of the literature in an attempt to answer the question
3. Evaluation of the data and data sources retrieved for methodologic rigor (i.e., data obtained as a result of randomized clinical trials as compared to data from anecdotal reports)
4. Analysis of the data uncovered to answer the question (Donald, 2002)

The limitations of EBP include the absence of organizational support and structure to properly utilize this decision-making framework; insufficient skills to frame the question, retrieve the data, or analyze the data; and gaps in the literature that make it impossible to sufficiently answer the question. In addition, some clinicians argue that EBP decreases or threatens clinical autonomy in decision making.

The role of the APN in EBP is continuing to expand. APNs, such as Marci in the opening scenario, are often relied on to be the clinical leaders of EBP. This leadership role includes continually researching and acquiring the most updated versions of BPGs or clinical guidelines; interpreting the guidelines for other staff and for patients and families; successfully implementing the recommendations of the guidelines; and conducting research to determine the effectiveness of the guidelines from clinical, quality, and cost perspectives after implementation. Chapter 12 contains additional information on EBP.

Summary

This chapter provides a basis for the APN to achieve understanding and appreciation for the utility of leadership and management theories in contemporary nursing practice. By virtue of their roles, APNs, such as Marci, are viewed as leaders and, as such, often have quite visible positions in organizations and the community.

Marci is in a position in which she needs to define her role. To be an effective leader, she must develop a leadership style that considers her personal strengths and weaknesses and fits the needs and personality of the unit. She will also need to use a number of management concepts and principles, particularly related to motivation and change, and must also be prepared to implement QI strategies that will affect the unit to improve client care.

Assimilation of strategies to improve leadership, motivation, change, decision making, and other concepts discussed in this chapter into the practice repertoire of the advanced practitioner in nursing is crucial to the viability and sustainability of the role.

Key Points

- Leadership and management, although closely related concepts, are different.
- Characteristics of both transformational leadership and transactional leadership are crucial to effective leadership.

- Fayol's principles of Classic Management Theory are still employed in organizations today.
- Higher levels of work environment empowerment and LMX result in greater personal transfer of knowledge in the practice setting by nurses.
- Individuals with high levels of personal resilience are valued by organizations, especially during times of turbulence and rapid change.
- QI empowers individuals and teams within systems to systematically examine processes in service delivery, to identify root causes of problems in the system, and to creatively propose and adopt solutions to the problems.
- Nurses value EBP and are ready to implement EBP.

Learning Activities

1. Analyze the leadership style of your current supervisor. Does the supervisor's leadership behavior vary from situation to situation? Would the supervisor be classified as a transformational, transactional, authentic, charismatic, servant, or other leader? Why?
2. Assess the organization in which you work today. Are Fayol's and Taylor's principles of management evident in this organization? Give examples.
3. Think back to the last time a major change occurred in your work environment. Was the change a planned change? What were the driving forces and restraining forces? Who was the change agent? Did the change occur as planned?
4. What QI initiatives are evident in your organization? How would you find out more about Lean/Six Sigma practices? Have any nurses in your organization served in the capacity as BBs or GBs? If so, what QI projects have they led or in which projects have they been involved?

REFERENCES

Adams, J. S. (1965). Inequity in social exchanges. In L. Berkowitz (Ed.), *Advances in experimental social psychology* (pp. 267–300). New York, NY: Academic Press.

Aguayo, R. (1990). *Dr. Deming: The American who taught the Japanese about quality.* New York, NY: Fireside.

American Nurses Credentialing Center. (2013). *History of the Magnet program.* Retrieved from http://www.nursecredentialing.org/MagnetHistory.aspx

Andel, C., Davidow, S. L., Hollander, M., & Moreno, D. A. (2012). The economics of health care quality and medical errors. *Journal of Health Care Finance, 39,* 39–50.

Avolio, B. J., & Gardner, W. L. (2005). Authentic leadership development: Getting to the root of positive forms of leadership. *The Leadership Quarterly, 16,* 315–338.

Avolio, B. J., Zhu, W., Koh, W., & Puja, B. (2004). Transformational leadership and organizational commitment: Mediating role of psychological empowerment and moderating role of structural distance. *Journal of Organizational Behavior, 25,* 951–968.

Banks, G. C., McCauley, K. D., Garner, W. L., & Guler, C. E. (2016). A meta-analytic review of authentic and transformational leadership: A test for redundancy. *The Leadership Quarterly, 27,* 634–652.

Bass, B. M., Avolio, B. J., Jung, D. I., & Berson, Y. (2003). Predicting unit performance by assessing transformational and transactional leadership. *The Journal of Applied Psychology, 88*(2), 207–218.

Bennis, W. (1984). The four competencies of leadership. *Training and Development Journal, 38*(8), 15–19.

Blanchard, K., & Hodges, P. (2003, May 12). The journey to servant leadership in work, life. *San Diego Business Journal,* p. A2.

Bolino, M. C. (2007, August). *What about us? Relative deprivation among out-group members in LMX relationships.* Paper presented at the Academy of Management Annual Meeting, Philadelphia, PA.

Bono, J. E., & Judge, T. A. (2003). Self concordance at work: Toward understanding the motivational effects of transformational leaders. *Academy of Management Journal, 46*(5), 554–571.

Borkowski, N. (2016). *Organizational behavior, theory, and design in health care* (2nd ed.). Burlington, MA: Jones & Bartlett Learning.

Buchbinder, S. B., & Shanks, N. H. (2017). *Introduction to health care management* (3rd ed.). Burlington, MA: Jones & Bartlett Learning.

Burns, J. M. (1978). *Leadership.* New York, NY: Harper & Row.

Caplan, E. (1971). *Management accounting and behavioral science.* Reading, MA: Addison-Wesley.

Carney, D. R., Cuddy, A. J. C., & Yap, A. J. (2010). Power posing: Brief nonverbal displays affect neuroendocrine levels and risk tolerance. *Psychological Science, 21*(10), 1363–1368.

Carson, P. P., Carson, K. D., & Roe, C. W. (1993). Social power bases: A meta-analytic examination of interrelationships and outcomes. *Journal of Applied Social Psychology, 23,* 1150–1169.

Cerasoli, C. P., Nicklin, J. M., & Ford, M. T. (2014). Intrinsic motivation and extrinsic incentives jointly predict performance: A 40-year meta-analysis. *Psychological Bulletin, 140*(4), 980–1008.

Chassin, M., & Loeb, J. M. (2011). The ongoing quality improvement journey: Next stop, high reliability. *Health Affairs, 30,* 559–568.

Chemers, M., Harp, R., Rhodewalt, F., & Wysocki, J. (1985). A person–environment analysis of job stress: A contingency model explanation. *Journal of Personality and Social Psychology, 49*(3), 628–635.

Conger, J. A., & Kanungo, R. N. (1988). Behavioral dimensions of charismatic leadership. In J. A. Conger & R. N. Kanungo (Eds.), *Charismatic leadership: The elusive factor in organizational effectiveness* (pp. 78–97). San Francisco, CA: Jossey-Bass.

Crosby, P. B. (1979). *Quality is free: The art of making quality certain*. New York, NY: McGraw-Hill.

Daft, R. L., & Marcic, D. (2015). *Understanding management* (9th ed.). Stamford, CT: Cengage Learning.

De Hoog, A., Den Hartog, D., & Koopman, P. (2005). Linking the Big Five-factors of personality to charismatic and transactional leadership: Perceived dynamic work as a moderator. *Journal of Organizational Behavior, 26,* 839–865.

de Koning, H., Verver, J. P. S., van den Heuvel, J., Bisgaard, S., & Does, R. J. M. M. (2006). Lean six sigma in healthcare. *Journal for Healthcare Quality, 28,* 4–11.

Deming, W. F. (1986). *Out of the crisis*. Cambridge, MA: MIT Press.

DeRue, S., & Ashford, S. (2010). Who will lead and who will follow? A social process of leadership identity construction in organizations. *Academy of Management Review, 35*(4), 627–647.

Donald, A. (2002). How to practice evidence-based medicine. *Medscape General Medicine, 5*(1). Retrieved from http://www.medscape.com/viewpublication/122_index

Drafke, M. (2009). *The human side of organizations* (10th ed.). Upper Saddle River, NJ: Prentice Hall.

DuBrin, A. J. (2007). *Fundamentals of organizational behavior* (4th ed.). Mason, OH: South-Western.

DuBrin, A. J. (2012). *Essentials of management* (9th ed.). Mason, OH: South-Western.

Fayol, H. (1949). *General and industrial management*. London, United Kingdom: Pitman & Sons.

Fiedler, F. (1967). *A theory of leadership effectiveness*. New York, NY: McGraw-Hill.

Fiedler, F. (1969). Style or circumstances: The leadership enigma. *Psychology Today, 2*(10), 38–43.

Fiedler, F., Chemers, M., & Mahar, L. (1976). *Improving leadership effectiveness: The leader match concept*. New York, NY: Wiley.

Ford, H., & Crowther, S. (1926). *Today and tomorrow*. Cambridge, MA: Productivity Press.

French, J., & Raven, B. (1959). *The bases of social power*. In D. Cartwright (Ed.), *Studies in social power* (pp. 259–269). Ann Arbor, MI: University of Michigan.

Georgopoulos, B., Mahoney, G., & Jones, N. (1957). A path-goal approach to productivity. *Journal of Applied Psychology, 41,* 345–353.

Gillem, T. (1988). Deming's 14 points and hospital quality: Responding to the consumer's demand for the best value health care. *Journal of Nursing Quality Assurance, 2*(3), 70–78.

Goleman, D., Boyatzis, R., & McKee, A. (2001). Primal leadership: The hidden driver of great performance. *Harvard Business Review, 79*(11), 42–51.

Graen, G., & Cashman, J. F. (1975). A role-making model of leadership in formal organizations: A developmental approach. In J. G. Hunt & L. L. Larson (Eds.), *Leadership frontiers* (pp. 143–165). Kent, OH: Kent State University Press.

Graen, G., & Uhl-Bien, M. (1995). Relationship-based approach to leadership: Development of the leader-member exchange (LMX) theory of leadership over 25 years: Applying a multi-level, multi-domain perspective. *Leadership Quarterly, 6,* 219–247.

Gray, E. R. (1978). The non-linear systems experience: A requiem. *Business Horizons, 21,* 31–36.

Green, J. P. (1981). People management: New directions for the 1980s. *Administrative Management, 42,* 22–26.

Harms, P. D., & Crede, M. (2010). Emotional intelligence and transformational and transactional leadership: A meta-analysis. *Journal of Leadership and Organizational Studies, 17*(1), 5–17.

Heineken, J., & McCloskey, J. (1985). Teaching power concepts. *The Journal of Nursing Education, 24*(1), 40–42.

Hellriegel, D., Jackson, S. E., & Slocum, J. W. (2008). *Management: A competency-based approach* (11th ed.). Mason, OH: South-Western.

Hersey, P., & Blanchard, K. (1977). *Management of organizational behavior: Utilizing human resources*. Englewood Cliffs, NJ: Prentice Hall.

Hersey, P., & Blanchard, K. (1982). *Management of organizational behavior: Utilizing human resources* (4th ed.). Englewood Cliffs, NJ: Prentice Hall.

Herzberg, F. (1966). *Work and the nature of man*. Cleveland, OH: World.

Hitt, M. A., Black, J. S., & Porter, L. W. (2011). *Management* (3rd ed.). Upper Saddle River, NJ: Prentice Hall.

House, R. (1971). A path-goal theory of leader effectiveness. *Administrative Science Quarterly, 16,* 321–338.

House, R. J. (1977). A 1976 theory of charismatic leadership. In J. G. Hunt & L. L. Larson (Eds.), *Leadership: The cutting edge* (pp. 189–207). Carbondale, IL: Southern Illinois University Press.

House, R. J. (1996). Path-goal theory of leadership: Lessons, legacy, and a reformulated theory. *The Leadership Quarterly, 7*(3), 323–352.

Institute of Medicine. (2001). *Crossing the quality chasm: A new health care system for the 21st century*. Washington, DC: National Academy Press.

Institute of Medicine. (2013). *Reports*. Retrieved from http://www.iom.edu/Reports.aspx

Judge, T. A., & Piccolo, R. F. (2004). Transformational and transactional leadership: A meta-analytic test of their relative validity. *The Journal of Applied Psychology, 89*(5), 755–768.

Jung, D. D., & Sosik, J. J. (2006). Who are the spellbinders? Identifying personal attributes of charismatic leaders. *Journal of Leadership and Organizational Studies, 12*(4), 12–26.

Juran, J. M. (1988). *Juran's quality control handbook*. New York, NY: McGraw-Hill.

Katz, N. H., & Lawyer, J. W. (1985). *Communication and conflict resolution skills*. Dubuque, IA: Kendall/Hunt.

Kay, A. (1973). Where being nice to workers didn't work. *Business Week, 1,* 98–100.

Kipnis, D. (1976). *The powerholders*. Chicago, IL: University of Chicago Press.

Kopelman, R. E., Prottas, D. J., & Davis, A. L. (2008). Douglas McGregor's theory X and Y: Toward a construct-valid measure. *Journal of Managerial Issues, 20*(2), 255–271.

Kotter, J. P. (1977). Power, dependence, and effective management. *Harvard Business Review, 55*(4), 125–136.

Kotter, J. P. (1995). Leading change: Why transformation efforts fail. *Harvard Business Review, 73,* 59–67.

Lewin, K. (1951). *Field theory in social science*. New York, NY: Harper & Row.

Lewin, K., & Lippitt, R. (1938). An experimental approach to the study of autocracy and democracy: A preliminary note. *Sociometry, 1,* 292–300.

Lindebaum, D., & Cartwright, S. (2010). A critical examination of the relationship between emotional intelligence and transformational leadership. *Journal of Management Studies, 47,* 1317–1342.

Malone, E. (1975). The non-linear systems experiment in participative management. *Journal of Business, 48,* 52–64.

Maslow, A. (1968). *Toward a psychology of being*. New York, NY: Nostrand Reinhold.

Maslow, A. (1971). *The farther reaches of human nature*. New York, NY: Viking.

Masters, M. L., & Masters, R. J. (1993). Building TQM into nursing management. *Nursing Economic$, 11*(5), 274–291.

McClelland, D. C. (1975). *Power: The inner experience*. New York, NY: Wiley.

Melnyk, B. M., & Fineout-Overholt, E. (2015). *Evidence-based practice in nursing and healthcare: A guide to best practice* (3rd ed.). Philadelphia, PA: Wolters Kluwer.

Minor, J. (1980). *Theories of organizational behavior*. Hinsdale, IL: Dryden.

Morse, J., & Lorsch, J. (1970). Beyond theory Y. *Harvard Business Review, 48*(3), 61–68.

O'Boyle, E. H., Jr., Humphrey, R. H., Pollack, J. M., Hawver, T. H., & Story, P. A. (2011). The relation between emotional intelligence and job performance: A meta-analysis. *Journal of Organizational Behavior, 32,* 788–818.

Peters, T. (1987). *Thriving on chaos*. New York, NY: Knopf.

Podsakoff, P. M., Bommer, W. H., Podsakoff, N. P., & Mackenzie, S. B. (2006). Relationships between leader reward and punishment behaviour and subordinate attitudes, perceptions, and behaviours: A meta-analytic review of existing and new research. *Organizational Behavior and Human Decision Processes, 99,* 113–142.

Port, O. (1991, October 25). Dueling pioneers. *Business Week,* p. 17.

Raven, B. H. (2008). The bases of power and the power/interaction model of interpersonal influence. *Analyses of Social Issues and Public Policy, 8*(1), 1–22.

Robbins, S. P., & Coulter, M. (2013). *Management* (12th ed.). Boston, MA: Pearson.

Robbins, S. P., & Judge, T. A. (2015). *Organizational behavior* (16th ed.). Boston, MA: Pearson.

Ross, T. K. (2014). *Health care quality management: Tools and applications.* San Francisco, CA: Jossey-Bass.

Rowold, J., & Heinitz, K. (2007). Transformational and charismatic leadership: Assessing the convergent, divergent, and criterion validity of the MLQ and the CKS. *Leadership Quarterly, 18,* 121–133.

Rue, L. W., & Byars, L. (1977). *Management: Theory and application.* Homewood, IL: Richard D. Irwin.

Schaubroeck, J., Lam, S. K., & Cha, S. E. (2007). Embracing transformational leadership: Team values and the impact of the leader behavior on team performance. *The Journal of Applied Psychology, 92*(4), 1020–1030.

Schriesheim, C. A., Castro, S. L., Zhou, X. T., & DeChurch, L. A. (2006). An investigation of path-goal and transformational leadership theory predictions at the individual level of analysis. *Leadership Quarterly, 17,* 21–38.

Schwartz, R. W., & Tumblin, T. (2002). The power of servant leadership to transform health care organizations for the 21st-century economy. *Archives of Surgery, 137*(12), 1419–1427.

Shamir, B., & Eilam, G. (2005). "What's your story?": A life-stories approach to authentic leadership development. *The Leadership Quarterly, 16,* 395–417.

Shirey, M. (2012). How resilient are your team members? *The Journal of Nursing Administration, 42*(12), 551–553.

Simon, H. A. (1965). *The shape of automation for man and management.* New York, NY: Harper & Row.

Small, A., Gist, D., Souza, D., Dalton, J., Magny-Normilus, C., & David, D. (2016). Using Kotter's change model for implementing beside handoff: A quality improvement project. *Journal of Nursing Care Quality, 31*(4), 304–309.

Snee, R. D., & Hoerl, R. W. (2004). *Six sigma beyond the factory floor.* Upper Saddle River, NJ: Pearson Education.

Stone, A. G., Russell, R. F., & Patterson, K. (2003). *Transformational versus servant leadership: A difference in leader focus.* Retrieved from http://www.regent/edu/acad/global/publications/sl_proceedings/2003/stone_transformation_versus.pdf

Tannenbaum, R., & Schmidt, W. H. (1973). How to choose a leadership pattern. *Harvard Business Review, 51,* 162–180.

Taylor, F. W. (1911). *The principles of scientific management.* New York, NY: Harper.

The Joint Commission. (2013). *Our history.* Retrieved from http://www.jointcommission.org/assets/1/6Joint_Commission_History.pdf

Thomas, K. W., & Kilmann, R. H. (1974). *The Thomas-Kilmann conflict mode instrument.* Tuxedo Park, NY: Xicom.

Tomey, A. M. (2009). *Guide to nursing management and leadership* (8th ed.). St. Louis, MO: Mosby.

Uhl-Bien, M., Riggio, R. E., Lowe, K. B., & Carsten, M. K. (2014). Followership theory: A review and research agenda. *The Leadership Quarterly, 25,* 83–104.

U.S. Department of Health and Human Services. (2016). *20 Million people have gained health insurance coverage because of the Affordable Care Act, new estimates show.* Retrieved from http://www.hhs.gov/about/news/2016/03/03/20-million-people-have-gained-health-insurance-coverage-because-affordable-care-act-new-estimates

Varkey, P., Reller, M. K., & Resar, R. K. (2007). Basics of quality improvement in health care. *Mayo Clinic Proceedings, 82*(6), 735–739.

Vecchio, R. P., Justin, J. E., & Pearce, C. L. (2008). The utility of transactional and transformational leadership for predicting performance and satisfaction within a path-goal theory framework. *Journal of Occupational and Organizational Psychology, 81,* 71–82.

Vroom, V. H. (1960). *Some personality determinants of the effects of participation.* Englewood Cliffs, NJ: Prentice Hall.

Vroom, V. H. (1964). *Work and motivation.* New York, NY: Wiley.

Vroom, V. H., & Jago, A. G. (1988). *The new leadership: Managing participation in organizations.* Englewood Cliffs, NJ: Prentice-Hall.

Vroom, V. H., & Jago, A. G. (2007). The role of situation in leadership. *The American Psychologist,* 17–24.

Vroom, V. H., & Yetton, P. W. (1973). *Leadership and decision-making.* Pittsburgh, PA: University of Pittsburgh Press.

Wagner, J. A., & Hollenbeck, J. R. (2014). *Organizational behavior: Securing competitive advantage* (2nd ed.). New York, NY: Routledge.

Walumbwa, F. O., Avolio, B. J., & Zhu, W. (2008). How transformational leadership weaves its influence on individual job performance: The role of identification and efficacy beliefs. *Personnel Psychology, 61,* 793–825.

Wang, H., Law, K. S., Hackett, R. D., Wang, D., & Chen, Z. X. (2005). Leader–member exchange as a mediator of the relationship between transformational leadership and followers' performance and organizational citizenship behavior. *Academy of Management Journal, 48*(3), 420–432.

Washington, R. R. (2007). Empirical relationships between theories of servant, transformational, and transactional leadership. *Academy of Management Proceedings,* 1–6.

Weber, M. (1970). Bureaucracy. In W. Sexton (Ed.), *Organization theories* (pp. 39–43). Columbus, OH: Merrill.

Williams, C. R. (2013). *Management* (7th ed.). Mason, OH: South-Western.

Winter, D. G. (1973). *The power motive.* New York, NY: Free Press.

18

Learning Theories

Evelyn M. Wills and Melanie McEwen

Barbara Davis is a family nurse practitioner working in a community clinic. Recently, she cared for Frank Young, a 65-year-old African American who came to the clinic at his wife's insistence because of recurring, severe headaches. Mr. Young reported that his headaches started about 6 months ago; he attributed them to stress caused by his recent retirement.

Mr. Young's physical findings indicated that he was about 50 lb overweight and that his blood pressure while sitting was 204/110 mmHg. His lower legs and feet were slightly edematous, and laboratory tests revealed a total cholesterol reading of 240 mg/dl. All other laboratory blood and urine results were normal.

Barbara explained to Mr. Young that he has high blood pressure and asked to discuss the problem with both him and his wife. She led the Youngs to a room in which they sat in comfortable chairs around a small table. Barbara began the discussion by asking if the couple had any experience with hypertension (HTN). After listening to their comprehension of the problem, she recognized the importance of giving them more current and concrete information. She corrected in plain words their ideas about HTN and explained the relationships among HTN, age, gender, and weight and described its prevalence among various ethnic groups. Realizing that learners can take in a limited amount of novel information at a time, she asked them if they would like to take a short break before going on to how the problem is treated.

When they reconvened, Barbara showed the Youngs a short video that used nonmedical terms to describe HTN and visually illustrated the physiologic changes that cause HTN. After the video, she questioned the Youngs to evaluate their level of understanding. A 15-minute discussion followed in which Barbara answered questions and described management strategies. She gave Mr. Young two prescriptions and explained what they were for and how to take them. Following the explanation, she had him repeat the information. To reinforce the information on HTN management, Barbara scheduled another meeting with the Youngs, this time at their home, where they would likely be less overwhelmed by the clinic atmosphere.

When Barbara visited with the Youngs, she reviewed the information they had already been given. Then they discussed the importance of limiting sodium and fat intake. She provided an illustrated booklet to describe varieties of foods. They discussed whether the sodium content was safe, high, or too high to consume. She included not only foods but also condiments with the allowed amounts. There were recipes for variations on favorite foods with lowered sodium and fat content; the booklet also included removable shopping lists to assist with decisions while grocery shopping. Learning that both Mrs. and Mr. Young enjoyed working and gaming on the computer, Barbara included websites with helpful hints on limiting sodium and fats and the URLs for "say NAYtoNA," a local Facebook support group page, and a Twitter site for social support.

At the end of the home visit, Barbara reviewed the medication and dietary information for HTN management and answered additional questions. Finally, she made a follow-up appointment for the following week to assess progress with his HTN control and encouraged Mrs. Young to accompany her husband to that meeting as well.

Teaching is one of the most important roles of professional registered nurses (RNs) and advanced practice nurses (APNs). Teaching performed by nurses at all levels is usually more informal than formal. That is, the nurse teaches clients and their families, or students and colleagues, more often on a one-to-one basis as the need arises, than in a formal, planned teaching session in a classroom setting. But teaching includes more than just providing information. Because someone has been told something does not mean that learning has occurred. Many factors are involved if learning is to be successful, and providing information is only one of them.

Health information can be unfamiliar, complex, and difficult to understand for patients and families, and the idea of health literacy as a component of health teaching is important in teaching patients/clients. Health literacy is defined as "the degree to which an individual has the capacity to obtain, communicate, process and understand basic health information and services to make appropriate health decisions" (Bastable, Meyers, & Poitevent, 2014, p. 261). Although health literacy is not an educational theory, health teaching depends on the ability of nurses to bring useful information and education to individuals and groups regardless of their educational level. Because many patients depend on someone else to help or to care for them, oftentimes, the caregivers must also be taught to provide assistance so that the patient may heal or live with chronic diseases or the effects of illness and trauma.

This chapter provides professional nurses with tools to facilitate learning for patients, families, and staff. Basic theories of learning can serve as a framework for the nurse in all teaching endeavors. Theories provide a way to organize information that will be communicated to other people. They may offer a mechanism whereby the instructor can look at a situation in a different way when current methods are not working, or they may provide a map for charting unfamiliar territory. In any event, facilitating learning is an essential objective of the professional nurse, and application of theories helps ensure that learning is optimized.

What Is Learning?

Learning has been defined as "a change in behavior (knowledge, attitudes, and/or skills) that can be observed or measured and that occurs at any time or in any place as a result of exposure to environmental stimuli" (Bastable & Gonzalez, 2016, p. 11) and "a relatively permanent change in behavior or in behavioral potentiality that results from experience" (Olson & Hergenhahn, 2012, p. 6). Learning occurs as individuals interact with their environment, incorporating new information into what they already know (Braungart, Braungart, & Gramet, 2014). Furthermore, if learning is to be permanent, it must be treated as a process that occurs over time rather than an isolated event. Often, time and repeated contacts are required for an individual to acquire new knowledge that is meaningful and significant.

Learning can be grouped into three categories: psychomotor learning (the acquisition and performance of skills), affective learning (a change in feelings, values, or beliefs), and cognitive learning (acquiring information). Examples of psychomotor learning would include a nursing student mastering certain patient care procedures (e.g., inserting an intravenous [IV] line or changing a sterile dressing) and a patient learning to self-inject insulin. Illustrations of affective learning include an alcoholic acquiring strategies to overcome addiction and a nurse developing cultural sensitivity when caring for immigrants. Cognitive learning generally involves the addition of new information, as when a new mother learns how to care for her infant or a novice nurse learns to recognize the signs and symptoms of heart failure. Although not always recognized, psychomotor learning tends to be more easily accomplished and measured than affective and cognitive learning (Rankin & Stallings, 2005). Nurses must understand all three types of learning and know how to facilitate each in patients and their families as well as among other nurses and ancillary staff.

The process of assimilating new knowledge into our daily lives makes all humans constant learners because learning is necessary for survival. Although all animals can learn, humans are capable of using their knowledge to be creative, predict the future, explain the past, or deal with the present. Indeed, learning is such an important human experience that it has created the desire or curiosity to discover how people learn. This search to understand how people learn has led to the development and formalization of learning theories.

What Is Teaching?

It must be recognized that although teaching and learning are interrelated, learning occurs as a separate and individual process apart from teaching. Teaching has been defined as "a system of directed and deliberate actions that are intended to induce learning through a series of directed activities" (Candela, 2012, p. 202). It refers to acts that communicate information to facilitate learning (Bastable & Alt, 2014). To accomplish this, teachers must be aware of the learning styles and learning needs of the individual and how capable that individual is of responding to the demands of instruction.

It is a common assumption that teaching is helping one to gain knowledge. Although that is certainly an important component of teaching, knowledge is seldom enough to elicit a change in behavior or thinking. Knowing what should be done and acting on that knowledge are two different things. For example, a patient with chronic renal failure may *know* that salt and potassium are to be avoided in the diet, but learning has not occurred until that knowledge has been incorporated as a change in behavior.

Anyone who teaches, including a mother or father teaching a child how to put away toys or a woman teaching a friend to crochet, has some belief regarding how learning occurs. Unfortunately, sometimes, the knowledge the teacher possesses about learning is simplistic: "I told you; therefore, you should know." An individual's beliefs about learning can influence that person's behavior regarding what should happen to make learning occur. By understanding basic theories of learning, the professional nurse will be better prepared to help the learner make the transition from acquiring knowledge to learning. This chapter presents some of the many theories of learning and describes how they are used to solve problems encountered in the teaching–learning process. These theories may be used by nurses in practice or education as well as for designing, implementing, and evaluating projects that involve education.

Categorization of Learning Theories

Some nurses might question why it is important to understand the process of learning and to know about some of the theories of learning. Learning theories describe the processes used to bring about changes in the ways individuals understand information and changes in the ways they perform a task or skill. Furthermore, learning theories can help provide a focus for creating an environment and conditions in which teaching can occur more effectively (Candela, 2016; Fisher, 2016). Kurt Lewin is credited with the adage, "There is nothing so practical as a good theory." A good theory enables one to make choices confidently and consistently and to explain or defend why choices were made. Thus, although nursing theory provides the framework for professional assessment of a client's condition or needs and the specific language the nurse uses when making a diagnosis or charting, learning theories explain *how* this information is assimilated and suggest effective ways to present it to the client as an intervention. Learning theory, then, combined with nursing theory, guides nurses as they interact with clients. This is particularly important for APNs and others prepared at the graduate level (Box 18-1, American Association of Colleges of Nursing [AACN] Essentials).

There are many different types of learning theories and only a few of the most commonly used in nursing are described in the following sections. The main categories as presented by Bigge and Shermis (1999) are the behavioral learning theories and the cognitive learning theories. Behavioral learning theories include the works of Pavlov, Skinner, and others. Cognitive learning theories include several subgroups including cognitive-field (Gestalt) theories, cognitive development or interaction theories, information-processing theories, humanistic learning theories, and Adult Learning Theory. Some of the major theories for each group will be discussed briefly, with examples of application from the nursing literature.

Behavioral Learning Theories

Behavioral theories were among the first to be widely recognized and used in education. Indeed, they were so pervasive in the American educational system in the 1950s and 1960s that many people still associate the term *learning theories* with behavioral theories. Behavioral learning theories served the growing American educational system well during the 20th century. They provided the rapidly expanding system with an organized, systematic approach.

Box 18-1	American Association of Colleges of Nursing Essentials and Learning Theories

Graduates of master's in nursing programs act as educators in almost all roles and settings, regardless of their specialty or type of practice. As outlined in Essential IX, all master's-prepared nurses should develop competencies to "apply learning theories and teaching principles to the design, implementation, and evaluation of health education programs for individuals or groups in a variety of settings."

Source: AACN (2011, p. 28).

Table 18-1   Comparison of Behavioral Learning Theories

Theorist	Theory Distinctions
Thorndike	Original stimulus–response framework; learners respond randomly to stimuli; learning is trial and error
Pavlov	Classical conditioning; responses are involuntary and based on experience
Skinner	Operant conditioning; learning produces a desirable behavior because it is reinforced or strengthened
Hull	Stimulus–response framework (based on Thorndike); includes reinforcement as a characteristic of learning

Overview

Behaviorism focuses on what is directly observable in learners. It is largely based on the works of Ivan Pavlov (1927) and Edward Thorndike (1932), who researched how both humans and animals learned, and their work became the basis for behavioral psychology (Candela, 2016; Olson & Hergenhahn, 2012). In behavioral theories, behavior (response) is viewed as the result of stimulus conditions. The behavioral learning theories that evolved from this perspective are sometimes referred to as the Stimulus–Response (S–R) Model of Learning. Some of the major behaviorist theorists include Thorndike (connectionism), Pavlov (classical conditioning), Skinner (operant conditioning), and Hull (reinforcement). Table 18-1 summarizes the assertions of each of these theorists.

Edward L. Thorndike (1874–1949) was one of the first theorists to attempt scientific studies to understand the learning process. He perceived that learners are empty organisms who respond to stimuli in a random manner. He provided the original S–R framework for behavioral psychology. For Thorndike, learning was the result of associations formed between stimuli and responses, and the S–R connections were formed through trial and error. Such associations or habits become strengthened or weakened by the nature and frequency of the S–R pairings. The hallmark of connectionism was that learning could be adequately explained without referring to any observable internal states (Thorndike, 1932).

In a well-known study, Pavlov (1849–1936) taught his dog to salivate when a tuning fork was rung by rewarding him with meat powder placed into his mouth. Soon, the dog would salivate when the tuning fork rang even though no meat powder was provided. This involuntary reaction is known as *conditioning*. Pavlov's work is labeled as *classical conditioning* to differentiate it from other types of S–R associations that deal with voluntary behavior (Braungart et al., 2014). Classical conditioning is what one sees in a child's response to the sight of a needle. The conditioned stimulus (the sight of the needle) is able to evoke the response (crying) formerly reserved for the unconditional stimulus (actual pain from an injection). Response to the sight of a needle is learned behavior based on experience.

To B. F. Skinner (1904–1990), the purpose of psychology is to predict and control the behavior of individuals. He defined learning as a change in probability of response and coined the term *operant conditioning*. An *operant* is a set of behaviors that constitutes an individual doing something. Operant conditioning is the learning process whereby a desirable behavior is made more likely to occur in the future or to occur more frequently because it is reinforced or strengthened (Olson &

Hergenhahn, 2012; Ormrod, 2016). When the desired response occurs, whether accidental or planned, a reward that is meaningful to the learner is provided, so recurrence of the desired response is increased. In the previously discussed classical conditioning, the person in question receives reinforcement no matter what he or she does, whereas in an operant conditioning situation, the individual's behavior causes the reward to happen.

Clark L. Hull (1884–1952) based his studies on Thorndike's work but included *reinforcement* as a major characteristic of learning. Reinforcement is a complex concept that is widely used in education today. Reinforcement is a consequence of an action that makes that action more likely to be repeated. Reinforcement may be internal/external, positive/negative, self-administered, social, or impersonal (Roberts, 1975). Reinforcement can be seen in many ways, from a simple smile (or frown) to aversion therapy (e.g., the "quit smoking" clinics that have individuals smoke one cigarette after another until they become sick). Problems can arise because the behavior the teacher intends to reinforce may not be the actual behavior that is reinforced.

Behaviorists are concerned with the observable and measurable aspects of human behavior. Basically, behaviorists believe that behavior can be controlled (thus demonstrating that learning has occurred) through rewarding desirable behavior and ignoring or punishing behavior that is undesirable. Reinforcing or strengthening the behavior increases the chance of its recurrence in the future. These theorists are concerned with behavior modification and make much use of the concepts of reflexes, reactions, objective measurement, quantitative data, sequence of behavior, and reinforcement schedules (Ormrod, 2016; Ozmon, 2011). Box 18-2 summarizes characteristics of behavioral learning theories.

Teachers who subscribe to this viewpoint are considered designers and controllers of students' behavior. The teacher is responsible for what students should learn and for evaluating how, when, and if they have learned. Teachers are expected to be content experts, transmit prescribed content, control the way learners receive and use the content, and then test to determine if they have received it (Knowles, 1981). Learning objectives (also called *behavioral objectives, instructional objectives*, or *performance criteria*) are broken down into a large number of very small tasks and reinforced one by one. The tasks are organized so that understanding develops progressively. This premise has led to the development of programmed texts and computer-assisted instruction. Tests are used in a classroom situation to measure the amount of knowledge a student has gained.

Use of behavioral theory encourages the development of clear behavioral outcomes and methods for evaluating those desired behaviors. It works well for many of the psychomotor skills that must be accomplished for both nurses and patients. Behavioral theory, however, is not without detractors. Because the learner assumes a relatively passive role, there is a possibility that old behaviors will be resumed once the learner is removed from the highly structured and controlled environments created by behaviorally based teaching methods. In other words, without the affective and cognitive components

Box 18-2   Characteristics of Behavioral Learning Theories

- Focuses on behavior modification, reflexes, reaction, and reinforcement
- Emphasizes observable and measurable aspects of human behavior
- Posits that behavior can be controlled through rewarding desirable behavior and ignoring or punishing undesirable behavior

of learning, there is no change in feelings or thinking for the learner. Once they are returned to the original environment that fostered and rewarded the undesirable behavior, chances are high that the original behavior will return. Many question whether behavioral techniques alone are capable of producing permanent changes in behavior.

Application to Nursing

Behaviorist principles are widely used by nurses, nursing educators, and staff developers. For example, learning contracts with clients are an outgrowth of this perspective. Likewise, nurses often use reinforcement when they comment on how well clients are following their treatment regimens and when they correctly repeat instructions. Also, much of nursing education is directed toward having students meet behavioral objectives, which is a hallmark of behavioral theories (see Chapter 22). Finally, grades can serve as either reinforcement or punishment—based on student performance, desires, and expectations.

Cognitive Learning Theories

In contrast to behavioral theories, which generally ignore the thoughts, feelings, and cognitive processes of the learner, cognitive learning theories emphasize the mental processes and activities that go on within the learner (Candela, 2016). Cognitive theorists do not view reward as a condition for learning, although they do not negate the role of reinforcement. The learner's own goals, thoughts, expectations, motivations, and abilities in the processing of information are seen as the foundations for learning (Braungart, Braungart, & Gramet, 2016).

Cognitive learning theories began to gain popular momentum in the 1960s when the recognition of the limitations of behavioral theories led to the development of more complete theories to frame and explain how people learn and how permanent changes in behavior are accomplished. One of the most important theorists in cognitive science, Jean Piaget, however, developed major components of his theory in the 1920s.

Cognitive theories focus on the operations of the mind and on how thoughts influence an individual's actions in relation to the environment (Candela, 2016). Several major subcategories of cognitive learning theories have evolved over time. Those described in the following sections include Gestalt (Cognitive-Field) Theories, cognitive development theories, social learning theories, psychodynamic theories, information-processing theories, and adult learning theories. Representative examples useful for nurses are presented in the following sections.

Cognitive-Field (Gestalt) Theories

A break with behaviorism occurred when the concept of "insight" learning was introduced into the gestalt theories. "Gestalt" is a German word that refers to the configuration or patterned organization of cognitive elements (Braungart et al., 2014).

Overview

The gestalt view of learning focuses on organization of a person's perceptual field to sort out and make sense of multiple parts. The scientific view underlying gestalt principles is field theory. Field theory espouses that a "field" is a dynamic, interrelated system in which any part can affect all other parts and that the whole is more than the sum of the parts (Olson & Hergenhahn, 2012). Gestalt Theory and field theory have become so closely associated that they are commonly referred to as *Cognitive-Field Theory*.

The cognitive-field psychologists consider learning to be closely related to perception. They define learning in terms of reorganization of the learner's perceptual or psychological world—his or her field. The field includes a simultaneous and mutual interaction among all the forces or stimuli affecting the person—the internal environment as well as the external environment. Experience is the interaction of a person and his or her perceived environment, whereas behavior is the result of the interplay of these forces. Consequently, perception and experiences of reality are uniquely individual, based on a person's total life experiences. Nothing exists in and of itself but only in relationship to something else. Learning, then, is the process of discovering and understanding the relationships among people, things, and ideas in the field. Learning is viewed as an active, goal-oriented process that is accomplished when information is processed and the "aha" moment is experienced. Transfer of information from the teacher to the student does not constitute learning. In order for learning to be accomplished, students must assume responsibility for learning and discover and assign their own meaning in order to understand and truly learn content. Through the learning process, the learner gains new insights or changes old ones. The purpose of learning is to think more effectively in a wide variety of situations and thus be able to solve problems.

Because cognitive-field theorists are concerned with the progressive development of the total person, they perceive self-actualization as the driving force that motivates all human behavior. Motivation involves the forces operating in a particular situation that cause the person to want to do something (as opposed to the behavioral theorists who think of motivation as a drive that reduces a perceived need). Growth and development are important in motivation and necessary for self-actualization to occur. As an individual matures, the forces operating to induce one to do something change.

Kurt Lewin (1890–1947), one of the major gestalt theorists, believed that humans have a basic need to bring order to a situation and that motivation to learn is stimulated by the ambiguity perceived in the situation. By involving students in the learning process, the instructor helps learners see the need to learn. Through the use of verbal explanations, showing pictures, drawing diagrams, and other teaching activities, the instructor helps the individual understand significant relationships so that the learner can organize the experience into a functional pattern and solve problems (Knowles, Holton, & Swanson, 2005).

Cognitive-field theorists believe people can learn information cognitively without changing their behavior and that motivation is the key. Motivation is an extremely difficult concept to implement. In health care, one often hears reports that an individual is noncompliant, when in actuality, the person is not motivated (for whatever reason) to do what the health care professionals perceive as the correct thing to do. Indeed, it often takes months and even years to find the right combination of factors that motivate an individual.

Mr. Young, from the opening case study, would probably rebel against changing his eating habits when he was a child, but he may be more likely to be motivated to do so as an adult because he understands the relationship between his diet and his headaches. Box 18-3 depicts characteristics of cognitive-field theories.

Application to Nursing

Barbara, the nurse in the case study, used Cognitive-Field Theory when she had the Youngs move into a room more conducive to learning. By controlling the external stimuli affecting the situation, she allowed the brain to focus more on the information she was presenting. By using visual models as well as her verbal explanation, she involved more senses in the learning process and thereby more of the whole person. Mr. Young's pain served as a good motivator, increasing his desire for relief and his willingness to participate in the learning process to prevent future episodes.

Box 18-3	Characteristics of Cognitive-Field Learning Theories

- Learning is related to perception.
- Perceptions of reality and experiences are uniquely individual and based on life experiences.
- Thoughts influence actions.
- Motivation is key to learning.
- Self-actualization is the main motivating force.

In reviewing recent nursing literature, Cognitive-Field Theory and/or Gestalt Theory was used several times. Kelly and Howie (2011), for example, presented an overview of Gestalt Theory and explained how it can be used by psychiatric nurses to promote self-knowledge, acceptance, self-responsibility, and personal growth. In another work, Shanley and Jubb-Shanley (2012) described how Gestalt Theory was one of several approaches they integrated into a system for mental health nurses to counsel people with serious and complex psychiatric needs. Lastly, Hanson and Stenvig (2008) used Cognitive-Field Theory/Gestalt Theory as a framework for a study of attributes of clinical nursing educators.

Cognitive Development or Interaction Theories

Cognitive development theories assume that behavior, mental processes, and the environment are interrelated. Also termed *interaction theories*, they are concerned with the progressive development and changes in thinking, reasoning, and perception of individual learners. A major assumption of cognitive development theories is that learning occurs as a sequential process. Learning takes place over time, as when a child explores and interacts with the environment.

The experiential learning model exemplifies the interaction theories, which postulate that individuals learn from their immediate experiences and that learning happens in all human settings (Kolb, 1984). Learning is how individuals adapt and cope with the environment (the world) in which they live. Because each person's experience is unique, individuals develop a preferred style for learning. Whereas behavioral objectives state what the student will learn, experiential learning focuses on the conditions of learning. The instructor's role is to create an environment for learning and the experiences that support student understanding of the whole rather than its separate parts (Braungart et al., 2014). This is achieved through activities such as group process, problem-solving activities, and simulation exercises. Some of the theories noted for this perspective are Piaget's Cognitive Development Theory, Gagne's Conditions of Learning, and Bandura's Social Learning Theories. Box 18-4 summarizes characteristics of cognitive development/interaction theories.

Box 18-4	Characteristics of Cognitive Development/Interaction Learning Theories

- Behavior, mental processes, and the environment are interrelated.
- Individuals learn from their experiences.
- Learning is how individuals adapt to and cope with their environment.
- Focus is on conditions that promote learning.

Piaget

Jean Piaget (1896–1980) is probably the best known of the cognitive development theorists. He believed that cognitive development occurs in stages and that the stages occur in a fixed order and are universal to persons everywhere. He identified the following stages: sensorimotor, preoperational, concrete operational, and formal operational.

Overview. According to Piaget, for learning to occur, an individual must be able to assimilate new information into existing cognitive structures or schemes; that is, the new experience must overlap with previous knowledge. Behavior becomes more intelligent as coordination between the reactions to objects becomes progressively more interrelated and complex. Cognitive development begins in the sensorimotor stage (which is evident from birth until about 2 years of age) with the baby's use of the senses and movement to explore its world. In the preoperational stage (from about 2 years old until about age 6 or 7 years), action patterns evolve into the symbolic but illogical thinking of the preschooler. In this stage, language ability grows rapidly (Berk, 2003). In the concrete operational stage, cognition is transformed into the more organized reasoning of the school-aged child (age 6 or 7 years until about 11 or 12 years). Abstract reasoning begins with the formal operational stage of the adolescent where youth are able to construct ideals and reason realistically about the future (Berk, 2003; Ormrod, 2016).

In Piaget's work, it is the schemes, or psychological structures, that change with age. Individuals build new schemes by adapting their experiences into previous knowledge. Assimilation and accommodation processes make up the adaptive process (Ormrod, 2016).

Many adults, however, have not developed complete formal operational thinking and need concrete examples before being presented with abstract ideas. Thus, it is important for the teacher to present information in a manner appropriate for the stage of development. The nurse usually has no formal means of testing an individual's cognitive development stage but must rely on the individual's verbal interaction during the assessment process. In the case study, Barbara could do this by using a familiar example of a clogged sink to explain what was occurring inside the blood vessels.

Application to Nursing. A few nursing articles can be found that use Piaget's theory either as a conceptual framework for a research study or to interpret or describe findings or actions. For example, Başkale and Bahar (2011) used Piaget's writings to develop a program to enhance nutritional education for preschool children. Another study used Piaget's theory as the conceptual framework in a cross-cultural examination of children's fears of medical experiences (Mahat, Scoloveno, & Cannella, 2004), and a third used Piaget's work to describe the processes children use to cope with disasters (Deering, 2000).

Gagne

Robert M. Gagne (1916–2002) believed that much of individual's learning (from sensorimotor to highly complex intellectual skills) requires different conditions for learning to be successful.

Overview. Gagne classified learning outcomes into five different categories: intellectual skills, verbal information, cognitive strategies, motor skills, and attitudes. Each category has subcategories and involves both internal and external conditions that contribute to, or interfere with, the learning process (Gagne, 1985). Gagne believed that there are eight different types of learning that proceed sequentially in a hierarchical order (Box 18-5).

| Box 18-5 | Gagne's Types of Learning |

1. *Signal learning*: An involuntary response occurs to a specific stimulus (based on Pavlov's conditioned response).
2. *Stimulus–response*: A voluntary response occurs to a specific stimulus (similar to Skinner's operant conditioning).
3. *Chaining*: Two or more stimulus–response (S–R) associations occur and a sequence of behaviors is learned.
4. *Verbal association*: A chain of verbal S–R connections is involved.
5. *Discrimination learning*: The learner responds to one stimulus but not a similar one.
6. *Concept learning*: The learner organizes different stimuli into a class and then responds to any member of that class in the same way.
7. *Principle or rule learning*: A chain of two or more concepts is constructed.
8. *Problem solving*: The combination of two or more principles or rules come together to form higher order thinking patterns.

Source: Gagne (1985).

For Gagne (1985), teaching means arranging the conditions that are external to the learner. When trying to get a client or patient to understand a concept (such as HTN in the case study), it is important not only to provide a definition of the concept but also to give many positive examples to illustrate the concept while at the same time giving negative examples to illustrate what the concept is not. The nurse can test clients' understanding of a concept by asking them to think of their own examples and applications.

Application to Nursing. Gagne's principles have been used in some nursing interventions. Shawler (2008) describes a strategy that uses standardized patients (actors instructed to simulate a set of symptoms) to teach graduate nursing students about complex mental disorders. In another example, Miner, Mallow, Theeke, and Barnes (2015) described how Gagne's theory was the framework for revision of the processes used for instruction in a medical-surgical nursing course. They reported that integration of Gagne's nine events—including gain attention, inform leaners of objectives, stimulate recall, and so forth—enhanced students' learning experiences.

Bandura

Albert Bandura's (1977b) Social Learning Theory (SLT) was based on the concept of reciprocal determinism and concerned with the social influences that affect learning (e.g., groups, culture, and ethnicity).

Overview. In SLT, environment, cognitive factors, and behavior interact with one another, so each variable affects the other two. For example, people learn from the continual bombardment of environmental stimuli without being aware that they are doing so.

Bandura's theory focuses on how people learn from one another and encompasses such concepts as observational learning, imitation, and modeling (Bandura, 1977b). Many behaviors that people exhibit have been acquired through observation and modeling of others. Individuals can imitate behaviors of someone they admire. For example, teenagers often imitate the behavior of their latest movie or rock star idol, or a nursing student may imitate the behaviors of an RN who exemplifies the student's concept of professionalism.

Learning by watching or listening to others (vicarious learning) can occur without imitating the behaviors observed. In this instance, people can verbally describe the behavior but may not demonstrate it until later, when there is a need to do so. The concept of vicarious learning is used frequently by schools of nursing. Because not all students can care for clients with the same condition, nursing schools have students share their clinical experiences in postconferences. Students learn from each other's experiences but may not have an opportunity to implement the learning until after they graduate.

In later years, Bandura focused more on the underpinnings of constructivism and social cognition. He stressed that the learner is actively involved with the environment through personal selection, intentionality, and self-regulation of the learning process based on his or her own "filter" of the world. People may actively select their own role models and regulate their own attitudes and actions regarding learning. An important finding of Bandura's research for health care professionals is that self-efficacy promotes learning and productive human function. This implies that nurses should promote patients' independence and confidence rather than simply accepting and endorsing dependent behaviors in order to facilitate learning and health promotion.

Application to Nursing. Numerous recent nursing articles cite using Bandura's theory to develop nursing interventions. For example, Chen, Wang, and Hung (2015) studied personal and environmental factors that predict health promoting and self-care behaviors in patients diagnosed as "prediabetic" using Bandura's SLT. Many examples of use of SLT to look at education of nurse can be found. In one example, Coulson and Harvey (2013) built on Bandura's theory in testing the use of a process called scaffolding to teach reflection as an independent learning means. They found that students go through a four-phase model which leads to a process of helping students make sense of an experiential learning opportunity. In this process, students are assisted by their faculty to learn to reflect and then use strategies of reflection to incubate their experiences as they are learning. In a second example, a literature review of various aspects of incivility among nurses was examined and evidence-based strategies to combat the incivility were proposed based on Bandura's theory (Lynette, Echevarria, Sun, & Ryan, 2016). Finally, Lin (2016) used SLT to study the relationship among organizational climate, self-efficacy, and outcome expectations with respect to cross-cultural competence of RNs. In the opening case study, Barbara was applying aspects of Bandura's SLT when she gave the Youngs the URLs for Facebook and Twitter sites of other people who were living with HTN. She understood that communicating with others living with a similar health situation forms a powerful support for learning and promotes self-efficacy.

Humanistic Learning Theory

Humanistic learning theories recognize that emotions can have a positive influence on the learning process. Humanistic psychologists, often referred to as "third force" psychologists, are concerned with human potential and are interested in helping individuals develop that potential. As individuals or groups achieve new abilities, the human potential improves; consequently, the individual is always "becoming." Human relations skills are one of the major human abilities that concerns humanistic educators. Humanistic educators want learners to have warm interpersonal relationships, to trust others and themselves, and to be aware of others' feelings. The teacher's role is to design experiences that help improve the learners' abilities to perceive, feel, wonder, sense, create, fantasize, imagine, and experience (Roberts, 1975). In addition, educators should strive to motivate others to develop their own potential and move toward self-actualization (Candela, 2016).

By redefining the role of the educator and focusing on the needs and feelings of the learner, humanistic theory has given health professionals a useful tool for development of student-centered teaching activities which promote students' experiences with learning. Humanistic theory is the foundation for many successful wellness programs, self-help groups, and palliative care (Braungart et al., 2014) and can be effectively applied in nursing education in strategies such as problem-based learning, service learning, and the flipped classroom.

Rogers

Carl Rogers (1902–1987), one of the leaders of the humanistic perspective, transferred his principles about "client-centered" therapy to "student-centered" teaching.

Overview. For Rogers (1983), the learner is in the process of becoming, the goal of education is to develop a "fully functioning person," and the teacher's role is to facilitate the process. He believed learning is a natural process, entirely controlled internally by the learner, in which the individual's whole being interacts with the environment as the learner perceives it. The learner has both the freedom to learn and to be self-directed (as opposed to teacher-directed). By providing problems real and meaningful to the learner, intrinsic motivation is stimulated to solve the problem. Rogers perceived the only truly educated person to be the one who learns how to learn, knows how to adapt to changing circumstances, and is continually seeking knowledge.

Application to Nursing. Nurses often use these principles in practice. For example, Missildine, Fountain, Summers, and Gosselin (2013) reported on their experiences with "flipping the classroom" to enhance student performance and satisfaction in an adult health undergraduate course. They noted improved learning with the flipped classroom but suggested that student satisfaction was less than comparison groups because the strategy required extra work. Hart (2015) reported on how service-learning projects can promote student engagement in a variety of learning activities in real-life situations; the result is development of leadership, social, and partnership skills. Vacek (2009) used concept mapping with students to promote critical thinking in a baccalaureate nursing program. The findings were that students using concept mapping experienced enhanced learning and critical thinking. Wong and colleagues (2008) adopted a problem-based learning approach in a clinical simulation. They found that the students learned best in a stable, safe environment and could experience the full range of learning issues without endangering themselves or their patients.

Information-Processing Models

Information-processing theories emerged in the 1970s. They arose from the field of artificial intelligence as researchers attempted to create computer systems to simulate human cognitive skills (Candela, 2016; Paas & Sweller, 2012). Learning theorists, such as Gagne, used these models to explain the process of acquiring information, storing it, remembering it, and using it for problem solving (Braungart et al., 2014; Byrnes, 2008).

Information-processing theories propose an elaborate set of internal processes to account for how learning and retention occur (Ormrod, 2016). In information-processing theories, human memory is thought to be composed of three stores: sensory store, short-term store, and long-term store. Information from the environment passes sequentially through the stores (Braungart et al., 2014). The sensory store (also known as the *sensory memory, iconic memory,* or *echoic memory*) holds incoming information long enough that preliminary cognitive processing can begin. Information stored in the sensory memory is stored basically in the form in which it was sensed—visual input is stored visually and auditory input in an auditory form. Although the sensory store has unlimited capacity, information is stored very briefly (Byrnes, 2008).

The short-term memory is the most active component of the memory systems. Thinking occurs within the short-term memory and determines which information will be attended to within the sensory memory. The short-term memory holds information while it is being processed from both the sensory memory and the long-term memory. Interpretation of newly received environment input is interpreted in the short-term memory.

The long-term memory is the most complicated of the memory systems and the one that has received the most research. Long-term memory is thought to have an unlimited capacity, but experts disagree regarding how long the information remains in storage. Some experts believe it is there forever, but others believe the information is lost through a variety of forgetting processes. Information is rarely stored in the long-term memory in the form in which it is received. What is stored is the "gist" of what was seen or heard rather than word-for-word sentences or precise mental images. Individuals organize the information that is stored in the long-term memory so related pieces of information are associated together (Ormrod, 2016).

In information-processing models, learning consists of strategies to transfer information from short-term storage to long-term storage. Information in the short-term memory (also known as the *working memory*) is lost within 5 to 20 seconds if action is not taken to reinforce it (Leahy & Sweller, 2016). For example, repeating the individual's name when introduced to a new person increases the ability to recall it at a later time. It is important for an instructor using this theory to present information in an organized manner, to overlap the information with previously learned knowledge, and to show the learner how the material is organized and how it relates to what was previously learned (Ormrod, 2016). External stimuli are thought to support several different types of ongoing internal processes involved in learning, remembering, and performing. Techniques such as visual imagery facilitate learning and the recall of information.

Going hand in hand with the question of how people remember is the question of why people forget. Three theories have been proposed to explain this phenomenon: decay, interference theories, and the loss of retrieval cues. Decay theory proposes that information weakens over time, if it is not practiced or used. This is similar to the "use it or lose it" theory of muscle strength. Interference theory postulates that something interferes between the information already in storage and the new information being learned. If the new information being learned interferes with previously stored information, it is called *retroactive inhibition*; if old information interferes with the learning of new information, it is called *proactive inhibition* (Ormrod, 2016). Loss of retrieval cues involves the weakening of associations among the retrieval cues and records (Byrnes, 2008). For example, a nurse frequently sees a colleague from another unit in the cafeteria. The nurse knows this person's name and recognizes him or her. When the nurse meets this same person in the grocery store in street clothes, however, the nurse knows she knows the person but may not recall from where or the name. Because the person is out of context, the associations are not readily available for recall.

Cognitive Load Theory

Cognitive Load Theory (CLT) is an example of an information processing theory based on the work of John Sweller, who began studying the idea in the 1980s. The major components of CLT include schemas: classifications of the material that the mind of the learner makes. A basic tenet of the theory is recognition that working memory can deal with only a few novel pieces of information at a time, but long-term memory allows the knowledge to be grouped together with already existing schemas to develop a huge amount of knowledge of specific fields.

Research in elements of CLT indicates that a single educational medium, rather than several types of presentations, is most productive of learning early in the educative process. Therefore, it is suggested that both lecture and readings and/or video productions not be used for very complex, new material. Rather, a single medium such as lecture be the first introduction to new material. Later, when the student has developed a basis for memory of the material, additional media can assist in providing schemas that will promote long-term memory (Leahy & Sweller, 2016; Paas & Sweller, 2012; van Merriënboer & Sweller, 2005).

Application to Nursing

Nurses in practice and research have used information-processing theories. In the opening case study, by asking the Youngs to repeat some actions they could take to assist in lowering Mr. Young's blood pressure, Barbara was helping the information to be stored in their long-term memory.

In examples from the nursing literature, using information processing theory, Hessler and Henderson (2013) found that five or fewer items of information were the maximum that should be presented at any one time to nursing students during computer simulation for optimum retention, especially if advanced cognitive skills such as critical thinking or analysis were required. In another work, Kaylor (2014) described how she used CLT as a framework for teaching pharmacology to undergraduate nursing students. In a third example, Ojeda (2016) piloted an educational program on carbohydrate counting for RNs and unlicensed personnel. She found that CLT was highly acceptable to the staff members and may be a promising framework for in-service education. The process of "mind mapping" was described by Rosciano (2015) as an active learning strategy nursing students can use to "build upon existing knowledge when new information is presented" (p. 93). Lastly, in a clinical situation, Li and Liu (2012) reported on their literature review of use of "errorless learning strategies," a process that promotes use of "implicit memory" and how it relates to long-term memory for patients with Alzheimer disease. They explained that the intent is to enhance memory rehabilitation in these patients.

Adult Learning

Malcolm Knowles (1913–1997), although not the first educator to study adult learning, is credited with popularizing the notion of andragogy in North America. *Andragogy* is concerned with a unified theory of adult learning, as opposed to *pedagogy*, which focuses on learning in children and youth.

Overview

For Knowles (Knowles et al., 2005), the single most important thing in helping adults to learn is to create a climate of physical comfort, mutual trust and respect, openness, and acceptance of differences. By responding to the needs of the learner and providing the learning resources required for learning, teachers facilitate learning. To be effective, presenters (teachers) need to "tell it like it is" and stress "how I do it" rather than telling the learner what to do. Through self-direction, learners are responsible for their own learning. Knowles and colleagues (2005) identified six assumptions regarding andragogy (Box 18-6).

| Box 18-6 | Knowles's Assumptions of Adult Learners |

1. *Need to know*: Adults need to know why they need to learn something.
2. *Self-concept*: As people mature, their self-concept moves from one of being dependent toward one of being self-directed.
3. *Experience*: As people mature, they accumulate a large amount of experience that can serve as a rich resource for learning.
4. *Readiness to learn*: Real-life problems or situations create a readiness to learn in the adult.
5. *Orientation to learning*: As a person matures, his or her time perspective changes from one of postponed application of knowledge to immediacy of application.
6. *Motivation*: Adults are primarily motivated by a desire to solve immediate and practical problems. As a person matures, motivation to learn is stimulated by internal stimuli rather than external stimuli.

Knowles and colleagues (2005) believed that adults need to know why they need to learn something. As a result, the teacher can help learners understand how the knowledge is important to their future or the quality of their lives. Second, Knowles recognized the importance of self-concept in the adult learner. He taught that as people mature, their self-concept moves from one of being dependent toward one of being self-directed. Adult learners want others to see them as being capable of self-direction and resent having someone else's will imposed on them. A self-directing teacher avoids "talking down" to the learner, provides information that enhances the adults' ability to solve problems, and encourages independence.

A third assumption revolves around experience. Knowles and colleagues (2005) explained that as people mature, they accumulate a large amount of experience that can serve as a rich resource for learning. Adults learn better when their own experiences are incorporated into the learning process. New experiences contribute to the learner's self-identity. Ignoring or devaluing this experience is perceived as rejecting them as a person.

The fourth assumption involves readiness to learn. Real-life problems or situations create a readiness to learn in the adult. Adults are problem-oriented learners, as opposed to subject-oriented learners; they want information that will help them solve a specific problem rather than an inclusive discussion of the subject. As a person matures, readiness to learn becomes increasingly oriented to the developmental tasks of social roles. Organizing learning activities around these life experiences facilitates the learning process. Readiness to learn can be created by exposing the individual to superior models, simulation exercises, and other techniques.

Similarly, the fifth assumption centers on orientation to learning. As a person matures, his or her time perspective changes from one of postponed application of knowledge to immediacy of application. Accordingly, the orientation toward self-learning shifts from one of subject centeredness to one of problem centeredness (Knowles et al., 2005).

Finally, motivation is the cornerstone of the adult learning theories. According to Knowles and colleagues (2005), adults are primarily motivated by a desire to solve immediate and practical problems. As a person matures, motivation to learn is stimulated by internal stimuli rather than external stimuli. The learner is self-directed, determines what is to be learned and how it is to be learned, and assumes the primary responsibility for learning. For example, some motivational force is exerted from external sources, such as a desire for a better paying job, but a stronger force arises from internal sources, such as job satisfaction.

Application to Nursing

There are a number of examples of the use of Knowles's theory in the nursing literature. A study by Nguyen, Miranda, Lapum, and Donald (2016), for example, concluded that andragogy, combined with drama, assisted undergraduate nursing students to understand the situations of their clients on a deeper level. In another work, the effectiveness of an interprofessional discharge planning process to promote patient and family engagement was examined by Knier, Stichler, Ferber, and Catterall (2015). They determined that their Adult Learning Theory–based model of care improved patient satisfaction after discharge. Curran (2014) discussed the value of nursing professional development specialists understanding and applying Adult Learning Theory principles to guide curriculum development and staff development activities. Finally, Clapper (2010) provided a detailed explanation of the importance of using Adult Learning Theory when developing and implementing simulations in nursing education, encouraging nursing faculty to go "beyond Knowles." The intent should be to develop self-directed, lifelong learners who understand and can use technology. See Link to Practice 18-1.

Summary of Learning Theories

As the previous discussions have illustrated, numerous learning theories have been posited over the past century. Table 18-2 summarizes the cognitive-focused theories described. Many other diverse areas of study have developed from both the

Link to Practice 18-1

Barbara Davis used Knowles's Adult Learning Theory to educate another client family—the Banzas—on care of Mr. Banza's new left ventricular assist device (LVAD) at home. In her planning, Barbara considered that because the Banzas were in their 70s, they might be relatively low in health literacy. She quickly learned that they were both motivated to learn and had the insight and experience of their years to call upon. Before retirement, Mr. Banza had owned his own successful home maintenance business and was a licensed and skilled electrician and plumber; therefore, he would be able to understand the implanted LVAD. Mrs. Banza, however, had only finished 10th grade. As a result, she had a fairly low literacy level and had never worked outside her home.

Barbara decided to work with the Banzas together and started by explaining the electronics and "plumbing" of the LVAD to Mr. Banza. Next, she discussed with both seniors the need for cleanliness and sterility when caring for abdominal and chest incisions. To avoid overwhelming them with information, Barbara organized her teaching in steps, beginning with what they needed to know immediately. She showed both Banzas the daily care of the LVAD and explained when and how Mrs. Banza was to summon assistance if there were problems or complications. In later sessions, Barbara gave the couple training on more complex elements of care.

Barbara saw the Banzas regularly for several months and less often for several years. They were successful in caring for Mr. Banza's device, and when Barbara saw them at their 5-year checkup, both let her know that they had organized a group of other patients with LVADs and that the support group was successful.

Table 18-2 Summary of Cognitive Learning Theories

Group of Theories	Key Principles	Examples of Theorists
Cognitive-Field (Gestalt) Theories	Learning relates to perception; motivation is key; behavior is related to perception and experience.	Lewin
Cognitive Load Theory	Learning is affected by many variables, including physical and mental ability, attitudes, interests, and values; learning interprets information based on previous knowledge and experiences; learning continues throughout life.	Piaget Maslow Erikson Havighurst
Cognitive development (interaction) theories	Individuals learn from their experiences; learning is how individuals adapt and cope with their environment.	Gagne Piaget Bandura
Information-processing theories (Cognitive Load Theory)	Memory is composed of sensory memory, short-term memory, and long-term memory; learning consists of strategies to transfer information from short-term memory to long-term memory.	Anderson Bahrick Sweller
Humanism	Reeducation of clients is important; focus is on human potential; emphasis is on collaboration in the learning process; recognizes that emotions can positively affect learning.	Rogers
Andragogy (Adult Learning Theory)	The process of learning rather than content is the focus; physical comfort, mutual trust and respect, openness, and acceptance are important concepts.	Knowles

behavioral and cognitive fields of learning theories. Examples include multiple intelligence (Gardner, 1999), whole brain learning (Maxfield, 1990), learning styles (Kolb, 1976), assimilation (Ausubel, 1978), proficiency (Knox, 1980), transformational learning (Brookfield, 1991; Mezirow, 1981), memory (Atkinson & Shiffrin, 1968), self-directed learning (Tough, 1967), self-efficacy (Bandura, 1977a), and problem solving (Newell & Simon, 1972).

Learning Styles

It is widely recognized that most individuals have a preferred style of learning. Learning style is a characteristic that allows individuals to interact with instructional circumstances in such a way that learning is produced. Learning style preference relates to the likes and dislikes a person has for certain sensory modes, learning conditions, and learning strategies. Most people have probably not thought about how they learn and if questioned would give an answer based on what they assume rather than what is correct.

By carefully listening to verbal comments of a patient, a nurse can obtain clues about the preferred learning style. For example, if the individual says something, such as "I hear what you're saying," the preferred learning style is most likely auditory. This individual learns best by hearing a discussion, presentation, audio device, and so forth. If, however, the response is "I see what you mean," the learning style is probably visual, and the person responds better to pictures, movies, or demonstrations. Tactual and kinesthetic learners make statements such as "I feel this is very important." These learners will learn best if able to manipulate or physically maneuver material with their hands. The availability of paper and pencils for taking notes, highlighter pens for marking important information, and picture puzzles will assist these types of learners (Morse, Oberer, Dobbins, & Mitchell, 1998).

In addition to age, gender also influences one's learning style. Men tend to be more visual, tactile, and kinesthetic than women. They are also more peer oriented and nonconforming and need the freedom to move around in an informal setting (Dunn & Dunn, 1992, 1993; Dunn & Griggs, 1995). In contrast, during learning situations, women tend to be more auditory, conforming, and authority oriented than men and are more able to sit passively (Pizzo, Dunn, & Dunn, 1990).

An important factor influencing learning is whether the individual tends to learn better analytically or globally. Analytic learners learn facts step by step in a logical progression building toward a whole. Global learners, by contrast, want to understand the whole before learning about the parts. Analytic learners will listen to all the facts as long as they believe they are heading toward a goal. Global learners need to know what they need to learn and why they need to learn it.

Different environments and different teaching strategies are required for global and analytic learners. Global learners learn better with intermittent periods of concentration and relaxation in a place with soft lighting, music, or other sound while sitting informally eating snacks. Short stories, anecdotes, humor, and illustrations can be used to capture the attention of global learners (Morse et al., 1998). Conversely, the analytic learner needs a quiet, well-lit formal setting with few or no interruptions and few or no snacks (Dunn & Griggs, 1998).

Principles of Learning

A common approach for teaching either individuals or groups is the use of learning principles. Principles of learning have been derived from multiple theories and are ideas that people can agree on no matter to which learning theory they subscribe. Whereas learning theories provide explanation about the underlying mechanisms involved in the learning process, principles identify specific elements that are important for learning and describe the particular effects of these variables on learning. The following are some other learning principles that may assist nurses as they attempt to provide health information to their clients.

- Learning is facilitated if information is provided from simple to complex, concrete to abstract, and known to unknown. This generally accepted learning principle recognizes the hierarchy in learning.
- Learning is facilitated if the information is personal and individualized. Learning occurs inside individuals and is activated by learners themselves. The client is more likely to remember what is taught if actively involved in the learning process.
- Learning is facilitated if it is relevant to the learner's needs and problems. What is relevant and meaningful is decided by the learner and must be discovered by him or her. Information that is meaningful is more easily stored and retrieved than information learned by rote memorization. What the nurse perceives as important to the health of the client may not be what the client perceives as important.
- Learning is facilitated if the individual is attentive. Attention is essential for learning. Attention is the process through which information moves into the short-term memory. Any internal (e.g., fear) or external factor (e.g., noise) that distracts the client can interfere with the learning process.

- Learning is facilitated when feedback is given close to the event rather than delayed.
- Learning is sometimes painful. This is true because learning is part of the growth process. Growth involves change, and change usually involves a certain amount of anxiety. Therefore, it is more comfortable for the individual to continue his or her ordinary behavior than to deal with the accompanying emotions required to change. What seems simple to a nurse giving information to a client may be a very complex process to the client.
- Learning is an emotional process as well as an intellectual process. The nurse needs to address the emotional aspects in the learning process as well as the knowledge aspects.
- The learning process is highly unique and individual. Simply put, people learn in different ways.

Application of Learning Theories in Nursing

Professional nurses and nurses in advanced practice must remember that no theory explains everything known about learning. There is not one theory that is best used for patient education or staff education. Depending on the learner and the given situation, certain theories may be more useful than others in designing instruction. The inherent value in the discussion of the theories in this chapter is that they give the nurse an opportunity to view patients and teaching through different frameworks and perspectives. It is suggested that the nurse use a broad knowledge of different theories rather than a specific theory alone to approach his or her teaching role. In the most pragmatic sense, the role of the nurse is to find what works best based on this broad knowledge and use it for the benefit of the client, whether that client is a patient, a colleague, or a student.

Learning theories are best contextually applied. Professional nurses must use the circumstances surrounding each different teaching situation to help decide the most useful and appropriate approach. To apply principles and adapt concepts to patient education, nurses need to ask themselves the following questions:

- How can I increase my effectiveness in teaching my clients?
- Which learning theories are most congruent with my own view of human nature and my purpose for teaching clients?
- Which techniques will be most effective for particular situations?
- What are the implications of the various learning theories for my own role and performance?
- Which learning theory should I use under what circumstances?

Many authors (Bastable & Alt, 2014; Fitzgerald & Keyes, 2014; Kitchie, 2016) have concluded that better learning outcomes are achieved when a variety of strategies, based on different learning theories, are used. By synthesizing elements from a variety of theories, the best approach for a given situation can be found.

Clients coming to nurses, however, are often in pain or frightened, factors that directly interfere with the learning process. This interference can be misinterpreted as "not paying attention" or noncompliance. During the assessment process, the nurse should be alert to any cognitive or physical problems that may interfere with learning. Potential problems include poor hearing, eyesight, or coordination as well as impaired thinking or memory. The person's personal and cultural beliefs should also be considered when trying to teach.

Theories from psychology and sociology (e.g., motivation, change, self-efficacy, health belief) can help the nurse determine the best learning approach. Although not directly related to learning, these theories do help explain human behavior and its impact on the learning process. Creative presentations, such as making up a rap song or an acronym for essential information, are often remembered longer than dialogue alone (Bruccoliere, 2000). Presenting too much information, too fast, and too soon can lead to learner frustration and failure. Furthermore, clients need feedback regarding what they are doing right as well as what they are doing wrong.

Nurses can also encourage clients to seek out information on their own. Many people today have access to the Internet, either at home or through their public library. By seeking answers to their own learning needs, individuals accept responsibility for their own learning; this can lead to greater self-confidence and a better self-image. The more self-confidence individuals have, the more likely they will be to take the actions necessary to correct health problems.

Summary

Professional nurses and nurses in advanced practice should study learning theories, principles, and concepts and use them to direct education efforts to best meet the needs of the learner. In the opening case study, Barbara's use of multiple techniques and interventions to work with her clients to enhance their understanding illustrates when and how learning theories can be used in nursing. The idea as discussed is learning that will result in behavior changes that will promote and maintain health.

As educational research has progressed, theorists have become interested in specific aspects of learning and have incorporated related concepts such as motivation, memory, and thinking into existing theories, or they have developed completely separate theories based on the works of others. In addition to the external environment, physical, emotional, and intellectual maturation have been recognized as affecting the learning process. The differences between child and adult learning have been explored, and new areas of learning are being investigated. As these areas are further developed, new theories regarding learning will emerge. Professional nurses must be aware of new developments in learning theory and be ready to apply new thoughts and concepts when caring for clients.

Key Points

- Learning theories provide background information on different ways people learn.
- Understanding different learning theories allows nurses to decide on a variety of strategies to use when providing meaningful education to clients.
- A number of different learning theories have been proposed by scholars both in psychology and in education.
- Using multiple theories can assist the nurse acting as educator to realize that different teaching methods may be needed at different times and for different health care situations.
- Learning is a personal and individual process and nurses must be able to use many different methods to assist patients and caregivers to promote or enhance patient education.

Learning Activities

1. Following the example of Barbara, the nurse from the opening case study, consider the patients you see each time you work or are in a clinical situation. Have you noticed whether they have had effective learning experiences to help them maintain their health? Using some of the cues in this chapter, decide what form of teaching would have complemented the learning styles of a particular patient or client, such that his or her health education would have been more effective?

2. Select a theory presented in this chapter. Review the nursing literature and identify nursing articles and studies describing how/when the theory is used in nursing. Organize the findings into a short paper.

3. Select one of the learning theories/learning principles/learning styles discussed in this chapter and research it in more depth. Use educational texts, original works, the Internet, or other sources. Write a one-page summary of the theory and how it could be applied to a population or a health problem that you routinely encounter in your practice.

4. Try to determine how you learn. Are you predominantly an auditory learner, visual learner, tactile learner, or some combination of these? How would you present learning materials to a client whose learning style differed from yours?

REFERENCES

American Association of Colleges of Nursing. (2011). *The essentials of master's education in nursing.* Retrieved from http://www.aacn.nche.edu/education-resources/MastersEssentials11.pdf

Atkinson, R. C., & Shiffrin, R. M. (1968). Human memory: A proposed system and its control processes. In K. W. Spence & J. T. Spence (Eds.), *The psychology of learning and motivation: Advances in research and theory* (Vol. 2, pp. 89–195). New York, NY: Academic Press.

Ausubel, D. P. (1978). *Educational psychology: A cognitive view* (2nd ed.). New York, NY: Holt, Rinehart and Winston.

Bandura, A. (1977a). Self-efficacy: Toward a unifying theory of behavioral change. *Psychological Review, 84,* 191–215.

Bandura, A. (1977b). *Social learning theory.* Englewood Cliffs, NJ: Prentice Hall.

Başkale, H., & Bahar, Z. (2011). Outcomes of nutrition knowledge and health food choices in 5- to 6-year-old children who received a nutrition intervention based on Piaget's theory. *Journal for Specialists in Pediatric Nursing, 16*(4), 263–279.

Bastable, S. B., & Alt, M. F. (2014). Overview of education in health care. In S. B. Bastable (Ed.), *Nurse as educator: Principles of teaching and learning for nursing practice* (4th ed., pp. 3–30). Burlington, MA: Jones & Bartlett Learning.

Bastable, S. B., & Gonzalez, K. M. (2016). Overview of education in health care. In S. B. Bastable (Ed.), *Essentials of patient education* (2nd ed., pp. 3–44). Burlington, MA: Jones & Bartlett Learning.

Bastable, S. B., Meyers, G. M., & Poitevent, L. B. (2014). Literacy in the adult client population. In S. B. Bastable (Ed.), *Nurse as educator: Principles of teaching and learning for nursing practice* (4th ed., pp. 255–311). Burlington, MA: Jones & Bartlett Learning.

Berk, L. E. (2003). *Child development* (6th ed.). Boston, MA: Allyn & Bacon.

Bigge, M. L., & Shermis, S. S. (1999). *Learning theories for teachers* (6th ed.). Boston, MA: Allyn & Bacon.

Braungart, M. M., Braungart, R. G., & Gramet, P. R. (2014). Applying learning theories to health care practice. In S. B. Bastable (Ed.), *Nurse as educator: Principles of teaching and learning for nursing practice* (4th ed., pp. 63–123). Burlington, MA: Jones & Bartlett Learning.

Braungart, M. M., Braungart, R. G., & Gramet, P. R. (2016). Applying learning theories to healthcare practice. In S. B. Bastable (Ed.), *Essentials of patient education* (2nd ed., pp. 45–76). Burlington, MA: Jones & Bartlett Learning.

Brookfield, S. D. (1991). *Developing critical thinkers.* San Francisco, CA: Jossey-Bass.

Bruccoliere, T. (2000). How to make patient teaching stick. *RN, 63*(2), 34–38.

Byrnes, J. P. (2008). *Cognitive development and learning in instructional contexts* (3rd ed.). Upper Saddle River, NJ: Pearson.

Candela, L. (2012). From teaching to learning: Theoretical foundations. In D. M. Billings & J. A. Halstead (Eds.), *Teaching in nursing: A guide for faculty* (4th ed., pp. 202–243). St. Louis, MO: Elsevier/Saunders.

Candela, L. (2016). Theoretical foundations of teaching and learning. In D. M. Billings & J. A. Halstead (Eds.), *Teaching in nursing: A guide for faculty* (5th ed., pp. 211–229). St. Louis, MO: Elsevier/Saunders.

Chen, M. F., Wang, R. H., & Hung, S. L. (2015). Predicting health-promoting self-care behaviors in people with pre-diabetes by applying Bandura social learning theory. *Applied Nursing Research, 28*(4), 299–304.

Clapper, T. C. (2010). Beyond Knowles: What those conducting simulation need to know about adult learning theory. *Clinical Simulation in Nursing, 6*(1), e7–e14.

Coulson, D., & Harvey, M. (2013). Scaffolding student reflection for experience-based learning: A framework. *Teaching in Higher Education, 18*(4), 401–413. doi:10.1080/13562517.2012.752726

Curran, M. K. (2014). Examination of the teaching styles of nursing professional development specialists, part I: Best practices in adult learning theory, curriculum development, and knowledge transfer. *Journal of Continuing Education in Nursing, 45*(5), 233–240.

Deering, C. G. (2000). A cognitive developmental approach to understanding how children cope with disasters. *Journal of Child and Adolescent Psychiatric Nursing, 13*(1), 7–16.

Dunn, R., & Dunn, K. (1992). *Teaching elementary students through their individual learning styles: Practical approaches for Grades 3–6.* Boston, MA: Allyn & Bacon.

Dunn, R., & Dunn, K. (1993). *Teaching secondary students through their individual learning styles: Practical approaches for Grades 7–12.* Boston, MA: Allyn & Bacon.

Dunn, R., & Griggs, S. A. (1995). *Multiculturalism and learning styles: Teaching and counseling adolescents.* Westport, CT: Greenwood Press.

Dunn, R., & Griggs, S. A. (1998). Learning styles: Link between teaching and learning. In R. Dunn & S. A. Griggs (Eds.), *Learning styles and the nursing profession* (pp. 11–23). New York, NY: NLN Press.

Fisher, M. L. (2016). Teaching in nursing: The faculty role. In D. M. Billings & J. A. Halstead (Eds.), *Teaching in nursing: A guide for faculty* (5th ed., pp. 1–14). St. Louis, MO: Elsevier/Saunders.

Fitzgerald, K., & Keyes, K. (2014). Instructional methods and settings. In S. B. Bastable (Ed.), *Nurse as educator: Principles of teaching and learning for nursing practice* (4th ed., pp. 469–515). Burlington, MA: Jones & Bartlett Learning.

Gagne, R. M. (1985). *The conditions of learning* (4th ed.). New York, NY: Holt, Rinehart and Winston.

Gardner, H. (1999). *Intelligence reframed: Multiple intelligences for the 21st century.* New York, NY: Basic Books.

Hanson, K. J., & Stenvig, T. E. (2008). The good clinical nursing educator and the baccalaureate nursing clinical experience: Attributes and praxis. *The Journal of Nursing Education, 47*(1), 38–42.

Hart, S. (2015). Engaging the learner: The ABC's of service-learning. *Teaching and Learning in Nursing, 10*(2), 76–79.

Hessler, K. L., & Henderson, A. M. (2013). Interactive learning research: Application of cognitive load theory to nursing education. *International Journal of Nursing Education Scholarship, 10*(1). doi:10.1515/ijnes-2012-0029

Kaylor, S. K. (2014). Preventing information overload: Cognitive load theory as an instructional framework for teaching pharmacology. *The Journal of Nursing Education, 53*(2), 108–111.

Kelly, T., & Howie, L. (2011). Exploring the influence of gestalt therapy training on psychiatric nursing practice: Stories from the field. *International Journal of Mental Health Nursing, 20*(4), 296–304.

Kitchie, S. (2016). Determinants of learning. In S. B. Bastable (Ed.), *Essentials of patient education* (2nd ed., pp. 79–115). Burlington, MA: Jones & Bartlett Learning.

Knier, S., Stichler, J. F., Ferber, L., & Catterall, K. (2015). Patient's perceptions of the quality of discharge teaching and readiness for discharge. *Rehabilitation Nursing, 40*(1), 30–39.

Knowles, M. (1981). *From teacher to facilitator of learning.* Westchester, IL: Follett. Reprinted in Knowles, M., Holton, E. F., & Swanson, R. A. (2005). *The adult learner: The definitive classic in adult education and human resource development* (6th ed., pp. 251–254). Burlington, MA: Elsevier.

Knowles, M., Holton, E. F., & Swanson, R. A. (2005). *The adult learner: The definitive classic in adult education and human resource development* (6th ed.). Burlington, MA: Elsevier.

Knox, A. B. (1980). Proficiency theory of adult learning. *Contemporary Educational Psychology, 5,* 378–404.

Kolb, D. A. (1976). *The Learning Style Inventory: Technical manual.* Boston, MA: McBer.

Kolb, D. A. (1984). *Experiential learning: Experience as the source of learning and development.* Englewood Cliffs, NJ: Prentice Hall.

Leahy, W., & Sweller, J. (2016). Cognitive load theory and the effects of transient information on the modality effect. *Instructional Science, 44*(1), 107–123. doi:10.1007/sl251-015-9362-9

Li, R., & Liu, K. P. Y. (2012). The use of errorless learning strategies for patients with Alzheimer's disease: A literature review. *International Journal of Rehabilitation Research, 35*(4), 292–298.

Lin, H. C. (2016). Impact of nurses' cross-cultural competence on nursing intellectual capital from a social cognitive theory perspective. *Journal of Advanced Nursing, 72*(5), 1144–1154.

Lynette, J., Echevarria, I., Sun, E., & Ryan, J. G. (2016). Incivility across the nursing continuum. *Holistic Nursing Practice, 30*(5), 263–268.

Mahat, G., Scoloveno, M. A., & Cannella, B. (2004). Comparison of children's fears of medical experiences across two cultures. *Journal of Pediatric Health Care, 18*(6), 302–307.

Maxfield, D. G. (1990). Learning with the whole mind. In R. M. Smith (Eds.), *Learning to learn across the life span* (pp. 98–122). San Francisco, CA: Jossey-Bass.

Mezirow, J. (1981). A critical theory of adult learning and education. *Adult Education, 32,* 3–27.

Miner, A., Mallow, J., Theeke, L., & Barnes, E. (2015). Using Gagne's 9 events of instruction to enhance student performance and course evaluations in undergraduate nursing course. *Nurse Educator, 40*(3), 152–154.

Missildine, K., Fountain, R., Summers, L., & Gosselin, K. (2013). Flipping the classroom to improve student performance and satisfaction. *The Journal of Nursing Education, 52*(10), 597–599.

Morse, J. S., Oberer, J., Dobbins, J. A., & Mitchell, D. (1998). Understanding learning styles: Implications for in-service educators. In R. Dunn & S. A. Griggs (Eds.), *Learning styles and the nursing profession* (pp. 27–40). New York, NY: NLN Press.

Newell, A., & Simon, H. A. (1972). *Human problem solving.* Englewood Cliffs, NJ: Prentice Hall.

Nguyen, M., Miranda, J., Lapum, J., & Donald, F. (2016). Arts-based learning: A new approach to nursing education using andragogy. *The Journal of Nursing Education, 55*(7), 407–410. doi:10.3928/01484834-20160615-10

Ojeda, M. M. (2016). Carbohydrate counting in the acute care setting: Development of an educational program based on cognitive load theory. *Creative Nursing, 22*(1), 33–44. doi:10.1891/1087.4535.22.1.33

Olson, M. W., & Hergenhahn, B. R. (2012). *An introduction to theories of learning* (9th ed.). New York, NY: Routledge.

Ormrod, J. E. (2016). *Human learning: Principles, theories, and educational applications* (7th ed.). Upper Saddle River, NJ: Pearson.

Ozmon, H. (2011). *Philosophical foundations of education* (9th ed.). Upper Saddle River, NJ: Pearson.

Paas, F., & Sweller, J. (2012). An evolutionary upgrade of cognitive load theory: Using the human motor system and collaboration to support the learning of complex cognitive tasks. *Educational Psychology Review, 24*(1), 27–45. doi:10.1007/s10648-011-9179-2

Pavlov, I. P. (1927). *Conditioned reflexes.* London, United Kingdom: Oxford University Press.

Pizzo, J., Dunn, R., & Dunn, K. (1990). A sound approach to reading: Responding to students' learning styles. *Journal of Reading, Writing, and Learning Disabilities International, 6,* 249–260.

Rankin, S. H., & Stallings, K. D. (2005). *Patient education in health and illness* (5th ed.). Philadelphia, PA: Lippincott Williams & Wilkins.

Roberts, T. B. (Ed.). (1975). *Four psychologies applied to education: Freudian, behavioral, humanistic, transpersonal.* New York, NY: Wiley.

Rogers, C. R. (1983). *Freedom to learn for the 80's.* Columbus, OH: Merrill.

Rosciano, A. (2015). The effectiveness of mind mapping as an active learning strategy among associate degree nursing students. *Teaching and Learning in Nursing, 10*(1), 93–99.

Shanley, E., & Jubb-Shanley, M. (2012). Coping focus counselling in mental health nursing. *International Journal of Mental Health Nursing, 21*(6), 504–512.

Shawler, C. (2008). Standardized patients: A creative teaching strategy for psychiatric-mental health nurse practitioner students. *The Journal of Nursing Education, 47*(11), 528–531.

Thorndike, E. L. (1932). *The fundamentals of learning.* New York, NY: Teachers College Press.

Tough, A. (1967). *Learning without a teacher.* Toronto, Canada: Ontario Institute for Studies in Education.

Vacek, J. E. (2009). Using a conceptual approach with concept mapping to promote critical thinking. *The Journal of Nursing Education, 48*(1), 45–48.

van Merriënboer, J. J. G., & Sweller, J. (2005). Cognitive load theory and complex learning: Recent developments and future directions. *Educational Psychology Review, 17*(2), 147–177. doi:10.1007/s1068-005-3951.0

Wong, F. K. Y., Cheung, S., Chung, L., Chan, K., Chan, A., To, T., et al. (2008). Framework for adopting a problem-based learning approach in a simulated clinical setting. *The Journal of Nursing Education, 47*(11), 508–514.

Application of Theory in Nursing

19

Application of Theory in Nursing Practice

Melanie McEwen

Emily Chan is an acute care nurse practitioner who coordinates a liver transplant program at a large medical center. In her position, she serves as the case manager for a number of individuals. Emily was assigned to work with Sarah Bishop, a 45-year-old high school teacher who had recently received a new liver after contracting hepatitis C from a blood transfusion more than a decade ago. Sarah is married and has two teenage children.

The management of liver transplant patients is highly complex; it is essential to consider multiple facets of care over an extended period of time. In designing a plan of care for Sarah, Emily conducted a lengthy assessment. She was pleased to discover that Sarah was well educated and knew a great deal about her illness. Sarah asked many informed questions and was anxious to learn all she could from Emily. During the time that Emily worked with Sarah, she used a number of principles and theories in care delivery. She explained physiologic principles related to chronic liver disease and liver failure to Sarah, and she combined that information with pharmacologic principles concerning the large number of medications required to prevent rejection. Complications of the disease, as well as side effects from the medications, were examined at length. For the educative processes, Emily used several different learning principles and theories and incorporated a variety of teaching techniques, including one-on-one time, printed materials, interactive computer programs, and videos.

To address the many psychosocial issues that Sarah and her family would face, Emily combined principles and concepts from different theories to plan interventions. She incorporated role theory, family theory, developmental theory, and others to help Sarah and her family understand how the illness might affect Sarah's roles as wife, mother, daughter, sister, and teacher. She encouraged family support and advocated for counseling for all family members and then referred Sarah to a support group. Emily also guided Sarah in addressing the spiritual issues involved in living with a chronic, life-threatening illness. Among other concepts discussed were hope, meaning, and transcendence.

Finally, a significant aspect of Sarah's care involved management of her finances. Emily carefully described the process of reimbursement and explained what services were covered. Incorporation of principles and concepts from management and economics was necessary for Emily to adequately understand and explain the financial aspects of Sarah's care.

Theory is considered to be both a process and a product. As a process, theory has numerous activities and includes four interacting, sequential phases (analyzing concepts, constructing relationships, testing relationships, and validating relationships) that are implemented in practice. As a product, theory provides a set of concepts and relationships that may be combined to describe, explain, predict, and prescribe phenomena of interest; this information is then used to guide nursing practice (Kenney, 2013). In a practice discipline such as nursing, theory and practice are inseparable. Indeed, development and application of theory affiliated with research-based practice is considered fundamental to the development of the profession and autonomous nursing practice.

Theory provides the basis of understanding the reality of nursing; it enables the nurse to understand why an event happens. To illustrate how theory is applied in practice at a basic level, Dale (1994) used the example of a nurse who knows theories and principles of the anatomy of soft tissues and the related physiologic concept of pressure. This knowledge allows the nurse to recognize how a pressure sore can develop. Armed with this knowledge, the nurse can take steps to prevent pressure sores.

To improve the practice of nursing, nurses need to search the literature, critically appraise research findings, and synthesize empirical and contextually relevant theoretical information to be applied in practice. Furthermore, nurses must continually question their practice and seek to find better alternatives (Litchfield & Jonsdottir, 2012). Nurses cannot afford to think of theory and research as intellectual pursuits separate from clinical performance; rather, nurses should be aware that theory and research provide the basis for practice (Marrs & Lowry, 2006; Risjord, 2010; M. C. Smith & Parker, 2015).

This chapter examines several issues related to the application of theory in nursing practice. First, the relationship between theory and practice and the concept of theory-based nursing practice are described. This is followed by a discussion of the perceived theory–practice gap that persists in nursing. Practice theories are then presented, including a discussion of how they interrelate to evidence-based practice (EBP). This chapter concludes with examples illustrating how theory is used and applied in nursing practice.

Relationship Between Theory and Practice

According to M. C. Smith and Parker (2015), the primary purpose of theory in nursing is to improve practice and thereby positively influence the health and quality of life of persons, families, and communities. In nursing, there should be a reciprocal relationship between theory and practice. Practice is the basis for nursing theory development, and nursing theory must be validated in practice. Theory is rooted in practice and refined by research, and it should be reapplied in practice. Box 19-1 shows the many ways in which theories influence nursing practice.

Theory provides nurses with a perspective with which to view client situations and a way to organize data in daily care. Theory allows nurses to focus on important information while setting aside less important, or irrelevant, data. Theory may assist in directing analysis and interpretation of the relationships among data and in predicting outcomes necessary to plan care. Furthermore, a theoretical perspective

| Box 19-1 | Ways in Which Theory Influences Nursing Practice |

- Identifies recipients/clients of nursing care
- Describes settings and situations in which practice should occur
- Defines what data to collect and how to classify the data
- Outlines actual and potential problems to be considered
- Assists in understanding, analyzing, and interpreting health situations
- Describes, explains, and sometimes predicts client's responses
- Clarifies objectives and establishes expected outcomes
- Specifies actions or interventions to be provided
- Determines standards for practice
- Differentiates nursing practice from practice of other health disciplines
- Promotes responsibility and accountability for nursing care
- Identifies areas for research

Sources: Fawcett (1992); Kenney (2013); M. C. Smith and Parker (2015).

allows the nurse to plan and implement care purposefully and proactively, and when nurses practice purposefully and systematically, they are more efficient, have better control over the outcome of care, and can better communicate that care with others (Masters, 2015; M. C. Smith & Parker, 2015). Thus, nurses need to use theoretical perspectives to help understand what information is important; how information, findings, and data are related; what can be predicted by relationships; and what interventions are needed to deal with special relationships.

For example, a nurse working in a postpartum maternity unit should be aware of the theoretical basis for the development of postpartum depression. That nurse should know risk factors for postpartum depression, its signs and symptoms, and various management strategies. Furthermore, if the nurse suspects postpartum depression in a teenage mother, he or she must know what additional data need to be gathered to address the complex issues created by the mother's special needs and circumstances. The additional information should be analyzed and interpreted based on an understanding of the specific problems and complications posed by teen pregnancy, and an appropriate plan of care for that young woman can be developed and goals and outcomes predicted.

Similarly, a nurse working in a pediatric clinic should understand the theoretical principles of immunity and disease prevention when explaining the importance of immunization to a new mother. If the mother expresses concerns about a potential complication of the vaccine, the nurse should gather additional information from the mother to understand her specific concerns. On learning that the mother had read reports that the measles/mumps/rubella vaccine might cause autism, the nurse must be able to articulate the rationale behind immunization and to direct the mother to sources of information about vaccine safety and potential complications, including the most recent and relevant research data. This information will allow the mother to make an informed decision about the care of her infant.

Theory-Based Nursing Practice

Theory-based nursing practice is the "application of various models, theories, and principles from nursing science and the biological, behavioral, medical and sociocultural disciplines to clinical nursing practice" (Kenney, 2013, p. 333). Nursing practice is complex, and theory informs the practitioner to do what is right and just (good practice). In nursing, practice without theory becomes rote performance of activities based on tradition, common sense, and following orders (Hanberg & Brown, 2006; Marrs & Lowry, 2006; Risjord, 2010).

Theory offers the practitioner a basis for making informed decisions that are based on deliberation and practical judgment. With increasing clinical experience, nurses are able to combine theoretical and clinical knowledge with critical thinking skills to make better clinical decisions and thereby improve practice. Nursing, like all practice disciplines, uses a special combination of theory and practice in which theory guides practice and the practice grounds theory. Nurses rely heavily on theoretical understanding, and practice will be improved not just by experience but by an understanding of a wide range of theories. As Cody (2003) pointed out, "One learns to practice nursing by studying nursing theories, and one learns to practice nursing very well by studying nursing theories very intensely" (p. 226).

Dreyfus and Dreyfus (1996) believe that as nurses gain knowledge, skills, and expertise, theory and practice intertwine in a mutually supportive process; however, only if both theory and research are encouraged and appreciated can full expertise in nursing practice be realized. Theory is needed to explain the ends and means of nursing practice, and the nurse who uses theory-based practice will be able to describe, explain, predict, and control nursing events and initiate preventive actions. Theory-based practice, therefore, is purposeful and controlled; it includes preventive action and can be explained by the nurse.

It is sometimes difficult to decide where, when, and how to apply theory in nursing practice. This may be particularly true for nursing students and novice nurses. The application of theory in practice requires an understanding of concepts and principles associated with the needs of a particular client, group of clients, or community and recognition of when and how to use these concepts and principles when planning and implementing nursing care. Chinn and Kramer (2015) suggested criteria for determining when theory should be applied in practice. These are shown in Table 19-1.

The Theory–Practice Gap

Despite the decades-long study of theory in nursing and the development and evolution of nursing theories, the notion that there is a "gap" between theory and practice is a common perception among nurses (Kellehear, 2014; Monaghan, 2015; M. C. Smith & Parker, 2015). Indeed, it has been observed that nurses in clinical practice rarely use the language of nursing theory, nursing diagnosis, or the nursing process unless mandated to do so by accrediting bodies or institutional practice policies (Liaschenko & Fisher, 1999).

Risjord (2010) explains that the gap arises when the body of knowledge is not used as it should be. Several reasons for this have been suggested. Historically, for example, theory development has been regarded as the domain of nurse educators and scholars rather than the concern of practitioners. Nursing theory and practice have been viewed as two separate nursing activities, with theorists seen as those who write and teach about the ideal, separated from those who implement care in reality.

Although most scholars believe that theory and practice are, or at least should be, reciprocal, to many, the relationship between theory and practice appears to be unidirectional and hierarchical. To those nurses, theory is seen as "above" practice and is positioned to direct practice; rarely does practice appear to affect theory. This has

	Table 19-1 Guidelines for Application of Theory in Nursing Practice	

Question	Process for Determining Application to Practice	Example
Are theory goals and practice goals congruent?	Examine the goal of the theory and compare it with the outcomes or goals of nursing practice (standards of practice, personal views of nursing).	A rehabilitation nurse developing a plan of care for a spinal cord injury must choose between a theory of coping and a theory of adaptation.
Is the context of the theory congruent with the practice situation?	Examine the theory to determine context for application and compare it with the context of the situation at hand.	A hospice nurse is concerned that a new agency policy on pain management is based on a theory for postsurgical pain relief.
Is there similarity between theory variables and practice variables?	Compare the theoretic variables (concepts) and the variables recognized to directly influence the practice situation to determine whether all essential concepts are addressed in the theory.	A nurse working with clients with AIDS believes a learning theory might not consider the health status of the learner (the learner is assumed to be healthy) on the outcome(s) of client education.
Are explanations of the theory sufficient to be used as a basis for nursing action?	Use expert judgment about nursing actions that are implied or explicit within the theory to determine sufficiency; examine correlation between theoretical and practice variables.	A theory of therapeutic touch may be intriguing to an oncology nurse, but sufficient study should be conducted to determine when and how to apply the intervention in an oncology unit.
Does research evidence support the theory?	Conduct a review of the literature for research support of the theory; critically examine study findings for validity and applicability to practice.	Before considering implementing expensive measures that might prevent nosocomial infection, the nurse manager of a surgical ICU conducts a literature review to learn how effective the measures have been in similar settings.
How can the theory influence nursing practice and the nursing unit?	Consider ways in which an approach will affect nursing practice and a nursing unit; plan changes including observation and recording of factors relevant to the theory's application.	A theory that partially explains medication errors is being incorporated into new policies and procedures on a general medical unit, and the unit supervisor wants to be sure that the procedures include data collection for outcomes evaluation.

Source: Adapted from Chinn and Kramer (2015).

caused confusion and apathy among practitioners who believe academic knowledge has little relevance in practice situations. Indeed, practitioners often complain that theory distorts practice, if it has any relevance to practice at all (Hanberg & Brown, 2006; Kellehear, 2014).

Language also contributes to the gap in theory and practice, as many theories contain concepts and constructs that must be explained and understood before they can be applied. Furthermore, in the ideal world of nursing theory, nursing practice is discussed as being performed as it ought to be rather than as how it is. As a result, many nurses believe that theory is irrelevant to practice because of the obscurity of academic language and focus on circumscribed, ideal situations (Hartrick Doane & Varcoe, 2005).

Finally, it has been noted that practice often develops without theory, and knowing theory is not a guarantee of good practice. Furthermore, many practices resist explanation. Practice changes and develops in the light of theory, but much of the knowledge of practice is different from theory.

A different view has been taken by some. Larsen, Adamsen, Bjerregaard, and Madsen (2002) conducted a study of nursing literature and determined that there is no inherent gap between theory and practice. They concluded that although theorists and practitioners are situated in different environments, they share common and implicit understandings related to knowledge development and implementation of that knowledge in practice. Furthermore, they contend that theoretical principles are applied daily in practice, although nurses do not always recognize their use of theory.

Closing the Theory–Practice Gap

Despite repeated calls to relate theory, practice, and research, the interaction remains fragmented or unrecognized. To promote nursing's ability to meet its obligations to society, there needs to be an ongoing, reciprocal relationship among nursing theory, nursing science, and nursing practice. This will help close the perceived gap between theory and practice.

Several factors that interfere in the reciprocal interrelationship of theory, practice, and research in nursing need to be addressed. These factors include educational issues, interaction between nursing researchers/scholars and practicing nurses, and problems or issues central to contemporary nursing practice.

Lack of exposure to theoretical principles during the basic educational program is a major impediment to closing the theory–practice gap. Because approximately half of nurses in the United States have been educated in associate degree or diploma schools of nursing, they are frequently not exposed to either theory or research, as is common among baccalaureate or master's programs. This lack of focus on theory has been recognized, and in recent years, there has been momentum in nursing education to enhance emphasis on research and knowledge development (Johnson & Webber, 2015; Risjord, 2010; Walker & Avant, 2011).

It is equally important to stress theoretical concepts and principles following completion of formal education because nurses are required to continually assimilate and synthesize a sizable amount of information into their practice. The professional growth of practicing nurses is vital, and fortunately, many practicing nurses read scholarly journals, research-based literature, and practice-based journals. It is imperative that all nurses in clinical practice also be encouraged to expand their knowledge through ongoing exposure to new theoretical concepts and nursing research in continuing educational offerings or formal educational programs. These critically viewed notions of enhanced education and training, as well as lifelong learning for all nurses, were key recommendations of the Institute of Medicine (IOM) in their widely acclaimed report on *The Future of Nursing* (IOM, 2011).

A second issue relates to the disparity between the world of nursing theorists and scholars and the world of practicing nurses. Unfortunately, many nurse theorists and nurse researchers have limited clinical involvement, and time constraints restrict their ability to develop relationships with clinically based nurses. Conversely, the majority of nurses in practice have little or no direct contact with nurse theorists or nurse researchers. To address this problem, those who propose theory and conduct research have recognized the need to be directly involved in clinical practice. Furthermore, many understand the importance of studying problems encountered in practice and using language and terminology that can be easily understood by clinical nurses who are working to implement these changes.

The final issue in closing the theory–practice gap relates to changes in health care delivery and the need to address current issues and practices from a theoretical perspective. Nurses face many challenges posed by changes in the health care delivery system. For example, the decrease in length of stay has dramatically reduced the time available for preoperative and postoperative teaching and discharge planning. Likewise, reimbursement mechanisms have dramatically influenced the availability of home health care and largely determined when and how nurses care for clients and what services are provided. These developments and anticipated changes designed to curb the inflation of health care costs may adversely affect care delivery and nursing care.

The demands of the changing health care system and attention to EBP, along with other anticipated problems, must be addressed from a practice, theory, and research perspective. These problems include chronic illnesses (e.g., heart disease, cancer), aging of the population, and the increase in the number of persons from a variety of racial and cultural backgrounds. These factors contribute to the growing need to integrate multiple concepts, principles, and theories into designing, planning, and implementing effective nursing care. Thus, as nursing continues to evolve to meet the challenges described, clinical practice will need to be more heavily based on theory and research and less reliant on routine, common sense, and tradition.

Situation-Specific/Practice Theories in Nursing

Earlier chapters described different types and levels of theory used in nursing. In addition to borrowed or shared theories, this book has described grand nursing theories and middle range nursing theories. This section provides information about the theories often termed *situation-specific* or *practice theories*, which are narrow, circumscribed theories proposed for a specific type of practice. It is important to stress that they are not the only theories applied in nursing practice.

Definition and Characteristics of Situation-Specific/Practice Theories

Practice theories are nursing theories used in the actual delivery of nursing care to clients. Several characteristics are common to practice theories. First, they are used to carry out nursing interventions and often include or lead to the performance of psychomotor procedures (e.g., dressing changes, venipuncture, medication administration) or are related to communication (e.g., education, counseling). Second, practice theories may be derived from grand or middle range theories, from clinical practice, and/or from research, including literature reviews, and may describe, explain, or prescribe specific nursing practices. Third, practice theories combine a set of principles or directives for practice and often have a role in testing theories. Finally, practice theories may benefit nursing practice and the development of nursing knowledge by allowing for an in-depth analysis of a particular nursing intervention or practice.

The term *situation-specific theory* is sometimes used to describe practice theory (Chinn & Kramer, 2015; Im, 2014; Im & Chang, 2012; Meleis, 2012). Practice theories are clinically specific and reflect a particular context that may include directions or blueprints for action. Furthermore, in comparison to grand or middle range theories, practice theories have a lower level of abstraction, are context specific, and are easily applied in nursing research and practice.

Practice theories often emerge from grounded theory research or from synthesizing and integrating research findings and applying this knowledge to a specific situation or population. Typically, the intent is to develop a framework or blueprint

Table 19-2 Types of Practice Theories Needed in the Discipline of Nursing	
Type of Practice Theory	**Examples**
Theories providing explanations about client problems	Theories of healing, airway patency, fatigue, and speech
Theories describing therapeutics for client problems	Theories of suctioning, wound care, rest, and learning
Theories providing the nurse with ideas about how to approach clients	Theories of caring, empowerment, and communication
Theories providing explanations or ideas about how the nurse makes or should make decisions	Theories of clinical inference and clinical decision making
Theories providing explanations about what happens in the actual delivery of nursing care	Theories describing outcomes of client care

Source: Kim (1994).

to understand that particular situation or group of clients. Many nursing scholars support developing theories that reflect nursing practice, thus ensuring that nursing practice is a source for theory development (Im, 2014; Im & Chang, 2012). Table 19-2 lists some areas that have been proposed for the development of practice theories for nursing.

Examples of Practice and Situation-Specific Theories From Nursing Literature

The nursing literature contains a growing number of examples of practice or situation-specific theories. In searching for illustrations, most theories that could be termed *practice theories* are those that were developed through grounded theory research or those developed through application of a grand theory or a borrowed theory to a specific aggregate or in a very defined set of circumstances. A few were identified that were reported to have resulted from quantitative research studies and literary synthesis. Also, as mentioned in Chapter 10, some of the theories that are termed by the author or others as *middle range* may be more appropriately labeled practice theories.

Examples of practice-level theories developed from qualitative, grounded theory studies include a work by Doering and Durfor (2011), who developed a theory of "persevering toward normalcy after childbirth." They identified the strategies and characteristics necessary to help manage fatigue and sleep deprivation that are key in the early weeks following childbirth. Also using grounded theory, Law (2009) developed a situation-specific theory entitled "Bridging Worlds," which is intended to provide a mechanism to help hospice nurses ensure that both the physical and emotional needs of dying patients are met. In another example, Riegel, Dickson, and Faulkner (2016) revised their "situation-specific theory of heart failure self-care" based on a review of the literature which cited the original theory; they updated it in three key areas based on the review.

An example of a practice theory based on a middle range theory is a work presented by Valek, Greenwald, and Lewis (2015) who applied concepts and linkages from Pender's Health Promotion Model to develop a theoretical framework to help nurse practitioners encourage maintenance of weight loss. A grand theory—Roy's Adaptation Model (RAM)—was used by Perrett and Biley (2013) to describe the development of a framework for "negotiating uncertainty," which was aimed at helping nurses recognize the process of adaptation to being HIV positive. Lastly, McLeod-Sordjan (2013) presented an excellent description of what she termed clinical application of a framework for "facilitated communication" at the end of life, with the goal of "death acceptance" (p. 390). This framework was based on Parse's Humanbecoming Theory. Additional examples of practice or situation-specific theories and information about each are presented in Table 19-3.

Situation-Specific Theory and Evidence-Based Practice

EBP and its relationship with nursing theory was discussed in Chapter 12. As mentioned, EBP has become widely accepted in nursing as an approach to problem solving in clinical practice because it consciously and intentionally applies the currently agreed upon "best" evidence to direct care for patients (LoBiondo-Wood & Haber, 2014). A typical process used to develop EBP guidelines includes identifying a clinical problem, conducting a comprehensive literature search for relevant information about the problem, evaluating the researched evidence critically, and determining appropriate interventions.

In many ways, this process and the desired outcome mirrors the process and intent of development and implementation of situation-specific theories. Both are research based and focused on a relatively small set or subset of patients in fairly narrowly defined situations. Similarly, the desired outcome of both is to develop nursing interventions that can be applied in clinical practice to improve the health of patients.

Table 19-4 presents selected definitions of situation-specific nursing theory (micro theory or practice theory) and evidence-based nursing practice guidelines taken from the recent nursing literature. Critical review of the definitions suggests several similarities. For example, both are developed to address specific situations or phenomena and to be applied in clinical situations. For EBP, the intent is to assist clinicians make decisions in specified conditions or situations; the same is true for situation-specific theories. Additionally, although the situation-specific theory definitions do not directly or explicitly explain the source or methods used in their development, a review of the information presented previously indicates that many of them—particularly the more recently published theories—were developed through comprehensive review of the relevant health care literature as well as through research studies, which is typically the basis or starting point for the development of EBP guidelines.

Thus, it appears that situation-specific theories and EBP guidelines, standards, and protocols have much in common. As nursing researchers and nurse theorists move forward in theory development, increasing attention needs to be given to the development of situation-specific theories, with consideration of how they might be more explicitly connected to EBP guidelines.

Application of Theory in Nursing Practice

A lack of understanding of theory leads to a failure to recognize the use of theory on a day-to-day, even minute-to-minute, basis in the practice of nursing. For example, the practice of washing hands prior to client contact is based directly on the principles of germ theory and the epidemiologic concepts of disease transmission and disease prevention. Barnum (1998) used the term *implied theory* to refer to those theories used by practicing nurses during routine client care. Examples of application of theory can be taken from several sources within practice-based nursing literature.

Table 19-3 Examples of Situation-Specific/Practice Theories and Models

Practice Theory or Model	Target Population	Development Process	Goal and Activities or Actions Prescribed
Anticipatory Grief (Shore, Gelber, Koch, & Sower, 2016)	Patients with advanced disease and their family members	Case study based on Roy Adaptation Model—extrapolation of assessment tools and management strategies	Enhance the care of patients and caregivers suffering from anticipatory grief.
Midlife Women's Attitudes Toward Physical Activity (MAPA) (Im, Stuifbergen, & Walker, 2010)	Midlife women	Review of the literature; other models (e.g., Attitude, Social Influence, and Self-Efficacy Model) and a study on women's attitudes toward physical activity	Directs nursing interventions and research related to increasing participation in physical activity
Health-related behaviors of Korean Americans (Lee, Fawcett, Yang, & Hann, 2012)	Korean Americans who have or are at risk for chronic hepatitis B virus (HBV) infection	Literature review of related research and the Network Episode Model	Explanation of correlates of health-related HBV behaviors of the population; used to develop and test nursing interventions to promote positive health behaviors
Transition to adulthood (Joly, 2016)	Young people with medical complexity	Systematic literature review; applications of Meleis's Transitions Theory	Support nursing interventions that aid young people with complex health conditions to promote positive outcomes during transition to adulthood.
Theory of Crisis Emergencies (Brennaman, 2012)	Invidious with severe, persistent mental illness	Integrative literature review, application of a middle range theory in the defined population	Theory for use by nurses in emergency department to distinguish between need for mental health crisis intervention or mental health emergency intervention
Well-being in refugee women experiencing cultural transition (Baird, 2012)	Refugee women from South Sudan immigrating to the United States	Research studies and application of Transitions Theory	Promotes culturally relevant interventions for nurses working with immigrant and refugee populations to foster well-being
Complexity of living with hepatitis C (MacNeil, 2012)	Patients with chronic hepatitis C virus infection	Hermeneutic dialectic qualitative research—interpreted through Newman's Theory of Expanding Consciousness	Identify patterns and themes to help patients move to higher level of consciousness through "transformative changes in their lives" (p. 261).
Situation-specific theory of self-care in diabetes mellitus (DM) (Song, 2010)	Individuals with DM	Adaption of another situation-specific theory and literature review	Describes use of health outcomes and patients' decision-making responses to signs and symptoms of DM; promote DM self-care to improve health outcomes
Situation-specific theory: "Moving Beyond Dwelling in Suffering" (Willis, DeSanto-Madeya, & Fawcett, 2015)	Adult males who had experienced childhood maltreatment (abuse and/or neglect)	Hermeneutic phenomenological study—interpreted through Rogers's Science of Unitary Human Beings	Identification of the facilitators and inhibiting processes help men move beyond suffering to well-being.

| Table 19-4 Definitions of Evidence-Based Nursing Practice Guidelines and Situation-Specific Nursing Theories ||
Evidence-Based Nursing Practice Guidelines	Situation-Specific Nursing Theories
Practice guidelines are "systematically developed statements to assist health care providers with making appropriate decisions about health care for specific clinical circumstances" (Schmidt & Brown, 2015, p. 542).	". . . theories that focus on specific nursing phenomena, that reflect clinical practice, and that are limited to specific populations or particular fields of practice" (Im, 2005, p. 298).
Evidence-based practice clinical guidelines ". . . systematically developed practice statements designed to assist clinicians [to] make health care decisions for specific conditions or situations" (LoBiondo-Wood & Haber, 2010, p. 11).	"Theory that is developed with the sensitive consideration of context; assumes that theory . . . [takes] into account important differences across populations; draws attention to the variables that significantly affect the successful use of theory" (Chinn & Kramer, 2015, p. 254).
Evidence-based practice " . . . tracking down and applying the best available knowledge related to any specific clinical process, which specifically meets patient needs and answers critical questions related to best practices" (Malloch & Porter-O'Grady, 2010, p. 4).	[Microrange theories] ". . . focus on specific nursing phenomena . . . and offer a blueprint that is more readily operational and/or has more accessible utility in clinical situations" (M. J. Smith & Liehr, 2013, pp. 21–22).
"Evidence-based clinical practice guidelines are specific practice recommendations . . . that are based on a methodologically rigorous review of the best evidence on a specific topic" (Melnyk & Fineout-Overholt, 2015, p. 604).	"Situation-specific theories are coherent representations and descriptions of a set of concepts, and explanation of the relationships between those concepts and prediction of outcomes related to these relationships . . . grounded in clinical, teaching, policy or administrative situations . . . focused on a specific set of phenomena, more subscribed situations, and has a limited set of conditions" (Meleis, 2012, pp. 420–421).

With few exceptions, as in real practice, the theoretical principles are implicit rather than explicit.

This section illustrates the application of a variety of theories, principles, and concepts in nursing journals and the Nursing Intervention Classification (NIC) system. The intent of this exercise is to show where and how nurses use theoretical principles in practice. For the most part, these theories are implied and extrapolated rather than explicitly stated in the works in question. Some readers may argue whether the theories/principles/concepts are addressed at all in the examples. Furthermore, the theories/principles/concepts discussed will most likely not be the only ones suggested in the work; indeed, there are probably countless others.

Theory in Nursing Taxonomy: Examples From the Nursing Intervention Classification System

To illustrate the use of theory in nursing taxonomies, two interventions from the NIC system are discussed. The NIC is a comprehensive list of 554 nursing interventions grouped into 30 classes and 7 domains. Nurses in all specialties and in all types of settings perform these interventions. The NIC includes physiologic, behavioral, safety, family, and community interventions, and there are interventions for illness treatment, illness prevention, and health promotion (Bulechek, Butcher, Dochterman, & Wagner, 2013).

The intervention of intermittent urinary catheterization is used to highlight the incorporation of theories and principles from biology, physiology, and medicine into nursing. In a second discussion, theories related to behavioral interventions (i.e., learning theories and psychosocial theories and principles) are examined in the intervention of patient contracting.

Urinary Catheterization: Intermittent

Intermittent urinary catheterization refers to the "regular periodic use of a catheter to empty the bladder" (Bulechek et al., 2013, p. 406). The procedure may be performed by the nurse, another caregiver, or the client and may be done in the home or in an institutional setting. The purposes are to eliminate residual urine in the bladder, reduce urinary infections, prevent incontinent episodes, regain bladder tone, achieve dilation of the urethra, increase client control of urinary elimination, and facilitate self-care.

The authors presented references to support the need and rationale for the intervention. The data presented in the references compared rates and are an example of the use of epidemiologic principles. Discussion of complications and side effects, including urinary tract infection and fistulas resulting from indwelling catheters, related to principles of anatomy and physiology as well as disease processes. Description of costs of alternative strategies implied the use of economic principles. Mention of reluctance to report incontinence suggested incorporation of psychosocial theories and encouraging self-care related to several nursing theories, such as those of Orem and Erickson, Tomlin, and Swain.

The activities that comprise the intervention of intermittent urinary catheterization largely focus on prevention and identification of infection and teaching needs related to the psychomotor skills used by nurses and others providing care. Table 19-5 lists a few of the activities for the intervention and suggests a broad theoretical basis for each.

Table 19-5 Intermittent Urinary Catheterization: Theoretical Basis for Activities

Activity	Possible Theory Base
Perform comprehensive urinary assessment, focusing on causes of incontinence.	Physiology, certain disease processes
Teach patient/family purpose, supplies, methods, and rationale of intermittent catheterization.	Teaching/learning principles and theories
Teach patient/family clean intermittent catheterization technique.	Germ theory (principles of asepsis)
Use clean or sterile technique for catheterization.	Germ theory (principles of asepsis)
Maintain client on prophylactic antibacterial therapy for 2–3 weeks at initiation as appropriate.	Pharmacology, health promotion/prevention strategies
Establish a catheterization schedule based on individual needs.	Developmental theory, role theory, needs theory
Teach patient/family signs and symptoms of urinary tract infection.	Principles of disease processes

Source: Bulechek et al. (2013).

Table 19-6 Patient Contracting: Theoretical Basis for Selected Activities	
Activity	**Possible Theory Base**
Encourage the individual to identify own strengths and abilities.	Role theory, developmental theory, needs theory
Assist the individual in identifying the health practice he or she wishes to change.	Self-determinism
Assist the client in identifying present circumstances that may interfere with achievement of goals.	Role theory, developmental theory, health beliefs, motivation theory
Encourage the individual to choose a reinforcement/reward that is significant enough to sustain the behavior.	Motivation theory

Source: Bulechek et al. (2013).

Patient Contracting

One of the many behaviorally focused NIC interventions is patient contracting. Patient contracting is defined as "negotiating an agreement with an individual which reinforces a specific behavior change" (Bulechek et al., 2013, p. 289). Patient contracting involves analyzing patient behaviors, setting goals, determining responsibilities of interested parties, and determination of consequences and reinforcement mechanisms. A written, signed contract with terms and dates may be developed.

The major theoretical basis of the intervention is principles from behavior modification and operant conditioning. The intervention also uses concepts and principles from other theories. These concepts include motivation, compliance/noncompliance, and risk factor management. In addition, patient contracting is based on the premise that all individuals have the right to self-determination to make their own choices and to be active in their own health care and that health care providers must offer treatments that empower patients to identify their own priorities, strengths, weaknesses, and goals. These are ethical principles, which are fundamental to professional nursing practice.

Bulechek and colleagues (2013) developed a long list of activities that might be used in patient contracting. Table 19-6 lists a few of these activities and identifies a possible theoretical basis for each.

Examples of Theory From Nursing Literature

The general nursing literature is replete with examples of how theories are applied in routine nursing practice. This section presents several examples of practice—application of borrowed or "implied" theories as described earlier as well as application of middle range and grand theories.

Application of "Borrowed" and "Implied" Theories in Nursing Practice

Examples of applying borrowed theories in practice are easily identified in the literature. For example, Blevins and Toutman (2011) looked at how several theories are applied in caring for patients with chronic renal disease. Within a general framework of "successful aging," they discussed multiple theories and concepts that should be applied when working with this population. Among them were physiologic and psychological changes in aging, developmental theory, spiritual concerns, and theories of aging. Other key concepts discussed within the "Theory of Successful Aging" included coping, adaptation, health promotion, and decision making. The authors concluded that the Theory of Successful Aging is useful for assisting nurses in providing comprehensive care and understanding the complexities of caring for older patients with chronic renal disease.

In another work, Cleveland, Minter, Cobb, Scott, and German (2008) explained the bases for recommendations for screening and strategies for managing lead exposure in pregnant women and children. This discussion included epidemiologic information describing risk factors and demographic data accounting for the disparities of distribution of high lead levels. Additionally, environmental concepts and theories of lead contamination and related prevention strategies were examined. Finally, the pathophysiology of lead absorption was explained, and this discussion included an overview of potential treatment for high lead levels (chelation therapy) and the related biomedical and pharmacological aspects of the therapy.

Another example of application of non-nursing theories in nursing practice comes from Adeola, Omorogbe, and Johnson (2016) who reported on the development and implementation of a health education program for teens to reduced distracted driving. She used the Health Belief Model (HBM) as a guide for a four-step intervention including a presentation on injury prevention, a video about driver distraction entitled "Get the Message," a tour of a trauma center, and crash survivors' testimonies of injuries and disabilities. In addition to HBM constructs, this program also illustrated application of other theories, models, and concepts, including learning theories, developmental theories, and epidemiology (prevention). Link to Practice 19-1 shows another example of applying non-nursing theories in nursing practice.

Application of Grand and Middle Range Theories in Nursing Practice

Articles showing how grand and middle range nursing theories have been applied in nursing practice can readily be found in the nursing literature (Link to Practice 19-2). For example, Seah and Tham (2015) used RAM to develop an intervention strategy for management of bulimia. Akyil and Ergüney (2013) also reported on use of the RAM for an effective educational intervention to assist patients adapt to chronic obstructive pulmonary disease (COPD).

Link to Practice 19-1

Application of "Shared" Theory in Nursing Practice

Phillips (2012) described an intervention that can be used by community health nurses who are working with older adults who smoke. She explained that because smoking is the most preventable cause of death, smoking cessation is a key public health goal. Her research-based guidelines can reduce smoking-related illness and promote health among older adults. Using Bandura's self-efficacy construct as well as the HBM as a framework, the author presented five different caring options for nurses working with elders who smoke. The options discussed were (1) brief intervention sessions in which the health provider presented advice, encouragement, and assessment; (2) weekly individual behavioral counseling; (3) group behavior therapy; (4) use of pharmacotherapies; and (5) provision of self-help materials.

Link to Practice 19-2

Application of Nursing Theory in Practice

Nursing care for mothers-to-be who experience nausea and vomiting was addressed by Isbir and Mete (2010). The authors explained how to develop a very comprehensive and theory-based plan of care for this population based on the RAM. With the primary goal of promoting adaptation, the authors first suggested evaluation of the adaptive system. It was thought that women with mild to moderate symptoms may have effective cognator and regulator systems and can cope with the symptoms and therefore would need minimal intervention, as they have adaptation at the compensatory level.

For women with severe and lasting symptoms, however, their compensatory processes are not adequate and the insufficient adaption levels need to be addressed. Nurses can help coordinate regulator and cognator processes and increase adaptation to compensatory levels. The authors continued to apply the RAM to other aspects of care for pregnant women experiencing nausea and vomiting. They examined relationships among the different modes (interdependence, role function, physiologic, and self-concept modes) and focal, contextual, and residual stimuli. They concluded by describing how nursing activities and interventions (e.g., counseling about nutrition, promoting social support, identifying stressors, and reducing stress levels) can positively influence the adaptive/coping systems.

In another work, Joly (2016) used Meleis's Transitions Theory to develop recommendations for pediatric nurses to assist young people with chronic health conditions during the process of transition to adulthood. She suggested development of programs to focus on health determinants, psychosocial concerns, and education to ease the transition for this vulnerable group.

In another example, the middle range theory of chronic sorrow was used to provide anticipatory guidance for parents with premature infants (Vitale & Falco, 2014). They explained how the theory can be used by nurses to recognize how chronic sorrow is a normal grief response, know how to assess chronic sorrow in parents of premature babies, and understand how to support parents experiencing chronic sorrow by applying evidence-based strategies to promote effective coping.

Examples of how the Synergy Model has been used in guiding nursing practice can readily be found in the literature. For example, Hardin (2012) described how the Synergy Model could be used to plan and provide care to older adults with hearing loss, allowing them to participate in decision making while in a critical care unit. Then, in another work, Schleifer, Carroll, and Moseley (2014) explained how the Synergy Model could be used to develop competencies for a tele-intensive care unit. Table 19-7 presents additional examples of how nurses can apply a variety of theories in their practice.

Summary

Many nursing scholars believe that theory-guided practice, often in the form of EBP or situation-specific theory, is the future of nursing. As nursing progresses into the 21st century, nurses must place theory-guided practice at the core of nursing, and

Table 19-7 Application of Theory in Nursing Practice: Examples From the Literature

Reference	Situation and/or Population	Theories/Concepts Applied
Martínez Pérez, G., & Turetsky, R. (2015). FGM Review: Design of a knowledge management tool on female genital mutilation. *Journal of Transcultural Nursing, 26*(5), 521–528.	Website that provides information for victims of female genital mutilation worldwide	Leininger's Culture Care Diversity Theory; informatics; health promotion; health education
Senn, J. F. (2013). Peplau's theory of interpersonal relations: Application in emergency and rural nursing. *Nursing Science Quarterly, 26*(1), 31–35.	Communication situations between nurses and patients in the emergency department and in rural settings	Peplau's Theory of Interpersonal Relations
Koren, M. E., & Papamiditriou, C. (2013). Spirituality of staff nurses: Application of modeling and role modeling theory. *Holistic Nursing Practice, 27*(1), 37–44.	Stresses the importance of self-care for both nurses and patients, considering that spirituality is foundational to nursing care	Modeling and Role-Modeling Theory; Erikson's Developmental Theory
Helman, S., Lisanti, A. J., Adams, A., Field, C., & Davis, K. F. (2016). Just-in-time training for high-risk low-volume therapies: An approach to ensure patient safety. *Journal of Nursing Care Quality, 31*(1), 33–39.	Staff nurses who care for patients undergoing risky, low-volume (infrequent) therapies	Synergy Model; quality and safety strategies
Mitchell, G. (2013). Selecting the best theory to implement planned change. *Nursing Management, 20*(1), 32–37.	How nursing managers can use theory to implement changes in their work settings	Lewin's Change Theory, leadership theories, Herzberg's Motivation Theory, Lippett's Change Theory
Darnell, L. K., & Hickson, S. V. (2015). Cultural competent patient-centered nursing care. *The Nursing Clinics of North America, 50*(1), 99–108.	Nurses who provide care to patients in the United States	Leininger's Culture Care Diversity Theory

they must integrate relevant outcome-driven practice with the art and science of caring and healing.

As pointed out in the opening case study, advanced practice nurses like Emily routinely use concepts, principles, and theories from many disciplines, including nursing, to meet the health needs of their clients. To provide comprehensive, holistic, and effective interventions, nurses should rely on sound theoretical principles to develop and implement the plan of care.

Beginning in their basic nursing education program, all nurses should be encouraged to recognize the theoretical basis for practice and seek ways to enhance the knowledge base that supports practice. In addition, there should be an increased emphasis on enhancing the reciprocal interaction among theory, research, and practice with a concerted effort to bridge the theory–practice gap. Through these efforts, nursing can continue to develop and use a unique knowledge base and further contribute to autonomous and professional practice.

Key Points

- Theory is both a process and a product. In the discipline of nursing, theory and practice are inseparable.
- To improve practice, nurses need to search the literature continually, critically appraise research findings, and synthesize empirical and contextually relevant theoretical information to be applied in practice.
- Theory-based nursing is the application of various models, theories, and principles from nursing science and the biologic, behavioral, medical, and sociocultural disciplines to clinical nursing practice.
- Despite the recognition of the importance of theory in nursing, there is a perceived gap between theory and practice.
- Theories may be developed by and for nurses (grand, middle range, or situation-specific nursing theories), may be shared with other disciplines, or may be implied (routinely used without being conscious processes).
- Nurses should promote and embrace theory-guided practice as the core of nursing. Nurses should recognize the theoretical basis for practice and seek ways to enhance the knowledge base that supports practice and bridges the theory–practice gap.

Learning Activities

1. Obtain a copy of the NIC (Bulechek et al., 2013). Select several interventions and try to identify the possible theoretical bases of each.
2. Debate the pros and cons of EBP with several classmates. Why would a focus on EBP be good for nursing? What are some drawbacks?
3. Obtain copies of recent mainstream nursing journals (e.g., *American Journal of Nursing, Nursing 2018*). Examine practice-focused articles and try to identify theories that affect the suggested nursing interventions and nursing implications.
4. Following the example of Emily, the acute care nurse practitioner in the opening case study, consider a complex patient or situation from your practice. Review theories and concepts described in previous chapters. Identify how they have been or could be applied while planning and implementing care for that patient/situation.

REFERENCES

Adeola, R., Omorogbe, A., & Johnson, A. (2016). Get the message: A teen distracted driving program. *Journal of Trauma Nursing, 23*(6), 312–320.

Akyil, R. Ç., & Ergüney, S. (2013). Roy's adaptation model-guided education for adaptation to chronic obstructive pulmonary disease. *Journal of Advanced Nursing, 69*(5), 1063–1075.

Baird, M. B. (2012). Well-being in refugee women experiencing cultural transition. *ANS. Advances in Nursing Science, 35*(3), 249–263.

Barnum, B. S. (1998). *Nursing theory: Analysis, application, evaluation* (5th ed.). Philadelphia, PA: Lippincott Williams & Wilkins.

Blevins, C., & Toutman, M. F. (2011). Successful aging theory and the patient with chronic renal disease: Application in the clinical setting. *Nephrology Nursing Journal, 38*(3), 255–260.

Brennaman, L. (2012). Crisis emergencies for individuals with severe, persistent mental illnesses: A situation-specific theory. *Archives of Psychiatric Nursing, 26*(4), 251–260.

Bulechek, G. M., Butcher, H. K., Dochterman, J. M., & Wagner, C. M. (Eds.). (2013). *Nursing Interventions Classification (NIC)* (6th ed.). St. Louis, MO: Elsevier.

Chinn, P. L., & Kramer, M. K. (2015). *Knowledge development in nursing: Theory and process* (9th ed.). St. Louis, MO: Mosby.

Cleveland, L. M., Minter, M. L., Cobb, K. A., Scott, A. A., & German, V. F. (2008). Lead hazards for pregnant women and children: Part 2: More can still be done to reduce the chance of exposure to lead in at-risk populations. *American Journal of Nursing, 108*(11), 40–47.

Cody, W. K. (2003). Nursing theory as a guide to practice. *Nursing Science Quarterly, 16*(3), 225–231.

Dale, A. E. (1994). The theory-theory gap: The challenge for nurse teachers. *Journal of Advanced Nursing, 20*, 521–524.

Doering, J., & Durfor, S. L. (2011). The process of "persevering toward normalcy" after childbirth. *MCN. The American Journal of Maternal Child Nursing, 36*(4), 258–265.

Dreyfus, H. L., & Dreyfus, S. E. (1996). The relationship of theory and practice in the acquisition of skill. In P. Benner, C. A. Tanner, & C. A. Chesla (Eds.), *Expertise in nursing practice: Caring, clinical judgment, and ethics* (pp. 29–47). New York, NY: Springer Publishing.

Fawcett, J. (1992). Conceptual models and nursing practice: The reciprocal relationship. *Journal of Advanced Nursing, 17*, 224–228.

Hanberg, A., & Brown, S. C. (2006). Bridging the theory–practice gap with evidence-based practice. *Journal of Continuing Education in Nursing, 37*(6), 248–249.

Hardin, S. R. (2012). Hearing loss in older critical care patients: Participation in decision making. *Critical Care Nurse, 32*(6), 43–50.

Hartrick Doane, G., & Varcoe, C. (2005). Toward compassionate action: Pragmatism and the inseparability of theory/practice. *ANS. Advances in Nursing Science, 28*(1), 81–90.

Im, E.-O. (2005). Development of situation-specific theories: An integrative approach. *ANS. Advances in Nursing Science, 28*(2), 137–151.

Im, E.-O. (2014). The status quo of situation–specific theories. *Research and Theory for Nursing Practice, 28*(4), 278–298.

Im, E.-O., & Chang, S. J. (2012). Current trends in nursing theories. *Journal of Nursing Scholarship, 44*(2), 156–164.

Im, E.-O., Stuifbergen, A. K., & Walker, L. (2010). A situation-specific theory of midlife women's attitudes toward physical activity (MAPA). *Nursing Outlook, 58*(1), 52–58.

Institute of Medicine. (2011). *The future of nursing: Leading change, advancing health.* Washington, DC: National Academies Press.

Isbir, G. G., & Mete, S. (2010). Nursing care of nausea and vomiting in pregnancy: Roy adaptation model. *Nursing Science Quarterly, 23*(2), 148–155.

Johnson, B. M., & Webber, P. B. (2015). *An introduction to theory and reasoning in nursing* (4th ed.). Philadelphia, PA: Wolters Kluwer.

Joly, E. (2016). Integrating transition theory and bioecological theory: A theoretical perspective for nurses supporting the transition to adulthood for young people with medical complexity. *Journal of Advanced Nursing, 72*(6), 1251–1262.

Kellehear, K. J. (2014). The theory–practice gap: Well and truly alive in mental health nursing. *Nursing & Health Sciences, 16*(2), 141–142.

Kenney, J. W. (2013). Theory-based advanced nursing practice. In W. K. Cody (Ed.), *Philosophical and theoretical perspectives for advanced nursing practice* (5th ed., pp. 333–351). Sudbury, MA: Jones & Bartlett Learning.

Kim, H. S. (1994). Practice theories in nursing and a science of nursing practice. *Scholarly Inquiry for Nursing Practice, 8*(2), 145–158.

Larsen, K., Adamsen, L., Bjerregaard, L., & Madsen, J. K. (2002). There is no gap "per se" between theory and practice: Research knowledge and clinical knowledge are developed in different contexts and follow their own logic. *Nursing Outlook, 50*(5), 204–212.

Law, R. (2009). 'Bridging worlds': Meeting the emotional needs of dying patients. *Journal of Advanced Nursing, 65*(12), 2630–2641.

Lee, H., Fawcett, J., Yang, J. H., & Hann, H. W. (2012). Correlates of hepatitis B virus health-related behaviors of Korean Americans: A situation-specific nursing theory. *Journal of Nursing Scholarship, 44*(4), 315–322.

Liaschenko, J., & Fisher, A. (1999). Theorizing the knowledge that nurses use in the conduct of their work. *Scholarly Inquiry for Nursing Practice, 13*(1), 29–41.

Litchfield, M. C., & Jonsdottir, H. (2012). A practice discipline that's here and now. In P. G. Reed & N. B. C. Shearer (Eds.), *Perspectives on nursing theory* (6th ed., 437–447), Philadelphia, PA: Lippincott Williams & Wilkins.

LoBiondo-Wood, G., & Haber, J. (2010). Integrating evidence-based practice. In G. LoBiondo-Wood & J. Haber (Eds.), *Nursing research: Methods and critical appraisal for evidence-based practice* (7th ed., pp. 5–26). St Louis, MO: Mosby.

MacNeil, J. M. (2012). The complexity of living with hepatitis C: A Newman perspective. *Nursing Science Quarterly, 25*(3), 261–266.

Malloch, K., & Porter-O'Grady, T. (2010). *Introduction to evidence-based practice in nursing and health care* (2nd ed.). Sudbury, MA: Jones & Bartlett Learning.

Marrs, J. A., & Lowry, L. W. (2006). Nursing theory and practice: Connecting the dots. *Nursing Science Quarterly, 19*(1), 44–50.

Masters, K. (2015). *Nursing theories: A framework for professional practice* (2nd ed.). Burlington, MA: Jones & Bartlett Learning.

McLeod-Sordjan, R. (2013). Human becoming: Death acceptance: Facilitated communication with low-English proficiency patients at end of life. *Journal of Hospice and Palliative Nursing, 15*(7), 390–395.

Meleis, A. I. (2012). *Theoretical nursing: Development and progress* (5th ed.). Philadelphia, PA: Lippincott Williams & Wilkins.

Melnyk, B. M., & Fineout-Overholt, E. (2015). Making the case for evidence-based practice and cultivating a spirit of inquiry. In B. M. Melnyk & E. Fineout-Overholt (Eds.), *Evidence-based practice in nursing and healthcare: A guide to best practice* (3rd ed., pp. 3–23). Philadelphia, PA: Wolters Kluwer.

Monaghan, T. (2015). A critical analysis of the literature and theoretical perspectives on theory–practice gap amongst newly qualified nurses within the United Kingdom. *Nurse Education Today, 35*(8), e1–e7.

Perrett, S. E., & Biley, F. C. (2013). A Roy model study of adapting to being HIV positive. *Nursing Science Quarterly, 26*(4), 337–343.

Phillips, A. (2012). Smoking cessation: Promoting the health of older people who smoke. *British Journal of Community Nursing, 17*(12), 606–611.

Riegel, B., Dickson, V. V., & Faulkner, K. M. (2016). The situation-specific theory of heart failure self-care: Revised and updated. *The Journal of Cardiovascular Nursing, 31*(3), 226–235.

Risjord, M. (2010). *Nursing knowledge: Science, practice, and philosophy.* Oxford, United Kingdom: Wiley-Blackwell.

Schleifer, S. J., Carroll, K., & Moseley, M. J. (2014). Developing criterion-based competencies for tele-intensive care unit. *Dimensions of Critical Care Nursing, 33*(3), 116–120.

Schmidt, N. A., & Brown, J. M. (2015). *Evidence-based practice for nurses: Appraisal and application of research* (3rd ed.). Burlington, MA: Jones & Bartlett Learning.

Seah, X. Y., & Tham, X. C. (2015). Management of bulimia nervosa: A case study with the Roy adaptation model. *Nursing Science Quarterly, 28*(2), 136–141.

Shore, J. C., Gelber, M. W., Koch, L. M., & Sower, E. (2016). Anticipatory grief: An evidence-based approach. *Journal of Hospice & Palliative Nursing, 18*(1), 15–19.

Smith, M. C., & Parker, M. E. (2015). Nursing theory and the discipline of nursing. In M. C. Smith & M. E. Parker (Eds.), *Nursing theories and nursing practice* (4th ed., pp. 3–18). Philadelphia, PA: F.A. Davis.

Smith, M. J., & Liehr, P. R. (2013). *Middle range theory for nursing* (3rd ed.). New York, NY: Springer Publishing.

Song, M. K. (2010). Diabetes mellitus and the importance of self-care. *The Journal of Cardiovascular Nursing, 25*(2), 93–98.

Valek, R. M., Greenwald, B. J., & Lewis, C. C. (2015). Psychological factors associated with weight loss maintenance: Theory-driven practice for nurse practitioners. *Nursing Science Quarterly, 28*(2), 129–135.

Vitale, S. A., & Falco, C. (2014). Children born prematurely: Risk of parental chronic sorrow. *Journal of Pediatric Nursing, 29*(3), 248–251.

Walker, L. O., & Avant, K. C. (2011). *Strategies for theory construction in nursing* (5th ed.). Upper Saddle River, NJ: Prentice Hall.

Willis, D. G., DeSanto-Madeya, S., & Fawcett, J. (2015). Moving beyond dwelling in suffering: A situation-specific theory of men's healing from childhood maltreatment. *Nursing Science Quarterly, 28*(1), 57–63.

20

Application of Theory in Nursing Research

Melanie McEwen

Peter Jacobson is in his second semester of a master's program in nursing. He is currently a supervisor on a general medical floor of a large teaching hospital and wants to advance in nursing administration after his graduation.

Peter's program requires that all students complete either a thesis or a formal research application project, and he wants to get an early start on developing this project. During a theory course in his first semester, Peter read about Pat Benner's (2001) work detailing the process of moving from novice to expert practice in nursing, and this work intrigued him. After talking about possible research topics with one of his professors, he decides that he wants to use concepts from her theory to develop and test an orientation schedule for new graduates using selected "expert" nurses as mentors.

To better conceptualize the research study, he obtains a copy of Benner's most recent work. He also collects articles from nursing journals describing application of the novice to expert framework in different situations, including nursing practice, nursing education, and nursing research. From this information, he is able to develop an outline for his research project that uses the model as the conceptual framework.

In any discipline, science is the result of the relationship between the process of inquiry (research) and the product of knowledge (theory). The purpose of research is to build knowledge in a discipline through the generation and/or testing of theory. To effectively build knowledge, the research process should be developed within some theoretical structure that facilitates analysis and interpretation of findings. This will ultimately result in development of scientific theory. When a study is placed within a theoretical context, the theory guides the research process; forms the research questions; and aids in design, analysis, and interpretation. Thus, a theory, conceptual model, or framework provides parameters for a research study and enables the scientist to weave the facts together.

For the past several decades, nursing leaders have called for research to develop and confirm nursing knowledge and for theory to organize it. They have recognized the need to link nursing research and theory because it has been observed that research without theory results in discrete information or data, which does not add to the accumulated knowledge of the discipline (Chinn & Kramer, 2015; Hardin, 2014).

However, it has been pointed out that the relationship between research and theory in nursing is not well understood. This may result from several factors, including the relative youth of the discipline and debates over philosophical worldviews (i.e., empiricism, constructivism, phenomenology) as described in Chapter 1.

There are also concerns regarding whether nursing should form a discrete body of knowledge without using theories from other disciplines. Nursing science is a blend of knowledge that is unique to nursing and knowledge that is imported from other disciplines (e.g., psychology, sociology, education, biology), but considerable debate continues about whether the use of borrowed theory has hindered the development of the discipline. This has contributed to problems connecting research and theory in nursing.

This chapter examines a number of issues related to the interface of research and theory in the discipline of nursing. Topics covered include the relationship between research and theory, types of theory and corresponding research, how theory is used in the research process, and the issue of borrowed versus unique theory for nursing. The chapter concludes with discussions of how theory should be addressed in a research report and the discipline's research agenda.

Historical Overview of Research and Theory in Nursing

In the discipline of nursing, research and theory were first integrated in the works of Florence Nightingale. In *Notes on Nursing*, she identified the need to organize nursing knowledge through observation, recording, and statistical inferences. Nightingale also supported her theoretical propositions through research, as statistical data, and prepared graphs were used to depict the impact of nursing care on the health of British soldiers (Dossey, 2010).

After Nightingale's time, for almost a century, reports of nursing research were rare. For the most part, research and theory developed separately in nursing. Blegen and Tripp-Reimer (1994) explained that between 1928 and 1959, only 2 of 152 studies published in nursing journals reported a theoretical basis for the research design.

The amount and quality of nursing research grew dramatically, however, beginning with the initial publication of *Nursing Research* in 1952. During the last half of the 20th century, the number of nursing journals focusing on research grew to include *Research in Nursing & Health*, *Western Journal of Nursing Research*, and *Advances in Nursing Science*. Many other nursing journals, both general (e.g., *Journal of Nursing Scholarship*, *Journal of Advanced Nursing*) and specialty based (e.g., *MCN: American Journal of Maternal Child Nursing*, *Heart & Lung: The Journal of Critical Care*, *AORN Journal*), also devote significant portions of each issue to nursing research.

In the early years, research in nursing focused on education and characteristics of nurses rather than on aspects of nursing practice and nursing interventions. However, by the 1990s, clinical studies comprised over 75% of articles in research journals (Blegen & Tripp-Reimer, 1994).

Beginning in the 1970s, nurse scholars encouraged researchers to provide a theoretical or conceptual framework for research studies. At about the same time, a growing number of nurse theorists were seeking researchers to explore ways to test their models in research and clinical application. As a result, there was a push to combine research and nursing models. This emphasis on using nursing models as the framework for research was proposed to provide research into the unique perspective of nursing (Chinn & Kramer, 2015).

Despite this encouragement, however, the vast majority of research studies in nursing do not test aspects of grand nursing theories or use them as a research framework. Rather, they examine concepts, principles, and theories from a number of theoretical perspectives and disciplines. This trend persisted throughout the 1990s and into the 21st century as the focus of research, and theory has moved more toward middle range, situation-specific/practice theories, and evidence-based practice (see Chapters 10, 11, 12, and 19). Finally, most nursing research still does not mention theory—either nursing or non-nursing. Indeed, according to Yarcheski, Mahon, and Yarcheski (2012), only about 22% of nursing research studies published in 2010 were theoretically based; this was down from about 31% in 1985.

Relationship Between Research and Theory

Knowledge development is cumulative, and knowledge generated from separate research studies should be integrated into a more comprehensive understanding of the subject or phenomenon being studied. The value of any research study is derived as much from how it fits with, and expands on, previous work as from the study itself. Thus, research gains its significance from the context within which it is placed—specifically from its theoretical context. The theoretical context, therefore, is the structure and system of important concepts, theoretical propositions, and theories that comprise the existing knowledge of the discipline (Chinn & Kramer, 2015; Fawcett & DeSanto-Madeya, 2013).

Moody (1990) explained that knowledge development in nursing science has lagged due to three major factors: (1) a limited theoretical base to guide practice; (2) an abundance of isolated studies that have not been tied to an integrating theoretical framework or placed in a theoretical context; and (3) inadequate efforts to link theory, measurement, and data interpretation during the research process. To further develop nursing science and strengthen the discipline, it is essential that nurse researchers and nurse scholars address these issues. This requires recognizing the relationship between research and theory and developing an understanding of how theory is used in, and developed through, research. The following sections describe this relationship.

Nursing Research

Research is the "systematic inquiry that uses disciplined methods to answer questions or solve problems" (Polit & Beck, 2017, p. 3). Research is conducted to describe, explain, or predict variables, and in a practice discipline such as nursing, research is assumed to contribute to the improvement of care. The research process consists of several essential steps that are followed in planning, implementing, and analyzing a research study (Box 20-1).

Nursing research has been defined as a "scientific process that validates and refines existing knowledge and generates new knowledge that directly and indirectly influences the delivery of evidence-based nursing" (Gray, Grove, & Sutherland, 2017, p. 2). It is concerned with the study of individuals in interaction with their environments and with discovering interventions that promote optimal functioning and wellness across the lifespan. In nursing, researchers have studied principles and laws governing life processes, the well-being and optimum functioning of human beings, patterns of

Box 20-1	Steps of the Research Process

- Identify the problem to be investigated and clarify the purpose of the study.
- Review the literature.
- Define the conceptual/theoretical framework and develop conceptual definitions.
- Formulate research questions or hypotheses.
- Select a research design.
- Determine methods of measurement (instruments/tools).
- Define the population sample to be studied.
- Address legal/ethical issues related to human/animal rights.
- Develop a plan for data collection and analysis.
- Collect the data.
- Analyze the data.
- Interpret findings.
- Identify conclusions and recommendations.
- Disseminate findings.

Sources: Gray et al., (2017); LoBiondo-Wood and Haber (2014); Polit and Beck (2017).

behavior as individuals interact with their environment during critical life situations (e.g., birth, loss, illness, death), and processes that bring about positive changes in a person's health status. Furthermore, nursing research measures the impact of nursing interventions on client outcomes to provide an informed basis for practice.

Purpose of Theory in Research

Theory is integral to the research process. It is important to use theory as a framework to provide perspective and guidance to a research study. Indeed, theoretical frameworks provide direction regarding selection of the research design, identify approaches to measurement and methods of data analysis, and specify criteria for acceptability of findings as valid (Fitzpatrick & Kazer, 2012).

Fitzpatrick (1998) summarized how theory can be used to guide the research process. In generating and testing phenomena of interest to nursing, theory can (1) identify meaningful and relevant areas for study, (2) propose plausible approaches to health problems to examine, (3) develop or reformulate middle range theory linked to research, (4) define concepts and propose relationships among concepts, (5) interpret research findings, (6) develop clinical practice protocols, and (7) generate nursing diagnoses based on research findings.

The Research Framework

As shown in Box 20-1, an essential step of the research process is selection of a theoretical or conceptual model that serves as a research framework. The investigator uses the conceptual model to view situations and events through a particular frame of reference, the researcher's perspective about how the concepts and variables of interest in the study fit together. The research framework describes the phenomena and problems to be studied as well as the purposes to be fulfilled by the research. It identifies the source of the data (e.g., individuals, groups, animals, documents, prior research) and the settings in which data are to be gathered. It contributes to selection of the research design and instruments, determines procedures to be used, and identifies the methods to be used for data analysis. Finally, the framework determines the contributions of the research to the advancement of knowledge by placing the findings within the context of previous knowledge.

LoBiondo-Wood and Haber (2014) believe that using a formal and explicit framework facilitates generalizing a study's findings. This can contribute to nursing science development and promote evidence-based practice. They explain that using a framework can simplify and provide direction to the research process. Unfortunately, in many published nursing research studies, especially studies involving clinical practice problems, a study's framework is implicit rather than explicit. It may be hidden or implied in the literature review, and the reader must "tease it out."

Types of Theory and Corresponding Research

As described in Chapter 2, theory is generally classified as descriptive, explanatory, or predictive. The research designs that generate and test these theories are descriptive, correlational, and experimental, respectively. Prescriptive theories or practice theories are also mentioned by a number of authors (Dickoff & James, 1968; Whall, 2016); these are sometimes referred to as situation-specific theories (Meleis, 2013). Table 20-1 shows the three primary types of theory described in nursing literature (descriptive, explanatory, and predictive) and provides additional examples from the nursing literature.

Descriptive Theory and Descriptive Research

A descriptive theory is an integrated set of concepts that focuses on dimensions, characteristics, situations, and commonalities of a phenomenon of interest (Meleis, 2013; Norwood, 2010).

Table 20-1 Types of Theory and Corresponding Research

Type of Theory	Type of Research	Examples From Nursing Literature
Descriptive	Descriptive or exploratory	Development of a model to address African Americans' spiritual needs during hospitalization (Hodge, Bonifas, & Wolosin, 2014) Development of the theory of strengthening capacity to limit intrusion (Ford-Gilboe, Merritt-Gray, Varcoe, & Wuest, 2011)
Explanatory	Correlational	Examination of the phenomenon of "Anger" among adolescents using the Roy Adaptation Model (Pullen et al., 2015) Development of a middle range Theory of Adaptive Spirituality from derived from research of the Roy Adaptation Model (Dobratz, 2016)
Predictive	Experimental	Comparison of motivational-interviewing coaching with standard treatment in managing cancer pain, based on the Transtheoretical Model (Thomas et al., 2012) Application of Orem's Self-Care Model to help reduce and prevent postpartum complications (Nazik & Eryilmaz, 2013)

Overview

A descriptive theory looks at a phenomenon and identifies its major elements or events. It may also note some relationships among the elements, but it generally only speculates about why the phenomenon occurs, how the elements relate to each other, or how changes in the elements affect each other (Barnum, 2005; Meleis, 2013).

Descriptive research involves observation of a phenomenon in its natural setting. Data are gathered by participant or nonparticipant observation and by open-ended or structured interview schedules or questionnaires. Data may be qualitative or quantitative or both. Descriptive research uses many different methods, including concept analysis, psychometric analyses, case studies, surveys, phenomenology, ethnography, grounded theory, and historical inquiry (McKenna & Slevin, 2008).

Descriptive research (exploratory research) answers questions such as: What are the characteristics of the phenomenon? What is the prevalence of the phenomenon? What is the process by which the phenomenon is experienced? Through systematic study of these or similar questions with a defined population or in a defined setting, a descriptive theory may result.

Nursing Studies

The nursing literature holds many excellent examples of descriptive theory and explanatory and descriptive research. For example, McAndrew and Leske (2015) developed a model for "end-of-life decision making as a balancing act" (p. 361) following a grounded theory study of the experiences of nurses and physicians working in critical care units. Their model illustrated how three interactive sub-themes of emotional responsiveness, professional roles and responsibilities, and intentional communication and collaboration provided the basic structure for the balance scale. The predicted outcomes were either balance, with positive end-of-life experience, or imbalance, leading to moral distress. Factors promoting balance for decision making were a team approach, shared goals, understanding perspectives, and knowing one's own beliefs. Factors causing imbalance were uncertainty, feeling powerless, difficult family dynamics, and recognizing suffering. The authors suggested development of support interventions for professionals involved in end-of-life decision making and efforts to improve communication and collaboration.

In a second example, Baumhover (2015) also used grounded theory methods to interview family member of intensive care unit (ICU) patients who had recently died to learn how they came to realize that their loved one was dying. Interviews with 14 family members resulted in a middle range theory termed "the process of death imminence awareness by family members of patient in adult critical care." Key categories leading to the process of family member awareness were the patient's awareness that they were near death, family members' recognition of "dying right in front of me," turning points in the patient's condition, a reported sense of "no longer the person I once knew," family member's desire to "do right by them," and the decision that it was "time to let go." Baumhover constructed the middle range theory from the findings to help provide more responsive and effective end-of-life care for both ICU patients and their family members.

Last, Strickland, Wells, and Porr (2015) conducted a grounded theory study of 18 mothers who were concluding treatment for cancer to assess their experiences of managing their role as mother during their "cancer journey." The result of the study was an explanatory model termed "safeguarding the children." The women described four strategies to protect their children—customizing exposure (determining how much to reveal about the cancer), reducing disruption to family life, finding new ways to be close, and increasing vigilance (maintaining the children's well-being). The researchers concluded that nurses can use the model to consider the needs of the whole family in order to better meet the concerns of young mothers during the cancer experience.

Explanatory Theory and Correlational Research

Explanatory theories specify relationships between dimensions or characteristics of individuals, groups, situations, or events. They explain why, and the extent to which, one phenomenon is related to another. Explanatory theories are composed of concepts and propositions (Norwood, 2010).

Overview

Explanatory theories are typically generated and tested by correlational research. Correlational research requires measurement of the dimensions or characteristics of phenomena in their natural states. Data are usually gathered by nonparticipant observation or a self-report instrument. Instruments can include fixed-choice, open-ended questionnaires, or interview schedules. Correlational research yields qualitative or quantitative data or both. Statistical analysis uses various nonparametric or parametric measures of association (LoBiondo-Wood & Haber, 2014).

Nursing Studies

One study (Ohlendorf, Weiss, & Oswald, 2015) used a correlational design to examine predictors and outcomes of postpartum mother's weight self-management behaviors using Meleis's Transitions Theory as the conceptual framework. In total, 66 women completed all phases of data collection for the 12-week study. The team determined that Transitions Theory was useful in conceptualizing the weight management after childbirth. They found that new mothers with "transition difficulty" have lower activation levels and were less likely to engage in weight self-management behaviors. Among their conclusions was a model illustrating the "proposed relationship between the study variables" (Ohlendorf et al., 2015, p. 1826) which explained the health outcome of "engagement in weight self-management behaviours."

In another example, Scoloveno (2015) conducted a correlational study of resilience in 311 middle adolescents (15 to 17 years). The intent of the study was to develop and test the "direct and indirect effects of resilience on hope, well-being, and health-promoting lifestyles" (Scoloveno, 2015, p. 342) among students at a public high school. The result was a beginning theoretical model which proposed propositions indicating that hope (belief in a personal future) is an outcome of resilience. Furthermore, resilience was predictive of both well-being and health-promoting lifestyles in this cohort.

Predictive Theory and Experimental Research

Predictive theories move beyond explanation to the prediction of relationships between characteristics or phenomena among different groups. Predictive theories are generated and tested by experimental research.

Overview

Experimental research involves the manipulation of some phenomenon to determine how it affects or changes some dimension or characteristic of another phenomenon. Experimentation encompasses many different designs, including pretest–posttest–noncontrol group design, quasi-experiments, time series analyses, and true experiments. Experimental research requires quantifiable data. Statistical analyses, involving various nonparametric and parametric tests, are used to measure differences. Qualitative data can be collected but generally must be coded to be tested statistically (LoBiondo-Wood & Haber, 2014).

Nursing Studies

Experimental research studies, and corresponding predictive theories, are relatively uncommon in nursing literature. Examples from recent nursing literature include a study by Dougherty, Thompson, and Kudenchuk (2012), which used a randomized experimental clinical trial comparing two interventions designed to improve outcomes for partners following receipt of an implantable cardioverter defibrillator (ICD). In a work guided by Bandura's Social Cognitive Theory, the researchers identified concerns and issues common to partners of patients who receive an ICD. Based on the ability to anticipate or predict common concerns, they designed and are currently testing nursing interventions to address them.

A second example using an experimental design is a study by Rogers, Keller, Larkey, and Ainsworth (2012). The team used Roy's Adaptation Model as a framework to study the efficacy of 12-week intervention employing "sign chi do" (SCD) exercises (meditative movements similar to tai chi) to promote physical activity among sedentary, community-dwelling older adults. Using a randomized experimental design with repeated measures, they examined the effect of SCD (intervention) on physiologic function adaptation and self-concept adaptation. Among the findings were that self-concept adaptation measures were not significantly different between the groups but that physiologic adaptation (balance and physical function) improved for the SCD group. This suggests that SCD is useful for improving physiologic functioning among sedentary older adults.

Then, a quasi-experimental design was used to test application of the Neuman Systems Model (Barutcu & Mert, 2016). In this study, the researchers tested the effectiveness of a support group intervention to improve the "burden" on caregivers of patients with heart failure. They concluded that the theory-based intervention improved caregiver burden overall—focusing on practical support, motivational support, emotional support, and personal care. All of the dimensions, except personal care showed to be statistically greater in the intervention group when compared with the control group. Depression symptoms, however, were not significantly different between the two groups.

How Theory Is Used in Research

Theory brings organization to the variables of interest and the concepts reflected in a study. It provides a guide for developing a study and allows the findings to be placed in, or linked to, a larger body of knowledge. Therefore, a theoretical perspective increases the scientific value of a study's findings.

Both nursing and non-nursing theories have relevance for problems studied by nursing researchers, and theories tend to show up in the research process in one of three ways. A theory can be generated as the outcome of a study. In other cases, a research project is undertaken for the specific purpose of testing a theory. Most frequently, a theory is used in a research framework as the context for a study (McEwen, 2014). Each of these three ways that theory is used in research is described in the following sections.

Theory-Generating Research

Research that generates theory (i.e., descriptive research) is designed to develop and describe relationships between and among phenomena without imposing preconceived notations of what these phenomena mean (Chinn & Kramer, 2015). It is inductive and includes grounded theory, field observations, and phenomenology. During the theory-generating process, the researcher moves by logical thought from fact to theory by means of a proposition stated as an empirical generalization.

Overview

Norwood (2010) explained several steps in the process of theory generation. First, the researcher identifies observations with shared characteristics or common themes in an identified group or in a particular setting. Second, the researcher translates these observations into more abstract concepts by determining what general phenomenon these observations represent. The third step involves identifying patterns of relationships between observations and concepts. Next, the researcher translates observations of relationships into propositional statements and finally weaves the concepts and propositions together into a framework or tentative theory. In some cases, the researcher may identify an existing theory that these concepts and relationships represent. Nursing Exemplar 1 analyzes a grounded theory study to further illustrate the steps involved in theory-generating research.

NURSING EXEMPLAR 1: THEORY-GENERATING RESEARCH

Hershberger, P. E., Sipsma, H., Finnegan, L., & Hirshfeld-Cytron, J. (2016). Reasons why young women accept or decline fertility preservation following cancer diagnosis. *Journal of Obstetric, Gynecologic, and Neonatal Nursing, 45*(1), 123–134.

The following study is a good example of theory generation using grounded theory research techniques. The study is analyzed using the steps described by Norwood (2010).

Identify Common Themes in an Identified Group: The researchers provided background information explaining the complex decision-making processes young women with cancer make with respect to fertility preservation. In the United States, many women delay pregnancy and childbearing until their 30s and 40s, and there is an increase in the number of women of childbearing age diagnosed with cancer who have not yet considered having children. Fertility preservation is defined as egg, embryo, or ovarian tissue cryopreservation. Young women with cancer are at risk for fertility loss, and egg and embryo cryopreservation are not considered standard in clinical practice. There are no studies to determine why young women choose fertility preservation.

Translate Observations Into Abstract Concepts: In-depth interviews were used to collect data from 27 participants between the ages of 18 and 42 years who had been diagnosed with cancer to determine how they made their decision about whether to accept or decline fertility preservation. Four "dimensions" for the decision-making process were defined from the interviews. These were cognitive appraisals (i.e., success rates, human risks and safety, financial costs, access, infertility risk), emotional responses (i.e., avoiding pain and suffering, fostering joy and happiness), moral judgments (i.e., embryo status, spirituality), and decision partners (i.e., family and friends, clinicians).

Patterns of Relationships Identified: The findings suggested, "Women who accepted fertility preservation often described a desire for motherhood or future children, and those who declined were often concerned with surviving cancer or minimizing cancer recurrence" (Hershberger, Sipsma, Finnegan, & Hirshfeld-Cytron, 2016, p. 123). Also, those who declined fertility preservation cited financial reasons, delay in cancer therapy, concerns over success rates, and lack of clinician support. For many, support—or lack of support—from family and friends contributed to decisions. Finally, some women who declined treatment reported mental and physical energy of preservation was too great.

Weave Concepts and Propositions Together Into a Framework or Rudimentary Theory: The four "dimensions" become the foundation for a developing theory of fertility preservation decision making. The model presented outlines the basic elements of the decision-making process; however, propositions and relational statements need additional development. The authors concluded that nurses aware of the reasons influencing fertility preservation decisions can use the information to help guide counseling and education.

Nursing Studies

Theory-generating research studies can readily be found in nursing literature. As mentioned, a number of nursing theories have been developed using grounded theory research techniques. Another method for theory generation is systematic literature review. For example, Roy (2014) constructed the middle range Theory of Coping from a review of quantitative nursing research studies examining adaptation and coping and describing how the findings from the studies could be interpreted and applied within the Roy Adaptation Model. She identified the major concepts that influence coping as focal stimuli (e.g., ageing and chronic pain, perceived stress of care giving), contextual stimuli (e.g., race, gender, caregiver burden), coping strategies (e.g., active, nonreligious, religious, passive avoidance), and outcomes (e.g., adaptive self-concept responses, spiritual well-being, adaptive role response) and outlined 12 propositions connecting various indicators. Finally, she described how the Theory of Coping can be applied in nursing practice.

Often, new theories are developed from existing theories. For example, Willis, DeSanto-Madeya, Ross, Sheehan, and Fawcett (2015) used four nursing theories (Neuman's Systems Model, Rogers's Science of Unitary Human Beings, the Roy Adaptation Model, and Watson's Theory of Human Caring) to explain the process of "spiritual healing in the aftermath of childhood maltreatment," and Dobratz (2011) developed the middle range theory "Psychological Adaptation in Death and Dying" based on aspects of the Roy Adaptation Model. In another example, the middle range Theory of Self-Care of Chronic Illness (Riegel, Jaarsma, & Strömberg, 2012) contained concepts and elements consistent with Orem's Grand Theory of Self-Care. Finally, Reimer and Moore's (2010) middle range Theory of "Flight Nursing Expertise" includes elements identified by Benner (2001).

Theory-Testing Research

Sometimes, a study is conducted for the purpose of testing a theory or assessing its explanatory value in a specific situation.

Overview

In theory-testing research, theoretical statements are translated into questions and hypotheses. Theory testing requires a deductive reasoning process that also follows several steps.

First, the researcher chooses a theory of interest and selects a specific propositional statement from the theory (rather than the entire theory) to be tested. Next, the researcher develops a hypothesis or hypotheses that must have specific measurable variables that reflect the propositional statement. The researcher conducts the study and interprets findings. The interpretation determines if the study supports or contradicts the propositional statement and, thus, the theory. Finally, the researcher determines if there are any implications for further use of the theory in nursing practice (LoBiondo-Wood & Haber, 2014; Norwood, 2010).

Examples of theory testing are fairly rare in nursing literature (Yarcheski et al., 2012). One reason for this is the lack of clarity about what constitutes theory testing. Silva (1986) pointed out that serious misconception exists among some researchers and theorists that if a conceptual model has been used as a theoretical framework for research, then this constitutes theory testing. It does not, however, because theory testing requires detailed examination of theoretical relationships and necessitates that the study be designed to accept or refute these relationships.

Another reason there has been little theory-testing research relates to interpretation and evaluation of the research. Acton, Irvin, and Hopkins (1991) developed criteria for evaluating theory-testing research (Box 20-2) that will help those who are interested in conducting this type of study as well as those using the criteria. In addition, Nursing Exemplar 2 gives an example of the evaluation of a theory-testing study using these criteria.

Box 20-2   Criteria for Evaluating Theory-Testing Research

- The purpose of the study is to examine the empirical validity of the constructs, concepts, assumptions, or relationship from the identified theory.
- The theory is explicitly described and summarized.
- The constructs and concepts to be examined are theoretically defined.
- An overview of the previous studies that are based on the theoretic framework, or that clearly show the derivation of the concepts being tested, must be included in the review of the literature.
- The research questions or hypotheses are logically derived from the definitions, assumptions, and propositions of the theory.
- The research questions or hypotheses are specific enough to put the theory at risk for falsification.
- The operational definitions are clearly derived from the theory.
- The design is congruent with the level of theory described.
- The instruments are theoretically valid and reliable.
- The theory guides the sample selection.
- The statistics used are the most robust possible.
- Data analysis provides evidence for supporting, refuting, or modifying the theory.
- The research report includes an interpretative analysis of the finding in relation to the theory being tested.
- The significance of the theory for nursing is discussed in the report.
- The researcher makes recommendations for further research on the basis of the findings.
- Researchers should identify theory-testing studies in their abstracts, publication titles, and library retrieval key words.

NURSING EXEMPLAR 2: THEORY-TESTING RESEARCH

Mefford, L. C., & Alligood, M. R. (2011). Testing a theory of health promotion of preterm infants based on Levine's conservation model of nursing. *The Journal of Theory Construction & Testing*, 15(2), 41–47.

The following is a review of an excellent example of theory-testing research. This study tested the Theory of Health Promotion for Preterm Infants based on Levine's Conservation Model of Nursing. Here, the research is evaluated using the criteria suggested in Box 20-2.

Purpose: "The purpose of this study was to perform an exploratory test of the middle range Theory of Health Promotion for Preterm Infants based on Levine's Conservation Model of nursing" (Mefford & Alligood, 2011, p. 41).

Explicit Summary of Theory: The theoretical framework, including goals of nursing care and subjects of nursing care (preterm infants and family), are discussed.

Definitions: Seven theoretical concepts (termed "latent variables") (physiologic immaturity at birth, structural immaturity at birth, neurologic immaturity at birth, family system characteristics at birth, etc.) are defined.

Previous Studies: The theoretical framework section described the process involved in development of the middle range theory and provided detail on both Levine's model and related information as well as a description of application and previous testing.

Hypotheses: Hypotheses were not specified. However, a path diagram model was provided that explained anticipated relationships among the latent variables in the theory to be used for statistical testing.

Operational Definitions: Operational definitions are clearly described as "measurement variables" for each of the theoretical concepts (latent variables).

Study Design: The design was a descriptive correlational ex post facto study using data collected from existing databases of a level III neonatal intensive care unit (NICU) and an associated intermediate care nursery.

Instruments: A number of measures were used for the study. Data were collected on such variables as "surfactant therapy," birth weight, Apgar scores, maternal age, prenatal care, and consistency of nursing caregivers. They also created a measure of "heath status" that assessed such indictors as postconceptual age at discharge, weight at discharge, and "morbidity score" (bronchopulmonary dysplasia, intraventricular hemorrhage, nosocomial infect, etc.).

Sample: The convenience sample included 235 infants with a gestational age at birth of less than 37 weeks who were treated in the study NICU.

Statistics: Measures of univariate and multivariate normality were submitted to LISREL program for structural equation modeling.

Data Analysis: The structural equation modeling carried out indicated that the "overall good fit of the model to the data . . . [had] a Goodness of Fit Index of 0.905" (Mefford & Alligood, 2011, p. 46). Each of the relationships originally posited were discussed, and most of the relationships presented in the original model were supported.

Research Report: The findings indicated that the middle range theory was supported as "the model fit and path directions and strengths were congruent with relational propositions of the theory" (Mefford & Alligood, 2011, pp. 46–47).

Significance of Theory for Nursing: The authors concluded that the findings validate the theoretical assertion that nursing care supports adaptive efforts of the infant and family and facilitates attainment of health. Furthermore, the researchers noted that consistency of nursing caregivers is very important to promoting health for preterm infants.

Recommendations: The study provided evidence that the Theory of Health Promotion for Preterm Infants holds promise as a theoretical framework to guide neonatal nursing practice and improve health outcomes of these tiny patients.

Nursing Studies

Some studies testing theories were found in recent nursing literature. Not surprisingly, most of those studies identified tested grand or middle range nursing theories or theories derived from grand nursing theories.

Research testing grand nursing theories included a study conducted by Gigliotti (2004). In this work, elements of Neuman's Systems Model were tested by examining maternal–student role stress. This study was designed to examine the moderating capabilities of the psychological and sociocultural variables in the flexible line of defense. In the study, 135 women were given questionnaires to measure role stress, maternal and student role involvement, and social support. It was concluded that the effect of student role involvement on maternal–student role stress is contingent upon low network support. Also, the effect of maternal role involvement on maternal–student role stress is significantly enhanced for women age 37 years and older.

Another example of research that tested theories or models derived from grand or middle range nursing theories was a work by Foli, South, and Lim (2014) which collected data on adoptive mothers' unrealistic/unmet expectations and experiences following adoption and to determined association with depression. Their findings were used to support and slightly refine Foli's (2010) middle range Theory of Depression in adoptive parents. Another example (Fawcett et al., 2011) tested multiple relationships within the Roy Adaptation Model examining women's perception of cesarean birth.

Theory as the Conceptual Framework or Context of a Study

The most common way of incorporating a theory into the research process is by using the theory to drive the entire study (McEwen, 2014). In these cases, the problem being investigated is fitted into an existing theoretical framework, which guides the study and enriches the value of its findings.

Overview

The process of using a theory as a conceptual framework also involves several steps. Typically, during the process of conducting the literature review, the researcher identifies an existing framework that can be meaningfully applied to the study or develops a conceptual framework that is unique to the study (Norwood, 2010). When a framework is used as the context, it is integrated into the study in a number of ways (Box 20-3). Nursing Exemplar 3 presents an evaluation of a published research study illustrating how a nursing theory is used as a conceptual framework.

If the conceptual framework used by the researcher is an existing framework, the process can be termed *theory fitting*. In theory fitting, the researcher formulates a research purpose or research question and then proceeds to the literature to search

Box 20-3	Use of a Theory as a Conceptual Framework in a Nursing Study

- The framework's concepts are used as variables in the study.
- The conceptual definitions are drawn from the framework.
- The data collection instrument is congruent with the framework.
- Findings are interpreted in light of explanations provided by the framework.
- The researcher identifies whether the study's findings support or challenge the framework.
- Implications for nursing practice are based on the explanatory power of the framework.
- Recommendations for further research address the concepts and relationships in the framework.

Source: Norwood (2010).

for a theory to guide the study. The theory that best fits the research study is then selected. There are potential problems with this practice, however. The concepts or relationships from the original theory may be incorrectly applied, the work may appear forced, or the study may fail to lead to meaningful conclusions. To be effective, theory fitting requires an extensive search of the literature and an understanding of theoretical progress in nursing and other fields (Moody, 1990).

NURSING EXEMPLAR 3: THEORY AS A CONCEPTUAL FRAMEWORK

Jackson, H., Yates, B. C., Blanchard, S., Zimmerman, L. M., Hudson, D., & Pozehl, B. (2016). Behavior-specific influences for physical activity among African American women. *Western Journal of Nursing Research*, *38*(8), 992–1011.

The following is a good example of using a nursing theory (Pender's Health Promotion Model [HPM]) as the conceptual framework for a research study. The criteria suggested in Box 20-3 were used to evaluate this work.

Research Problems Consistent With the Framework: The purpose of this study was to "describe physical activity (PA) behaviors and physical functioning of prehypertensive and Stage I hypertensive African American Women (AAW) and to examine the relationship between PA behavior, physical functioning, personal factors, and behavior-specific influences" (Jackson, et al., 2016, p. 992). The HPM was cited as the framework for the study, and the major concepts are consistent with those of the HPM.

Conceptual Definitions Derived From the Framework: Concepts studied were prehypertension, perceived barriers to PA, and interpersonal (social) support for PA. The major concepts were defined and explained within the context of the HPM.

Instruments Congruent With the Framework: The research instruments were described in detail. They included a demographic questionnaire, "personal factors" (defined as systolic and diastolic blood pressure, body mass index, and waist circumference), physical functioning (a timed 400-m walk test). Concepts from the HPM included physical activity behaviors and social support. These were measured by the International Physical Activity Questionnaire, the Exercise Barriers Scale, and the Social Support for Exercise Scale.

Findings Interpreted Based on the Framework: The findings for PA and social support for PA were interpreted based on explanations of the HPM. Notably, moderate levels of barriers to exercise (e.g., lack of time, fatigue) were identified. Also, it was determined that social support from family and friends for PA was minimal.

Relationship of Findings to Framework: The researchers described the findings in relation to the HPM. They determined that behavior-specific influences demonstrating positive physical activity behaviors and physical functioning were fewer barriers to PA and more family and friend support.

Implications for Nursing: It was concluded that nursing interventions for prehypertensive African American women "should focus on removing barriers and improving social support for PA" (Jackson et al., 2016, p. 1007) in order to improve their levels of physical activity among and improve their overall health.

Recommendations for Future Research: The researchers noted that further inquiry should be conducted with a larger sample.

Nursing Studies

A number of current studies using both nursing and non-nursing theories as the research framework were identified. For example, a group led by Wong (Wong, Ip, Choi, & Lam, 2015) conducted a correlational study of 531 secondary school girls to examine their self-care behaviors in coping with dysmenorrhea using Orem's Self-Care Deficit Nursing Theory as the framework. In other examples, Virginia Henderson's Needs Theory was the framework to develop a study to assess the effectiveness of a "delirium prevention bundle" in decreasing the incidence of delirium in an intensive care unit (Smith & Grami, 2017), and Hart, Hardin, Townsend, and Mahrle-Henson (2013) used American Association of Colleges of Nursing (AACN) Synergy Model as the framework for their correlational study which explored the satisfaction of patient's families and nurses with visitation guidelines in the ICU. Lastly, a qualitative study that examined factors that influence health behaviors among active duty Air Force personnel was conducted by Hatzfeld, Nelson, Waters, and Jennings (2016) who interpreted the findings based on Pender's Health Promotion Model.

Non-nursing theories are frequently used as conceptual frameworks, and numerous examples are found throughout the nursing literature. For example, Richards and colleagues (2016) used the Theory of Reasoned Action (Theory of Planned Behavior) as their conceptual framework in a study of the factors involved in women's intentions to undergo contralateral prophylactic mastectomy, although they are considered to be "low risk" for developing breast cancer. Chen, Wang, and Hung (2015) used Bandura's Social Cognitive Theory as the framework for their study to identify personal and environmental factors that help predict health promotion and self-care behaviors among people with prediabetes, and Vanden Bosch, Robbins, and Anderson (2015) studied the correlates of physical activity in middle-aged women with and without diabetes using a framework that combined elements of both Social Cognitive Theory and the Theory of Planned Behavior. Finally, Tonlaar and Ayoola (2014) combined a nursing theory (Pender's Health Promotion Model) and a non-nursing theory (Bandura's Social Cognitive Theory) as the conceptual framework for their descriptive study on pregnancy intention and use of contraceptive methods among low-income women.

Nursing and Non-Nursing Theories in Nursing Research

As explained in previous chapters, there has been significant debate in the discipline of nursing regarding the source of the theories used in nursing research. Some scholars have emphasized the importance of using only nursing theories for research to ensure that what results is, indeed, nursing research. But it has also been shown that nurses depend on and use knowledge drawn from various sources in developing nursing research and that this practice does not negate the importance of the findings to nurses.

Rationale for Using Nursing Theories in Nursing Research

Some nursing theorists and nursing researchers believe that it is essential to use only nursing theories and models in nursing research. They assert that only nursing models truly deal with the scope and direction of nursing interventions; therefore, they provide a sound conceptual framework for nursing research. Additionally, their use as frameworks for research is one way of ensuring that the study will be relevant to the discipline (Fawcett & DeSanto-Madeya, 2013).

Proponents argue that conceptual models of nursing and nursing theories can be used to guide all forms of nursing research. They believe that nursing theories help nurse researchers identify the phenomena of central interest to the discipline and assist in designing studies that reflect nursing's distinctive perspective of people and their environment in matters of health. Fawcett (2000), in particular, questioned whether using a theory from another discipline resulted in nursing research, even if a nurse conducted the research. To address her concerns about using theories and concepts from other disciplines, she challenged researchers to base studies in the context of conceptual models of nursing and nursing theories.

One common criticism regarding the use of nursing models to direct research is a practice used by the editors of many nursing journals. It has been reported that if a nursing theory is used as a conceptual framework, the authors are often asked (by the journal's editors) to rewrite an article to delete the notation of the nursing theory component. Roberts (1999) concluded that it appears that "editors and reviewers of clinical specialty journals are anxious to protect the reader from nursing theory . . . to make the article more readable" (p. 300).

Concerns Over Reliance on Nursing Models to Direct Nursing Research

In response to repeated calls to focus research only on nursing theories and models, Brink (2000) wrote that many manuscripts that include a nursing theory or conceptual model treat the model or theory as an appendage. She pointed out that, in many cases, reporting of the conceptual framework consists of a single-paragraph description of the model, which often has nothing to do with the rest of the manuscript. She explained that the theory does not direct the literature review, the models, or the problem under study and never relates to the conclusions, and the author is asked to delete the paragraph. Brink argued that borrowed theories or practice theories can readily be used to describe and explain phenomena that affect nursing and concluded that to limit nurses to using only nursing theories in nursing research is shortsighted.

Tripp-Reimer (1984) described the difference between theories *of* nursing and theories *for* nursing. She believed that grand theories are theories *of* nursing and describe the nature and scope of the discipline to assist nurses in their general approach to care. On the other hand, theories *for* nursing identify what nurses should do to achieve the best client care. She noted that too often, superimposing a grand theory as a conceptual framework is confusing, and theories or concepts that are being studied do not underlie the nursing models, even though they may be congruent with them. Although the theories are congruent with the nursing models, they do not underlie the models; thus, the relationship appears forced.

Tripp-Reimer (1984) wrote that research should develop and test theories *for* nursing practice. Research should focus on testing which interventions work best with certain types of clients in specific clinical situations. This is being accomplished with the increasing interest in the development and testing of middle range nursing theories (see Chapters 10 and 11) and practice/situation-specific theories (see Chapter 12).

Other Issues in Nursing Theory and Nursing Research

To enhance understanding of the use of theory in nursing research, other issues should be addressed. Two significant issues are:

1. Recognizing the importance of adequately describing the theory in the research report
2. Examining how theory fits into the discipline's research agenda

The Research Report

To clearly illustrate the impact of the theoretical framework in developing the research study and to show the context within which the findings should be interpreted, discussion of the theoretical framework should be incorporated into several sections of the research report (Norwood, 2000). First, the framework should be introduced and briefly described in the problem statement.

Second, the framework is usually described in detail under its own heading at the end of the literature review. In this section, the description of the theory or concepts should be drawn from primary sources. The concepts should be clearly defined, and proposed relationships need to be described. A model or diagram that depicts both the framework and how it is being translated or applied to the present study may be added. Additionally, if the study is using an existing framework, the section should describe previous research application of the framework.

Third, how the framework is operationalized should be delineated in the methodology section. This will explain how the framework influences or is reflected in the study's design, data collection strategies, and data analysis methods. If an instrument has been developed for the study, the specific items that are used as indicators of the concepts in the framework need to be identified (Norwood, 2000).

Fourth, the framework needs to be referred to in the discussion section of the research report. The findings should be discussed in terms of how they illustrate, support, challenge, or contradict the framework.

Finally, suggestions for changing nursing practice or conducting further research that are consistent with the framework's concepts and propositions should be offered in the report's conclusion (Norwood, 2000). Box 20-4 presents an outline for inclusion of the theoretical framework in the research report.

Nursing's Research Agenda

There is a need for nurses to increase research that addresses significant clinical problems and adds to the knowledge base of the discipline. To accomplish this, research themes must be significant to the discipline's theory and practice, and research must

Box 20-4	Guidelines for Writing About a Research Study's Theoretical Framework

In the Study's Problem Statement

■ Introduce the framework.
■ Briefly explain why it is a good fit for the research problem area.

At the End of the Literature Review

■ Thoroughly describe the framework and explain its application to the present study.
■ Describe how the framework has been used in studies about similar problems.

In the Study's Methodology Section

■ Explain how the framework is being operationalized in the study's design.
■ Explain how data collection methods (such as questionnaire items) reflect the concepts in the framework.

In the Study's Discussion Section

■ Describe how study findings are consistent (or inconsistent) with the framework.
■ Offer suggestions for practice and further research that are congruent with the framework's concepts and propositions.

Source: Norwood (2000).

build on previous knowledge to lead to knowledge accumulation. Recommendations for future nursing research are to move beyond descriptive studies to explanatory and predictive studies, to promote study replication, and to conduct meta-analyses in areas where experimental studies have been conducted. Finally, it is important that nurses explicate the theoretical perspective of the research design in the research report to demonstrate how the study fits into the current body of knowledge.

The National Institute of Nursing Research (NINR) began as a center within the National Institutes of Health in 1986 and became an institute in 1993. The NINR supports clinical and basic research to establish a scientific basis of the care of individuals across the lifespan. This includes caring for individuals during illness and recovery, reduction of risks for disease and disability, promotion of healthy lifestyles, promotion of quality of life in those with chronic illness, and care for individuals at the end of life. Research priorities of the NINR (2011) are:

■ Enhance health promotion and disease prevention.
■ Improve quality of life by managing symptoms of acute and chronic illness.
■ Improve palliative and end-of-life care.
■ Enhance innovation in science and practice.
■ Develop the next generation of nurse scientists.

See Link to Practice 20-1 for more information.

To build the body of nursing knowledge, nurses must consider these issues from a theoretical perspective and must avoid looking at them in isolation.

In a well-supported essay, Hinshaw (2000) identified "areas of evolving nursing science" (p. 119) that should be targeted for directed nursing research (Box 20-5). These areas should receive priority attention in nursing theory and nursing research in the 21st century. Additionally, according to Hinshaw, research programs should

Link to Practice 20-1

The NINR (see www.ninr.nih.gov) provides significant funding for nursing research. Graduate students and potential nurse researchers should review the research priorities set by the NINR to understand its major areas for funding priorities. The NINR has indicated that it will invest in basic clinical and translation research to:

1. Enhance health promotion and disease prevention.

   - Develop innovative behavior interventions to promote health and prevent illness in diverse populations.
   - Study the behavior of systems that promote the development of personalized interventions.
   - Translate scientific advances to effect positive health behavioral change.

2. Improve quality of life by managing symptoms of acute and chronic illness.

   - Improve knowledge of biologic and genomic mechanisms associated with symptoms and symptom clusters.
   - Study the multiple factors that influence management of symptoms.
   - Develop strategies to assist individuals and their caregivers in managing chronic illness.

3. Improve palliative and end-of-life care.

   - Study complex issues and choices in palliative and end-of-life care.
   - Develop and test biobehavioral interventions that provide palliative care.
   - Determine the impact of providers trained in palliative and end-of-life care on health care outcomes.

4. Enhance innovation in science and practice.

   - Develop new technologies and informatics-based solutions to promote health.
   - Use genetic and genomic technologies to advance knowledge.

5. Develop the next generation of nurse scientists.

   - Support ongoing development of investigators at all stages of their research careers.
   - Facilitate more rapid advancement from student to scientist.
   - Expand research knowledge through established infrastructure (NINR, 2011).

Box 20-5   Areas of Evolving Nursing Science

- Critical health needs of communities and vulnerable populations
- Practice strategies and outcomes
- Family health and transitions
- Health promotion/risk reduction
- Biobehavioral manifestations of health and illness
- Women's health
- Health and illness of older adults
- Environments for optimizing client outcomes
- Genetics research
- End-of-life research
- Evidence-based practice

Table 20-2 Examples of Research Priorities in Nursing Practice, Nursing Administration/Management, and Nursing Education

Nursing Practice	Nursing Administration and Management	Nursing Education
Client needs related to health and illness (e.g., health promotion/illness prevention, symptom management, enhancing quality of life)	Development and evaluation of new patient care delivery models	Use of instructional technology (e.g., new approaches to laboratory and simulated learning)
Providing and testing nursing care interventions and measuring outcomes of care	Provision and maintenance of healthful work/practice environments	Development, implementation, and evaluation of new pedagogies
Evidence-based nursing practice (multiple areas)	Development of provider and patient safety guidelines	Development, implementation, and evaluation of flexible curriculum designs
Identification, prevention, and management of common health problems/threats in specific community-based settings (e.g., worksites, homes, schools)	Implementation and evaluation of use of technology to complement patient care	Development of new models for teacher preparation and faculty development
Reducing health disparities (e.g., delivery of culturally competent care, enhancing access to and utilization of health care)	Evaluation of outcomes of care related to cost effectiveness and quality	Methods for teaching evidence-based practices
Enhancing nursing care provision related to specific health problems or issues (by specialty area, setting, or other category) (e.g., pain management, reducing incidence of low–birth-weight infants, improving immunization compliance, prevention of nosocomial infection, reduction of HIV infection, prevention of lower back strain)	Program planning, implementation, and evaluation	Evaluation of processes for grading, testing, and evaluation of students, faculty, and curricula
Examination of appropriate application of genetics information and knowledge in nursing practice	Strategies to improve nurse retention and satisfaction	Strategies to enhance community-based learning and service strategies

Sources: Websites of American Association of Colleges of Nursing; American Organization of Nurse Executives; International Council of Nurses; and National League for Nursing; American Association of Operating Room Nurses.

focus on intervention research to provide a stronger, more predictable base for nursing practice.

Hinshaw (2000) also called for interdisciplinary collaboration and multidisciplinary research partners. She wrote that this will more effectively address complex problems and provide a global perspective for care. However, it is important to recognize that interdisciplinary and multidisciplinary research will necessitate familiarity with theories, concepts, and principles of other disciplines.

In addition to the research priorities listed in Box 20-5, nursing knowledge must be developed that will direct nursing practice, nursing administration and management, and nursing education. Table 20-2 gives suggestions for further research in these three areas that will be beneficial for the development of the discipline.

Summary

The relationship between research and theory is undeniable, and it is important to recognize the impact of this relationship on the development of nursing knowledge.

This chapter has provided details on the interface of theory and research and given examples of when, where, and how theory and research interface.

In the discipline of nursing, research may be theory generating or theory testing. Or, as in the opening case scenario, a theory may be used as the conceptual framework that drives the study. The source of the theory for a research study may be unique to nursing (such as using Benner's Novice to Expert Model by the student in the case scenario) or borrowed from another discipline, but the theoretical base should be explicit and appropriate.

As an evolving science, nurses should avoid research in isolation. It is imperative that nursing research respond to important questions and issues from nursing practice, administration and management, and education. This will provide a sound base of knowledge, which will further strengthen the discipline.

Key Points

- The purpose of research is to build knowledge through generation and/or testing of theory.
- Nursing research is the "scientific process that validates and refines existing knowledge and generates new knowledge that directly and indirectly influences nursing practice" (Gray et al., 2017).
- One of the essential steps of the research process is the selection of a theoretical or conceptual model that serves as a research framework.
- Several types of theory and corresponding research are commonly found in nursing. Among them are (1) descriptive theory and descriptive research, (2) explanatory theory and correlational research, and (3) predictive theory and experimental research.
- Theory is typically used in nursing research in one of three ways: (1) as an outcome or product of research (the research generates theory), (2) the research is undertaken to test a theory, and (3) theory is used as a framework or context for the research.
- Both nursing and non-nursing theories are useful in directing nursing research.
- Research priorities for nursing should include theoretical bases or foundations.

Learning Activities

1. Following the example of Peter, the nurse in the opening case study, outline a research study using a theory, a framework, or a research study that tests a theory. Determine how the theory will guide the study including definition and measurement of key terms or concepts, identification of potential relationships, and how the research will contribute to the body of nursing knowledge. Discuss the potential research with classmates.
2. Find a research article from a recent journal that purports to test a theory. Use the guidelines from Box 20-2 to evaluate the research study (see the example in Nursing Exemplar 2).
3. Find a research article from a recent nursing journal that uses a grand or middle range theory as a conceptual framework. Use the guidelines from Box 20-3 to evaluate how well the conceptual framework is used to guide the research project (see the example in Nursing Exemplar 3).

REFERENCES

Acton, G. J., Irvin, B. L., & Hopkins, B. A. (1991). Theory-testing research: Building the science. *ANS. Advances in Nursing Science, 14*(1), 52–61.

Barnum, B. S. (2005). *Nursing theory: Analysis, application, evaluation* (5th ed.). Philadelphia, PA: Lippincott Williams & Wilkins.

Barutcu, C. D., & Mert, H. (2016). Effect of support group intervention applied to the caregivers of individuals with heart failure on caregiver outcomes. *Holistic Nursing Practice, 30*(5), 272–282.

Baumhover, N. C. (2015). The process of death imminence awareness by family members of patients in adult critical care. *Dimension of Critical Care Nursing, 34*(3), 149–160.

Benner, P. (2001). *From novice to expert: Excellence and power in clinical nursing practice* (Commemorative Edition). Englewood Cliffs, NJ: Prentice Hall.

Blegen, M. A., & Tripp-Reimer, T. (1994). The nursing theory–nursing research connection. In J. C. McCloskey & H. K. Grace (Eds.), *Current issues in nursing* (4th ed., pp. 87–91). St. Louis, MO: Mosby.

Brink, P. J. (2000). A response to Fawcett. *Western Journal of Nursing Research, 22*(6), 653–655.

Chen, M. F., Wang, R. H., & Hung, S. L. (2015). Predicting health-promoting self-care behaviors in people with pre-diabetes by applying Bandura social learning theory. *Applied Nursing Research, 28*(3), 299–304.

Chinn, P. L., & Kramer, M. K. (2015). *Knowledge development in nursing: Theory and process* (9th ed.). St. Louis, MO: Elsevier.

Dickoff, J., & James, P. (1968). A theory of theories: A position paper. *Nursing Research, 17*(3), 197–203.

Dobratz, M. C. (2011). Toward development of a middle-range theory of psychological adaptation in death and dying. *Nursing Science Quarterly, 24*(4), 370–376.

Dobratz, M. C. (2016). Building a middle-range theory of adaptive spirituality. *Nursing Science Quarterly, 29*(2), 146–153.

Dossey, B. (2010). *Florence Nightingale: Mystic, visionary, healer.* Philadelphia, PA: F.A. Davis.

Dougherty, C. M., Thompson, E. A., & Kudenchuk, P. J. (2012). Development and testing of an intervention to improve outcomes for partners following receipt of an implantable cardioverter defibrillator in the patient. *ANS. Advances in Nursing Science, 35*(4), 359–377.

Fawcett, J. (2000). But is it nursing research? *Western Journal of Nursing Research, 22*(5), 524–525.

Fawcett, J., Abner, C., Haussler, S., Weiss, M., Meyers, S. T., Hall, J. L., et al. (2011). Women's perceptions of caesarean birth: A Roy international study. *Nursing Science Quarterly, 24*(40), 352–362.

Fawcett, J., & DeSanto-Madeya, S. (2013). *Contemporary nursing knowledge: Analysis and evaluation of nursing models and theories* (3rd ed.). Philadelphia, PA: F.A. Davis.

Fitzpatrick, J. J. (1998). *Encyclopedia of nursing research.* New York, NY: Springer Publishing.

Fitzpatrick, J. J., & Kazer, M. W. (2012). *Encyclopedia of nursing research* (3rd ed.). New York, NY: Springer Publishing.

Foli, K. J. (2010). Depression in adoptive parents: A model of understanding through grounded theory. *Western Journal of Nursing Research, 32*(3), 379–400.

Foli, K. J., South, S. C., & Lim, E. (2014). Maternal postadoption depression: Theory refinement through qualitative content analysis. *Journal of Research in Nursing, 19*(4), 303–327.

Ford-Gilboe, M., Merritt-Gray, M., Varcoe, C., & Wuest, J. (2011). A theory-based primary health care intervention of women who have left abusive partners. *ANS. Advances in Nursing Science, 34*(3), 198–214.

Gigliotti, E. (2004). Etiology of maternal–student role stress. *Nursing Science Quarterly, 17*(2), 156–164.

Gray, J. R., Grove, S. K., & Sutherland, S. (2017). *Burns and Grove's: The practice of nursing research: Appraisal, synthesis and generation of evidence* (8th ed.). St. Louis, MO: Elsevier.

Hardin, S. R. (2014). History and philosophy of science. In M. R. Alligood (Ed.), *Nursing theorists and their work* (8th ed., pp. 114–122). St. Louis, MO: Mosby.

Hart, A., Hardin, S. R., Townsend, A. P., & Mahrle-Henson, A. (2013). Critical care visitation: Nurse and family preferences. *Dimensions of Critical Care Nursing, 32*(6), 289–299.

Hatzfeld, J. J., Nelson, M. S., Waters, C. M., & Jennings, B. M. (2016). Factors influencing health behaviors among active duty Air Force personnel. *Nursing Outlook, 64*(5), 440–449.

Hinshaw, A. S. (2000). Nursing knowledge for the 21st century: Opportunities and challenges. *Journal of Nursing Scholarship, 32*(2), 117–123.

Hodge, D. R., Bonifas, R. P., & Wolosin, R. J. (2014). Develop a model to address African Americans' spiritual needs during hospitalization. *Clinical Gerontologist, 37*(3), 386–405.

LoBiondo-Wood, G., & Haber, J. (2014). Integrating evidence-based practice. In G. LoBiondo-Wood & J. Haber (Eds.), *Nursing research: Methods, critical appraisal, and utilization* (8th ed., pp. 5–26). St. Louis, MO: Elsevier.

McAndrew, N. S., & Leske, J. S. (2015). A balancing act: Experiences of nurses and physicians when making end-of-life decisions in intensive care units. *Clinical Nursing Research, 24*(4), 357–374.

McEwen, M. (2014). Theoretical frameworks for research. In G. LoBiondo-Wood & J. Haber (Eds.), *Nursing research: Methods, critical appraisal, and utilization* (8th ed.). St. Louis, MO: Elsevier.

McKenna, H. P., & Slevin, O. D. (2008). *Nursing models, theories and practice.* Oxford, United Kingdom: Blackwell.

Meleis, A. I. (2013). *Theoretical nursing: Development and progress* (5th ed.). Philadelphia, PA: Lippincott Williams & Wilkins.

Moody, L. E. (1990). Developing a theoretical design for research. In L. E. Moody (Ed.), *Advancing nursing science through research* (pp. 211–248). Newbury Park, CA: Sage.

National Institute of Nursing Research. (2011). *Bringing science to life: NINR strategic plan.* Retrieved from https://www.ninr.nih.gov/sites/www.ninr.nih.gov/files/ninr-strategic-plan-2011.pdf

Nazik, E., & Eryilmaz, G. (2013). The prevention and reduction of postpartum complications: Orem's model. *Nursing Science Quarterly, 26*(4), 360–364.

Norwood, S. L. (2000). *Research strategies for advanced practice nurses.* Upper Saddle River, NJ: Prentice Hall.

Norwood, S. L. (2010). *Research essentials: Foundations for evidence-based practice.* Upper Saddle River, NJ: Prentice Hall.

Ohlendorf, J. M., Weiss, M. E., & Oswald, D. (2015). Predictors of engagement in postpartum weight self-management behaviours in the first 12 weeks after birth. *Journal of Advanced Nursing, 71*(8), 1833–1846.

Polit, D. F., & Beck, C. T. (2017). *Nursing research: Generating and assessing evidence for nursing practice* (10th ed.). Philadelphia, PA: Wolters Kluwer.

Pullen, L., Modrcin, M. A., McGuire, S. L., Lane, K., Kearnely, M., & Engle, S. (2015). Anger in adolescent communities: How angry are they? *Pediatric Nursing, 41*(3), 135–143.

Reimer, A. P., & Moore, S. M. (2010). Flight nursing expertise: Towards a middle-range theory. *Journal of Advanced Nursing, 66*(5), 1183–1192.

Richards, I., Tesson, S., Porter, D., Phillips, K.-A., Rankin, N., Musiello, T., et al. (2016). Predicting women's intentions for contralateral prophylactic mastectomy: An application of an extended theory of planned behaviour. *European Journal of Oncology Nursing, 21*(1), 57–65.

Riegel, B., Jaarsma, T., & Strömberg, A. (2012). A middle-range theory of self-care of chronic illness. *ANS. Advances in Nursing Science, 35*(3), 194–204.

Roberts, K. L. (1999). Through a looking glass: Nursing theory and clinical nursing research. *Clinical Nursing Research, 8*(4), 299–301.

Rogers, C. E., Keller, C., Larkey, L. K., & Ainsworth, B. E. (2012). A randomized controlled trial to determine the efficacy of Sign Chi Do exercise on adaptation to aging. *Research in Gerontological Nursing, 5*(2), 101–113.

Roy, C. (2014). Synthesis of a middle range theory of coping. In C. Roy (Ed.), *Generating middle range theory: From evidence to practice.* New York, NY: Springer Publishing.

Scoloveno, R. (2015). A theoretical model of health-related outcomes of resilience in middle adolescents. *Western Journal of Nursing Research, 37*(3), 342–359.

Silva, M. C. (1986). Research testing nursing theory: State of the art. *ANS. Advances in Nursing Science, 9*(1), 1–11.

Smith, C. D., & Grami, P. (2017). Feasibility and effectiveness of a delirium prevention bundle in critically ill patients. *American Journal of Critical Care, 26*(1), 19–27.

Strickland, J. T., Wells, C. F., & Porr, C. (2015). Safeguarding the children: The cancer journey of young mothers. *Oncology Nursing Forum, 42*(5), 534–541.

Thomas, M. L., Elliott, J. E., Rao, S. M., Fahey, K. F., Paul, S. M., & Miaskowski, C. (2012). A randomized, clinical trial of education or motivational-interviewing-based coaching compared to usual care to improve cancer pain management. *Oncology Nursing Forum, 39*(1), 39–49.

Tonlaar, Y. J., & Ayoola, A. B. (2014). Pregnancy intention and contraceptive use among low income women. *Journal of Obstetric, Gynecologic, and Neonatal Nursing, 43*(Suppl. 1), S71–S71.

Tripp-Reimer, T. (1984). Commentaries. *Western Journal of Nursing Research, 6*(2), 195–197.

Vanden Bosch, M. L., Robbins, L. B., & Anderson, K. (2015). Correlates of physical activity in middle-aged women with and without diabetes. *Western Journal of Nursing Research, 37*(12), 1581–1603.

Whall, A. L. (2016). Philosophy of science positions and their importance in cross-national nursing. In J. J. Fitzpatrick & A. L. Whall (Eds.), *Conceptual models of nursing: Global perspectives* (5th ed., pp. 8–28). Boston, MA: Pearson.

Willis, D. G., DeSanto-Madeya, S., Ross, R., Sheehan, D. L., & Fawcett, J. (2015). Spiritual healing in the aftermath of childhood maltreatment: Translating men's lived experiences utilizing nursing conceptual models and theory. *ANS. Advances in Nursing Science, 38*(3), 162–174.

Wong, C. L., Ip, W. Y., Choi, K. C., & Lam, L. W. (2015). Examining self-care behaviors and their associated factors among adolescent girls with dysmenorrhea: An application of Oren's self-care deficit nursing theory. *Journal of Nursing Scholarship, 47*(3), 219–227.

Yarcheski, A., Mahon, N. E., & Yarcheski, T. J. (2012). A descriptive study of research published in scientific nursing journals form 1985 to 2010. *International Journal of Nursing Studies, 49*(9), 1112–1121.

21

Application of Theory in Nursing Administration and Management

Melinda Granger Oberleitner

Greta Martin is a family nurse practitioner who has been employed for several years as part of a multiphysician practice. Most of her practice has been focused on managing the care of adults with chronic illnesses, such as heart failure, arthritis, and diabetes.

Although she enjoys her work very much, Greta has always been interested in exploring one of the entrepreneurial opportunities that a career in nursing has to offer. Recently, she has focused on combining her interests in computers and technology with her expertise as an advanced practice nurse (APN). Along with several investors, she is in the process of creating an Internet-based disease management company. As envisioned, the company will focus on the needs of seniors and will engage APNs and other registered nurses (RNs) to provide clinical services and to serve as case managers for plan members diagnosed with chronic illnesses.

As she began the planning process for the project, Greta found that she had much to learn in regard to applying management and administration principles. In particular, she needed to learn more about organizational design. As the company is established, she must examine issues such as chain of command, control, authority, and responsibility. The group must determine how the company will be structured and who will be responsible for day-to-day operations.

The group is also looking at case management models to select or modify one that is appropriate for use with its anticipated clientele and the method of delivery. Finally, Greta realized that she should learn about her leadership style and develop her leadership abilities to direct the new company. Recognizing her deficiencies in administration and management, Greta sought information from a number of sources to learn about administration theories and how to apply them in her new enterprise.

Nursing practice, including advanced nursing practice, occurs within a larger context that is shaped by traditional and prevailing theories, models, and frameworks of administration and management. Even if only one nurse is employed by an organization, that nurse's practice is influenced by models and principles of leadership, management, and administration used by the leaders of the organization. To be most effective, all nurses should be able to recognize and adapt to the specific characteristics that define the organization in which she or he practices.

This chapter expands on concepts and principles presented in Chapter 17. It explores application of administration and management theories, models, and frameworks in nursing and health care. These concepts include organizational design; shared governance; transformational leadership; patient care delivery models; case management; disease/chronic illness management; quality management (QM)/performance improvement processes, tools, and techniques; and evidence-based practice (EBP).

Organizational Design

The structure of an organization provides a formal framework in which management processes occur. This formal framework historically serves many purposes, including provision of a chain of administrative command or authority that should be evident to all employees, a formal system of communication between management and staff, and a method to accomplish the work of the organization effectively and efficiently. The right structure enables the organization to reach its organizational goals.

Six elements of structure that were formulated by management theorists in the 1900s still provide a guide to the design of organizations in the 21st century. These six elements are listed in Box 21-1, and each is discussed briefly in the following sections (Robbins & Judge, 2014).

Work Specialization

Work specialization is having each step of the work process performed by a different individual rather than the whole process being done by one person. Proponents of work specialization argue that it makes the most efficient use of worker skills, attributes, and characteristics. Medication administration can be used to illustrate the concept of work specialization. Physicians determine the need for a medication order and decide on the composition of that order; hospital pharmacists then review the order and fill the prescription as directed by the physician. The nurse on the unit administers the medication ordered by the physician and prepared by the pharmacist. In the traditional hospital structure, pharmacists work in an isolated group to prepare all medications to be delivered by nurses to patients in the facility.

| Box 21-1 | Elements of Organizational Structure |

1. Work specialization
2. Chain of command
3. Span of control
4. Authority and responsibility
5. Centralization versus decentralization
6. Departmentalization

The usual configuration of APNs is an excellent representation of work specialization. For example, a certified registered nurse anesthetist (CRNA) would not be considered interchangeable with a certified nurse midwife (CNM) because of the obvious degree of work specialization in the two roles. Both the CRNA and the CNM are educationally prepared as experts in a specific specialty area and are not considered generalists.

In recent years, recognition that work specialization can contribute to boredom, low productivity, and poor quality has led to a reexamination of the concept. In many cases, this has resulted in assigning employees a variety of activities to accomplish and encouraging employees to work in teams. In some hospitals, a clinical pharmacist is part of a team of health care workers assigned to accomplish the work of the unit and resides, along with the traditional nursing staff, on the clinical unit. Some unit-based clinical pharmacists engage in tasks, such as medication administration, which was once considered the exclusive domain of nursing.

Chain of Command

Fayol (1949), Weber (1970), and Taylor (1911) (see Chapter 17) advocated that an employee should be administratively responsible to, or report to, only one supervisor. This arrangement is termed *the chain of command*. Chain of command refers to formal lines of communication and authority and can usually be determined by looking at an organizational chart. However, as organizations have become increasingly complex, individuals in organizations may find themselves administratively responsible to more than one individual (Mancini, 2015).

Although the nurse working on the 7 pm to 7 am shift in the intensive care unit (ICU) is ultimately administratively responsible to the ICU director, there is usually a different chain of command on the night shift; this may include the night charge nurse and the night house supervisor.

Similarly, APNs in today's health care organizations may be administratively responsible to a variety of individuals, some of whom may not be nurses, such as product or service line managers. Some APNs may also assume managerial roles, as in the case of a CRNA who is administratively in charge of a group of nurse anesthetists.

Span of Control

The third element of management, span of control, can also be determined from the organizational chart. Span of control refers to the number of employees directed by a manager (Mancini, 2015). The classical management theorists recommended narrow spans of control for workers performing complex jobs. There is no consensus regarding the optimal number of employees one manager should have in his or her span of control—suggested ranges are from 3 to 50 employees. Several contingencies play a role in the variability of the range of numbers of employees in span of control. These contingencies include the quality and experience of the manager, the abilities and maturity of the employees, the complexity of the task, and, in some cases, the geographic location of the work setting. Research results indicate a significant level of improvement in nurse engagement when the manager is responsible for 50 or fewer direct reports (Cathcart et al., 2004). Wider spans of control in health care organizations have been shown to produce negative effects on effective leadership styles and are detrimental to staff and patient satisfaction (Meyer et al., 2011).

Recent decrease in reimbursement levels for health care services has resulted in restructuring and downsizing in health care institutions. In some organizations, this has led to the elimination or decrease in nurse manager positions and increased span of control for retained managers (Wong et al., 2015). The expanded nurse manager role in acute care facilities includes significant financial, operational, and human resources responsibilities for professional, multidisciplinary, and unlicensed employees in one or more service lines.

Research on effects of increasing spans of control for nurse managers include serious negative consequences on nurse turnover rates, staff empowerment, and time for professional development of staff, which in turn can have deleterious impacts on patient care and patient satisfaction. For example, Havaei, Dahinten, and MacPhee (2015) examined the influence of perceived organizational support, which was defined as employees' perceptions of how much they are valued by the organization, span of control, and leadership rank on the organizational commitment of nurse leaders who were considered to be novices. They determined that organizational support is linked to nurse satisfaction and loyalty to the organization; the higher the perceived support from the organization by the nurse, especially in times of downsizing or restructuring, the higher the satisfaction with and loyalty to the work institution by the nurse. In addition, organizational support also positively influenced organizational commitment.

Factors which should be considered when contemplating altering managerial span of control on nursing units include skill mix and expertise of the unit staff, duties of first-level managers (i.e., charge nurses) when the middle-level manager is not present, potential savings in salary expenses, and impact on nurse turnover and on nurse and patient satisfaction (Havaei et al., 2015; Jones, McLaughlin, Gebbens, & Terhorst, 2015). Link to Practice 21-1 presents how one health care organization developed a tool to measure aspects of span of control and its effects.

Link to Practice 21-1

Measuring Scope and Span of Control

Nurse administrators affiliated with the University of Pittsburgh Medical Center, an integrated health system composed of 22 hospitals, developed a measurement tool to determine the varying scope and span of control of nurse managers in their system. Implementation of the tool has enabled collection of quantifiable data in five areas central to the nurse manager role: head count, department workload, hours of operation, number of cost centers, and controllable expenses exclusive of salaries. Outcomes associated with implementation included a significant decrease in nurse manager separation rates and transfer of nurse managers out of leadership roles by the end of the first year of implementation, recognition that the nurse manager role should be compensated comparably to others on the leadership pay structure in the organization, and the recognition that "scope creep" occurs as additional responsibilities are added to the nurse manager roles.

Jones, D., McLaughlin, M., Gebbens, C., & Terhorst, L. (2015). Utilizing a scope and span of control tool to measure workload and determine supporting resources for nurse managers. *The Journal of Nursing Administration, 45*(5), 243–249.

Authority and Responsibility

Line authority and *staff authority* are two distinctions that describe formal relationships in an organization. When looking at an organizational chart, line authority refers to chain of command, superior–subordinate, and leader–follower relationships. For example, the chief nursing officer (CNO) delegates authority to the unit manager, who then delegates to a subordinate, the charge nurse. The command relationship is a direct "line" between supervisor and subordinate.

In larger organizations, managers can be designated as top-level, middle-level, or first-level managers. Top-level managers include the organization's chief executive officer (CEO) and the highest nursing administrator. Middle-level managers, as the name implies, coordinate management activities between the top management level and first-level managers. Middle-level managers are usually involved in long-range planning and in policy decisions that affect one unit or multiple units. This manager is usually responsible for day-to-day activities of the units. Titles in nursing that represent middle-level managers include nurse managers, unit managers, unit directors, and unit supervisors. First-level managers are assigned to one unit and are concerned with that specific unit's work. First-level managers, such as charge nurses, team leaders, and primary care nurses, are crucial to the success of the unit's work. APNs are most often administratively responsible to either top-level or middle-level managers. APNs who assume administrative responsibilities in the organization may be top-level or middle-level managers.

In some organizations, APNs are in *staff* positions as opposed to *line* positions. Staff authority supports the work of the line manager without having any line authority or responsibility. Employees in staff positions support, assist, and advise those in line authority positions. In a staff position, the APN is not responsible for the hiring, firing, directing, or disciplining of other employees. This lack of authority could be a disadvantage to the APN in accomplishing the tasks of the role because the APN often must work through others to accomplish goals. Even when the APN is in a staff position, the APN is responsible to a line manager, who is either a top-level or middle-level manager.

Centralization Versus Decentralization

Centralization and *decentralization* are degrees of how decision making is dispersed or diffused throughout the organization. In organizations with centralized decision making, decisions are made by one individual or a small group of individuals at the top of the organizational structure. Decentralization refers to decision making that occurs at the lowest levels feasible. Most of today's organizations are really neither totally centralized nor decentralized but are a combination of the two. With the advent of performance improvement initiatives over the past 30 to 40 years, the trend in American organizations has been toward decentralization in an effort to involve employees directly responsible for the work product in the decision-making process. In nursing, organizational designs, such as shared governance, have gained popularity as a method to empower and engage staff in the decision-making process.

Departmentalization

The primary purpose of *departmentalization* is to subdivide the work of the organization so that specialization of the work can be accomplished. Departmentalization emphasizes specialization of skills. Hospitals have historically implemented departmentalization with traditional departments, such as central supply, pastoral care, and patient care departments, among others. A typical manufacturing plant, although different from a hospital, is probably organized in much the same way as the hospital. For example, both probably have marketing, accounting, and human resources departments. Grouping activities in this manner is known as functional departmentalization.

Other types of departmentalization include product, customer, geographic, and process departmentalization. Today, hospitals and other organizations use cross-disciplinary teams to accomplish the organization's performance initiatives that transcend traditional departmental boundaries to better focus on customer needs (Robbins & Judge, 2014).

Shared Governance

Shared governance is "a structural model through which nurses can express and manage their own practice with a higher level of professional autonomy" (Porter-O'Grady, 2003, p. 251). Nursing shared governance, an organizational structure and process, was introduced in the late 1970s as an alternative to traditional or industrial bureaucratic organizational design (Laschinger & Finegan, 2005). In this design, professional nurses use self-directed work teams at the unit level to make professional practice decisions and to accomplish the work of the unit.

Porter-O'Grady, Hawkins, and Parker (1997) described the major components of shared governance as the creation of partnerships, equity, accountability, and ownership. Much of the effort directed at restructuring the nursing organization to implement shared governance was done to empower nurses to join with each other and with other health care decision makers to better confront issues affecting the practice of professional nursing. In the shared governance model, staffs, not managers, are empowered to make patient care decisions at the staff level (Mancini, 2015).

Implementation of shared governance is usually accompanied by the simultaneous implementation of participation and decentralization. Participation and decentralization are not substitutes for shared governance and should not be used synonymously with the term *shared governance*. Participative models call for employees to be involved in the decisions that involve them. However, management still determines the breadth and depth of employee participation. Decentralization allows employees at lower levels of the hierarchical structure to have greater involvement in decision making and to have some authority to implement the decisions, but management usually retains the real authority and power in terms of which decisions are to be implemented. In short, both participation and decentralization rely on management discretion to determine the amount of employee involvement in decision making, whereas shared governance does not (Marquis & Huston, 2012).

Nursing shared governance models have always focused on nurses controlling their professional practice. To be able to control practice, nurses must have control over resources that impact professional practice and they must also have influence over themselves as a professional group (Bieber & Joachim, 2016; Mancini, 2015).

Porter-O'Grady (2012) advanced the idea that in order for true interprofessional team-based models of accountability to thrive in health services organizations, five principles govern the practice and relationships of the teams and are needed to sustain shared governance:

- Professions are driven by practice and practitioners—the locus of control for decision making in terms of what constitutes professional practice, quality, competence, and knowledge generation must be retained by the practitioner. The farther away the decision making is from the knowledge worker (the professional), the lower the decision quality and the higher the cost of the decision.

- Structure is key—there must be direct alignment between organizational structure and intended behaviors and outcomes. Organizational structures that are ineffective in producing the most effective outcomes for knowledge workers such as RNs include traditional bureaucratic structures such as vertical, hierarchical structures in which management has ultimate control of decision and policy making.
- Accountability is central to professional practice—true accountability by professionals can only thrive in environments in which the organizational structure is such that accountability is within the control of the practitioner at the point of practice.
- Control of accountability must be purposefully designed into the shared governance structure—shared governance facilitates distributive decision making. In a true shared governance model, practitioners retain control over professional practice—not management.
- Leadership by management is crucial to the effectiveness of shared governance—the competencies of managers and leaders in shared organization are different than in traditional organizations. These competencies include distributive decision making, effective servant leadership, and assisting practice peers to create work environments in which knowledge workers can practice to the fullest extent (Porter-O'Grady, 2012).

Three general models of shared governance are:

1. Councilor model—the most common model; utilizes a coordinating council to integrate decisions made by staff and managers in subcommittees that report to the coordinating council
2. Administrative model—the organizational chart is split to resemble two tracks—a management track and a clinical track; membership in both tracks includes managers and staff
3. Congressional model—uses a democratic process to empower nurses to vote on issues

Structure of the models is not important; what is important is control over practice that leads to improved patient, nurse, and organizational outcomes (Anthony, 2004; Bieber & Joachim, 2016).

Research-based studies have attempted to evaluate the outcomes of shared governance from the perspectives of the organization, the nurse, and the patient. From an organizational perspective, in general, research supports the finding of an improved financial posture for the organization after implementation of shared governance. The improved finances stem from either cost savings or cost reductions. Reported examples of cost savings and reductions range from a decrease in overall meeting time for staff to multimillion dollar reductions in the use of temporary or agency nurses once shared governance has been fully implemented. Research studies indicate implementation of shared governance has resulted in improving the work environment of nurses, which leads to increased nurse satisfaction and ultimately to improved nurse retention (Joseph & Bogue, 2016).

In one recent example, Kutney-Lee and team (2016) examined the relationships between shared governance, specifically nurse engagement, and impact on nurse and patient outcomes in 425 nonfederal acute care hospitals in the United States. They determined that hospitals which provide nurses with the ability to be the most actively involved in institutional decision making are more likely to be institutions in which nurses cultivate better patient experiences resulting in superior levels of care and increased patient and nurse satisfaction levels. Indeed, increased nurse engagement in institutional decision making is critical in an era focused on value-based purchasing and cost containment. It also has strong impact on the health care institution's financial picture in terms of significant losses, financial and other, associated with nurse turnover.

Detractors of the shared governance model point to the expense of introducing and maintaining the model, the longer time it takes to arrive at decisions using the model, and the fact that not all nurses want to have a role in decision making or want accountability for decisions.

Transformational Leadership in Nursing and in Health Care

Historically, nursing and health care organizations were built on old paradigm beliefs of hierarchical structures with an emphasis on rationality and logical decision making. The old paradigm is evolving to a new paradigm that values mutuality, affiliation, co-operation, networking, and an emphasis on human relations. In nursing, the shift has led to decentralization, participative management and decision making, and shared governance.

In transformational leadership, the leader and the follower have the same purpose. Barker (1994) proposed that it is easier to study the *results* of transformational leadership than the *process*. Transformational leadership is moral and philosophical leadership rather than technical leadership. Bennis and Nanus (1985) conceptualized four strategies for transformational leadership: (1) creating a vision, (2) building a social architecture that provides the framework for generating commitment to the vision and for establishing an organizational identity, (3) developing and sustaining organizational trust, and (4) attending to the self-esteem of others in the organization. Cottingham (1988) proposed six strategies for a transformational leader (Box 21-2).

Porter-O'Grady (1992) suggested that transformational nursing leaders should focus on relationships and develop personal skills such as paradigm assessment, process ambiguity, staff decision making, and shared governance. Transformational leadership is not leading and controlling; rather, it is coordinating, integrating, and facilitating. Transformational leaders should strive to build coalitions and networks among

---

Box 21-2   Strategies for a Transformational Leader

Know the people you work with: Find out about their interests outside of the work environment; be visible and accessible.

Help people to learn and develop: Expose them to new ideas and methods; encourage attendance at seminars to help team members learn as much as possible about their roles.

Provide frequent feedback about performance: Give feedback quickly rather than waiting for a formal evaluation meeting. Feedback should be specific enough to enable the person to correct deficiencies; criticism should be positive rather than negative.

Award responsibility and status to coworkers: Give them the opportunity to participate in work projects that will allow for growth and increased responsibility. Recognize the potential in others and give them the opportunity to realize that potential.

Reward coworkers for a job well done: Monetary rewards should be as high as possible within the framework of the organization.

Make information available to all involved: Involve coworkers in decision making and problem solving and support their efforts.

disciplines and departments by bringing diverse groups together toward a shared vision or goal while at the same time managing the complexity of the organization.

One essential element of the Magnet recognition model is evidence of transformational leadership in the organization. Clavelle, Drenkard, Tullai-McGuinness, and Fitzpatrick (2012) explored leadership practices of CNOs in Magnet facilities. The results of this study revealed increased education and experience of the CNO was positively correlated with transformational leadership characteristics. Older CNOs and those with doctoral degrees scored significantly higher in the transformational leadership practices of inspiring a shared vision and challenging the process. Key practices identified by the study were enabling others to act and modeling the way for others.

In a recently published work, Fischer (2016) analyzed the concept of transformational leadership and provided defining attributes specific to the nursing context. She identified a set of competencies associated with it. These competencies are emotional intelligence, communication, collaboration, coaching, and mentoring. Application of competencies provides a foundation for developing transformational leaders for practice and in academic environments.

Patient Care Delivery Models

Nursing care in the acute care setting is delivered most often utilizing a group practice model. The group practice model provides the structure and context for the delivery of care. Practice models range from those that are based on patient assignments (such as team nursing), accountability systems (primary nursing), and managed care (case management) to models that are designed to incorporate professional practice concepts of autonomy, decision making, participation, and professional values (shared governance model) (Anthony, 2004; Marquis & Huston, 2012).

Assignment systems for nursing staff or patient care delivery models change in response to changing needs. For example, in the 1920s, the *case method* and *private duty nursing* models of total patient care were the systems most often implemented. By the 1950s, *functional nursing* was introduced as a response to a shortage of nurses. *Team* or *modular nursing* was also introduced in the 1950s to capitalize on the expertise of professional nurses and to use nonprofessional team members in the provision of nursing care. *Primary nursing*, a shift back to care of individual patients by professional nurses, was commonly used in the 1960s and 1970s. The method that has most recently appeared in the literature is *patient-focused care* (PFC).

Each of the delivery methods has inherent advantages and disadvantages. These patient care delivery methods are used primarily in hospitals, but they can be adapted for use in other settings. Factors to consider prior to implementation of a particular method or system include type and acuity of patients, complexity of the tasks to be performed, availability or supply of RNs, skill and expertise of the staff, and the economic resources of the organization.

Total Patient Care (Functional Nursing)

Total patient care, the oldest delivery method, was accomplished by nurses in the home and hospital settings. Most of the patients were assigned to nurses as cases; one nurse attended to all of the patient's needs during the course of the nurse's shift. The major disadvantage of this method is cost, particularly in times of nursing shortages.

Evolving as a result of the nursing shortage that occurred during World War II, the functional method of providing patient care was derived from the principles of scientific management, that is, emphasis on efficiency, division of labor, and rigid controls (Marriner-Tomey, 2009). In this method, the patient's physical needs are attended to primarily by unlicensed workers (i.e., nursing aides), with RNs responsible primarily for managerial functions. The focus of this method was on the completion of certain tasks, such as administering medication or performing treatments, rather than on meeting all of the needs of the patient by one nurse, as was accomplished in total patient care methods (Sportsman, 2015).

Although patient care appears to be delivered efficiently and there would appear to be little confusion regarding responsibilities for tasks and assignments with this method, functional nursing has several disadvantages. These disadvantages include the need for greater coordination of care, fragmentation of care, the majority of care being provided by nonprofessional and unlicensed workers, de-emphasis on the psychological needs of the patient, and the repetitive nature of the work. In times of nursing shortages, health care administrators often return to a hybrid of functional nursing, including the use of unlicensed health care workers or unlicensed assistive personnel (UAP) (Marquis & Huston, 2012; Sportsman, 2015).

Team Nursing

Team nursing was developed after World War II in an effort to alleviate the fragmented care associated with functional care. In the team nursing approach, a professional or technical nurse is the team leader of a group of other health care workers that may include other professional and technical nurses and unlicensed personnel such as nursing assistants. The team is responsible for the provision of care to a group of patients on a nursing unit.

The team leader is the coordinator of the group and is responsible for assigning team members to specific patient assignments. The team leader may or may not have a patient assignment. The team leader is responsible for knowing about the conditions and needs of all of the patients assigned to the team and for communicating with physicians. Duties that cannot be performed by other team members because of lack of skill, expertise, or licensure are performed by the team leader. Team members report to the team leader, who in turn reports to the unit manager.

Advantages of team nursing are the democratic nature of the method, the focus on the entire patient rather than on specific tasks to be accomplished, the autonomy provided to the team to accomplish the work, and increased satisfaction with the method by workers and patients. Disadvantages of team nursing include the high degree of coordination and planning required and the dependence on the unique skills of the team leader to make the concept work efficiently and effectively. Team nursing has rarely been implemented in its purest form. Instead, a combination of team and functional nursing has most frequently been implemented (Marquis & Huston, 2012).

Primary Nursing

Primary nursing was initiated in the late 1960s and early 1970s in response to professional nurses who decried the lack of personal contact with patients and who were unhappy with the provision of fragmented care. Primary nursing uses some of the concepts on which total patient care was based (i.e., during work hours, the primary nurse, an RN, would be responsible for planning care and providing total patient care to a group of patients). When the primary nurse was not on duty, an associate nurse (another RN) would provide care to the patients based on a care plan developed by the primary nurse. However, the primary nurse retained responsibility for the assigned patient load 24 hours a day while the patient was hospitalized (Sportsman, 2015).

Job satisfaction is high in primary nursing because of the high degree of autonomy and responsibility afforded to the primary nurse. Continuity of care is greatly facilitated by the primary nursing model. Disadvantages to primary nursing include the number of RNs required to implement primary nursing and the high degree of coordination and professional nursing expertise required for the role. Primary nurses who are inadequately trained or incompetent to implement the role may be incapable of fulfilling the primary nurse role.

Patient-Focused Care/Patient-Centered Care

The PFC model was developed in an effort to decrease the cost of providing health care while improving the quality of the service and was focused on the inpatient care experience (Myers, 1998). The principles of PFC are derived from total QM/continuous quality improvement (QI) in that PFC brings patient care needs as close as possible to the bedside. A goal of PFC is to decrease the number of health care workers needed while simultaneously increasing the time nurses would have to spend with patients. Theoretically, the cost of care should decrease while quality of care increases.

Mang (1995) described principles of implementation of PFC. These principles are summarized in Box 21-3 and are discussed briefly in the following text. *Patient redeployment* involves placing patients with similar needs and diagnoses in the same geographic location. The optimal number of patients with similar needs and diagnoses on a unit should be between 50 and 100 to create an economy of scale and to ensure predictable census and workload. *Decentralization of support services* refers to relocation of ancillary services (i.e., pharmacy, radiology, admissions, and laboratory) closer to the patient to allow for more efficient use of personnel.

Creation of *multiskilled workers*, or cross-trained workers, is accomplished by combining appropriate types of tasks. For example, the multiskilled worker would be responsible for housekeeping, food service, and other unskilled tasks for a group of patients. The goal of creating the multiskilled worker is to decrease the number of workers the typical patient comes in contact with by up to 75% (Clouten & Weber, 1994).

Now a key indicator of high-quality care as defined by the Institute of Medicine (IOM), patient-focused, patient-centered care evolved into a model in which patients and families are active participants in decision making about care. Four concepts are associated with contemporary patient- and family-centered care models: dignity and respect, information sharing, participation, and collaboration (Johnson et al., 2008). Indeed, in this model, patients must be well informed and included in all decision making related to the plan of care. In addition, *task simplification* would be applied to every aspect of the patient's care to allow for greater efficiency and time savings, which results in earlier discharge for the patient.

Box 21-3   Principles of Patient-Focused Care

- Patient redeployment
- Support services decentralization
- Worker cross-training
- Creation of multidisciplinary teams
- Patient involvement
- Task simplification

The goals of PFC are to (1) transform the health care organization into a customer-focused organization; (2) improve continuity of care for patients; (3) improve professional relationships among doctors, nurses, and other caregivers; (4) minimize the movement of patients throughout hospitals; (5) increase the proportion of direct care activities as compared to other activities in the organization; (6) reconfigure the clinical environment to truly meet the needs of the patients; and (7) empower direct caregivers to plan and implement work in ways that are most responsive to the needs of patients (Zarubi, Reiley, & McCarter, 2008). The results of studies evaluating the PFC model indicate that patient and staff satisfaction improve after implementation of PFC, as does physician satisfaction in relationship with nursing staff. In terms of savings, some institutions reported a decrease in time of the admission process, a decrease in inventory, and an improvement in costs. Quality indicators, such as direct patient care time, patient satisfaction, continuity of care, and nosocomial infection rates, revealed positive trends after implementation of PFC.

Some health care organizations have extended the patient- and family-centered care model by engaging former patients and family members in an advisory capacity to assist the organization with patient satisfaction, quality, and safety concerns (Cunningham & Walton, 2016; Warren, 2012). These advisors relate their experiences from past care encounters in the organization or facility with the goal of improving the care experiences of other patients and families in the future. Patient and family advisors have assisted health care facilities with making changes to policies, the physical environment, and aspects of clinical care delivery as well as with staff education and development.

There is considerable interest in patient- and family-centered care models as a result of provisions of the Patient Protection and Affordable Care Act (ACA). These models focus on patient satisfaction and which have the potential to significantly impact reimbursement for care provided in health care organizations. For example, The Hospital Consumer Assessment of Healthcare Providers and Systems (HCAHPS) initiative provides a mechanism for health care facilities to benchmark patient satisfaction trends in their facilities with expected national outcomes; outcomes are tied to financial incentives for health care institutions (Cropley, 2012). Implementation of patient- and family-centered care models may lead to improved patient/family experiences, which results in increased satisfaction scores and financial incentives for the institution providing the care.

Also included in provisions of the 2010 ACA, the Patient-Centered Outcomes Research Institute (PCORI) was established to fund research efforts focused on comparing patient-centered clinical effectiveness research. A central tenet of PCORI is that including the patient perspective in health research is valuable and should result in the acceleration of the integration of research findings into clinical practice to the ultimate benefit of patients (Frank, Basch, & Selby, 2014).

Use of Patient Care Delivery Models Today

Rarely do pure forms of any of the patient care delivery methods described earlier exist in practice today. Typically, components of several of the methods, or a combination of the methods, are used to accomplish patient care. Delivery methods usually differ between inpatient and outpatient areas and from unit to unit, depending on the nature of the patient care unit and the skill mix of the licensed and unlicensed staff assigned to the unit.

The Nursing Work Index-Revised (Aiken & Patrician, 2000) has been used to measure attributes of the work environment of professional nurses that support professional clinical practice. These attributes include organizational support for nursing practice, specifically, adequacy of resources to support the practice of professional nursing, including adequate RN staffing, autonomy for nurses, nurse control of nursing practice, and collegial nurse–physician relationships. When these attributes are present to a sufficient degree, nurse job satisfaction is higher and burnout rates and physical disability rates are lower. Improved patient-related outcomes such as decreased adverse events, lower mortality, and higher levels of patient satisfaction with care are noted.

Aiken, Clarke, Sloane, Sochalski, and Silber (2002) were some of the earliest researchers to explicate the evidence linking nurse staffing to patient outcomes. In a study based on an analysis of outcomes of many thousands of patients in 168 Pennsylvania hospitals over a 20-month period, risk of death following common surgical procedures increased by 7% for each patient added to the nurse's workload over a nurse-to-patient ratio of 1:4. The result is that nurses employed by hospitals which enforce large patient loads are significantly less likely to save the life of a patient who develops a serious complication. In addition, increased needlestick injuries for nurses, increased patient and family complaints, falls with injuries, medication errors, and hospital-acquired infections are more likely to occur when the nurse-to-patient ratio is higher (Aiken, Clarke, & Sloane, 2002; Cho, Ketefian, Barkauskas, & Smith, 2003).

Higher patient-to-nurse ratios are also associated with increased emotional exhaustion, turnover intention, and job dissatisfaction (Gabriel, Erickson, Moran, Diefendorff, & Bromley, 2013). Recently, Cimiotti, Aiken, Sloane, and Wu (2012) documented a significant association between patient-to-nurse ratio and incidence of urinary tract and surgical site infections. When using a statistical model that controlled for patient severity and nurse and hospital characteristics, only RN burnout was significantly associated with urinary tract and surgical site infections. These findings become even more significant when examined in light of provisions associated with the Patient Protection and Accountable Care Act, which included loss of reimbursement to health care organizations for facility-acquired conditions such as urinary tract and surgical site infections (Andel, Davidow, Hollander, & Moreno, 2012).

In 1999, California became the first state in the United States to pass legislation to enforce minimum nurse staffing levels in hospitals to improve the quality of care for patients. Spetz (2008) conducted a study to examine whether nurses who work in hospitals in California were more satisfied with staffing levels and other job attributes since minimum staffing levels were enacted. The results indicated that nurse satisfaction did increase between 2004 and 2006.

Other studies failed to substantiate a relationship between increased nurse staffing levels and improved patient outcomes (Burnes Bolton et al., 2007; Donaldson et al., 2005; Hickey, Gauvreau, Jenkins, Fawcett, & Hayman, 2011). However, a study conducted by Aiken and colleagues (2010) concluded that mandatory staffing levels in California were associated with lower patient mortality and with improved nurse retention. Furthermore, Tellez and Seago (2013) explored the effect of California's minimum staffing legislation on changes to the California RN workforce, particularly the direct care nurse in the acute care setting, and concluded there was improvement in nurse satisfaction.

In a final example, Aiken and colleagues (2011) attempted to determine the conditions under which the impact of three variables—nurse–patient staffing ratios, nurse educational level, and work environment—are associated with patient outcomes, such as inpatient mortality rate and failure-to-rescue rates.

The results of this study revealed that lowering the patient-to-nurse ratio by one patient per nurse in hospitals with good work environments significantly improved patient outcomes, slightly improved outcomes in hospitals with average practice environments, but had no effect in hospitals with poor environments. Increasing by 10% the numbers of nurses with the bachelor of science in nursing (BSN) degree led to a 4% decrease in patient death, which confirms previous findings by Aiken, Clarke, Cheung, Sloane, and Silber (2003).

According to the American Nurses Association (2015), as of December 2015, 14 states (California, Connecticut, Illinois, Maryland, Minnesota, Nevada, New Jersey, New York, Ohio, Oregon, Rhode Island, Texas, Vermont, and Washington) have enacted legislation specific to nurse staffing levels. Attempts to enact legislation at the federal level to require staffing plans based on unit needs and RN-to-patient staffing ratios have been unsuccessful to date.

American Nurses Credentialing Center Magnet Recognition Program

The Magnet Recognition Program originated as a result of a 1983 landmark policy study (McClure, Poulin, Sovie, & Wandelt, 1983) conducted by the American Academy of Nursing to identify characteristics common to hospitals with environments of nurse recruitment and retention. At that time, during a national nursing shortage, 41 hospitals became the focus of intensive research efforts. The characteristics identified were referred to as the "Forces of Magnetism" (Wolf, Triolo, & Ponte, 2008).

The Magnet Recognition Program was developed by the American Nurses Credentialing Center (ANCC) in the early 1990s to recognize health care organizations that provide exemplary nursing care and that uphold the traditions within nursing of professional nursing practice. The program also serves as a method or means to disseminate successful best practices and strategies in nursing among institutions. Magnet hospitals have incorporated proven solutions to address nurse recruitment and retention and to foster nursing leadership (Clavelle, Porter O'Grady, & Drenkard, 2013).

After undergoing some research-based modifications to the program in 2005 (Triolo, Scherer, & Floyd, 2006; Wolf et al., 2008), the model for Magnet was adopted in 2008. The new model consolidated the 14 Forces of Magnetism into five components which lead to empirically derived, quality outcomes. Overarching the five components is the concept of global issues in nursing and health care. The five components are presented in Box 21-4 (ANCC, 2008).

The Magnet Recognition Program is based on quality indicators and standards of nursing practice as originally defined in the American Nurses Association's (2004) *Scope and Standards for Nurse Administrators.* The Magnet designation process includes the appraisal of both qualitative and quantitative factors in nursing. As of mid 2017, a total of 469 health care organizations in the United States, as well as 3 organizations in Australia, 1 in Canada, 1 in Lebanon, and 2 in Saudi Arabia, have achieved Magnet designation (ANCC, 2017).

Box 21-4   Components of the Magnet Model

- Transformational leadership
- Structural empowerment
- Exemplary professional nursing practice
- New knowledge, innovations, and improvements
- Empirical quality results

Considerable research has been done on the effect of the Magnet designation. Indeed, when compared to non-Magnet hospitals, Magnet hospitals have:

- Better patient outcomes and lower mortality rates (McHugh et al., 2013)
- Reduced incidence of hospital-acquired pressure ulcers (Ma & Park, 2015)
- Lower central line-associated bloodstream infection rates (Barnes, Rearden, & McHugh, 2016)
- Lower nurse turnover rates (Park, Gass, & Boyle, 2016)
- Better overall working environment (Clavelle et al., 2013)
- More involvement in decision making by staff nurses (Houston et al., 2012)

Lastly, Stimpfel, Sloane, McHugh, and Aiken (2016) examined the relationship between nursing excellence, with Magnet recognition as an indicator of excellence, and patients' experiences as reported in the HCAHPS. The results of this study indicated that patients admitted to Magnet hospitals rated their overall experiences higher, had more favorable perceptions of their communications with nurse caregivers, and were more likely to recommend the hospital to others. These findings are important because patient experience ratings are integral and significant in determining financial incentives and reimbursements to health care facilities under value-based purchasing initiatives endorsed by the Centers for Medicare & Medicaid Services (CMS) and support a business case for Magnet recognition (Jayawardhana, Welton, & Lindrooth, 2014).

Case Management

The Case Management Society of America (CMSA) defines *case management* as "a collaborative process that assesses, plans, implements, coordinates, monitors, and evaluates options and services to meet an individual's health needs through communication and available resources to promote quality cost-effective outcomes" (Yamamoto & Lucey, 2005). Case management is a role developed in the late 1980s and early 1990s in response to the prospective payment system and diagnosis-related groups (DRGs). An expansion of the total patient care system, case management originated in outpatient settings. For example, community and public health nurses carry a caseload of patients for which they plan, coordinate, and evaluate care. Rarely do these nurses implement the care personally; however, they retain responsibility for patient outcomes.

As a result of the proliferation of managed care in hospitals, case management was also adopted in inpatient facilities, which is sometimes referred to as "within the walls" case management (Yamamoto & Lucey, 2005). Most inpatient case management systems are based on one of two models: the New England Medical Center Model, which focuses primarily on managing patient care to control resources, or the St. Mary's (or Carondelet) Model, in which the role of the case manager is to control or lower costs associated with patient stays while simultaneously reducing the length of stay and producing optimal patient outcomes (Sportsman, 2015).

The minimal recommended educational requirement for nurse case manager roles is the baccalaureate degree in nursing. However, although not all case managers may need to perform case management duties at the advanced level, many organizations prefer advanced educational preparation and specialization for nurses in the role of case manager. Advantages of the APN as opposed to the BSN in the case management role include recognition of the APN as expert practitioner, change agent, researcher, manager, teacher, and consultant.

Although case management implementation varies from institution to institution and location to location, one variation is to assign a case manager to a group of high-risk patients within a specific population. For example, one hospital, health care organization, or insurance company may have case managers in pediatrics, neuroscience, oncology, cardiovascular, orthopedics, and other specialty areas. The case manager does not coordinate the care of all the patients in a specialty. Instead, coordination of care by a case manager occurs only for those patients who have been designated as "high risk" because of age, comorbidities, and other factors that would place that patient at risk for greater consumption of resources or prolonged length of stay.

Ideally, the case manager coordinates the care of the patient from preadmission to the time of discharge and perhaps beyond discharge. This coordination of care requires interdisciplinary collaboration and cooperation. The case manager's role in this model transcends geographic or unit boundaries. The neuroscience case manager, for example, may first meet the patient in the neurosurgery clinic or at the neurosurgeon's office and would play a role in coordinating preadmission testing. Following surgery, the case manager would track the progress of the patient from the ICU, to an intermediate care unit, to the neurology floor, and then to a rehabilitation unit if required. The case manager would then be involved in establishing postdischarge home care if necessary (Sportsman, 2015).

Case managers are employed not only by hospitals but also by health maintenance organizations (HMOs), other managed care organizations (MCOs), insurance companies, and disease management companies. Case managers serve as the liaison between patients and families, health plans, care providers, and purchasers to determine the extent of coverage and probable costs and to coordinate treatment at a lower cost and outside of inpatient care if possible.

As an example of the integral role that case managers play in coordinating care outside of inpatient facilities, a joint venture between Banner Health and Blue Cross Blue Shield of Arizona Advantage provides at least one home visit by a case manager for members who qualify for case management services. Patients who qualify for the visits are typically no longer eligible for home health and are recovering at home from major conditions or chronic illnesses such as stroke, heart attack, heart failure, and/or chronic obstructive pulmonary disease (COPD). The program also targets individuals who were admitted following fractures and related health problems resulting from a fall. The home visit is focused on conducting a home assessment to decrease the client's risk for subsequent falls. The primary goal of the home visit initiative is to reduce readmission rates into acute care facilities. Since the program was established, readmission rates for all age groups have dropped by 13% (AHC Media, 2013). Although RNs constitute the largest professional group in case management, the role is becoming increasingly multidisciplinary, with social workers, respiratory therapists, physical therapists, and other health care professionals joining organizations as case managers. However, many recognize the unique capabilities of the RN in optimizing the role of case manager.

Disease/Chronic Illness Management

The onset and eventual progression of many chronic illnesses is considered by many to be preventable. *Disease management* has been defined in the literature as a patient care approach that emphasizes comprehensive, coordinated care along a disease continuum and across health care delivery systems (Ellrodt et al., 1997). Disease management is the redirection of patient care services from inpatient to outpatient settings

Box 21-5	Criteria for Evaluating Need for Disease Management Services

- A high percentage of complications associated with the disease are preventable.
- The effect of a disease management program would be evident within 1–3 years after implementation.
- The conditions that are manifested can be managed in a nonsurgical, outpatient setting.
- There is a high rate of noncompliance with treatment protocols; however, the noncompliance is amenable to change.
- Practice guidelines are available (or there is potential to develop such guidelines) that outline optimal treatments of the disease.

and is viewed as a proactive rather than a reactive approach to providing health care services. In essence, disease management programs use medical, prescription drug, and other health-related data to identify individuals with chronic illnesses who are at high risk for experiencing serious health problems and to provide early intervention to avoid or minimize those problems (Marquis & Huston, 2012).

People diagnosed with chronic illnesses (e.g., asthma, diabetes mellitus, congestive heart failure [CHF], AIDS, lower back pain, and certain forms of cancer) are potential candidates for disease management interventions. Kongstvedt (2013) offered a set of criteria by which to evaluate what types of chronic illnesses are appropriate for disease management (Box 21-5).

The potential of disease management to reduce health care costs associated with common chronic illnesses seems significant. With the aging of the large "baby boomer" cohort of the population, a precipitous rise in the incidence of chronic illnesses, such as diabetes and CHF, seems to be a foregone conclusion. At current rates, the economic burden related to the treatment of just five of the most costly and preventable chronic conditions (heart disease, cancer, COPD/asthma, diabetes, and hypertension) in the United States is staggering at over $347 billion dollars or about 30% of total health care spending in 2010 (American Public Health Association, 2017).

Disease Management Models

Historically, disease management programs were developed by pharmacy benefits management (PBM) organizations, which were mainly owned by pharmaceutical companies that had a financial stake in management of diseases. The theory was that if disease management programs were successful, the drug manufacturing company sponsoring the program would sell more drugs to the individual. As interest in disease management has grown, PBMs, as disease management program sponsors, represent only a small segment of the business. Other more recent sponsors and advocates of disease management programs include managed care companies, individual state Medicaid agencies, provider organizations, and independent vendors. Independent disease management vendors are the most rapidly growing segment in the disease management arena because of the potential for profitability. Many of the independent vendors are web-based providers of disease management services.

Managed care and MCOs evolved in an attempt to control costs associated with traditional fee-for-service insurance reimbursement practices. MCOs are held clinically and financially responsible for health outcomes of their enrolled members on

492 Unit IV Application of Theory in Nursing

a capitated fee basis. Many MCOs have implemented disease management and wellness programs that utilize a case management approach to improve clinical outcomes. The method of disease management implementation in Medicaid and other state programs varies by state and is becoming more widely used, with states reporting disease management programs to cover asthma, diabetes, CHF, and other chronic illnesses.

Clinical outcomes have been tracked using disease management indicators since the inception of the program. Examples of disease management indicators related to patients with CHF, for example, include tracking the percentage of patients with appropriate use of drugs, such as angiotensin-converting enzyme (ACE) inhibitors and beta-blockers, inappropriate use of calcium channel blockers and nonsteroidal anti-inflammatory drugs (NSAIDs), hospital admission rates, use of emergency departments, and regular primary care or cardiology visits as well as other indicators.

Among the most notable outcomes of this disease management program are increases in the percentages of patients with improved glycated hemoglobin (HbA1c) levels and improved low-density lipoprotein (LDL) levels and the increased use of aspirin in the diabetic population. Clinical improvements were also observed in the CHF population, in patients with asthma, and in patients with HIV. Cancer-related screening practices also improved including increased use of mammography, Papanicolaou (PAP), and prostate-specific antigen (PSA) testing (Horswell et al., 2008).

Increasingly, APNs such as nurse practitioners (NPs) are assuming greater roles and responsibilities in disease management programs in recognition of the equal or superior quality outcomes of NP care at costs which are often lower than physician-provided care for similar services. A recently conducted analysis of Medicare claims data from 2012 sought to determine whether primary care type 2 diabetes management for a subset of Medicare beneficiaries differed in outcomes by provider type—physician or NP. The analysis revealed patients in the NP-only group had significantly improved outcomes in terms of health care service utilization and in most clinical outcomes at lower costs when compared to care received by patients from primary care physicians (Lutfiyya et al., 2017).

Population Health Accountable Care Organizations and Medical Home Models of Care

Newer initiatives in health care include the formation of accountable care organizations (ACOs) and patient-centered medical homes (PCMHs) models of care coordination. Population health, which is viewed as an extension of public health, arose as part of the Institute for Healthcare Improvement's strategy to transform the American health care system (Fox & Grogan, 2017). This strategy, referred to as *Triple Aim*, is focused on improving care to individuals and improving the health of populations while reducing health care costs. Identifying and directing resources to combat the three major known causes of most chronic illnesses—poor nutrition, lack of physical exercise, and substance abuse—is the major focus of Triple Aim.

Triple Aim became a priority of the CMS during the Obama administration. Organizations seeking designations as ACOs from CMS were required to integrate the three aims into their programs. Other population health initiatives were incorporated into aspects of the ACA. For example, the ACA mandated tax-exempt hospitals to perform a community health needs assessment at least every 3 years. The assessments serve as a basis for the development of strategies which focus on the health care needs of lower income, medically underserved, or minority populations. Monetary penalties and loss of tax-exempt status can result if hospitals fail to comply with the regulations. As a result, there has been expansive growth of ACOs and other similar organizations fostering implementation of Triple Aim initiatives in many areas of the country (Fox & Grogan, 2017).

According to the CMS (2017), "ACOs are groups of doctors, hospitals, and other health care providers, who come together voluntarily to give coordinated high quality care to the Medicare patients they serve" (para. 1). The goal of ACOs is well-coordinated care for defined population groups which is accomplished across care settings and which facilitates partnerships between providers, payers, and patients/families. At the federal level, financial incentives have been established through the Medicare Shared Savings Program to reward ACOs which are able to meet quality performance standards and metrics while simultaneously decreasing costs of care provision.

The first ACO in the United States was formed in New Hampshire in 2012 by NPs in collaboration with Anthem Blue Cross/Blue Shield. In this ACO, patients are managed in NP-owned and NP-operated clinics. In a recent analysis, patients managed by the NPs met or exceeded all quality standards, including sustaining some of the lowest hospitalization rates in the state while achieving costs savings compared with physician-managed care (Wright, 2017).

Some challenges associated with implementation of ACOs include enhancing the collaboration, communication, and teamwork skills of physicians and other providers. Although many medical, nursing, and other health sciences curricula now include content, such as the situation, background, assessment, recommendation (SBAR) communication technique, older physicians and nurses may not have been exposed to these techniques and skills and will require professional development in these areas (Press, Michelow, & MacPhail, 2012).

The goals of PCMHs include improving health care by promoting care coordination while reducing costs associated with care. PCMHs emphasize preventive care and primary care and were first introduced in the care of pediatric patients in the 1960s. The PCMH approach is focused on increased coordination of care, which results in enhanced patient outcomes, as opposed to the more common volume-based models of care in which providers are reimbursed based on the numbers of patients seen and the numbers of procedures for which they are able to bill. PCMHs seem to hold promise in providing effective chronic disease management at lower costs (DeVries et al., 2012).

The growing need to manage chronic illnesses is creating an unprecedented opportunity for nurses, particularly APNs, who by virtue of their educational credentials and clinical expertise, are uniquely positioned to become leaders in disease management. Roles for APNs include coordination of care for persons with chronic illnesses in for-profit and not-for-profit health care organizations in which APNs provide an array of direct services to plan members. APNs use published practice guidelines to manage and coordinate care of individuals with chronic illnesses across health care settings.

Quality Management

In 2001, the IOM released the publication, *To Err Is Human*. The release of this document, which asserted that medical errors were responsible for between 44,000 and 98,000 deaths annually in the United States, spurred demands for greater accountability and quality in the U.S. health care system (Kohn, Corrigan, & Donaldson, 2000). Since that time, many QI or QM initiatives have been undertaken in health care systems and organizations that directly impact the discipline of nursing.

Although there is some variation in the emphasis placed on specific aspects of QM between organizations, seven key principles or elements are viewed as integral components of all QM programs. These elements include focus on the customer, process improvement, variance analysis, leadership, employee involvement, scientific method, and benchmarking (Baker & Gelmon, 1996).

In the QM environment, quality is defined in terms of what is acceptable to the customer; that is, the customer determines expectations of quality. Comprehensive knowledge of the customer's needs and expectations is integral to providing the best in quality customer service. There are two types of customers: customers who are external to the organization and customers who are internal. In health care, for example, external customers are patients, families, physicians not employed by the organization, payers, and communities. Internal customers are staff members employed by the organization to provide a service to external customers. For example, the staff on a nursing unit is a customer of pharmacy services. The nursing staff relies on the pharmacy staff to provide accurate medications in a timely fashion to the nursing unit to enable the external customer, the patient, to receive medications appropriately and on time (Folse, 2015; Marquis & Huston, 2012).

Process improvement involves scrupulously examining work processes involved in achieving a work product. For example, in a hospital setting, the process of transferring a patient from an orthopedic unit to a rehabilitation unit may have 20 or more steps and may involve five or six different departments. The more steps (and people) involved, the greater the likelihood that the transfer will be delayed or that an error will be made during the transfer, which leads to increased costs. Process improvement dictates that every aspect of patient transfer must be examined to determine whether each step in the process is really needed to accomplish the transfer. Members of each department or unit involved in the transfer are included on a process improvement team to examine the process for redundancies and lapses in service and to streamline the process.

Monitoring and analysis of variation in processes is crucial, particularly in health care organizations. There are two types of variation: common cause variation, which occurs no matter how well a system operates, and special cause variation. Special cause variation is variation that occurs outside of what is to be expected and can be caused by employee error and equipment or systems failure. The scientific method used to distinguish between common cause and special cause variation is statistical control (Varkey, Reller, & Resar, 2007).

Leadership in a QM environment has two components: comprehensive knowledge and an understanding of concepts and techniques of QI and personal involvement. Leaders must be familiar with the terminology, the concepts, and the statistical techniques used in QM. Essential roles and responsibilities of leaders in QM include being personally committed to the philosophy, providing resources that include training others in the philosophy, reviewing progress on a regular basis, giving recognition, and managing resistance while empowering others.

To initiate and sustain a successful, meaningful QI program, all members of the organization should have education and training related to QM. Employees should come away from the training with a clear understanding of their individual roles and responsibilities related to QI. A broad range of employees should be encouraged to participate on QI teams to design and improve work processes. Organizations that have been successful in implementing QM have empowered employees at all levels to search for better ways to redesign work processes to achieve customer satisfaction.

True QI activities are based on scientific and statistical methods rather than on trial-and-error approaches to problem identification and problem solving. The scientific method is a precise, systematic, orderly, planned, and organized method of problem solving that can be replicated and understood by employees of the organization. Several problem-solving methods can be used by health care organizations, including the most commonly used approach for rapid improvement in health care, the plan-do-stay-act (PDSA) cycle (Varkey et al., 2007). Other QI methods utilized in contemporary health care organizations are Six Sigma and lean strategies. Problem analysis tools (also called statistical process control tools) used in the problem-solving process include flow charts, cause-and-effect diagrams, and run charts.

Benchmarking, a process originally implemented by the Xerox Corporation in 1979 (Camp & Tweet, 1994), is the identification, adaptation, and dissemination of best practices among competitors and noncompetitors that lead to their superior performance. In other words, quality can be improved in an organization by analyzing and then copying the methods of leaders in a field such as health care. Effective benchmarking involves identifying specific key indicators of a process (i.e., length of endotracheal intubation in postoperative patients), comparing this process with other organizations, determining the best process, and then using knowledge of the best process internally to design new processes or improve existing ones (Baker & Gelmon, 1996).

As described previously, there has been intense effort among government (CMS) and other payers in elevating quality outcomes in the American health care sector, including, but not limited to, application of financial incentives and penalties. Since passage of the ACA, there has been a decided shift in balancing the value (cost) of health care in addition to measuring quality of care in an effort to rein in ever-escalating national health care costs (Shiver & Cantiello, 2016). Many governmental, public, and private groups are working to make health care rankings and information available to consumers. For example, using the websites HealthCare.gov and Medicare.gov, Medicare enrollees and other consumers can search for and compare the quality of physicians, hospitals, nursing homes, home health agencies, and dialysis facilities. Comparisons of hospitals include patient satisfaction survey results, timely and effective care results, readmission, complications and death rates, and number of Medicare patients by diagnosis type treated in the facility. From these sites, a prospective patient can determine areas of the hospital's performance that need improvement and can compare the hospital's performance in some categories with state and national results (benchmarking data).

As a result of these Internet-based rating mechanisms, health care consumers are becoming increasingly savvy about checking quality "report cards" of health care facilities and providers. Institutions that are implementing best practices and continually striving to improve performance while decreasing costs will be the biggest winners in the competitive health care environment of the future. Link to Practice 21-2 presents how one health care facility used a QI to ensure greater safety.

Evidence-Based Practice

Health care consumers expect quality care, and most health care practitioners want to provide quality care. Pressure for cost containment compels providers to demonstrate that interventions produce cost-effective outcomes that do not sacrifice the quality of health care. Furthermore, selected interventions must be not only effective but also justified and congruent with acceptable standards.

EBP is a problem-solving approach that enables clinicians to provide the highest quality of care to patients and their families by integrating the following approaches:

- Critical appraisal and critique of the most recent and relevant research (evidence)
- Considering the clinician's own clinical expertise
- Considering preferences and values of the patient (Melnyk & Fineout-Overholt, 2015)

Link to Practice 21-2

Quality Improvement to Promote Safety

Occurrence of a major adverse event in a patient care setting often serves as the impetus for change in terms of quality improvement. After a patient safety issue was identified at a children's hospital related to the use of "smart pumps" in the administration of intravenous medications, a performance improvement team was assembled to increase use of medication safety software by nurses. The quality improvement team utilized the Deming Cycle performance improvement method to increase adherence and compliance with intravenous medication delivery software. Strategies implemented by the team to improve compliance included improved communication with nurses who were direct caregivers, staff education related to safety software specifics, acquisition of additional technology, and implementation of the medication safety champion role. Adherence monitoring was also incorporated. Following implementation of the performance improvement strategies, nurse adherence improved dramatically from 28% at baseline to greater than 85%, an adherence rate that exceeded nationally accepted benchmark adherence rates.

Gavriloff, C. (2012). A performance improvement plan to increase nurse adherence to use of medication safety software. *Journal of Pediatric Nursing, 27*(4), 375–382.

For EBP to take root and flourish in an organization, there must be institutional support and commitment from administrators. This support stems from the mission, goals, and culture of the organization. Without this support, necessary resources and infrastructure components, such as access to databases, dedicated personnel, and computer support, which are integral to a successful EBP program, may not be allocated or made fully available and accessible (Melnyk & Fineout-Overholt, 2015).

APNs must make clinical decisions on the best evidence available. They must also select interventions that are linked to cost-effective outcomes. This integrated approach allows the APN to use critical thinking skills to determine whether scientific evidence and clinical practice guidelines are relevant and consistent with the applicable health care situation and with the patient's values, preferences, and life context.

In one example, an inpatient asthma education QI program at Children's Hospital in Boston utilizes evidence-based guidelines and a team approach of an inpatient asthma nurse practitioner (IANP), other APNs, and unit-based RNs to provide patient and family education using individualized asthma action plans. The education is based on 2007 National Heart, Lung, and Blood Institute/National Asthma Education and Prevention Program guidelines, which recommend that care providers teach and reinforce asthma self-management techniques during every care encounter. Acute care encounters are especially valuable as parents and other caregivers are likely to want to participate in activities that prevent further emergency room visits and inpatient stays (McCarty & Rogers, 2012).

Chapter 12 contains additional information about EBP. See also Link to Practice 21-3 for a novel approach to encouraging EBP.

Link to Practice 21-3

Promoting Evidence-Based Practice

Nursing administrators in a hospital district in Houston hosted a Sacred Cow Contest as a strategy to promote a culture that values clinical inquiry and to stimulate nurse interest in EBP. As part of the contest, nurses were encouraged to challenge the routines inherent in clinical practice, such as changing bed linens daily, performing "routine" vital signs, and the necessity for all nurses to listen to shift report on all patients on a given unit. Nurses were asked to consciously think of activities and procedures they performed daily and to question why the activity or procedure was necessary. When a practice was questionable, the nurses were asked to consider if it may be a sacred cow and were asked to submit entries challenging the practice. Sample entry categories for the contest were cash cow, mad cow, holy cow, and put the cow out to pasture, among others. More than 100 Sacred Cow Contest entries were received from inpatient and outpatient settings and from individual nurses as well as teams of nurses. After winning entries were named, a message communicating contest follow-up actions was sent to the nursing staff. Nurses were asked to adopt a sacred cow and were offered support and resources to establish EBP workgroups on the nursing units to address the sacred cow issue identified.

Mick, J. (2011). Promoting clinical inquiry and evidence-based practice: The sacred cow contest. *The Journal of Nursing Administration, 41*(6), 280–284.

Summary

This chapter has provided examples of the application of specific theories, models, and frameworks in nursing administration and management. The models, which were described along with related historical and contemporary applications, should provide the APN with a foundation for navigating the complex, ever-changing environment of health care organizations today and in the future.

Health care organizations of the future hold great promise for APNs, such as Greta from the opening case study, who are willing to assume entrepreneurial and intrapreneurial roles in providing cost-effective quality health care. A more detailed understanding of some of these models will be necessary in certain circumstances (e.g., as in the case study), but it is hoped that this chapter has provided a basis for further investigation for those who need more detailed information.

Key Points

- Organizational structure and design are key elements in determining efficiency and effectiveness of work processes and quality of outcomes in health care organizations.
- Shared governance is imperative to nurses controlling professional practice.
- Transformational leaders bring a competitive advantage to an organization and play an important role in cultivating healthy professional work environments.
- Nursing care in the acute care setting is most often delivered using a group practice model. Attributes of the work environment such as nurse staffing ratios and

nurse educational level have significant and direct impact on patient outcomes such as infection, failure-to-rescue, and mortality rates.

■ Implementation of concepts associated with patient- and family-centered care models, including dignity and respect, information sharing, participation, and collaboration, lead to improved patient and staff satisfaction.

■ Case management, disease management, and population health initiatives play crucial roles in acute care facilities and in other models of coordinated and integrated health care models such as HMOs, MCOs, ACOs, and PCMHs.

■ QI and EBP are concepts that are inextricably linked in today's highest performing health care organizations.

Learning Activities

1. Interview a middle-level manager in a hospital to determine recent changes in span of control. Has the span of control for the manager decreased or increased in the past 2 to 3 years? What impact has the manager noticed related to decreased or increased span of control? What is the manager's preference in terms of numbers of employees in his or her span of administrative control?

2. Have health care organizations in your area participated in mergers and acquisitions in recent years as part of newly configured integrated systems? If so, what APN roles, if any, have been created as a result?

3. What are the roles of APNs employed by health care organizations in QI activities in your community? Are APNs the leaders of QI teams? What significant contributions have occurred as a result of APN involvement on QI teams?

4. Talk with APNs who are employed in hospitals in your area. Determine the following:
   a. Are the APNs unit-based? If so, what is the method of patient care delivery on the unit, that is, primary nursing, team nursing, PFC? What are the advantages and disadvantages to the APN role related to each of the different delivery methods?
   b. Do the APNs have staff or line authority? What are the advantages and disadvantages to the role of each type of authority?
   c. Administratively, do the APNs report to a senior or middle-level manager?
   d. Do any of the APNs work in a shared governance environment?

5. What roles do nurses, especially APNs, play in integrated health systems such as HMOs, MCOs, ACOs, and PCMHs in your area? Are these nurses in case management roles? Do they work independently or are they part of an interdisciplinary team of case managers?

6. What EBP activities have APNs in your area spearheaded? Have health care consumers benefited?

REFERENCES

AHC Media. (2013). Home visit help to reduce Medicare readmissions. *Case Management Advisor, 24*(2), 15–16.

Aiken, L. H., Cimiotti, J. P., Sloane, D. M., Smith, H. L., Flynn, L., & Neff, D. M. (2011). Effects of nurse staffing and nurse education on patient deaths in hospitals with different nurse work environments. *Medical Care, 49*(12), 1047–1053.

Aiken, L. H., Clarke, S. P., Cheung, R. B., Sloane, D. M., & Silber, J. H. (2003). Educational levels of hospital nurses and surgical patient mortality. *JAMA, 290*, 1617–1623.

Aiken, L. H., Clarke, S. P., & Sloane, D. M. (2002). Hospital staffing, organization, and quality of care: Cross-national findings. *International Journal for Quality in Health Care, 14*(1), 5–13.

Aiken, L. H., Clarke, S. P., Sloane, D. M., Sochalski, J., & Silber, J. H. (2002). Hospital nurse staffing and patient mortality, nurse burnout, and job dissatisfaction. *JAMA, 288*(16), 1987–1993.

Aiken, L. H., & Patrician, P. (2000). Measuring organizational traits of hospitals: The revised Nursing Work Index. *Nursing Research, 49*(3), 146–153.

Aiken, L. H., Sloane, D., Cimiotti, J. P., Clarke, S. P., Flynn, L., Seago, J. A., et al. (2010). Implications of the California nurse staffing mandate for other states. *Health Services Research, 45*(2), 904–921.

American Nurses Association. (2004). *Scope and standards for nurse administrators* (2nd ed.). Silver Spring, MD: Author.

American Nurses Association. (2015). *Nurse staffing.* Retrieved from http://www.nursingworld.org/MainMenuCategories/Policy-Advocacy/State/Legislative-Agenda-Reports/State-Staffing PlansRatios

American Nurses Credentialing Center. (2008). *Announcing a new model for ANCC's Magnet Recognition Program.* Retrieved from http://www.nursecredentialing.org/MagnetModel.aspx

American Nurses Credentialing Center. (2017). *Find a magnet hospital.* Retrieved from http://www.nursecredentialing.org/Magnet/FindaMagnetFacility

American Public Health Association. (2017). *Public health and chronic disease: Cost savings and return on investment.* Retrieved from https://www.apha.org/~/media/files/pdf/factsheets/chronic diseasefact_final.ashx

Andel, C., Davidow, S. L., Hollander, M., & Moreno, D. A. (2012). The economics of health care quality and medical errors. *Journal of Health Care Finance, 39*(1), 39–50.

Anthony, M. K. (2004). Shared governance models: The theory, practice, and evidence. *Online Journal of Issues in Nursing, 9*(1), 7. Retrieved from http://www.nursingworld.org/MainMenuCategories/ANAMarketplace/ANAPeriodicals/OJIN/TableofContents/Volume92004/No1Jan04/SharedGovernanceModels

Baker, G. R., & Gelmon, S. B. (1996). Total quality management in health care. In J. A. Schmele (Ed.), *Quality management in nursing and health care* (pp. 66–87). Albany, NY: Delmar.

Barker, A. M. (1994). An emerging leadership paradigm: Transformational leadership. In E. C. Hein & J. M. Nicholson (Eds.), *Contemporary leadership behavior: Selected readings* (4th ed., pp. 81–86). Philadelphia, PA: J.B. Lippincott.

Barnes, H., Rearden, J., & McHugh, M. D. (2016). Magnet® hospital recognition linked to lower central line-associated bloodstream infection rates. *Research in Nursing & Health, 39*(2), 96–104.

Bennis, W., & Nanus, B. (1985). *Leaders: Strategies for taking charge.* New York, NY: Harper & Row.

Bieber, P., & Joachim, H. (2016). Shared governance: A success story. *Nurse Leader, 14*(1), 62–66.

Burnes Bolton, L., Aydin, C. E., Donaldson, N., Brown, D. S., Sandhu, M., Fridman, M., et al. (2007). Mandated nurse staffing ratios in California: A comparison of staffing and nursing-sensitive outcomes pre- and postregulation. *Policy, Politics & Nursing Practice, 8*(4), 238–250.

Camp, R. C., & Tweet, A. G. (1994). Benchmarking applied to health care. *The Joint Commission Journal on Quality Improvement, 20*(5), 229–238.

Cathcart, D., Jeska, S., Karnas, J., Miller, S. E., Pechacek, J., & Rheault, L. (2004). Span of control matters. *The Journal of Nursing Administration, 34*(9), 395–399.

Centers for Medicare & Medicaid Services. (2017). *Accountable care organizations (ACOs): General information.* Retrieved from https://innovation.cms.gov/initiatives/ACO/

Cho, S. H., Ketefian, S., Barkauskas, V. H., & Smith, D. G. (2003). The effects of nurse staffing on adverse events, morbidity, mortality, and medical costs. *Nursing Research, 52*(2), 71–79.

Cimiotti, J. P., Aiken, L. H., Sloane, D. M., & Wu, E. S. (2012). Nurse staffing, burnout, and health care-associated infection. *American Journal of Infection Control, 40*, 486–490.

Clavelle, J. T., Drenkard, K., Tullai-McGuinness, S., & Fitzpatrick, J. J. (2012). Transformational leadership practices of chief nursing officers in Magnet® organizations. *The Journal of Nursing Administration, 42*(4), 195–201.

Clavelle, J. T., Porter O'Grady, T., & Drenkard, K. (2013). Structural empowerment and the nursing practice environment in Magnet® organizations. *The Journal of Nursing Administration, 43*(11), 566–573.

Clouten, K., & Weber, R. (1994). Patient-focused care . . . playing to win. *Nursing Management, 25*(2), 34–36.

Cottingham, C. (1988). Transformational leadership: A strategy for nursing. *Today's OR Nurse, 10*(6), 24–27.

Cropley, S. (2012). The relationship-based care model: Evaluation of the impact on patient satisfaction, length of stay, and readmission rates. *The Journal of Nursing Administration, 42*(6), 333–339.

Cunningham, R., & Walton, M. K. (2016). Partnering with patients to improve care: The value of patient and family advisory councils. *The Journal of Nursing Administration, 46*(11), 549–551.

DeVries, A., Li, C.-H., Sridhar, G., Hummel, J. R., Breidbart, S., & Barron, J. J. (2012). Impact of medical homes on quality, healthcare utilization, and costs. *The American Journal of Managed Care, 18*(9), 534–544.

Donaldson, N., Bolton, L. B., Aydin, C., Brown, D., Elashoff, J., & Sandhu, M. (2005). Impact of California's licensed nurse-patient ratios on unit-level nurse staffing and patient outcomes. *Policy, Politics & Nursing Practice, 6*, 198–210.

Ellrodt, G., Cook, D. J., Lee, J., Cho, M., Hunt, D., & Weingarten, S. (1997). Evidence-based disease management. *JAMA, 278*(20), 1687–1692.

Fayol, H. (1949). *General and industrial management.* London, United Kingdom: Pitman & Sons.

Fischer, S. A. (2016). Transformational leadership in nursing: A concept analysis. *Journal of Advanced Nursing, 72*(11), 2644–2653.

Folse, V. N. (2015). Managing quality and risk. In P. S. Yoder-Wise (Ed.), *Leading and managing in nursing* (6th ed., pp. 361–382). St. Louis, MO: Elsevier.

Fox, D. M., & Grogan, C. M. (2017). Population health during the Obama administration: An ambitious strategy with an uncertain future. *American Journal of Public Health, 107*(1), 32–34.

Frank, L., Basch, E., & Selby, J. V. (2014). The PCORI perspective on patient-centered outcomes research. *JAMA, 312*(15), 1513–1514.

Gabriel, A. S., Erickson, R. J., Moran, C. M., Diefendorff, J. M., & Bromley, G. E. (2013). A multilevel analysis of the effects of the Practice Environment Scale of the Nursing Work Index on nurse outcomes. *Research in Nursing & Health, 36*(6), 567–581.

Havaei, F., Dahinten, V. S., & MacPhee, M. (2015). The effects of perceived organisational support and span of control on the organisational commitment of novice leaders. *Journal of Nursing Management, 23*, 307–314.

Hickey, P. A., Gauvreau, K., Jenkins, K., Fawcett, J., & Hayman, L. (2011). Statewide and national impact of California's staffing law on pediatric cardiac surgery outcomes. *The Journal of Nursing Administration, 41*(5), 218–225.

Horswell, R., Butler, M. K., Kaiser, M., Moody-Thomas, S., McNabb, S., Besse, J., et al. (2008). Disease management programs for the underserved. *Disease Management, 11*(3), 145–152.

Houston, S., Leveille, M., Luquire, R., Fike, A., Ogola, G. O., & Chando, S. (2012). Decisional involvement in Magnet®, Magnet-aspiring, and non-Magnet hospitals. *The Journal of Nursing Administration, 42*(12), 586–591.

Jayawardhana, J., Welton, J. M., & Lindrooth, R. C. (2014). Is there a business case for magnet hospitals? Estimates of the cost and revenue implications of becoming a magnet. *Medical Care, 52*(5), 400–406.

Johnson, B., Abraham, M., Conway, J., Simmons, L., Levitan, S. E., Sodomka, P., et al. (2008). *Partnering with patients and families to design a patient- and family-centered health care system. Recommendations and promising practices.* Bethesda, MD: Institute for Family-Centered Care and Institute for Healthcare Improvement. Retrieved from http://www.hqontario.ca/Portals/0/modals/qi/en/processmap_pdfs/articles/partnering%20with%20patients%20and%20families%20to%20design%20a%20patient-%20and%20family-centered%20health%20care%20system.pdf

Jones, D., McLaughlin, M., Gebbens, C., & Terhorst, L. (2015). Utilizing a scope and span of control tool to measure workload and determine supporting resources for nurse managers. *The Journal of Nursing Administration, 45*(5), 243–249.

Joseph, M. L., & Bogue, R. J. (2016). A theory-based approach to nursing shared governance. *Nursing Outlook, 64*(4), 339–351.

Kohn, L. T., Corrigan, J. M., & Donaldson, M. S. (Eds.). (2000). *To err is human: Building a safer health system.* Washington, DC: National Academy Press.

Kongstvedt, P. R. (2013). *Essentials of managed health care* (6th ed.). Burlington, MA: Jones & Bartlett Learning.

Kutney-Lee, A., Germack, H., Hatfield, L., Kelly, S., Maguire, P., Dierkes, A., et al. (2016). Nurse engagement in shared governance and patient and nurse outcomes. *The Journal of Nursing Administration, 46*(11), 605–612.

Laschinger, H. K., & Finegan, J. (2005). Empowering nurses for work engagement and health in hospital settings. *The Journal of Nursing Administration, 35*(10), 439–449.

Lutfiyya, M. N., Tomai, L., Frogner, B., Cerra, F., Zismer, D., & Parente, S.(2017). Does primary care diabetes management provided to Medicare patients differ between primary care physicians and nurse practitioners? *Journal of Advanced Nursing, 73*(1), 240–252.

Ma, C., & Park, S. H. (2015). Hospital Magnet status, unit work environment, and pressure ulcers. *Journal of Nursing Scholarship, 47*(6), 565–573.

Mancini, M. E. (2015). Understanding and designing organizational structures. In P. S. Yoder-Wise (Ed.), *Leading and managing in nursing* (6th ed., pp. 136–152). St. Louis, MO: Elsevier.

Mang, A. L. (1995). Implementation strategies of patient-focused care. *Hospital & Health Services Administration, 40*(3), 426–435.

Marquis, B. L., & Huston, C. J. (2012). *Leadership roles and management functions in nursing* (7th ed.). Philadelphia, PA: Lippincott Williams & Wilkins.

Marriner-Tomey, A. (2009). *Guide to nursing management and leadership* (8th ed.). St. Louis, MO: Mosby Elsevier.

McCarty, K., & Rogers, J. (2012). Inpatient asthma education program. *Pediatric Nursing, 38*(5), 257–262.

McClure, M. L., Poulin, M. A., Sovie, M. D., & Wandelt, M. A. (1983). *Magnet hospitals: Attraction and retention of professional nurses.* Washington, DC: American Nurses Association.

McHugh, M. D., Kelly, L. A., Smith, H. L., Wu, E. S., Vanak, J. M., & Aiken, L. H. (2013). Lower mortality in Magnet hospitals. *The Journal of Nursing Administration, 43*(10 Suppl.), S4–S10.

Melnyk, B. M., & Fineout-Overholt, E. (2015). *Evidence-based practice in nursing and healthcare: A guide to best practice* (3rd ed.). Philadelphia, PA: Wolters Kluwer.

Meyer, R. M., O'Brien-Pallas, L., Doran, D., Streiner, D., Ferguson-Paré, M., & Duffield, C. (2011). Front-line managers as boundary spanners: Effects of span and time on nurse supervision satisfaction. *Journal of Nursing Management, 19*(5), 611–622.

Myers, S. (1998). Patient-focused care: What managers should know. *Nursing Economics, 16*(4), 180–188.

Park, S. H., Gass, S., & Boyle, D. K. (2016). Comparison of reasons for nurse turnover in Magnet® and non-Magnet hospitals. *The Journal of Nursing Administration, 46*(5), 284–290.

Porter-O'Grady, T. (1992). Transformational leadership in an age of chaos. *Nursing Administration Quarterly, 17*(1), 17–24.

Porter-O'Grady, T. (2003). Researching shared governance: A futility of focus. *The Journal of Nursing Administration, 33*(4), 251–252.

Porter-O'Grady, T. (2012). Reframing knowledge work: Shared governance in the postdigital age. *Creative Nursing, 18*(4), 152–159.

Porter-O'Grady, T., Hawkins, M., & Parker, M. (1997). *Whole systems shared governance: Architecture for integration.* Gaithersburg, MD: Aspen.

Press, M. J., Michelow, M. D., & MacPhail, L. H. (2012). Care coordination in accountable care organizations: Moving beyond structure and incentives. *The American Journal of Managed Care, 18*(2), 778–780.

Robbins, S. P., & Judge, T. A. (2014). *Organizational behavior* (16th ed.). Upper Saddle River, NJ: Prentice-Hall.

Shiver, J., & Cantiello, J. (2016). *Managing integrated health systems.* Burlington, MA: Jones & Bartlett Learning.

Spetz, J. (2008). Nurse satisfaction and the implementation of minimum nurse staffing regulations. *Policy, Politics & Nursing Practice, 9*(1), 15–21.

Sportsman, S. (2015). Care delivery strategies. In P. S. Yoder-Wise (Ed.), *Leading and managing in nursing* (6th ed., pp. 232–254). St. Louis, MO: Elsevier.

Stimpfel, A. W., Sloane, D. M., McHugh, M. D., & Aiken, L. H. (2016). Hospitals known for nursing excellence associated with better hospital experience for patients. *Health Services Research, 51*(3), 1120–1134.

Taylor, F. W. (1911). *The principles of scientific management.* New York, NY: Harper.

Tellez, M., & Seago, J. A. (2013). California nurse staffing law and RN workforce changes. *Nursing Economics, 31*(1), 18–26.

Triolo, P. K., Scherer, E. M., & Floyd, J. M. (2006). Evaluation of the Magnet Recognition Program. *The Journal of Nursing Administration, 36*(1), 42–48.

Varkey, P., Reller, M. K., & Resar, R. K. (2007). Basics of quality improvement in health care. *Mayo Clinic Proceedings, 82*(6), 735–739.

Warren, N. (2012). Involving patient and family advisors in the patient and family-centered care model. *Medsurg Nursing, 21*(4), 233–239.

Weber, M. (1970). Bureaucracy. In W. Sexton (Ed.), *Organization theories* (pp. 39–43). Columbus, OH: Charles E. Merrill.

Wolf, G., Triolo, P., & Ponte, P. R. (2008). Magnet recognition program: The next generation. *The Journal of Nursing Administration, 38*(4), 200–204.

Wong, C. A., Elliott-Miller, P., Laschinger, H., Cuddihy, M., Meyer, R. M., Keatings, M., et al. (2015). Examining the relationships between span of control and manager job and unit performance outcomes. *Journal of Nursing Management, 23*(2), 156–168.

Wright, W. (2017). New Hampshire nurse practitioners take the lead in forming an accountable care organization. *Nursing Administration Quarterly, 41*(1), 39–47.

Yamamoto, L., & Lucey, C. (2005). Case management "within the walls": A glimpse into the future. *Critical Care Nursing Quarterly, 28*(2), 162–178.

Zarubi, K. L., Reiley, P., & McCarter, B. (2008). Putting patients and families at the center of care. *The Journal of Nursing Administration, 38*(6), 275–281.

22

Application of Theory in Nursing Education

Melanie McEwen and Evelyn M. Wills

Linda Washington is a supervisor on a surgical floor of a large teaching hospital. Her responsibilities require her to work closely with the faculty from two area nursing schools and help place students with preceptors. Because of her enjoyment in working with students and faculty, Linda decided that she would like to become a nursing educator and enrolled in a master's degree program. This semester, she is taking a course titled "Curriculum Development and Evaluation," and she is learning a great deal about how nursing programs are structured and the underlying rationale. The course requires a project in which a small group of students designs a nursing program that will meet the changing needs of the health care system and the emerging profile of nursing students in the 21st century. Initially, this project seemed daunting for Linda and her colleagues, and they were unsure where to begin.

During one class period, Linda's professor explained how the curriculum of a nursing program is derived from the faculty's philosophy of nursing and nursing education. She explained that a conceptual framework is then developed from the philosophy, and it is from this framework that the curriculum is built. The students also learned that in most nursing programs, the conceptual framework is an eclectic blend of concepts and processes, although some programs use grand nursing theories as their basis.

In a brainstorming session, Linda and her group agreed on a philosophy of nursing education, describing what they saw as the interplay of the metaparadigm concepts and concepts and processes of teaching and learning. But there was considerable discussion and significant differences among group members about what other concepts or theories should be used as the basis for the curriculum framework. In addition, there was disagreement on what would be the best teaching strategies to meet the needs of older nursing students and students from diverse backgrounds. Some members of the group favored a structured, traditional type of program in which the faculty member was responsible for directing learning experiences, whereas other group members preferred to focus on less rigid instructional techniques and incorporate more web-based options and simulation.

The discussions were enlightening, and finally, Linda's group compromised. They would use "caring" as a central concept and draw heavily from Jean Watson's (1996) work to structure the curriculum. They would also incorporate adult learning principles and technologically based instructional strategies into their program. With these parameters in place, the group began to describe courses, write objectives, outline course sequencing, discern outcome measures, identify teaching strategies, and set up evaluation methods.

The health care delivery system has changed dramatically during the past 15 years. Nursing practice has also changed, requiring it to adapt to transitioning from institution-based, acute care to more community-based care with an enhanced focus on caring for older adults and individuals with chronic conditions as well as understanding the importance of cultural differences. Nursing education, too, must adapt to changes and anticipated trends in health care and education. Furthermore, nursing leaders and nursing organizations who believe that "it is the responsibility of nursing education, in collaboration with practice settings, to shape practice, not merely respond to changes in the practice environment" (American Association of Colleges of Nursing [AACN], 1999, p. 60).

The literature is awash with buzzwords for nursing education. Problem-based learning, lifelong learning, informatics, evidence-based education, quality/performance improvement, competency-based curricula, culturally relevant care, service learning, interpersonal communication, and excellence are only a few. Furthermore, new trends for curricula reflect increased emphasis on evidence-based practice, population diversity, patient outcomes, health promotion, genetics, and informatics (Mueller, 2016; Pressler & Kenner, 2015; Speziale & Jacobson, 2005). Other evolving emphases in nursing education include a greater focus on economics of health care, increasing use of simulation, along with more attention to interprofessional educational collaborations and distance education (Institute of Medicine [IOM], 2011; Keating, 2015a; O'Neil, 2015).

In general terms, theoretical principles, concepts, and models are used in two major ways in nursing education. First, they are used to determine the content and organization and structure of a program's curriculum. Second, they are used to determine the instructional processes and strategies used by faculty to teach students. Both of these contributions of theory to nursing education are discussed in this chapter.

Theoretical Issues in Nursing Curricula

Curriculum refers to the content and processes by which learners gain knowledge and understanding; develop skills; and alter attitudes, appreciation, and values under the auspices of a given school or program. The curriculum of a school of nursing typically includes philosophy and mission statements; an organizational or conceptual framework; lists of outcomes, competencies, and objectives for the program; individual courses, course outlines and syllabi; educational activities; and evaluation methods (Sullivan, 2016). Furthermore, most nursing curricula specify essential nursing content and means of application in clinical practice (Keating, 2015b). Specific components of the curriculum of a given program of study are summarized in Box 22-1.

Several issues that relate to the incorporation of theoretical principles and frameworks into nursing curricula are reviewed in this section. These include basic curriculum design, the impact of regulating organizations on nursing curricula, components

| Box 22-1 | Components of a Curriculum |

- A defined philosophy or mission statement
- An organizing framework
- Anticipated outcomes, competencies, and/or objectives to be achieved
- Selected content with specific sequencing of the content
- Educational activities and experiences to facilitate learning
- Means of evaluation

Source: Sullivan (2016).

of curricular conceptual/organizational frameworks, and the processes involved in designing and organizing nursing curricula. The section concludes with a short discussion of current issues in nursing curriculum development.

Curriculum Design in Nursing Education

A *curriculum* is a "formal plan of study that provides the philosophical underpinnings, goals, and guidelines for the delivery of a specific educational program" (Keating, 2015a, p. 1). The curriculum provides faculty with a means of conceptualizing and organizing the knowledge, skills, values, and beliefs critical to the delivery of a coherent program of study that facilitates the achievement of the desired outcomes (Ruchala, 2015; Sullivan, 2016).

The curricula of most nursing programs are based on the Tyler Curriculum Development Model, which was published in 1949. Bevis (1989a, 1989b) stated that the incorporation of the Tyler model within nursing curricula began in the 1950s and continued throughout the 1960s and 1970s. According to Bevis (1989b), introduction of Tyler's concepts in the 1950s, along with her first book on curriculum development (Bevis, 1973) and Mager's (1962) publication of *Preparing Instructional Objectives*, led to the development of Tyler-type curricula throughout nursing education. Eventually, the Tyler model became the primary model used in developing nursing curricula for all levels of nursing education—diploma, associate degree, and baccalaureate.

The Tyler model begins with identification of the educational purposes or objectives for the program. It then differentiates what learning experiences should be selected to attain the objectives. The third issue addressed by the Tyler model is how to organize learning experiences for effective instruction. Finally, the model focuses on evaluation of behaviors to determine if objectives have been met (Bevis, 1989b). The Tyler model values effectiveness, efficiency, and predictability, and it emphasizes individualism and competition. It assumes that knowledge consists of facts, generalizations, principles, and theories and that events or phenomena can be explained by cause-and-effect relationships that can be deductively examined.

Nursing Curricula and Regulating Bodies

The impact of the Tyler model on nursing curricula and nursing education cannot be overstated; it has directly influenced not only the state boards of nursing but also the accreditation process. State boards of nursing set rules and requirements regarding nursing educational programs and curricula; these boards eventually based criteria for licensure of nursing programs on the Tyler model (Bevis, 1987; Rentschler & Spegman, 1996).

According to Bevis (1989b), the Tyler-based curriculum development process has been translated into essential curricular components, and without evidence of these components, state boards will not grant program approval. The rules and regulations set by state boards of nursing typically specify content areas that must be covered, minimum hours that must be spent by all students in clinical settings, and competencies or skills that all students must possess at the completion of the nursing program (Boland & Finke, 2012).

Similar to the impact on state board criteria, the Tyler model has heavily influenced the framework for accreditation by the National League for Nursing (NLN). Through the accreditation process, the NLN has had a great impact on the development, implementation, and evaluation of undergraduate nursing curricula (Boland & Finke, 2012). The first NLN accreditation visits were in 1939, and soon NLN accreditation requirements became the standard for nursing education (Bevis, 1989a; Ervin, 2015). Beginning in 1972, the NLN criteria for bachelor's (bachelor of science in nursing [BSN]) programs included a criterion requiring that the curriculum be based on a conceptual framework that was consistent with the stated philosophy, purposes, and objectives of the program (Kelley, 1975; NLN, 1972; Wu, 1979). Likewise, in the 1970s, accreditation requirements for associate degree in nursing (ADN) programs required that the "conceptual framework of the program of learning is clearly stated and implemented" (NLN, 1977, p. 14).

Meleis (2012) observed that the recognition of the potential of nursing theories to be used as guidelines for the conceptual frameworks of nursing curricula and programs in the 1960s and 1970s coincided with the development of most of the nursing theories. Indeed, nursing education promoted theory development in the search for a coherent presentation of nursing to guide and structure curricula.

Over the ensuing years, accreditation criteria changed somewhat. During this time, "the requirements for a conceptual framework were a major source of confusion and concern among nurse educators" (Tanner, 1989, p. 8). Because of this confusion, guidelines were changed, and since the mid-1980s, they have been more flexible. Most recently, the Accreditation Commission for Education in Nursing's (ACEN) accreditation standards, for example, state that the curriculum must "incorporate established professional standards, guidelines and competencies . . . clearly articulate student learning outcomes and program outcomes consistent with contemporary practice" (ACEN, 2017, p. 4). Thus, although not explicitly requiring a defined conceptual framework, some type of specific organizational strategy must be used to structure the program.

Since the mid-1990s, the AACN's Commission on Collegiate Nursing Education (CCNE) has also been accrediting baccalaureate and master's nursing programs. In its accreditation standards, like the ACEN, the CCNE does not specify an organizing framework per se. Rather, the need for a curricular framework is implied as Standard III states that the "curriculum is . . . logically structured to achieve expected individual and aggregate student outcomes" (CCNE, 2013, Standard III-C). See Link to Practice 22-1.

Conceptual/Organizational Frameworks for Nursing Curricula

A well-developed and articulated theoretical or organizational framework gives a nursing program the perspective that shapes the content and the methods that guide students' learning; eventually, the content and methods presented will have an impact on nursing practice (Iwasiw & Goldenberg, 2015; Keating, 2015a). A theoretical basis provides the foundation that helps nursing students define their professional

Link to Practice 22-1

Application of Theoretical Information for Nursing Educators

Linda, the nurse from the opening case study, was surprised at the organizational structure of nursing education as she studied the elements of teaching and of curriculum. She perused the baccalaureate essentials of the CCNE (AACN, 2008) to learn more about requirements for BSN education. As the nursing program she was attending was preparing for accreditation, she asked to be allowed to attend faculty meetings to gain more insight into the process. The chair of the committee welcomed Linda to the accreditation preparation meetings, and her attendance formed an informative learning experience regarding curriculum design and instructional strategies.

Access the CCNE website at http://www.aacn.nche.edu/education-resources /essential-series to learn more.

philosophies and values. It identifies and describes essential concepts and significant problems and suggests approaches to structure and methods that the student may use in continuing to develop their knowledge. Additionally, the theoretical framework or model for the nursing program can influence the means by which material is presented and the methods by which learning is evaluated. Barnum (1998) wrote that theoretical principles drawn from a number of sources directly affect a curriculum whether faculty members recognize it or not. Indeed, a nursing curriculum conveys a theory (or theories) of nursing by virtue of the content selected.

As mentioned previously, the conceptual or organizational framework of a nursing program should be an outgrowth of the philosophy of the faculty, which typically reflects the faculty's philosophical beliefs about the metaparadigm concepts (Keating, 2015b; Sullivan, 2016). The interrelationship of these concepts is the basic organizational framework of the curriculum, and as the concepts are further defined within the framework, the curriculum becomes established. Additional concepts and theories selected to comprise the conceptual framework are likewise taken from the philosophy (Sullivan, 2016).

According to Bevis (1989a), a curriculum conceptual framework is an "interrelated system of premises that provides guidelines or ground rules for making all curricular decisions—objectives, content, implementation, and evaluation" (p. 26). The conceptual framework may be referred to as the curriculum framework, the framework for curriculum development, the conceptual system, the curriculum theory, a theory of education, or the theoretical framework, but regardless of the name, it is the conceptualization and articulation of concepts, facts, propositions, postulates, theories, and variables relevant to the specific nursing program.

Purposes of the Conceptual Framework

The conceptual or organizational framework for a curriculum serves several purposes. First, it allows faculty to determine what knowledge is important to nursing (i.e., the concepts, principles, skills, and theories to be covered) and how that knowledge should be defined, categorized, and linked with other knowledge. It also helps explain how these ideas or concepts apply to nursing practice. Second, the conceptual framework facilitates the sequencing and prioritizing of knowledge in a way that is logical and internally consistent. Thus, organizing frameworks provide faculty with a blueprint for construction of a cohesive curriculum to give students the essential learning experiences which will allow them to achieve the desired educational outcomes (Sullivan, 2016).

Designing a Curriculum Conceptual Framework

Sullivan (2016) stated that there are two approaches to determining or developing an organizational framework for a nursing curriculum. Faculty members may choose a single, specific nursing theory or model on which to build the framework, or they may choose a more eclectic approach, selecting concepts from multiple theories or models. She explained that use of a single theory to develop the conceptual framework helps by providing a single image with a defined vocabulary that is shared by both the learner and the teacher. Newman (2008) agreed and wrote that using nursing models as the framework for baccalaureate nursing education would assist with identification of the essential knowledge of the discipline and strengthen the purposefulness of nursing knowledge in education and practice. When a single theory is used as the framework, the faculty will adopt and perhaps adapt the theory and use its definitions and relationships to structure and organize content.

Several articles in the nursing literature describe the use of nursing theories as the basis for the curriculum framework of nursing programs. In one example, Berbiglia (2011) provided a detailed explanation of how Orem's Self-Care Deficit Theory (SCDT) can be used as the conceptual framework in BSN programs. Also focusing on Orem's SCDT, Secrest (2008) described the process of tool development in an Orem-based curriculum and the role of faculty in bringing a curriculum revision to fruition. Beckman, Boxley-Harges, and Kaskel (2012) discussed the processes used by faculty at their nursing program as their program transitioned from an associated degree program to a BSN program using the Neuman Systems Model as the curricular framework.

To avoid being constrained by a single nursing theory or model, most faculty choose an eclectic approach that combines many theories and concepts in framework development (Keating, 2015b; Sullivan, 2016). Often, two or three organizing themes are used to build a curriculum grid. These themes can be variables, such as life phases, body systems, and the nursing process.

If the eclectic approach is taken, a combination of many theories, concepts, or processes is used, and borrowed concepts must be specifically defined for the program. Relationships between and among the concepts must also be explained. On the other hand, an advantage to an eclectic approach is the ability to incorporate concepts and definitions that best fit the faculty's beliefs and values (Sullivan, 2016).

Several years ago, McEwen and Brown (2002) completed a large-scale, nationwide study that examined the curricular frameworks of BSN, ADN, and diploma nursing programs. The findings illustrated trends at that time in structuring the conceptual frameworks of nursing curricula. In general, the nursing process was the most commonly used component of conceptual frameworks for nursing curricula, being used by 55% of all programs. Simple-to-complex organization (37% of all programs), a biopsychosocial model (36% of all programs), and nursing theorists (33% of all programs) were the other most frequently reported components. Of those identifying a nursing theory as part of the conceptual framework, the most commonly reported nursing theorists were Orem, Roy, Watson, Neuman, and Benner. The most commonly used non-nursing theories reported were systems theory, Maslow's and Erickson's theories, and adaptation.

Components of the Curricular Conceptual Framework

The two major areas to be addressed during development of a curriculum framework are as follows: (1) What concepts will be covered? (2) What will be the structure, ordering, or sequencing for introducing the concepts and delineating the relationships between and among them?

Curriculum Concepts. Once a conceptual framework for a nursing program is agreed on, the task is to identify the major elements or concepts that will appear and reappear as "threads" at each level of the curriculum and thus provide a basis for the organization and sequencing of content. Most undergraduate nursing conceptual frameworks minimally describe the concepts of health, person, environment, and nursing. Other concepts, such as caring, self-care, growth and development, nursing process, and adaptation, may be added to expand or clarify the framework. Each of the central concepts should be defined, and the linkages between and among the concepts should be explained to unify or interrelate the details.

The conceptual framework may then use additional constructs or devices to help structure or organize the material. It may use developmental stage, acute/chronic concepts, health/illness continuum, settings, or the nursing process as the chief organizer. In addition, "process threads" or themes are usually present throughout the curriculum. These might include the nursing process, problem solving, interpersonal relationships, communication, research, change, and teaching. Each of these constructs or devices should also be defined and explained.

Curriculum Structure or Sequencing. The curriculum is designed to provide a sequence of learning experiences that will enable students to achieve desired educational outcomes. Content may be structured or organized based on such variables as location (e.g., hospital, clinics, community), developmental stage (e.g., infant, child, adolescent, adult, older adult), or physiologic systems (e.g., musculoskeletal, gastrointestinal, cardiovascular, reproductive). Factors to be considered in sequencing the curriculum include consideration of the relationships among the concepts and the sequences in which the content should be ordered so that the organization supports the selected relationships. The conceptual properties (attributes) of the concepts to be learned, and the sequence in which the content is ordered, should be logically consistent. Table 22-1 gives examples of how sequencing can be used to organize courses based on several parameters (i.e., metaparadigm concepts, attributes of the person, subconcepts, activities, and complexity).

In most programs, sequencing moves from concepts that are relatively simple to concepts that are more complex or from wellness to progressively serious illnesses (Keating, 2015b). It has been noted that both of these organizational strategies can be problematic because the self-evident needs of the ill client(s) may be easier for the novice nurse to recognize and understand than the more subtle health needs of the well client(s) (Scales, 1985).

Patterns of Curricular Conceptual Frameworks

There are two common patterns of curriculum organization in nursing programs. Probably the more common one is that of *blocking* course content. When courses are blocked, content is generally structured around a particular clinical specialty area, client population, or body systems. In this organizational scheme, content can be organized according to specific practice settings (e.g., medical-surgical nursing, mental health nursing, critical care nursing), developmental stages (birth, infancy, childhood, adulthood, older adult), or body systems (e.g., respiratory system, circulatory system, digestive system). This approach produces a curriculum that is highly structured (Sullivan, 2016).

Table 22-1 Methods for Sequencing Used in Nursing Curricula

Basis of Sequencing	Beginning Level	Intermediate Levels	Final Level
Sequencing based on metaparadigm concepts	Introduction to the concepts and discussion that there are interrelationships	Focus on relationship between person(s) and nursing; move toward focus on interrelationships of person(s), nursing, and health	Focus on interrelationship of all concepts (persons, nursing, health, environment)
Sequencing based on the attributes of person(s)	Concept of personhood established (individual, family, community)	Focus on individual; move to focus on family and groups	Focus on community
Sequencing based on relationships of concepts	Person (individual, family, community) identified; nursing focused on restoration, maintenance, or promotion; health on a continuum; environment is controlled.	Focus on relationship of individual and the nursing goal of health restoration; environment is controlled. Move to focus on nursing of family and/or groups and the goal of health maintenance; environment is less controlled.	Focus on relationship of community and the nursing goal of health promotion; environment is open and less confined.
Sequencing based on activities	Student is an observer.	Student is an observer-participant.	Student is a participant-practitioner.
Sequencing based on complexity	Examines health care environments with few variables	Examines health care environments with many variables	Examines health care environments with complex variables

Source: Scales (1985).

Sullivan (2016) explained that blocking has some advantages because it facilitates course assignments and complements faculty expertise. Also, in a blocked course design, it is easy to trace placement of content within the curriculum. However, there are some concerns. Blocking of content often causes the content to become isolated from previous or following courses. This may impede the student's ability to integrate knowledge and to transfer concepts, information, and expertise across courses. Another concern is that each area is self-contained and based on a different set of premises because every major block of study is derived from a different theoretical base. For example, Barnum (1998) explained that fundamentals of nursing focuses on skills, medical-surgical nursing focuses on body systems, obstetrics is a life event–based specialty, psychiatric nursing is based on client behavior, and public health nursing is based on principles of epidemiology.

The second curriculum pattern is that of integrating or *threading* course content. Integrating course content is a more conceptual approach to curriculum design. In the integrated curriculum, faculty members identify concepts considered core to nursing practice and then integrate or thread these concepts throughout the curriculum. A nursing theory, for example, may be used to define core concepts across the program. Concepts that are frequently integrated include life span development, nutrition, and pharmacology (Sullivan, 2016).

Current Issues in Curriculum Development

There have been several recent shifts in nursing curricula. First, increasingly, community-based and population-focused components are being added to basic curricula. This has been encouraged by changes in the health care delivery system that has moved much

Box 22-2	Concepts and Content Areas to Enhance in Nursing Education

- Geriatrics/gerontology
- Patient-centered care
- Evidence-based practice
- Cultural diversity and health disparities
- Spiritual care
- Technology (informatics, electronic medical records, telehealth)
- Globalization of health problems (threat of spread of diseases)
- Alternative or complementary therapies
- Genetics and genomics
- Palliative care/end-of-life care
- Population health
- Health care reform and reimbursement
- Health policy and regulation issues
- Safety/quality
- Leadership
- Ethics

of patient care out of the acute care hospital. With that shift, there has been a growing tension between curricula that focus on technology and pathophysiology and those that focus on a more humanistic, holistic concept of nursing. Other recent changes in nursing education involve less focus being given to skills and tasks, with a corresponding increased focus on the integration of content and problem-solving strategies and concept-based curricula (Cannon & Boswell, 2012; Duncan & Schulz, 2015; Hardin & Richardson, 2012).

Nursing educators recognize that the content, concepts, principles, and theories taught in nursing programs should be regularly updated. For example, there has been attention given to strengthening nursing curricula, particularly in the areas of spiritual care (Burkhart & Schmidt, 2012; Taylor, Testerman, & Hart, 2014), safety and quality (Bednash, Cronenwett, & Dolansky, 2013; Monsivais & Robinson, 2016; Pauly-O'Neill, Cooper, & Prion, 2016; Ross & Bruderle, 2016), genetics (Fater, 2014; Giarelli & Reiff, 2012; Jenkins & Calzone, 2014), gerontology (Gray-Miceli et al., 2014; Skiba, 2012), informatics (Choi & De Martinis, 2013; Weiner, Trangenstein, Gordon, & McNew, 2016), and end-of-life care/palliative care (AACN, 2016; Josephsen & Martz, 2014). A number of areas in which enhanced content in nursing programs should be addressed to meet current and future health care needs have been identified in the nursing literature (Lewis, 2012; Stokowski, 2011). Box 22-2 summarizes these.

Theoretical Issues in Nursing Instruction

To accommodate changing student profiles and address the needs of students from different generations (e.g., baby boomers, generation X, millennial), students from a variety of cultural backgrounds, students with family responsibilities, and students from remote or rural areas, nursing educators have observed that changes or modifications in methods of instruction are warranted. To this end, new teaching strategies, based on sound educational theories and research, should be developed and promoted.

What is taught in nursing programs can be divided into three categories: (1) cognitive content, (2) psychomotor tasks, and (3) application of content and skills in nursing practice. Cognitive content refers to all of the information the nurse learns as background for functioning (e.g., anatomy, physiology, pathology, psychology, medical procedures, nursing techniques). Psychomotor tasks are the acts or skills nurses perform according to a given rationale by applying accepted techniques (e.g., administering medications, changing dressings, inserting intravenous lines). Application of cognitive knowledge and skills involves recognizing and interpreting phenomena in the clinical setting and adapting care based on the interpretation.

Teaching strategies are different for each of the three areas. Cognitive content is easily transmitted through a variety of means: lectures, discussions, programmed learning, or reading assignments. Acquisition of cognitive content can be achieved in the absence of skilled teaching if another source of information (i.e., a textbook) is available. Psychomotor skills require demonstration, return demonstration with corrective feedback, and skill development through practice. Learning to apply cognitive knowledge and psychomotor skills in practice is the most complex learning task and takes time as learning accumulates from multiple clinical experiences in varied settings. Increasingly, simulation is being utilized to develop and refine psychomotor skills.

The following sections examine two major issues in nursing instruction. These are incorporation of multiple theory-based strategies in teaching and the use of technology in nursing education. Use of multiple teaching strategies is important to enable nursing students to attain cognitive content and psychomotor skills and, most importantly, enable them to apply these in clinical settings. Technologic instruction is included because it is becoming increasingly important in nursing education, and the use of distance education methods has become commonplace in nursing education, particularly in graduate programs (Russell, 2015).

Theory-Based Teaching Strategies

To best meet the learning needs of students at the beginning of the 21st century, nursing educators are encouraged to move beyond reliance on traditional techniques of lecture and reading assignments to incorporate other teaching strategies that are based on sound theoretical principles. Some theoretically based strategies suggested by Barnum (1998) are dialectic learning, problem-based learning, operational instruction, and logistic teaching. Each of these strategies is presented in this section, along with examples from the nursing literature showing how they have been applied in education.

Dialectic Learning

Traditional dialectic teaching leads students to develop and expand their own thoughts on a given subject, primarily through the use of well-constructed questions. Questioning can lead to demonstration of inconsistencies in, or contradictions to, the student's position. In dialogue, the student moves from a narrow conception of the subject matter to a broader and more comprehensive understanding that encompasses more events and more complexities. Dialogue often results in self-revelation because the student is required to think through issues while considering answers to complex questions (Barnum, 1998).

Application to Nursing. Dialectic teaching is used frequently in nursing education. For example, it is commonly used in clinical situations and postclinical conferences. Dialectic teaching has shown to be effective in updated examples of clinical postconferences as described by Schams and Kuennen (2012) and Yehle and Royal (2010).

In other examples of dialectic strategies, Brown and Schmidt (2016) explained how a service-learning project used dialogue to develop critical thinking in postconferences, and Kowalski and Horner (2015) reported on the effectiveness of discussions when using a "flipped classroom" approach rather than a lecture format.

Problem-Based Learning Strategies

Problem-based learning (PBL) involves the use of predefined clinical situations and case studies to enhance or stimulate students to acquire specific skills, knowledge, and abilities (Phillips, 2016). Simulated clients may be used, or the student might be given a real problem in an actual clinical case; the objective of PBL is to determine how to manage the person's care.

PBL allows the instructor to manipulate multiple variables to add increasingly complex issues or circumstances that must be considered in problem resolution. For beginner students, the teacher may identify the problems but let the students seek solutions. Or the teacher may use the case as a problem-seeking exercise, teaching students how to find the important facts among the array of available data (Barnum, 1998).

In addition, PBL encourages self-direction, interpersonal communication, and use of information technology. Typically, small groups of students work together in self-directed teams; the case studies challenge them to improve their critical thinking capabilities, learn self-evaluation strategies, and promote communication among peers (Bentley, 2004; Phillips, 2016). Although it is an effective learning strategy, PBL can be time-intensive to implement because it requires faculty to develop realistic scenarios that usually focus on problems encountered by a single individual and/or family in a changeable clinical situation (Bentley, 2004).

Application to Nursing. PBL techniques are commonly used in nursing education. For example, Hodges and Massey (2015) explored the effects of PBL on an interprofessional course looking at the interdependence of nurses and pharmacists. They determined that the PBL activities allowed the students the "opportunity to explore professional interdependence while mastering fact-based content" (Hodges & Massey, 2015, p. 205). In another example, Atherton (2015) used PBL activities in teaching mental health nursing students, concluding that PBL should be considered as an alternative to the usual didactic teaching processes. Finally, Martyn, Terwijn, Kek, and Huijser (2014) found that PBL-based learning activities enhanced beginning nursing student's readiness for critical thinking.

Operational Teaching Strategies

Operational teaching strategies focus on presenting various perspectives regarding an agent or issue. A symposium that uses speakers with different perspectives on the same subject matter or a debate is an example. Other operational strategies focus on providing different or atypical activities for the learner. Using educational games or viewing nonmedical videos for illustration is considered to be operational teaching activities (Barnum, 1998).

Application to Nursing. Many nursing faculty use operational teaching techniques to make learning more interesting and enjoyable and to provide a different perspective on a particular topic (Herrman, 2011; Robb, 2012). Use of games to enhance students' decision making, critical thinking, and teamwork was described by Stanley and Latimer (2011). In other examples, Thomas and Schuessler (2016) used games and humor along with case studies to improve nursing student outcomes in a pharmacology course. Similarly, a group led by Day-Black, Merrill, Konzelman, Williams, and

Hart (2015) used "serious games" as one strategy for teaching students in an online community health nursing course. Use of movies, films, and television as a method to engage nursing students was described by several nursing educators (McAllister, 2015; Oh, De Gagné, & Kang, 2013; Wilson, Blake, Taylor, & Hannings, 2013).

Logistic Teaching Strategies

Logistic teaching strategies are based on the concept of mastery of sequential learning. Logistic teaching techniques generally divide the material to be learned into learning sequences, where acquisition of one section of the material is a necessary prerequisite to acquisition of another component. Logistic strategies teach the student clearly defined components and provide for reinforcement and testing of each component as the program progresses. As sections of the material are added and related to each other, knowledge accumulates (Barnum, 1998).

Formative testing is a logistic teaching strategy because a course is conceived as consisting of separate and definite units and tests are constructed to measure attainment of each unit. Other strategies include use of self-instructional modules and portfolios; these are typically logistic in nature because they follow a pattern of assembling information that is built on previously explained material (Phillips, 2016).

Application to Nursing. Logistic or sequential teaching is common in nursing curricula and has been effective because courses are sequenced and must be passed, and objectives or outcomes met, before students can progress to the next course or level. Examples from recent nursing literature include a work by Wassef, Riza, Maciag, Worden, and Delaney (2012), which described a mechanism in which graduate students were required to maintain and periodically submit electronic portfolios to document academic progress. Also describing how portfolios can be used effectively as summative assessment for nursing student progression were Hill (2012) and Smith and McDonald (2013). Use of modules to promote learning was described in several situations. Examples include using a modular format to teach ethics to undergraduate BSN students (Hsu & Hsieh, 2011), graduate students about complementary and alternative therapies (Swanson et al., 2012), and disaster management for public health nurses (Chiu, Polivka, & Stanley, 2012).

Use of Technology in Nursing Education

The use of technology-based distance learning methods, such as the Internet and interactive videoconferencing, has become widespread in nursing programs. In addition, computer-assisted instruction, which has been available since the early 1990s, is becoming more sophisticated and much more widely used in nursing education.

Three main types of technology-based educational methods are available to nursing educators. Interactive distance learning includes the use of two-way video and audio broadcasts carried over telephone lines. Internet courses with interactive video classrooms now are broadcast from colleges and universities to which students in widely dispersed geographic locations can participate. This technology, called *synchronous delivery*, requires that teacher and student be available to each other simultaneously (Friesth, 2016). Another interactive distance learning technique uses virtual classrooms that are available to students who have Internet carriers. These interactive virtual classrooms are available at all hours via a server. Finally, computer-based virtual reality simulations allow students under the guidance of the nursing educator to rehearse psychomotor interventions in realistic nursing situations prior to placing the patient into the learning situation as what happens in a practicum (Cannon & Boswell, 2012).

Familiarity with both synchronous (immediate or real-time access) and asynchronous (delayed access) technology makes it possible to use multiple teaching strategies. Virtual classrooms may combine both synchronous and asynchronous technology. Synchronous technology (e.g., videoconferencing, chat rooms, and real-time online classrooms) allows students to have personal contact with the instructor with immediate feedback, similar to face-to-face instruction, although the depth of the discussion may suffer. Asynchronous technology permits students to fit learning into their busy lifestyles. Asynchronous methods allow students to answer in greater depth because they have time to consider an answer.

Synchronous methods, such as videoconferencing, offer slightly more traditional pedagogy than strict reliance on Internet delivery, as the instructor is seen and heard and, through multiple media, can present a broad and diverse lecture format. Depending on the depth and difficulty of the materials, students may respond less frequently in the video classroom than on a chat facility in the virtual classroom. Use of both synchronous and asynchronous methods supports adult learning more effectively than any single method alone.

Virtual reality simulation is an innovation in clinical skills education and often employs use of high-fidelity human patient simulators. Some of these computerized mannequins produce motion and sounds that allow realistic situations as students practice assessing, planning, and carrying out interventions. The faculty preprogram the simulator with clinical situations to allow students to practice skills in a patient-safe environment (Cannon & Boswell, 2012; Jeffries, Swoboda, & Akintade, 2016).

High-fidelity patient simulation is the closest thing to virtual reality currently being widely used in nursing education. High-fidelity simulation typically consists of a mannequin and the apparatus within, which is programmed and accessed using a laptop, desktop, or handheld computer. Several current models simulate patients of all ages providing students with opportunities to assess heart, lung, and bowel sounds and initiate interventions to deal with multiple situations and patient responses (Bussard, 2016; Jeffries, 2012; Jeffries et al., 2016).

Issues in Technology-Based Teaching

Several issues should be considered when applying technologic innovations in nursing instruction. Instructors who use distance education by electronic modalities should be familiar with the technology at the user level and must carefully design courses for students involved in self-paced, independent study. Furthermore, faculty using electronic educational methods should be familiar with principles of adult learning (Knowles, 1980) when constructing the curricula and the course work for electronic delivery.

Institutional issues include the provision of the technology, software, and facilities for its use (Thompson, 2016). Faculty responsibilities include design or modification of the curriculum and the course content to reflect technology-based delivery. Other faculty concerns are the type of media to be used, faculty–student interaction, technology management, student evaluation, and faculty and course evaluation (Cannon & Boswell, 2012; Horsley & Wambach, 2015; Jeffries, 2012; Lubbers & Rossman, 2017; Woda, Gruenke, Alt-Gehrman, & Hansen, 2016).

Debriefing is considered to be an essential part of the clinical simulation learning process. During debriefing, students and educators can review what went on in the simulation, and the educator can correct any missed information or give positive feedback to the students (Padden-Denmead, Scaffidi, Kerley, & Farside, 2016; Page-Cutrara & Turk, 2017).

Numerous platforms are available to educators that permit multiple methods of interface between the teacher and student. These programs allow students to gain access to the course materials on their own schedule and to have real-time experiences with the instructor, such as is found in a chat facility or on a synchronous and telephone-based format such as Skype. Some also allow testing and provide security parameters to authorize only the teacher and student to have access to the student's records. E-mails, blogs, Twitter feeds, wikis, and social media formats permit messages between instructor and students and among students or groups of students through password-protected means. It is incumbent to mention that any information that should not be distributed to the public should not be shared through these media.

To take advantage of electronic teaching methods, the instructor must become proficient in multiple methods of conveying content and should be prepared to apply appropriate learning theories. Technology-based education embraces adult educational principles. Indeed, the content is presented in useful form, the immediacy of the student's need for knowledge is supported, and the student's ability to rely on previous knowledge base to provide a foundation for his or her questioning are all present in the typical interactive web-based classroom. The use of multiple ways of presenting the material in a course conducted using interactive technology-based education/learning creates the stimulus for learning and expands the educator's abilities in conveying course content.

Although the rewards of teaching by electronic methods are many, there are also issues of which faculty who are teaching online courses should be made aware. For example, distance methods such as web-based teaching may require more time than in-class, face-to-face strategies (Andersen & Avery, 2008; McAfooes, 2016). The necessary time to spend on this activity is becoming more recognized but has still not been adequately addressed by educational administrators. Preparation time expands including the time necessary to learn new electronic teaching methods. Indeed, the time that instructors invest in teaching online courses can be overwhelming to both novices and experienced educators.

The advantage of web-based instruction is that communication can be carried on all hours of the day, 7 days weekly, by web-based classroom, virtual chat, discussion boards, e-mail, fax, and telephone (McAfooes, 2016). Although the educator becomes a facilitator of adult education and the strategies are organized to take advantage of the self-directed, independent nature of the learners, the educator soon learns it is important to manage time to avoid becoming overwhelmed (Friesth, 2016; McAfooes, 2016). Educators who are contemplating using web-based teaching–learning strategies should consult with seasoned faculty mentors. They should be encouraged to take advantage of their experience with the methods of delivery for electronic education, peruse the literature about the issues of time and recognition, and negotiate from a position of knowledge to obtain the required time and promise of recognition.

Application to Nursing. Although technology-based instruction in nursing is relatively new, an increasing number of examples have appeared in the literature describing how technology is being used in nursing education and discussing successes and lessons learned. Because simulation has become widely used, the literature is full of examples describing how it can be used in many aspects of nursing education. For example, Burbach, Barnason, and Thompson (2015) used a "Think Aloud" strategy with baccalaureate nursing students to capture their clinical reasoning as they took part in a clinical simulation. Their findings suggested that simulation was an excellent way to assess students' clinical reasoning as they performed skills in a simulated clinical environment. In another example, Strickland and March (2015) used an experimental design to quantify the impact of simulation on didactic learning and high stakes examination outcomes. They found that examination scores of the students who had participated in the simulation were higher than of those who had not.

In a third example, Dame and Hoebeke (2016) developed an end-of-life-care simulation in which they measured pre- and post-simulation attitudes toward care of the dying of sophomore nursing students. They found that student attitudes toward caring for dying patients improved after the simulation. Bussard (2016), in a qualitative descriptive study, found that videotaped high-fidelity simulations assisted students in self-reflection on their practice. Video-recorded simulations benefitted the students in their developing clinical judgment.

Finally, McPherson and MacDonald (2017) blended simulation-based learning with interpretive pedagogy in a leadership course and found that students moved from merely knowing theories to more effectively applying leadership principles in action.

Through these research studies and many others, it is evident that many iterations and combinations of integrated, participatory simulated experiences are effective teaching strategies in nursing. As these educational experiences are developed, however, faculty must ensure that they use appropriate learning theories and recognized and evidence-based teaching strategies.

Summary

This chapter has presented two major areas relevant to the use of theoretic principles and models in nursing education: curriculum design and instruction. In the opening case study, Linda and her classmates learned that it is necessary to have a sound, identified theoretical base to serve as the framework for a nursing program. They also recognized that it is important to select multiple teaching strategies to deliver the material in a manner that will best support student learning.

Likewise, it is essential that all nurse educators be aware of how theoretical principles are used in education. They should be able to articulate the conceptual framework of their program and recognize how the framework shapes the program. Nursing educators should also use multiple strategies and techniques for instruction to enable students to develop their knowledge base and to develop critical thinking abilities and problem-solving skills.

Finally, nursing educators should recognize that technology will play an increasingly important role in nursing education and be prepared to incorporate tested distance education methods and virtual reality simulation into instruction.

Whether the focus is continuing education of practicing nurses or fundamental education of students of the discipline at any level, modern teaching and learning methods make educational efforts more available to a wide variety of individuals with a variety of educational and learning needs, at times when the students are most available, in widely distributed areas of the country. It is therefore imperative that nursing educators understand relevant principles and theories to address these needs.

Key Points

- Curricula are created by faculty to fulfill their ideals of nursing education and to provide the community with effective, safe, well-educated nurses.
- Curricula are best organized around a guiding principle, be it a nursing theory or a collection of nursing and shared theories; the outcome is to provide the students with intellectual and clinical development as professional nurses.
- Nursing programs are evaluated and accredited by several bodies, including the state boards of nursing, the AACN's CCNE, and the ACEN.

- Teaching methods should be theory- and evidence-based to enhance learning.
- Innovations such as critical thinking, PBL, and simulation are part of many nursing curricula.
- Learning environments have evolved. Today, they include fully face-to-face, in-class learning; hybrid models in which some content is presented via web-based methods; and totally web-based courses in which all of the content is presented online.

Learning Activities

1. Following the example of Linda, the nurse from the opening case study, work with other students to outline the curriculum for an undergraduate, prelicensure nursing program or a program to prepare advanced practice nurses. Start with development of a curricular framework and identification of the key concepts and content for the curriculum.

2. Select one of the courses in a nursing program and modify it to be delivered using some type of distance learning (e.g., Internet delivery, such as podcasting, or other innovative online methods). How will presentation of the material be accomplished? How will students interact with each other and with the instructor? What activities will be added? What activities will be deleted?

3. Search recent nursing literature for research on technology-based nursing education. Do these techniques appear to be as effective as traditional class work in ensuring that students achieve the goals or competencies of the nursing program? What are the strengths and weaknesses of the research you have found?

4. Discuss the use of patient simulators in clinical nursing staff education. Consider the cost and upkeep of the equipment for simulators and faculty training and education and the need for technical support of the equipment.

REFERENCES

Accreditation Commission for Education in Nursing. (2017). *Standards and criteria for baccalaureate programs.* Retrieved from http://www.acenursing.net/manuals/sc2017_B.pdf

American Association of Colleges of Nursing. (1999). A vision of baccalaureate and graduate nursing education: The next decade. *Journal of Professional Nursing, 15*(1), 59–65.

American Association of Colleges of Nursing. (2008). *The essentials of baccalaureate education for professional nursing practice.* Retrieved from http://www.aacnnursing.org/Portals/42/Publications/BaccEssentials08.pdf

American Association of Colleges of Nursing. (2016). CARES: Competencies and recommendations for educating undergraduate nursing students: Preparing nurses to care for the seriously ill and their families. *Journal of Professional Nursing, 32*(2), 78–84.

Andersen, K. M., & Avery, M. D. (2008). Faculty teaching time: A comparison of web-based and face-to-face graduate nursing courses. *International Journal of Nursing Education Scholarship, 5*, 2.

Atherton, H. (2015). Problem-based learning in pre-registration mental health nursing: The student experience. *Mental Health Practice, 19*(1), 28–33.

Barnum, B. S. (1998). *Nursing theory: Analysis, application, evaluation* (5th ed.). Philadelphia, PA: Lippincott Williams & Wilkins.

Beckman, S. J., Boxley-Harges, S. L., & Kaskel, B. L. (2012). Experience informs: Spanning three decades with the Neuman systems model. *Nursing Science Quarterly, 25*(4), 341–346.

Bednash, G. P., Cronenwett, L., & Dolansky, M. A. (2013). QSEN transforming education. *Journal of Professional Nursing, 29*(2), 66–67.

Bentley, G. W. (2004). Problem-based learning. In A. J. Lowenstein & M. J. Bradshaw (Eds.), *Fuszard's innovative teaching strategies in nursing* (3rd ed., pp. 83–106). Sudbury, MA: Jones & Bartlett Learning.

Berbiglia, V. A. (2011). The self-care deficit nursing theory as a curriculum conceptual framework in baccalaureate education. *Nursing Science Quarterly, 24*(2), 137–145.

Bevis, E. O. (1973). *Curriculum building in nursing: A process.* St. Louis, MO: Mosby.

Bevis, E. O. (1987). History of curriculum development. In *Curriculum revolution: Mandate for change* (pp. 27–40). New York, NY: National League for Nursing Press.

Bevis, E. O. (1989a). *Curriculum building in nursing: A process* (3rd ed.). New York, NY: National League for Nursing Press.

Bevis, E. O. (1989b). Illuminating the issues: Probing the past, a history of nursing curriculum development—the past shapes the present. In E. O. Bevis & J. Watson (Eds.), *Toward a caring curriculum: A new pedagogy for nursing* (pp. 13–35). New York, NY: National League for Nursing Press.

Boland, D. L., & Finke, L. M. (2012). Curriculum designs. In D. M. Billings & J. A. Halstead (Eds.), *Teaching in nursing: A guide for faculty* (4th ed., pp. 119–137). St. Louis, MO: Elsevier.

Brown, J. M., & Schmidt, N. A. (2016). Service-learning in undergraduate nursing education: Where is the reflection? *Journal of Professional Nursing, 32*(1), 48–53. doi:10.1016/j.profnurs.2015.05.001

Burbach, B., Barnason, S., & Thompson, S. A. (2015). Using "Think Aloud" to capture clinical reasoning during patient simulation. *International Journal of Nursing Education Scholarship, 12.* doi:10.1515/ijnes-2014.0044

Burkhart, L., & Schmidt, W. (2012). Measuring effectiveness of a spiritual care pedagogy in nursing education. *Journal of Professional Nursing, 28*(5), 315–321.

Bussard, M. E. (2016). Self-reflection of video-recorded high-fidelity simulations and development of clinical judgment. *Journal of Nursing Education, 55*(9), 522–527. doi:10.3928/01484834-20160816-06

Cannon, S., & Boswell, C. (2012). *Evidence-based teaching in nursing: A foundation for educators.* Sudbury, MA: Jones & Bartlett Learning.

Chiu, M., Polivka, B. J., & Stanley, S. A. R. (2012). Evaluation of a disaster-surge training for public health nurses. *Public Health Nursing, 29*(2), 136–142.

Choi, J., & De Martinis, J. E. (2013). Nursing informatics competencies: Assessment of undergraduate and graduate nursing students. *Journal of Clinical Nursing, 22*(13–14), 1970–1976.

Commission on Collegiate Nursing Education. (2013). *Standards for accreditation of baccalaureate and greater nursing education programs.* Washington, DC: American Association of Colleges of Nursing. Retrieved from http://www.aacnnursing.org/Portals/42/CCNE/PDF/Standards-Amended-2013.pdf?ver=2017-06-28-141019-360

Dame, L., & Hoebeke, R. (2016). Effects of a simulation exercise on nursing students' end-of-life care attitudes. *Journal of Nursing Education, 55*(12), 701–705. doi:10.3928/01484834-20161114-07

Day-Black, C., Merrill, E. B., Konzelman, L., Williams, T. T., & Hart, N. (2015). Gamification: An innovative teaching-learning strategy for the digital nursing students in a community health nursing course. *The ABNF Journal, 26*(4), 90–94.

Duncan, K., & Schulz, P. S. (2015). Impact of change to a concept-based baccalaureate nursing curriculum on student and program outcomes. *Journal of Nursing Education, 54*(3 Suppl.), S16–S20.

Ervin, S. M. (2015). History of nursing education in the United States. In S. B. Keating (Ed.), *Curriculum development and evaluation in nursing* (3rd ed., pp. 5–32). New York, NY: Springer Publishing.

Fater, K. H. (2014). Introducing genomics to novice baccalaureate nursing students. *Journal of Nursing Education, 53*(9 Suppl.), S119–S120.

Friesth, B. M. (2016). Teaching and learning at a distance. In D. M. Billings & J. A. Halstead (Eds.), *Teaching in nursing: A guide for faculty* (5th ed., pp. 342–356). St. Louis, MO: Elsevier.

Giarelli, E., & Reiff, M. (2012). Genomic literacy and competent practice: Call for research on genetics in nursing education. *Nursing Clinics of North America, 47*(4), 529–545.

Gray-Miceli, D., Wilson, L. D., Stanley, J., Watman, R., Shire, A., Sofaer, S., et al. (2014). Improving the quality of geriatric nursing care: Enduring outcomes from the geriatric nursing education consortium. *Journal of Professional Nursing, 30*(6), 447–455.

Hardin, P. K., & Richardson, S. J. (2012). Teaching the concept curricula: Theory and method. *Journal of Nursing Education, 51*(3), 155–159.

Herrman, J. W. (2011). Keeping their attention: Innovative strategies for nursing education. *Journal of Continuing Education in Nursing, 42*(10), 449–456.

Hill, T. L. (2012). The portfolio as a summative assessment for the nursing students. *Teaching and Learning in Nursing, 7*(1), 140–145.

Hodges, H. F., & Massey, A. T. (2015). Interprofessional problem-based learning project outcomes between prelicensure baccalaureate of science in nursing and doctor of pharmacy programs. *Journal of Nursing Education, 54*(4), 201–206. doi:10.3928/01484834-20150318-03

Horsley, T. L., & Wambach, K. (2015). Effect of nursing faculty presence on students' anxiety, self-confidence, and clinical performance during a clinical simulation experience. *Clinical Simulation in Nursing, 11*, 4–10. doi:10.1016/j.ecns.2014.09.012

Hsu, L. L., & Hsieh, S. I. (2011). Effects of a blended learning module on self-reported learning performances in baccalaureate nursing students. *Journal of Advanced Nursing, 67*(11), 2435–2444.

Institute of Medicine. (2011). *The future of nursing: Leading change, advancing health.* Washington, DC: National Academies Press.

Iwasiw, C. L., & Goldenberg, D. (2015). *Curriculum development in nursing education* (3rd ed.). Burlington, MA: Jones & Bartlett Learning.

Jeffries, P. R. (2012). *Simulation in nursing education: From conceptualization to evaluation.* New York, NY: National League for Nursing.

Jeffries, P. R., Swoboda, S. M., & Akintade, B. (2016). Teaching and learning using simulations. In D. M. Billings & J. A. Halstead (Eds.), *Teaching in nursing: A guide for faculty* (5th ed., pp. 304–323). St. Louis, MO: Elsevier.

Jenkins, J., & Calzone, K. A. (2014). Genomics nursing faculty champion initiative. *Nurse Educator, 39*(1), 8–13.

Josephsen, J., & Martz, K. (2014). Faculty and student perceptions: An end-of-life nursing curriculum survey. *Journal of Hospice & Palliative Nursing, 16*(8), 474–481.

Keating, S. B. (2015a). Overview of nursing education: History, curriculum development processes, and the role of faculty. In S. B. Keating (Ed.), *Curriculum development and evaluation in nursing* (3rd ed., pp. 1–4). New York, NY: Springer Publishing.

Keating, S. B. (2015b). The components of the curriculum. In S. B. Keating (Ed.), *Curriculum development and evaluation in nursing* (3rd ed., pp. 185–228). New York, NY: Springer Publishing.

Kelley, J. (1975). The conceptual framework in nursing education. In *Curriculum development, part VI: Curriculum revision in baccalaureate nursing education* (pp. 15–20). New York, NY: National League for Nursing Press.

Knowles, M. S. (1980). *The modern practice of adult education: From pedagogy to andragogy* (2nd ed.). New York, NY: Cambridge Books.

Kowalski, K., & Horner, M. D. (2015). Preparing educators to implement flipped classrooms as a teaching strategy. *Journal of Continuing Education in Nursing, 46*(8), 346–347. doi:10.3928/00220124-20150721-14

Lewis, D. Y. (2012). Incorporating national priorities into the curriculum. *Journal of Professional Nursing, 28*(2), 105–109.

Lubbers, J., & Rossman, C. (2017). Satisfaction and self-confidence with nursing clinical simulation: Novice learners, medium-fidelity, and community settings. *Nurse Education Today, 48*, 140–144. doi:10.1016/j.nedt.2016.10.010

Mager, R. F. (1962). *Preparing instructional objectives.* Belmont, CA: Fearon.

Martyn, J., Terwijn, R., Kek, M. Y., & Huijser, H. (2014). Exploring the relationships between teaching, approaches to learning and critical thinking in a problem-based learning foundation nursing course. *Nurse Education Today, 34*(5), 829–835. doi:10.1016/j.nedt.2013.04.023

McAfooes, J. (2016). Teaching and learning in online learning communities. In D. M. Billings & J. A. Halstead (Eds.), *Teaching in nursing: A guide for faculty* (5th ed., pp. 357–383). St. Louis, MO: Elsevier.

McAllister, M. (2015). Connecting narrative with mental health learning through discussion and analysis of selected contemporary films. *International Journal of Mental Health Nursing, 24*(4), 304–313.

McEwen, M., & Brown, S. C. (2002). Conceptual frameworks in undergraduate nursing curricula: Report of a national survey. *Journal of Nursing Education, 41*(1), 5–14.

McPherson, C., & MacDonald, C. (2017). Blending simulation-based learning and interpretative pedagogy for undergraduate leadership competency development. *Journal of Nursing Education, 56*(1), 49–54. doi:10.3928/01484834-20161219-10

Meleis, A. I. (2012). *Theoretical nursing: Development and progress* (5th ed.). Philadelphia, PA: Lippincott Williams & Wilkins.

Monsivais, D. B., & Robinson, K. (2016). Developing students as future researchers using QSEN competencies as a framework. *Nursing Forum, 51*(4), 238–245.

Mueller, C. (2016). Service learning: Developing values, cultural competence, social responsibility, and global awareness. In D. M. Billings & J. A. Halstead (Eds.), *Teaching in nursing: A guide for faculty* (5th ed., pp. 197–209). St. Louis, MO: Elsevier.

National League for Nursing. (1972). *Criteria for the appraisal of baccalaureate and higher degree programs in nursing.* New York, NY: National League for Nursing Press.

National League for Nursing. (1977). *Criteria for the evaluation of educational programs in nursing leading to an associate degree* (5th ed.). New York, NY: National League for Nursing Press.

Newman, D. M. (2008). Conceptual models of nursing and baccalaureate nursing education. *Journal of Nursing Education, 47*(5), 199–200.

Oh, J., De Gagné, J. C., & Kang, J. (2013). A review of teaching-learning strategies to be used with film for prelicensure students. *Journal of Nursing Education, 52*(3), 150–156.

O'Neil, C. (2015). Teaching in online learning environments. In M. H. Oermann (Ed.), *Teaching in nursing and role of the educator: The complete guide to best practice in teaching, evaluation and curriculum development* (pp. 103–116). New York, NY: Springer Publishing.

Padden-Denmead, M. L., Scaffidi, R. M., Kerley, R. M., & Farside, A. L. (2016). Simulation with debriefing and guided reflective journaling to stimulate critical thinking in prelicensure baccalaureate degree nursing students. *Journal of Nursing Education, 55*(11), 645–650. doi:10.3928/01484834-20161011-07

Page-Cutrara, K., & Turk, M. (2017). Impact of prebriefing on competency performance, clinical judgment and experience in simulation: An experimental study. *Nurse Education Today, 48*(1), 78–83. doi:10.1016/j.nedt.2016.09.012

Pauly-O'Neill, S., Cooper, E., & Prion, S. (2016). Student QSEN participation during an adult medical-surgical rotation. *Nursing Education Perspectives, 37*(3), 165–167.

Phillips, J. M. (2016). Strategies to promote student engagement and active learning. In D. M. Billings & J. A. Halstead (Eds.), *Teaching in nursing: A guide for faculty* (5th ed., pp. 245–262). St. Louis, MO: Elsevier.

Pressler, J. L., & Kenner, C. A. (2015). Reasoning back, looking ahead. *Nurse Educator, 40*(1), 5–6.

Rentschler, D. D., & Spegman, A. M. (1996). Curriculum revolution: Realities of change. *Journal of Nursing Education, 35*(9), 389–393.

Robb, M. K. (2012). Managing a large class environment: Simple strategies for new nurse educators. *Teaching and Learning in Nursing, 7*(1), 47–50.

Ross, J. G., & Bruderle, E. (2016). Student-centered teaching strategies to integrate the quality and safety education for nurses competency, safety, into a nursing course. *Nurse Educator, 41*(6), 278–281.

Ruchala, P. L. (2015). Curriculum development and approval processes in changing educational environments. In S. B. Keating (Ed.), *Curriculum development and evaluation in nursing* (3rd ed., pp. 3–48). New York, NY: Springer Publishing.

Russell, B. H. (2015). The who, what, and how of evaluation within online nursing education: State of the science. *Journal of Nursing Education, 54*(1), 13–21. doi:10.3928/01484834-20141228-02

Scales, F. S. (1985). *Nursing curriculum: Development, structure, function.* Norwalk, CT: Appleton-Century-Crofts.

Schams, K. A., & Kuennen, J. K. (2012). Clinical postconference pedagogy: Exploring evidence-based practice with millennial-inspired "building blocks." *Creative Nursing, 18*(1), 13–16.

Secrest, J. (2008). The role of tool development in an Orem-based curriculum. *Self-Care, Dependent-Care & Nursing, 16*(2), 25–33.

Skiba, D. J. (2012). Technology and gerontology: Is this in your nursing curriculum? *Nursing Education Perspectives, 33*(3), 207–209.

Smith, C. M., & McDonald, K. (2013). Transition to an electronic professional nurse portfolio: Part II. *Journal of Continuing Education in Nursing, 44*(8), 340–341.

Speziale, H. J., & Jacobson, L. (2005). Trends in registered nurse education programs 1998–2008. *Nursing Education Perspectives, 26*(4), 230–235.

Stanley, D., & Latimer, K. (2011). "The ward": A simulation game for nursing students. *Nurse Education in Practice, 11*(1), 20–25.

Stokowski, L. A. (2011). *Overhauling nursing education.* Retrieved from http://www.medscape.com/viewarticle/736236

Strickland, H. P., & March, A. L. (2015). Longitudinal impact of a targeted simulation experience on high-stakes examination outcomes. *Clinical Simulation in Nursing, 11*(7), 342–347. doi:10.1016/j.ecns.2015.04.006

Sullivan, D. T. (2016). An introduction to curriculum development. In D. M. Billings & J. A. Halstead (Eds.), *Teaching in nursing: A guide for faculty* (5th ed., pp. 89–117). St. Louis, MO: Elsevier.

Swanson, B., Zeller, J. M., Keithley, J. K., Fung, S. C., Johnson, A., Suhayda, R., et al. (2012). Case-based online modules to teach graduate-level nursing students about complementary and alternative medical therapies. *Journal of Professional Nursing, 28*(2), 125–129.

Tanner, C. A. (1989). An analysis of the historical and political background of the revision of the NLN's criteria for the appraisal of baccalaureate and higher degree programs. In N. Diekelmann, D. Allen, & C. Tanner (Eds.), *The NLN criteria for appraisal of baccalaureate programs: A critical hermeneutic analysis* (pp. 3–10). New York, NY: National League for Nursing Press.

Taylor, E. J., Testerman, N., & Hart, D. (2014). Teaching spiritual care to nursing students: An integrated model. *Journal of Christian Nursing, 31*(2), 94–99.

Thomas, V., & Schuessler, J. B. (2016). Using innovative teaching strategies to improve outcomes in a pharmacology course. *Nursing Education Perspectives, 37*(3), 174–176.

Thompson, B. W. (2016). The connected classroom: Using digital technology to promote learning. In D. M. Billings & J. A. Halstead (Eds.), *Teaching in nursing: A guide for faculty* (5th ed., pp. 324–341). St. Louis, MO: Elsevier.

Wassef, M. E., Riza, L., Maciag, T., Worden, C., & Delaney, A. (2012). Implementing a competency-based electronic portfolio in a graduate nursing program. *Computers, Informatics, Nursing, 30*(5), 242–248.

Watson, M. J. (1996). Watson's theory of transpersonal caring. In P. H. Walker & B. Neuman (Eds.), *Blueprint for use of nursing models: Education, research, practice, & administration* (pp. 141–184). New York, NY: National League for Nursing Press.

Weiner, E., Trangenstein, P., Gordon, J., & McNew, R. (2016). Integrating informatics content into the nursing curriculum. *Studies in Health Technology and Informatics, 225*, 302–306.

Wilson, A. H., Blake, B. J., Taylor, G. A., & Hannings, G. (2013). Cinemeducation: Teaching family assessment skills using full-length movies. *Public Health Nursing, 30*(3), 239–245.

Woda, A. A., Gruenke, T., Alt-Gehrman, P., & Hansen, J. (2016). Nursing student perceptions regarding simulation experience sequencing. *Journal of Nursing Education, 55*(9), 528–532. doi:10.3928/01484834-20160816-07

Wu, R. R. (1979). Designing a curriculum model. *Journal of Nursing Education, 18*(3), 13–21.

Yehle, K. S., & Royal, P. A. (2010). Changing the postclinical conference: New time, new place, new methods equal success. *Nursing Education Perspectives, 31*(4), 256–258.

Future Issues in Nursing Theory

Melanie McEwen

Rebecca Jackson will graduate from a master's program in nursing in only a few weeks. She has learned a great deal about nursing practice, research, administration and management, and education from the various courses she has taken, and she is enthusiastic about the career opportunities she is considering. When she started the program, she was confident that she wanted to become a nurse administrator, but midway through her studies, she decided to focus on research. She ultimately wants to get a doctorate and become an educator and researcher.

Currently, Rebecca is working as a clinical supervisor at the public health department in a major metropolitan area. In the 10 years Rebecca has been with the health department, she has witnessed tremendous growth in the diversity of the population served. There are immigrant families from several Spanish-speaking countries as well as from the Southeast Asian countries of Cambodia, Laos, Vietnam, and Philippines. Recently, there has been an influx of refugees from Iraq, Syria, Bosnia, and Eastern Africa. Rebecca is intrigued by these groups' divergent perceptions of health and ways to promote health. Furthermore, she is concerned with communication issues and how to motivate health promotional practices. She has determined that this is particularly important in working with children and in teaching parents ways to improve their health.

In her position, Rebecca has had several opportunities to be involved in funded research. At present, she is working with a sociologist, an anthropologist, a clinical psychologist, and an epidemiologist to write a grant for a research project that will examine and compare health beliefs, health practices, and health promotional behaviors among various cultural groups in the city. The study will have multiple levels and phases and will incorporate both quantitative and qualitative data collection techniques and analysis.

Rebecca helped develop the conceptual framework for the study, which combines aspects of the Health Belief Model and Leininger's Culture Care Diversity Theory (McFarland & Wehbe-Alamah, 2015). The framework identifies cultural beliefs, practices, and values and incorporates them with knowledge of health threats and perceptions of illness severity, seriousness, and value for taking action. The researchers expect that the information provided by the study will allow the health department to develop a series of health programs that are sensitive to the needs, beliefs, and practices of the many cultural groups in the department's catchment area.

During the last two decades, a number of shifts occurred in the demographic patterns of the United States. This has been coupled with major changes in the health care delivery system and changes in the causes of illness, disability, and death. The Patient Protection and Affordable Care Act of 2010 (ACA) has contributed to the growing emphasis on health care financing, community-based care, health promotion, and access to care. Additionally, further legislative efforts to "repeal and replace" or radically "overhaul" the ACA are under consideration. Significant cost reductions, restructuring of health care services, and growth in integrated health care systems using managed care strategies are anticipated. Concurrently, the increased severity of illness among persons in inpatient facilities and the increased incidence of chronic illnesses, particularly in the growing number of older adults, have taxed the health care system. Box 23-1 describes current and future health care challenges that the discipline of nursing and nursing science must recognize, understand, and address (Institute of Medicine [IOM], 2011, 2016).

In the face of system-wide changes associated with implementation and revision of the ACA and other initiatives, major problems remain and must be addressed. For example, the health care system is not designed to provide convenient care to all who need it. The system is organized according to physicians' specialties and schedules, not according to the needs of their patients. Hospitals are used inappropriately, with access to care, supplemental insurance, and home care services still unevenly distributed.

Box 23-1   The Future of Nursing—Health Care Challenges

In *The Future of Nursing*, the Institute of Medicine (IOM, 2011) identified five major "health care challenges" facing the U.S. health care system in the 21st century. These are:

- Chronic conditions (e.g., diabetes, hypertension, arthritis, cardiovascular disease, and mental health conditions): Prevalence of these conditions is expected to increase and to be exacerbated by growing rates of obesity.
- Aging population: The proportion of the U.S. population aged 65 years and older is expected to grow from 12.7% in 2008 to 19.3% in 2030. This will dramatically affect the demand for health care services.
- Diverse population: Minority groups are projected to increase from about a third of the U.S. population to 54% by 2042. Diversity involves various ethnic and racial groups, language, immigrant status, socioeconomic status, and other cultural features.
- Health disparities: Inequities in the burden of disease, injury, or death experienced by socially disadvantaged groups. Health disparities are not only partially caused by deleterious socioenvironmental conditions and behavior risk factors but may also be influenced by bias that results in unequal, inferior treatment.
- Limited English proficiency: Related to the increasingly diverse population is the problem of limited English proficiency. To be effective, health information must be accessible, understandable, and culturally relevant. Limited English proficiency and varying cultural and health practices contribute to the complex challenges that health care providers must address.

There is also a growing need for health care providers, including nurses, who can meet the challenges of the changing system and evolving health and illness patterns. Nurses of the future must be capable of ensuring access to care and promoting high-quality outcomes. The American Association of Colleges of Nursing (AACN, 2008) has described the skills and practice capabilities currently expected for nurses (Box 23-2). In short, essential competencies include critical thinking and clinical judgment skills, ability to work in a variety of health care settings and with patients who have complex health problems, effective organizational and teamwork skills, understanding of evidence-based care, recognition of the influence of culture on health and ability to care for individuals from diverse backgrounds and across the life span, and a commitment to personal accountability and professional development.

The IOM's (2011) publication on *The Future of Nursing* has been viewed as a challenge and strategy to (1) make quality health care accessible to the diverse populations of the United States, (2) intentionally promote wellness and disease prevention, (3) improve health outcomes, and (4) provide compassionate care across the life span. The IOM describes a future health system in which:

■ Primary care and prevention are central drivers.
■ Interprofessional collaboration and coordination are the norm.
■ Payment for services rewards value rather than volume.
■ Quality care is affordable for individuals and society.

To plan for the future health care system, the discipline of nursing should give increasing attention to related theories, concepts, and models. Among these are primary health care (as opposed to "illness care"), health promotion, health protection, motivation, health as a resource for everyday life, health economics, patient safety, and quality of life. Frameworks for practice will embrace community-based and community-focused care, changing identification of the client (population/ aggregate/group vs. individual), interprofessional collaboration, noninstitutional care settings, innovation, technology transformation, and multiple levels of decision-making authority (Bodenheimer & Grumbach, 2016; IOM, 2016; Porter-O'Grady & Malloch, 2015).

This chapter describes the current state and some of the anticipated changes that will affect the discipline of nursing during the next decade and examines how these changes will influence theory and knowledge development. Topics covered include

---

Box 23-2 Competencies and Skills Needed by Generalist Nurses

Practice from a holistic, caring framework.
Practice from an evidence base.
Promote safe, quality patient care.
Use clinical/critical reasoning to address simple to complex situations.
Assume accountability for one's own and delegated nursing care.
Practice in a variety of health care settings.
Care for patients across the health–illness continuum.
Care for patients across the life span.
Care for diverse populations.
Engage in care of self in order to care for others.
Engage in continuous professional development.

Source: AACN (2008).

future issues in nursing science and future issues in theory development. This is followed by an exploration of future theoretical issues related to nursing practice, research, administration and management, and education.

Future Issues in Nursing Science

Nursing science is concerned with answering questions of interest to the profession and adding to its body of knowledge. Knowledge development is accomplished through the study of concepts, relationships, and theories relevant to the discipline and generally occurs within the broad domain of one of the major worldviews of the discipline.

As discussed in Chapter 1, a paradigm is a pattern, model, or global concept accepted by most people in an intellectual community; it is a set of systematic beliefs or a worldview. Paradigms provide scientists with a general orientation to phenomena, a way of organizing perceptions, criteria for selecting problems, guidelines for investigations and methods, and limitations on possible solutions. The paradigm, or worldview, provides a guiding framework for resolving problems, conducting research, and deriving theories and laws in the discipline.

Nursing science has two predominant paradigms, broadly classified as empiricist and constructivist, which hold fundamentally opposing views of knowledge development and reality. Chapter 1 described the ongoing debate within the scientific nursing community about the appropriateness of the two philosophies and methodologies for directing and conducting research as well as identifying questions of relevance to the discipline.

Most in the profession today find the philosophical debate inconclusive, frustrating, and not particularly germane to promoting nursing. Many scholars believe that nursing should emphasize the benefits of inquiry per se, rather than the supremacy of one paradigm over the other, because neither method is more scientific than the other, and the process of inquiry is the same despite the methods used to acquire knowledge (Chinn & Kramer, 2015; Melnyk & Fineout-Overholt, 2015; Polit & Beck, 2017; Risjord, 2010).

In the 21st century, nursing science should work to eliminate obstacles to nursing research and promote acceptance of multiple methods of inquiry and use of research findings—or "translation"—in practice (White, Dudley-Brown, & Terhaar, 2016). Because the problems of nursing are so diverse and complex, use of differing viewpoints and paradigms is needed to help answer questions and provide solutions to questions of interest. Because multiple perspectives encourage appreciation of the uniqueness of individuals, use of various perspectives will encourage identification of answers to important problems. Also, applying different viewpoints provides new insights that can help nurses formulate new ideas for study.

Combining or triangulating methods can maximize the strengths and minimize the weaknesses of each method and should be encouraged. Integration of qualitative and quantitative methods has been suggested as one way to advance nursing science because research traditions from both paradigms are complementary, although the approaches are different. Qualitative methods can describe phenomena of interest in nursing and generate theories that propose relationships between identified concepts. Quantitative methods can test the relationships of qualitatively developed theories and suggest whether the theory should be accepted or revised (Bekhet & Zauszniewski, 2012; Polit & Beck, 2017). Indeed, Chinn and Kramer (2015) observed that blending and using a variety of research processes and techniques in knowledge development indicates growing maturity in nursing scholarship. Nurses should be encouraged to be pragmatic regarding research methodology and use the right method for the task.

Future Issues in Nursing Theory

According to the AACN (2006, 2011), nurses in advanced practice should be prepared to critique, evaluate, and use theory. Nurses should be able to integrate and apply a wide range of theories from nursing and other sciences into a comprehensive and holistic approach to care. Thus, in addition to nursing theories, nurses prepared at the graduate level should be exposed to relevant theories from a wide range of fields, including natural sciences, social sciences, biologic sciences, and organizational and management concepts. Basic theoretical knowledge and skills proposed by the AACN are listed in Box 23-3.

As explained in Chapter 2, the discipline of nursing is currently in the "integrated knowledge stage" of theory development. In this stage, there is an increasing emphasis on conducting research that will produce knowledge to support practice. Additionally, in this stage, there has been a shift in focus to application of "evidence" from across all health-related sciences (translational research). It is anticipated that the importance of middle range and situation-specific/practice theories will continue to be emphasized, and there will be less attention given to grand theories and conceptual frameworks. See Chapters 10, 11, 12, and 19 for detailed discussions of middle range, situation-specific theories, and evidence-based practice (EBP) guidelines.

Implications for Theory Development

The discipline of nursing has recognized several new trends for theory development. These include development of middle range theories, situation-specific (practice) theories, and EBP protocols/procedures as the latest steps in knowledge development.

There has been broad acceptance of the need to develop middle range theories to support nursing practice (Chinn & Kramer, 2015; Meleis, 2012; Peterson & Bredow, 2017; Roy, 2014; Smith & Liehr, 2014). This call for development of middle range theory is consistent with a desire to focus increased attention on substantive knowledge development. In the future, as additional middle range theories are developed, there will be a growing need to consider their analysis and evaluation (whether formal or informal). Indeed, nurses should direct considerable effort toward developing, testing, evaluating, and refining middle range theories to develop the discipline's substantive knowledge base.

Box 23-3	Theoretical Knowledge and Skills for Doctor of Nursing Practice

The doctor of nursing practice (DNP) program prepares the graduate to:

1. Integrate nursing science with knowledge from ethics and the biophysical, psychosocial, analytical, and organizational sciences as the basis for the highest level of nursing practice.
2. Use science-based theories and concepts to:
   a. Determine the nature and significance of health and health care delivery.
   b. Describe actions and advanced strategies to enhance, alleviate, and ameliorate health and health care and deliver phenomena as appropriate.
3. Evaluate outcomes. Develop and evaluate new practice approaches based on nursing theories and theories from other disciplines.

Source: AACN (2006, p. 9).

In recent years, there has been enhanced attention to the application of theory in practice and the relationship of theory, practice, and research. Development of situation-specific (practice) theories and EBP models has consequently become increasingly emphasized (Chinn & Kramer, 2015; Dahnke & Dreher, 2016; Im, 2014; Meleis, 2012). Furthermore, many nurse researchers use theories from other disciplines in their studies, and as a result, more emphasis and discussion should be given to "borrowed" or "shared" theory, along with recognition that this practice does not negate the findings or make them less valuable to nursing.

It is important that nurses understand the interrelationship between theory, research, and practice and recognize the importance of this reciprocal relationship to the continuing development of nursing as a profession. In a practice discipline such as nursing, theory and practice are inseparable, and development and application of theory affiliated with research-based practice have been seen as fundamental to the development of professionalism and autonomous practice. Despite repeated calls to merge theory, practice, and research, there remains a confusing and fragmented mix. Progress has been made, however, because there has been increased emphasis on the interchange and interaction among research, clinical practice, and theory development. This trend should continue.

Theoretical Perspectives on Future Issues in Nursing Practice, Research, Administration and Management, and Education

With accessibility, cost containment, and provision of quality care driving health care reform, the discipline of nursing must anticipate how these forces will affect nursing within the changing health care system. With implementation of the ACA and pending major revisions to it, along with other health system changes in the near future, nurses are expected to assume a central role in helping to achieve cost-effective, quality health services (IOM, 2016). How these changes and related theoretical implications will affect nursing practice, nursing research, nursing administration and management, and nursing education are examined separately.

Future Issues and Nursing Practice

A transformation is occurring in nursing practice. This has been driven by socioeconomic factors as well as by developments in health care delivery. Many nursing leaders have identified relevant factors. Among these are changing demographics and increasing racial and ethnic diversity and related health disparities, the explosion of technology and information systems, globalization of the world's economy, more educated consumers, increasing acceptance and use of alternative therapies, explosion of genomic information, a shift to population-based care, potential shortage of nurses, proliferation of medical errors, increasing complexity of care, and concerns over end-of-life issues (Huston, 2017; IOM, 2011, 2016; Porter-O'Grady & Malloch, 2016; Stokowski, 2011).

Increasingly, nurses are finding employment in home health and other ambulatory settings in which they provide care for well or chronically ill clients. These trends will most likely continue throughout the near future, and in response, nursing interventions will focus more on comprehensive assessment and care planning, case management, and client teaching to achieve the goals of health promotion, health maintenance, and disease prevention. Furthermore, in the future, nurses will routinely use diagnosis and intervention databases, as well as expert systems, to assist with decision making.

Table 23-1 Nursing Practice Competencies for Today's Health Care System	
Competency	**Examples of Activities**
Health promotion—activities to enable clients to improve health, maximize health potential, and enhance well-being	Teach prevention and health promotion activities. Educate patients about lifestyle and its effect on health. Use community resources to enhance care. Advocate for policy change to promote health.
Supervision—ability to coordinate the implementation of the plan of nursing care by ancillary or subordinate members of the health care team	Supervise ancillary nursing staff. Delegate and monitor work tasks of ancillary staff. Assume responsibility for personnel under direct supervision.
Interpersonal communication—use relationship skills to work effectively on an interdisciplinary team	Organize daily routine in an efficient manner. Function as a participating member of the health care team. Function effectively in problem-solving situations. Apply effective communication skills. Collaborate with other members of the health care team.
Direct care—appropriately use psychomotor and/or technical skills in delivering patient care	Administer medications. Perform activities of daily living (ADL) for assigned patients. Perform major care tasks (e.g., catheterization, Levine tube insertion).
Computer technology—ability to use electronic and technologic equipment to access, retrieve, and store information that assists in the delivery of effective care	Demonstrate computer literacy. Access and retrieve electronic data necessary for patient care. Use information technology to facilitate communication, manage data, and solve patient care problems.
Caseload management—ability to coordinate care of a number of clients	Organize care for a group of 2–10 patients (depending on the nurse's experience and responsibilities, patient needs, and patient acuity)—involves direct care, time management, and resource management.

Source: Utley-Smith (2004).

Nurses, particularly advanced practice nurses (APNs), need to be prepared to function in some type of community-based health care system. They must be able to collaborate and cooperate within a multidisciplinary team and to demonstrate critical thinking and decision-making capabilities. They will be asked to resolve conflicts and effect health care at both the individual and aggregate level. Nurses must also have at least a basic knowledge of several disciplines, including public health, biostatics, and behavioral sciences. In addition, they must possess management and administrative skills. Specific nursing practice competencies needed for today's health care system are shown in Table 23-1.

Theoretical Implications for Nursing Practice
Based on current and anticipated changes, a number of models, concepts, and theories need to be developed and applied in nursing practice and then studied and refined. New models should be based on community-based practice, population focus, case management, and interprofessional and interagency collaboration. Concepts and theories should be developed that focus on cultural competence, resource management, health promotion, risk reduction, motivation, management of chronic diseases, normal aging, maternal–child welfare, and social epidemics, among others.

The concept of EBP has grown dramatically and will help fill the gap among research, theory, and practice (Chinn & Kramer, 2015; Jensen, 2015; McEwen, 2014;

Walker & Avant, 2011). This focus on EBP should assist in the integration of research findings into clinical practice. As discussed in Chapter 12, EBP is relatively new in nursing because many nursing practices are based on experience, tradition, intuition, common sense, and untested theories. Although the encouragement to move to EBP is growing, implementation has been stalled somewhat. This is attributed to the delay in implementation of nursing research findings in practice. More effort will be needed to identify and define "best practices" and to communicate them to both providers and consumers of health care. As the conceptualization of EBP becomes more established within nursing, however, the relationship between EBP and theory must become more explicit. Nursing theorists and scholars should focus attention on melding middle range theory and EBP and turn attention to recognizing the association between EBP and situation-specific or prescriptive theories.

Future Issues and Nursing Research

The new century challenges nursing research with many critical imperatives for improving health care. Health and illness challenges of the 21st century will necessitate reshaping health research as well as health care delivery. Likewise, the changes in the nation's population, its health needs and expectations, and changes in the health care financing will have a dramatic impact on the direction of nursing research. Changes in technology and hospital systems, changes in staffing patterns, and scientific emphasis in areas such as genetics must also be addressed in nursing research. Furthermore, greater emphasis must be placed on reporting nursing research activities and findings to other researchers, clinicians, the media, and the public (National Institute of Nursing Research [NINR], 2016).

During the last three decades, there has been a significant increase in the amount and quality of nursing research. In the last 10 years, research priorities focused on topics such as end-of-life/palliative care, chronic illness experiences (e.g., managing symptoms, avoiding complications of disease and disability, supporting family caregivers, and promoting health behaviors), quality of life, and quality of care. Additional areas of interest related to these themes as well as additional ones have been identified by the NINR (2016) for more focused study in the future (Table 23-2).

Theoretical Implications for Nursing Research

With the identification and promotion of these nursing research priorities, a number of concepts and theories should be studied and further developed over the next decade. These include such phenomena as transitions, quality of life, motivation, changing lifestyle habits, health promotion, symptom management, palliative care, economics of care, caregiver support, disparity, vulnerability, gender differences, informatics, telehealth, genetics, decision making and self-determination, and family interactions.

To improve health care and ultimately promote nursing science, nurses should continue developing and testing middle range and practice theories. They should test conceptual relationships and combine the study of concepts and relationships from various theories. Use of techniques such as meta-analysis and triangulation to synthesize findings will become increasingly important.

Future Issues and Nursing Leadership and Administration

A number of issues and developments will dramatically affect nursing leadership and administration in the future (Box 23-4). Concerns about health care costs affect nursing by determining how work is organized and treatment planned and influencing clients' perception of, and participation in, care. Calls for significant change

Table 23-2 Future Areas for Nursing Research Emphasis

Themes	Examples Targeted for Future Study
Symptom science: Promoting personalized health strategies	Develop, test, and disseminate novel symptom management interventions, including nonpharmacologic interventions to improve health outcomes and quality of life. Determine common biobehavioral, mechanistic pathways that change symptom trajectory from acute to chronic. Determine key interceding points in symptom management that can alter the trajectory of chronic conditions. Demonstrate how biomarkers can be used to understand symptom expression and variability, develop personalized symptom management and prevention strategies, and better manage physical and psychological symptoms in persons with chronic conditions.
Wellness: Promoting health and preventing disease	Integrate scientific advances in precision medicine, mobile health, and "omics" science to develop interventions to promote health and wellness. Determine the complex relationships between physical activity, nutrition, and environment. Prevention, development, and trajectory of communicable and noncommunicable illnesses and acute trauma Develop nurse-led collaborative initiatives focused on innovative and sustainable strategies to prevent chronic conditions across the life span and in underrepresented minority populations. Determine and improve the personal and social pathways that can be translated into health promotion and illness prevention. Employ research approaches to determine the most feasible and effective biobehavioral interventions to reduce or eliminate health disparities.
Self-management: Improving quality of life for individuals with chronic illness	Identify basic mechanisms that influence successful self-management that impacts adherence to treatment or that impacts interventions. Examine effects of interventions integrating environmental factors, caregivers, and health care professionals to promote functional health and well-being. Incorporate personalized decision making, health, disability, and social factors in interventions to maintain health and quality of life. Develop innovative technologies, devices, and biobehavioral interventions to promote health and improve access to health care in those with chronic conditions. Apply data science to validate existing self-management measures to predict intervention outcomes.
End-of-life and palliative care: The science of compassion	Develop strategies to optimize integrated and coordinated care transitions, interventions, and treatments to improve patient-centered outcomes of hospice and palliative care across diverse care settings, populations, and cultural contexts. Determine the theoretical and causal mechanisms that underlie complex issues and choices in end-of-life and palliative care. Develop effective ways to screen, assess, monitor, and treat the needs of individuals at the end of life. Develop, test, and implement personalized, culturally congruent, and evidence-based palliative and hospice interventions. Discover the unique palliative characteristics of advanced symptoms with the goal of developing personalized and targeted interventions to alleviate or manage symptoms.

(continued)

Table 23-2 Future Areas for Nursing Research Emphasis (Continued)

Themes	Examples Targeted for Future Study
Promoting innovation: Technology to improve health	Identify essential components of successful, evidence-based, innovative interventions that are easily tailored to diverse populations across health care settings. Support interprofessional research and develop infrastructures by building partnerships with technical developers to design and test new technologies in various settings. Develop technologies to maximize the use of innovative methodologies that capture community and cultural context to promote positive health behaviors and management of chronic conditions. Explore a wide range of technologic formats that can be used to improve health interventions and support clinical decisions to improve health.
The 21st century nurse scientists: Innovative strategies for research careers	Identify novel and modifiable biologic and behavioral contributors to the psychology of symptom risk, severity, duration, and response to treatment. Improve the understanding of key biologic, environmental, cultural, and other measures to influence wellness. Develop innovative research methods and technologies to address chronic illness trajectory, particularly among those with disparate health outcomes. Identify and develop interventions to assist individuals, families, and health care professionals in managing symptoms of limiting conditions and planning for end-of-life decisions.

Source: NINR (2016).

in health care financing will dramatically change reimbursement mechanisms. With implementation and potential revision of the ACA, there have been increased regulations related to costs, care coordination, and managed care, and states will continue to define, measure, and assess quality and serve as contractors for corporate entities while enforcing accountability of health care providers, insurance companies, and health care organizations.

Focus on cost containment and attention to preventive care will lead to greater levels of interprofessional and collaborative practice. Addressing problems related to the anticipated nursing shortage and the essential need to promote integration of care through systems thinking and collaboration among health teams and changes in practice models to promote autonomy, empowerment, and professional development

Box 23-4   Issues Affecting Nursing Administration and Management in the Future

- Cost of health care
- Challenge of managed care
- Impact of health policy and regulation
- Interdisciplinary education for collaborative practice
- Nursing shortage
- Opportunities for lifelong learning and workforce development
- Significant advances in nursing science and research

Source: Roy (2000).

are particularly important issues facing nursing administrators (Ellis & Hartley, 2012; Huston, 2017; Porter-O'Grady & Malloch, 2016).

In nursing administration, collaboration and care coordination will be increasingly important with enhanced efforts to contain the costs associated with managing complex client needs, particularly within the context of implementation and revision of the ACA. As a result, there should be some degree of interdisciplinary competence in all health professions. This will necessitate corresponding changes in leadership and management priorities that promote unity and collaboration. Competencies needed by future nurse managers include leadership skills, financial/budgeting knowledge, business acumen, communication skills, technology understanding, and human resource and labor relations skills as well as collaboration and team building skills.

Nursing administrators must be able to identify institutional strengths and weaknesses and to assess human resources and environmental issues. Nursing administrators should also focus on maximizing human potential and accountability and work to encourage growth and development of employees. There is a need to use proven motivational techniques to encourage both staff and clients. The challenge is to integrate services in an efficient and effective way to improve care outcomes while managing costs and meeting satisfaction needs.

Theoretical Implications for Nursing Administration and Management

For the future, models of care delivery must be developed that will achieve desired client outcomes and contribute to staff satisfaction, retention, and productivity. Furthermore, these models must contribute to the financial integrity of the organization for which they are developed because there is a need to make the system efficient and cost-effective while ensuring quality care. Data management and processing of information are essential in every area, and administrators must be able to quantify changes in client acuity and to provide exact information about clients.

Models of care should provide greater integration of health services, more intense management of services, an increase in outcome-oriented management, and an increase in ambulatory and community-based health care. There will also be an increased emphasis on bioinformatics and communication skills, and health care financing will continue to be of paramount importance. Concepts to be developed and examined in nursing administration and management include cost, value, competency, utilization, quality measurement, productivity, innovation, integration, civility, safety, and outcomes (Porter-O'Grady & Malloch, 2016; Rutherford, 2008). Quinless and Elliot (2000) recommended that nursing students and administrators learn to apply basic economic theories and concepts and be aware of the costs involved in providing complex health care for the growing population. They also suggested that nurses understand how to balance care and cost and design cost-effective health care delivery. Finally, all nurses should constantly consider the ethical considerations that underlie health services.

Future Issues and Nursing Education

In the past, nursing education supported passive learning using structured, professional instruction and supervised practice. Nursing students have been socialized using mechanistic, rigid standards, where faculty demands that they meet the minimum standards of objective-based learning. To survive in the highly complex, challenging, and rapidly changing health care system, however, it will be increasingly important for nurses to use and apply creative and critical thinking skills. Nursing leaders have recognized that significant changes are needed in nursing education to promote these skills.

Furthermore, issues such as the shortage of nursing faculty, coupled with a serious shortage of nurses educated to teach nursing, the growing acceptance of virtual education and simulation, the increase in nontraditional students, the explosion of accelerated programs, and the widespread acceptance of the doctor of nursing practice (DNP) degree have challenged previous nursing education models and traditions (Billings & Halstead, 2016; Dahnke & Dreher, 2016; IOM, 2011, 2016; Stokowski, 2011).

In recent years, nurse educators have been called to review old assumptions and methods for educating nurses. Because nurses must be able to think critically and independently, content and learning experiences must be revamped to produce graduates with the competencies needed for current and future practice. A nationwide study for nursing education programs (Speziale & Jacobson, 2005) identified several content areas that will need enhanced emphasis now and in the future. These include diversity, informatics, and EBP. Furthermore, nursing educators expect to place greater emphasis in use of distance education, case studies, active learning strategies, concept mapping, computer-assisted instruction, and virtual reality simulations in nursing programs in the future. Other teaching strategies or modalities that will be used increasingly in the future include web-based courses, including massive open online courses (MOOCs), problem-based learning, simulation, concept-based curricula, mentoring, and videoconferencing.

To support these changes, nursing educators need to teach thinking skills as well as content. They should use active learning strategies to foster student responsibility for learning. They may restructure clinical experiences and modify content to place less emphasis on hospital experiences and narrow medical specialty areas to de-emphasize illness care and emphasize wellness care. In addition, nursing students must learn to evaluate the effectiveness of nursing interventions.

Suggestions for curricular changes in future nursing education include increased emphasis on the process and procedure of learning (Benner, Sutphen, Leonard, & Day, 2010; Iwasiw & Goldenberg, 2015; Keating, 2015). Among the recommendations are these: Integrate teaching and learning in classroom and clinical settings more effectively, shift to competency-based curricula, focus on "knowledge management," and promote interprofessional education. Other suggestions to broaden understanding include encouraging the use of group work to promote communication and social skills and increasing use of projects that require months to complete to enhance understanding of the complexity of the real world as well as providing greater diversity in clinical experiences. The Link to Practice 23-1 presents recommendations of the IOM of changes in nursing education to meet current and future health care needs.

Theoretical Implications for Nursing Education

Rather than teach traditional specialties (e.g., maternity nursing, pediatrics, psychiatric nursing), nursing educational programs in the future should stress essential concepts, theories, and models. These should include issues such as aging and care of older adults, aspects of pharmacology, human growth and development, vulnerable populations, genetics, complementary and alternative therapies, environmental health issues, health policy, palliative care, and culture. Models should incorporate high-tech care, EBP, quality, and patient safety. Pathophysiology of chronic illnesses, health promotion, disease prevention, self-care, community health care, decision making, change processes, and management and leadership models should also be part of nursing curricula (AACN, 2008; Benner et al., 2010; IOM, 2011, 2016; Stokowski, 2011).

Curricula should shift from being primarily content-driven and controlled by the faculty to being outcome-driven and focused on the needs of the learner, the profession, and the public. A diversity of theoretical and practice experiences should be encouraged,

Link to Practice 23-1

Recommendations From the Institute of Medicine

Transforming Nursing Education

- Nursing education needs to provide understanding of, and experience in, care management, quality improvement methods, systems change management, and reconceptualized roles of nurses in a reformed health care system.
- Nursing education should serve as a platform for continued lifelong learning and include opportunities for seamless transition to higher degree programs.
- Accrediting, licensing, and certifying organizations need to mandate demonstrated mastery of core skills and competencies to complement the completion of degree programs and written board examinations.
- The nursing student body must become more diverse in response to underrepresentation of racial and ethnic minority groups and men in the nursing workforce.
- Nurses should be educated with physicians and other health professionals as students and throughout their careers.

Transforming Nursing Practice

Among the recommendations from the IOM with regard to practice are the following. Nurses can:

Improve access to primary care—APNs can be utilized to build the primary care workforce as access to coverage, service settings, and services increase under the ACA.

Improve quality of care—Nurses are crucial in preventing medication errors, reducing infection, and facilitating transition from hospital to home.

Create new opportunities for nurses in new and expanded capacities. Suggestions include:

- Accountable care organizations—a group of primary care providers, a hospital, and perhaps some specialists who share the risk and rewards of providing care at a fixed reimbursement rate
- Medical/health homes—a specific type of primary care practice that coordinates and provides comprehensive care; promotes a relationship between patient and provider; and measures, monitors, and improves quality of care
- Community health centers—clinics that provide high-value, quality primary and preventive care in poor and underserved areas
- Nurse-managed health centers—clinics run by nurses and including other professionals such as physicians, social workers, health educators, and outreach workers as part of a collaborative team. Services include primary care, family planning, mental/behavior care, and health promotion.
- Information technology—develop technology to aid providers to plan, deliver, document, and review clinical care

Source: IOM (2011)

and experiences should include involvement in discharge planning, caring for clients in outpatient and ambulatory care settings, assisting families in well-baby clinic visits, and assisting individuals in gaining access to community resources. Furthermore, interprofessional learning and collaborative practice experiences are essential.

Content for nursing education in the future should include leadership development, critical thinking and problem-solving skills, EBP, clinical competency in a variety of settings, collaboration and communication, outcomes focus, cultural competence, and appreciation of research directed toward practice and educational evaluation. Other concepts to be stressed in nursing education programs are safety, teaching and learning, health promotion, illness prevention, lifelong learning, and professional development.

Experiential knowledge and active participation in learning can lead to the development of a knowledge base and a better ability to think critically and independently. Contemporary educational systems must provide opportunities for students to practice and use critical and creative processes within their basic nursing education. Programs should emphasize group and resource management, organizational and leadership skills, clinical management and coordination, technologic capabilities, and professional judgment.

Summary

Increasingly, nurses will be coordinators of teams of care, where they will manage multiskilled workers and share accountability for clinical and financial outcomes. They will need to become adept at care coordination, delegation, interprofessional collaboration, standards setting, and outcomes monitoring across the continuum of care. For the future, it is important that the discipline continue to develop the broad knowledge base of nursing and work to understand the integration of theory, research, and practice. Additionally, the discipline should recognize how this reciprocal arrangement affects nursing practice, administration and management, and education.

Rebecca, the nurse in the opening case study, recognized some of the changes described in this chapter (e.g., increasing cultural diversity, the need to focus on health promotion, communication challenges) and wanted to address them in her practice and research. She also understood that to respond to these changes, she had much to learn about issues in nursing practice, research, administration and management, and education, particularly related to theory and development of nursing science.

Nurses are committed to a holistic view of the person, and as the health profession with the largest number of providers, nursing has the potential to have the greatest impact on health and health care delivery. But to prepare for the future, nurses must more clearly identify and communicate what they do. Ongoing development, application, analysis, and evaluation of concepts, principles, theories, and models are vital to this process; nurses must be encouraged to continue these activities to develop the discipline.

Key Points

- As the health care delivery system changes and evolves in response to changes in demographics, health care needs, and health care financing, the discipline of nursing must respond.
- The IOM's landmark report, *The Future of Nursing*, provides guidelines and recommendations for nursing to meet the health needs of individuals, families, groups, and populations in the future.

- In the future, nursing theory will increasingly focus on development, application, and testing of middle range theories, situation-specific theories, and EBP protocols as the latest steps in knowledge development.
- Nursing practice will be dramatically influenced by changes in the health system subsequent to full implementation of the ACA as well as other system changes. Practice models will increasingly be community-based and population-focused. Interprofessional collaboration will be encouraged. Attention will be on concepts/needs including health promotion, resource management, informatics, and case management.
- Nursing research will focus more on "mixed methods" or combining or triangulating research methods that will more completely and accurately address the complex issues and clients found in contemporary health care. Themes for enhanced research and related theory development include interventions for health promotion, symptom management, end-of-life issues, effective use of technology, and development of future nursing scientists.
- Nursing leadership and administration will need to address such pressing issues as quality and safety, cost management, collaboration, and the need to effectively integrate care. Cultivation of communication skills, leadership skills, technology acumen, and knowledge of human resources and economics are vital.
- Nursing education for the future will incorporate changes in modes of delivery including increasing use of simulation and better, more focused integration of clinical and classroom learning. Competency-based curricula, lifelong learning, and seamless academic progression will all be stressed.
- In the future, nurses must more clearly identify and communicate what they do through development, application, analysis, and evaluation of concepts, principles, theories, and models.

Learning Activities

1. Like Rebecca, the nurse from the opening case study, seek out opportunities to partner with other health care professionals to develop research projects, interventions to improve practice, or joint educational opportunities. Consider what can be done to promote collaboration and overcome barriers to interprofessional care delivery?
2. Talk to a nurse administrator, a nurse educator, a nurse researcher, and an APN (nurse practitioner or clinical nurse specialist) about future issues in nursing and health care delivery. What changes do they anticipate in the next few years? How should currently practicing nurses prepare for future changes?
3. Select a nursing journal that deals primarily with education, research, or administration (e.g., *Journal of Nursing Education, Nursing Research, Journal of Nursing Administration*) and review issues from the past 3 years to analyze trends. What are the "hot topics"? Can any predictions be made for future issues?
4. Select a nursing journal that primarily discusses scholarly issues or topics related to nursing science (e.g., *Advances in Nursing Science, Journal of Nursing Scholarship*) and review issues from the past 3 years to analyze trends. What are the "hot topics"? Can any predictions be made for future issues?
5. Select a nursing specialty journal (e.g., *MCN: The American Journal of Maternal Child Nursing, Pediatric Nursing, Journal of Community Health Nursing*) that is primarily concerned with practice and review issues from the past 3 years to analyze trends. What are the "hot topics"? Can any predictions be made for future issues.

REFERENCES

American Association of Colleges of Nursing. (2006). *The essentials of doctoral education for advanced nursing practice*. Washington, DC: Author. Retrieved from http://www.aacnnursing.org/Portals/42 /Publications/DNPEssentials.pdf

American Association of Colleges of Nursing. (2008). *The essentials of baccalaureate education for professional nursing practice*. Washington, DC: Author. Retrieved from http://www.aacnnursing .org/Portals/42/Publicaations/BaccEssentials08.pdf

American Association of Colleges of Nursing. (2011). *The essentials of master's education in nursing*. Washington, DC: Author. Retrieved from http://www.aacnnursing.org/Portals /42/PublicationsMastersEssentials11.pdf

Bekhet, A., & Zauszniewski, J. (2012). Methodological triangulation: An approach to understanding data. *Nurse Researcher, 20*(2), 40–43.

Benner, P., Sutphen, M., Leonard, V., & Day, L. (2010). *Educating nurses: A call for radical transformation*. San Francisco, CA: Jossey-Bass.

Billings, D. M., & Halstead, J. A. (2016). *Teaching in nursing: A guide for faculty* (5th ed.). St. Louis, MO: Elsevier.

Bodenheimer, T., & Grumbach, K. (2016). *Understanding health policy: A clinical approach* (7th ed.). New York, NY: McGraw-Hill.

Chinn, P. L., & Kramer, M. K. (2015). *Knowledge development in nursing: Theory and process* (9th ed.). St. Louis, MO: Elsevier.

Dahnke, M. D., & Dreher, H. M. (2016). *Philosophy of science for nursing practice: Concepts and applications* (2nd ed.). New York, NY: Springer Publishing.

Ellis, J. R., & Hartley, L. (2012). *Nursing in today's world: Trends, issues & management* (10th ed.). Philadelphia, PA: Lippincott Williams & Wilkins.

Huston, C. J. (2017). *Professional issues in nursing: Challenges and opportunities* (4th ed.). Philadelphia, PA: Wolters Kluwer.

Im, E.-O. (2014). The status quo of situation-specific theories. *Research and Theory for Nursing Practice, 28*(4), 278–298.

Institute of Medicine. (2011). *The future of nursing: Leading change, advancing health*. Washington, DC: National Academies Press.

Institute of Medicine. (2016). *Assessing progress on the Institute of Medicine report: The future of nursing*. Washington, DC: National Academies Press.

Iwasiw, C. L., & Goldenberg, D. (2015). *Curriculum development in nursing education* (3rd ed.). Sudbury, MA: Jones & Bartlett Learning.

Jensen, E. (2015). Linking theory, research, and practice. In N. A. Schmidt & J. M. Brown (Eds.), *Evidence-based practice for nurses: Appraisal and application of research* (3rd ed., pp. 133–149). Burlington, MA: Jones & Bartlett Learning.

Keating, S. B. (2015). *Curriculum development and evaluation in nursing* (3rd ed.). New York, NY: Springer Publishing.

McEwen, M. (2014). Theoretical frameworks for research. In G. LoBiondo-Wood & J. Haber (Eds.), *Nursing research: Methods and critical appraisal for evidence-based practice* (8th ed., pp. 75–91). St. Louis, MO: Elsevier.

McFarland, M. R., & Wehbe-Alamah, H. B. (2015). *Leininger's culture care diversity and universality: A worldwide nursing theory* (3rd ed.). Burlington, MA: Jones & Bartlett Learning.

Meleis, A. I. (2012). *Theoretical nursing: Development and progress* (5th ed.). Philadelphia, PA: Lippincott Williams & Wilkins.

Melnyk, B. M., & Fineout-Overholt, E. (2015). *Evidence-based practice in nursing & healthcare: A guide to best practice* (3rd ed.). Philadelphia, PA: Wolters Kluwer.

National Institute of Nursing Research. (2016). *The NINR strategic plan: Advancing science, improving lives*. Retrieved from https://www.ninr.nih.gov/sites/www.ninr.nih.gov/files /NINR_StratPlan2016_reduced.pdf

Peterson, S. J., & Bredow, T. S. (2017). *Middle range theories: Application to nursing research and practice* (4th ed.). Philadelphia, PA: Wolters Kluwer.

Polit, D. F., & Beck, C. T. (2017). *Nursing research: Generating and assessing evidence for nursing practice* (10th ed.). Philadelphia, PA: Wolters Kluwer.

Porter-O'Grady, T., & Malloch, K. (2015). *Quantum leadership: Building better partnerships for sustainable health* (4th ed.). Burlington, MA: Jones & Bartlett Learning.

Porter-O'Grady, T., & Malloch, K. (2016). *Leadership in nursing practice: Changing the landscape of health care* (2nd ed.). Burlington, MA: Jones & Bartlett Learning.

Quinless, F. W., & Elliot, N. L. (2000). The future in health care delivery: Lessons from history, demographics, and economics. *Nursing and Health Care Perspectives, 21*(2), 84–89.

Risjord, M. (2010). *Nursing knowledge: Science, practice, and philosophy*. Oxford, United Kingdom: Wiley-Blackwell.

Roy, C. (2000). A theorist envisions the future and speaks to nursing administrators. *Nursing Administration Quarterly, 24*(2), 1–12.

Roy, C. (2014). *Generating middle range theory: From evidence to practice*. New York, NY: Springer Publishing.

Rutherford, M. M. (2008). The how, what, and why of valuation and nursing. *Nursing Economics, 26*(6), 347–352.

Smith, M. C., & Liehr, P. R. (2014). Preface. In M. J. Smith & P. R. Liehr (Eds.), *Middle range theory for nursing* (3rd ed., pp. xiii–xvi). New York, NY: Springer Publishing.

Speziale, H. J. S., & Jacobson, L. (2005). Trends in registered nurse education programs 1998–2008. *Nursing Education Perspectives, 26*(4), 230–235.

Stokowski, L. A. (2011). *Overhauling nursing education*. Retrieved from http://www.medscape.com/viewarticle/736236

Utley-Smith, Q. (2004). 5 competencies needed by new baccalaureate graduates. *Nursing Education Perspectives, 25*(4), 166–170.

Walker, L. O., & Avant, K. (2011). *Strategies for theory construction in nursing* (5th ed.). Upper Saddle River, NJ: Pearson Education.

White, K. M., Dudley-Brown, S., & Terhaar, M. F. (2016). *Translation of evidence into nursing and health care* (2nd ed.). New York, NY: Springer Publishing.

Adaptation   The ability of the body to incorporate different ways of working as a result of changes in bodily makeup, chemistry, or the environment.

Agent   In epidemiology, refers to those factors, such as biologic organisms, chemical agents, or physical factors, whose presence or absence can result in disease in the host.

Andragogy   Description of Knowles's theory of adult learning. Knowles believed that the most important thing in helping adults to learn is to create a climate of physical comfort, mutual trust and respect, openness, and acceptance of differences.

Antecedent   That which necessarily goes before; a cause that must precede an effect. For example, the presence of food on the table is antecedent to dinner.

Assumptions   Beliefs about phenomena one must accept as true to accept a theory about the phenomenon as true; they cannot be empirically testable.

Autonomy   Bioethical principle that focuses on respect for persons; that is, the rights of individuals to make informed choices about their health care. It is based on the conviction that the patient or subject is the ultimate authority on what is best for his or her well-being, and health care professionals should *always* provide *all* of the relevant information to the person about his or her health, illness, and treatment options in order to empower him or her to make an informed decision.

Beck's Postpartum Depression Theory   Proposes interventions to alert nurses to the incidence and impact of postpartum depression. The model stresses the importance of identifying new mothers who might be suffering from postpartum depression and suggested interventions.

Behavioral learning theories   Referred to as the Stimulus–Response (S–R) Models of Learning. Some of the major behaviorist theorists include Thorndike (connectionism), Pavlov (classical conditioning), Skinner (operant conditioning), Watson (behaviorism), and Hull (reinforcement).

Behavioral System Model   Dorothy Johnson's human needs–based model.

Belmont Report   Developed following the infamous Tuskegee airmen experiments. The Belmont Report outlined three basic ethical principles—respect for persons, beneficence, and justice (nonmaleficence was added later)—to serve as an analytical framework to guide the resolution of ethical problems arising from research involving human subjects.

Beneficence   Bioethical principle that refers to doing what is in the patient's best interest and involves balancing benefits and burdens.

Benner's Model of Skill Acquisition in Nursing   Patricia Benner's theoretical model, which outlines and explains five stages of skill acquisition in nursing: novice, advanced beginner, competent, proficient, and expert.

Bioethical principles   Set of ethical principles to be used to make decisions in situations involving health and health care delivery. A system of bioethical principles has been proposed consisting of four main ideologies: autonomy, beneficence, nonmaleficence, and justice.

Bioethics   The systematic study of how to provide the best possible care in the health care delivery system by evaluating the impact of biologic and technologic advances on humans and what is permissible.

Change   In a system, a state of flux which can elicit feeling of uncertainty, anxiety, and upheaval.

Chaos Theory   is the study of unstable, aperiodic behavior in deterministic (nonrandom) nonlinear dynamical systems; dynamical refers to the time-varying behavior of a system and aperiodic is the non-repetitive but continuous behavior that results from the effects of any small disturbance.

Cognitive-behavioral theory (Beck)   Behavior theory based on the observation that biased cognitions are faulty; these thoughts are labeled *cognitive distortions*.

Cognitive development theories (interaction theories)   Assume that behavior, mental processes, and the environment are interrelated. Cognitive development theories are concerned with the progressive development and changes in thinking, reasoning, and perception of individual learners. A major assumption of cognitive theories is that learning is experiential and occurs as a sequential process, over time. Major cognitive development theorists include Piaget, Gagne, and Bandura.

Cognitive distortions   Habitual errors in thinking that are formed in the conscious mind. These distorted cognitions create a false basis for beliefs, particularly regarding the self; influence one's basic attitude about the self; and may lead to inaccurate conclusions about the self.

Cognitive-field (Gestalt) theories   View that considers learning to be closely related to perception. In Gestalt theory, learning is seen in terms of reorganization of the learner's perceptual or psychological world—his or her field. The field includes a simultaneous and mutual interaction among all the forces or stimuli affecting the person. Experience is the interaction of a person and his or her perceived environment, whereas behavior is the result of the interplay of these forces. Consequently, perception and experiences of reality are uniquely individual, based on a person's total life experiences. Learning is the process of discovering and understanding the relationships among people, things, and ideas in the field.

Cognitive learning theories   Group of theories that explains that learning relies on the assimilation of facts and information that can be tested by having the person repeat the facts, steps, reasons, and information back to the teacher and act on the knowledge gathered.

Cognitive restructuring   The process of changing cognitive distortions.

Comfort Theory   Katherine Kolcaba's theory, which explains that patients experience needs for comfort in stressful health care situations. These needs are identified by the nurse, who then seeks to implement interventions to meet them.

Complex Adaptive Systems (CAS)   A collection of individual agents (or components within the system) with freedom of behaviors that may not be predictable.

Complexity Science   Application of principles of physics and mathematics to explain the relationship among variables that allow for variation and emergent behaviors that are not fully predictable. Complexity Science focuses on finding the underlying order in the apparent disorder of natural and social systems and understanding how change occurs in nonlinear, dynamical systems over time.

Concept   A word or term that refers to phenomena that occur in nature or thought; formulated in words that enable people to communicate meaning about reality in the world.

Concept analysis   Explores the meaning of concepts to promote understanding.

Concept development   The rigorous process of bringing clarity to the definition of concepts used in science.

Conceptual framework   A set of interrelated concepts that symbolically represents and conveys a mental image of a phenomenon.

Conceptual model   A set of interrelated concepts that symbolically represents and conveys a mental image of a phenomenon.

Conflict theories   Centered on the observation that in human societies, elements of inequality, power/authority, domination/subjugation, interests, and conflict are common. These elements result in "conflicts" that may potentially change the society.

Consequence   The result or outcome of a situation or action.

Conservation Model   Myra Levine's model, which focuses on the interactions of nurse and client and considers multiple factorial interactions to produce predictable results using probability as the reality.

Construct   A complex concept composed of more than one concept and typically built or "constructed" to fit a purpose.

Critical Social Theory   Uses societal awareness to expose social inequalities that keep people from reaching their full potential. Proponents of critical social theory maintain that social exchanges will stimulate the evolution to a more just society.

Cultural bias   Interpreting and judging phenomena in relation to one's own culture (e.g., racism, sexism, classism, and ageism).

Culture Care Diversity and Universality Theory   Madeline Leininger's theory, which recognizes and demonstrates to nurses the importance of considering the impact of culture on health and healing. Major concepts of the model are culture, culture care, and culture care differences (diversities) and similarities (universals) pertaining to transcultural human care.

Curriculum   The content and processes by which learners gain knowledge and understanding; develop skills; and alter attitudes, appreciation, and values under the auspices of a given school or program.

Curriculum conceptual framework   An interrelated system of premises that provides guidelines or ground rules for making all curricular decisions—objectives, content, implementation, and evaluation.

Declaration of Helsinki   A set of rules and requirements for research involving human subjects built on the Nuremberg Code. It includes the need to obtain assent from those not able to consent themselves. It established the standard for submitting research protocols to an independent review board for approval of the research prior to initiation and addresses issues such as the requirement to publish negative benefits and to report sources of funding and declaring potential conflicts of interest.

Deontology   Refers to a system of duty-based laws, with duty implying absolute, nonnegotiable requirements. Immanuel Kant was the main early source for deontology, and he explained that rational beings are obligated to act first and foremost from a sense of duty—irrespective of the consequences.

Descriptive theories   Theories that describe, observe, and name concepts, properties, and dimensions but don't generally explain the interrelationships among the concepts or propositions.

Discipline   Distinctions between bodies of knowledge found in academic settings; a branch of education instruction or a department of learning or knowledge.

Disease causation   A force or factor that contributes to a condition that disturbs the normal functioning of an organism; failure of an organism to respond to or adapt to its environment, leading to a disease state.

Driving forces   In Planned Change Theory, driving forces encourage or facilitate movement to a new direction, goal, or outcome.

Dynamical   In Chaos Theory, it refers to the time-varying behavior of a system.

Dynamical system   In Complexity Science, a system whose state evolves over time according to a rule and initial conditions.

Emotional intelligence (EI)   Refers to the ability to manage one's self and one's relationships effectively. EI includes understanding one's own feelings, sensitivity, and empathy for others and the regulation of emotions.

Empiricism   Philosophical school of thought that values observation, perception by senses, and experience as sources of knowledge. Empiricism is founded on the belief that what is experienced is what exists; these experiences must be verified through scientific methodology.

Empowerment   The transfer or delegation of responsibility and authority from managers to employees; the sharing of power, vision, mission, knowledge, expertise, decision making, and resources necessary for employees to reach organizational goals.

Environment   In grand nursing theory, the external elements that affect the person; internal and external conditions that influence the organism; significant others with whom the person interacts; and an open system with boundaries that permit the exchange of matter, energy, and information with human beings.

Environment/environmental factors   In the epidemiologic triangle, refers to events, physical elements or properties, biologic entities (e.g., animals, plants), or social/economic considerations that may influence whether an individual will develop a disease.

Epidemiologic Triangle   Classic epidemiologic model frequently used to illustrate the interrelationships among the host, agent, and environment with regard to disease causation. A change in any of the three components can result in the disease process.

Epistemology   Study of knowledge or ways of knowing; how people come to have knowledge.

Ethics   A branch of philosophy that involves the systematic study of how one should best live his or her life and treat others; the formal study of morality from a wide range of perspectives.

Evidence   The facts that lead to the belief in the truth about a situation.

Evidence-based nursing   The integration of nursing theory with the best available research evidence as well as the expertise of the nurses, the available resources including professional expertise along with patient-family preferences, and quality improvement findings.

Evidence-based practice   An approach to problem solving that conscientiously uses the current "best" evidence in the care of patients. Evidence-based practice involves identifying a clinical problem, searching the literature, critically evaluating the research evidence, and determining appropriate interventions.

Exchange theories Theories based on utilitarianism, which supports the notation that maximization of each individual's satisfaction automatically leads to maximum satisfaction of the wants of all. In exchange theories, individuals are motivated to maximize material benefits from exchanges with others.

Exemplar An item that is exactly what a concept or idea is about; a true example of the concept.

Exhaustion Final stage of the stress response in Selye's work in which the body has exhausted all its resources and a diseased state can occur.

Explanatory theories Theories that relate concepts to one another and describe and specify associations or interrelations between and among concepts.

Feminist theories Based on the observation that gender differences and subordination have traditionally been viewed as both natural and inevitable. A core assumption in feminist theories is that women are oppressed and that gender is socially constructed and tends to justify the subordination and exploitation of women.

Fight-or-flight response First stage of stress response in Selye's work; alarm reaction that mobilizes the body's defense forces, putting the body in a state of disequilibrium.

Gate Control Theory (GCT) Theory that posits that a gating mechanism occurs in the spinal cord. Pain impulses are transmitted from the periphery of the body by nerve fibers, and the impulses travel to the dorsal horns of the spinal cord, specifically to the area of the cord called the *substantia gelatinosa*. The cells of the *substantia gelatinosa* can inhibit or facilitate pain impulses, and if the activity of the transmission cells is inhibited, the gate is closed and impulses are less likely to be conducted to the brain. The GCT suggests that if pain medication is administered before the onset of pain (i.e., before the gate is opened), it will help keep the gate closed longer and fewer pain impulses will be allowed to pass through.

General Adaptation Syndrome (GAS) Selye's work that explains the physiologic responses to stress in three stages: "fight-or-flight syndrome," resistance, and exhaustion.

General Systems Theory (GST) A "grand" theory that explains that systems are composed of both structural and functional components that interact within a boundary that filters the type and rate of exchange with the environment. Input, throughput, output, and feedback are common to systems. One basic tenet of GST is that systems are composed of subsystems, each with its own function systems. Also, systems contain energy and matter and may be open or closed.

Germ Theory Early theory of disease infection proposed by Louis Pasteur. Pasteur theorized that a specific organism (i.e., a germ) was capable of causing an infectious disease.

Grand theories Theories that are composed of relatively abstract concepts that are not operationally defined and attempt to explain or describe very comprehensive aspects of human experience and response; may incorporate numerous other theories.

Great Man Theory A trait theory that asserts that leaders possess certain characteristics (i.e., physical or personality traits and talents) that nonleaders do not.

Health In grand nursing theory, the ability to function independently; successful adaptation to life's stressors; achievement of one's full life potential; and unity of mind, body, and soul.

Health as Expanding Consciousness Margaret Newman's nursing theory, which posits that persons are identified by pattern and organization and are consciousness rather than merely having consciousness. Health is a pattern of the individual.

Health Belief Model A widely used social psychology theory that explains health behavior in terms of several constructs: perceived susceptibility of the health problem, perceived severity, perceived benefits, perceived barriers, self-efficacy, and cues to action.

Health literacy Describes how well an individual can read, interpret, and comprehend health information for maintaining an optimal level of wellness.

Health Promotion Model Nola Pender's framework for integrating nursing and behavioral science perspectives on factors that influence health behaviors. The model may be used as a guide to explore the biopsychosocial processes that motivate individuals to engage in behaviors directed toward health.

Homeodynamics   The idea that health is achieved through continuous interaction of human and environmental energy systems.

Host/host factors   In the epidemiologic triangle, refers to factors (e.g., age, gender, race/ethnicity, marital status, economic status, state of immunity, lifestyle factors) that may influence whether an individual develops a disease.

Humanbecoming Paradigm   Rosemary Parse's theory, which states that humanbecoming is a separate paradigm of nursing in which nurses guide patients in choosing the possibilities in changing health process through intersubjective processes.

Human Caring Science   Jean Watson's theory of nursing that incorporates spiritual dimensions of nursing with the ideals of the unitary process theories but reflects the interactive processes of nursing.

Human needs theory   Maslow's description of the hierarchy of dynamic processes that are critical for human development and growth. There are six incremental stages: physiologic needs, safety needs, love and belonging needs, self-esteem needs, self-actualizing needs, and self-transcendent needs. The goal of Maslow's theory is to attain the sixth level or stage: self-transcendent needs. Motivation is the key to Maslow's theory because individuals are seen as striving for self-actualization.

Human science   The study of human life by valuing the lived experience of persons and seeking to understand life in its matrix of patterns of meaning and values. Knowledge is created to provide understanding and interpretation of phenomena.

Immune system   Refers to a complex, coordinated group of systems that produces physiologic responses to injury or infection. The purpose of the immune system is to neutralize, eliminate, or destroy microorganisms that invade the body. Extensive interactions affect the manufacture of products that alter the structure and function of cells.

Immunity   State or process of being immune to a disease state; involves specific recognition of what is designated as an antigen, memory for particular antigens, and responsiveness on reexposure.

Implied theory   Refers to those theories used by practicing nurses during routine client care without conscious consideration.

Informed consent   Concept is derived from the principle of autonomy. To obtain informed consent, patients and potential research subjects should receive information on the risks and benefits of treatment or research. This information needs to include not only the risks and benefits of the potential treatments, interventions, or trials but also all available reasonable alternatives. Additionally, to give consent, the person needs to be able to comprehend the information, the information should be presented in a format and with language that the receiver can understand, and the choice needs to be voluntary—free of coercion or undue influence.

Intention   Main determinant in the Theory of Reasoned Action/Theory of Planned Behavior; the cognitive representation of the individual's readiness to perform a behavior and is determined by attitude, subjective norms, and perceived behavioral control.

Interpersonal theory   Sullivan's developmental theory based on the premise that an individual cannot exist apart from his or her relationships with other people. Development is dependent on interpersonal situations which continue throughout the person's life. The sequence of interpersonal events to which a person is exposed from infancy to adulthood and ways in which these situations occur contribute to the individual's development.

Intersystem Model   Barbara Artinian's model explaining the interactions between patient and nurse systems. These become more complex when the interaction is between and among community systems and health care systems.

Justice   Bioethical principle that focuses on fairness in both treatment and research. Justice obligates health care professionals to provide necessary treatment for all members of society.

Knowledge   The awareness or perception of reality acquired through insight, learning, or investigation. In a discipline, knowledge is what is collectively seen to be a reasonably accurate understanding of the world perceived by members of the discipline.

Learning   A relatively permanent change in behavior that results from experience. Learning occurs as individuals interact with their environment, incorporating new information into what they already know.

Learning styles   The many ways a person may learn including preferences for learning formats. Some people learn best by reading, some by being told, others by being shown; many learners need a motor component to the learning, and others prefer computer learning methods.

Maternal Role Attainment/Becoming a Mother Ramona Mercer's work on identification of the factors that influence the development and evolution of relationships between key maternal and infant variables that determine maternal role attainment.

Metatheory A theory about theory; focuses on broad issues such as the processes of generating knowledge and theory development.

Methodology The means of acquiring knowledge.

Middle range theories Theories that are substantively specific and encompass a limited number of concepts and a limited aspect of the real world.

Model A graphic or symbolic representation of phenomena or reality. Models objectify and present certain perspectives or points of view about nature or function or both.

Modeling and Role-Modeling (MRM) Theory A deductive theory developed by Erickson, Tomlin, and Swain that focuses on the interpersonal interactions between nurse and client.

Morality An accepted set of cultural beliefs about what is right and wrong, involving personal values, character, or conduct of individuals or groups.

Motivation–Hygiene Theory (Herzberg's Two-Factor Theory) Explains differences between factors that are true motivators for individuals (i.e., recognition for a job well done, opportunities for promotion or advancement, challenging and rewarding work) and hygiene or maintenance factors (e.g., salary, quality of supervision, interpersonal relationships with co-workers, and good working conditions).

Natural History of Disease Model A model that explains the progression of a disease process in an individual over time using two stages: prepathogenesis and pathogenesis. The model also describes the three levels of prevention—primary prevention, secondary prevention, and tertiary prevention.

Neuman Systems Model Betty Neuman's systems-based approach focused on human needs and relief from stress in the nursing care of vulnerable patients.

Nonlinear dynamics Application of mathematics (nonlinear algebra) to examine patterns of a system over time.

Nonmaleficence Bioethical principle that relates to the Hippocratic principle of "first, do no harm." Health care professionals have an obligation to avoid causing bodily harm and death to patients and to minimize pain and suffering.

Nuremberg Code Developed in the years following World War II to describe the basic principles of ethical human experimentation. The Nuremberg Code was widely praised and rapidly accepted as the guideline for research using human subjects.

Nursing In grand nursing theory, a science, an art, and a practice discipline that involves caring. Goals of nursing include caring for the well, caring for the sick, assisting with self-care activities, helping individuals attain their human potential, and discovering and using nature's laws of health. The purposes of nursing care include placing the client in the best condition for nature to restore health, promoting the adaptation of the individual, facilitating the development of an interaction between the nurse and the client in which jointly set goals are met, and promoting harmony between the individual and the environment.

Nursing metaparadigm A worldview or global perspective of the discipline. Nursing's metaparadigm is generally thought to consist of the concepts of person, environment, health, and nursing.

Nursing philosophy The belief system of the profession; provides perspective for nursing practice, scholarship, and research.

Nursing research A scientific process that validates and refines existing knowledge and generates new knowledge that directly and indirectly influences nursing practice. Nursing research is concerned with the study of individuals in interaction with their environments and with discovering interventions that promote optimal functioning and wellness across the life span.

Nursing science The substantive, discipline-specific knowledge that focuses on the human-universe-health process articulated in nursing frameworks and theories. The system of relationships of human responses in health and illness addressing biologic, behavioral, social, and cultural domains.

Nursing: What it is and what it is not Florence Nightingale's organized definition of professional nursing. Nightingale's work served as the basis for modern nursing by focusing on the needs of vulnerable patients for nursing care.

Ontology The study of being; what is or what exists; nature of reality.

Operant Conditioning B. F. Skinner's term for the manipulation of selected reinforcers. According to Skinner, an individual performs a behavior (discharges an operant) and receives a consequence (reinforcer) as a result of performing the behavior. The consequence is either positive or negative, and the consequence will most likely determine whether the behavior will be repeated.

Operational definition The actual measurement of a concept, term, or phenomenon for a research study.

Paradigm A worldview or overall way of looking at a discipline and its science. It is an organizing framework that contains concepts, theories, assumptions, beliefs, values, and principles that form the way a discipline interprets the subject matter with which it is concerned. Paradigm shift occurs when the traditional theories no longer describe the world as newer information has been learned.

Parsimony That which is as constrained as possible so that only those elements that are needed are included.

Path–Goal Theory An expectancy theory in which situational factors (i.e., nature and scope of the task, the employee's perceptions and expectations, and the role of the leader) are examined. The leader is responsible for helping the employee determine and clarify the path the worker is to take to reach the goal and to provide motivation and reward. The leaders also must identify and remove obstacles from the path of the worker to enable him or her to successfully attain the goal.

Pathogenesis Second stage of the Natural History of Disease Model. After exposure or interaction, the stage moves from early pathogenesis to the disease course to resolution—either death, disability, or recovery.

Patient-Centered Approaches to Nursing Abdellah's grand theory based on the human needs of patients and focused on education and practice of nursing care of the patients with illness at home or hospital.

Person In grand nursing theory, a being composed of physical, intellectual, biochemical, and psychosocial needs; a human energy field; a holistic being in the world; an open system; an integrated whole; an adaptive system; and a being who is greater than the sum of his parts.

Phenomenology The study of phenomena; emphasizes the appearance of things as opposed to the things themselves. In phenomenology, understanding is the goal of science, and it recognizes the connection between one's experience, values, and perspectives.

Phenomenon That which may be sensed or not but which exists in the real world.

Philosophy A study of problems that are ultimate, abstract, and general. These problems are concerned with the nature of existence, knowledge, morality, reason, and human purpose. A statement of beliefs and values about human beings and the world.

Planned change theory Lewin's theory describing change process that occurs by design (rather than spontaneously or by chance). There are two forces involved in change: *driving forces* and *restraining forces*. Change is a move from the status quo that results in a disruption in the balance of forces or disequilibrium between opposing forces and often leads to feelings of uneasiness, uncertainty, and loss of control. In planned change, driving forces should be identified and accentuated, and restraining forces should be identified and minimized to achieve the desired outcome or change. Effective change is the return to equilibrium as a result of balancing opposing forces. Three phases must occur if planned change is to be successful: unfreezing the status quo, moving to a new state, and refreezing the change to make it permanent.

Positivism A term often equated with empiricism. Positivism supports mechanistic, reductionist principles where the complex can best be understood in terms of its basic components.

Postmodern theory A philosophical reaction to the underlying assumptions and universalizing tendency of the doctrine of positivism and scientific objectivity characterized by "modernity."

Power The influence wielded by an individual or group of individuals to change behaviors and attitudes and to sway decisions; implies a dependency relationship.

Practice (or applied) science A science that uses the knowledge of basic science for a practical end. Research is largely clinical and action-oriented.

Practice-based evidence Evidence from large practice databases that include findings not only from research studies but also from benchmarking data, clinical expertise, data from cost-effectiveness and quality improvement studies, infection control, medical re-cords, and national standards of care as well as patient and family preferences.

Predictive theories   Theories that describe precise relationships between concepts; are able to describe future outcomes consistently and include statement of causal or consequential relatedness.

Prepathogenesis   First stage of the Natural History of Disease Model occurring prior to interaction of the disease agent and human host when the individual is susceptible.

Prescriptive theories   Theories that prescribe activities necessary to reach defined goals. In nursing, prescriptive theories address nursing therapeutics and predicate the consequence of interventions.

Problem-based learning (PBL)   The use of pre-defined clinical situations and case studies to enhance or stimulate students to acquire specific skills, knowledge, and abilities. PBL allows the instructor to manipulate multiple variables to add increasingly complex issues or circumstances that must be considered in problem resolution.

Profession   A learned vocation or occupation that has a status of superiority and precedence within a division of work.

Psychic energy   Term used by Freud to explain how the human as an energy system is composed of instincts, whereby instincts are the sole energy source for human behavior.

Psychoanalytic Theory   Theory developed by Freud in which behavior is the product of an interaction among the three major systems of the personality: the id, ego, and superego.

Psychodynamic theories   Theories that attempt to explain the multidimensional nature of behavior and understand how an individual's personality and behavior interface; also provide a systematic way of identifying and understanding behavior.

Psychosocial Developmental Theory   Erikson's theory, which describes eight stages of a person's life that are formed by social influences that interact with the physical/psychological, maturing organism. The first four stages occur in infancy and child-hood, the fifth stage occurs in adolescence, and the last three stages occur during the adult years. Erikson believed that each stage of development builds on the next, thus contributing to the formation of the total person.

Quality improvement (QI)   The commitment and approach used to scrupulously examine and continuously improve every process in every part of an organization. The ultimate intent of QI is meeting and exceeding customer expectations.

Randomized, controlled clinical trials   Research studies in which an intervention is tested against another intervention. The interventions are randomly assigned to the subjects who are in the study to form at the minimum two groups: a research group and a control group. The data are collected and statistically analyzed to indicate the results of the research.

Rational Emotive Theory   Ellis's theory, which describes the interconnectedness between thoughts, feelings, and actions. The underlying premise is that an individual has the cognitive ability to think, decide, analyze, and do and that the individual thinks either rationally or irrationally. The repetition of irrational thoughts reinforces dysfunctional beliefs, which, in turn, produce dysfunctional behaviors. These dysfunctional beliefs lead to self-defeating behaviors. Ellis posited that if behaviors are learned, they can be unlearned.

Research   The systematic inquiry that uses disciplined methods to answer questions or solve problems. Research is conducted to describe, explain, or predict variables, and in a practice discipline such as nursing, research is assumed to contribute to the improvement of care.

Resistance   The second stage of the stress response in Selye's work; the body's physiologic responses to regain homeostasis.

Restraining forces   In the planned change theory, restraining forces block or impede progress toward a goal.

Role theory   A theory that contends that normative expectations and requirements, such as culturally defined behavioral rules, are attached to positions (status) in social organizations (e.g., family, corporation, society). Roles can be assumed to carry rights and privileges as well as duties and obligations.

Roy Adaptation Model (RAM)   Callista Roy's model, which focuses on assisting the client to adapt to and overcome the stresses of illness and environmental factors.

Science A way of explaining observed phenomena as well as a system of gathering, verifying, and systemizing information about reality (i.e., it is both a process and a product).

Science of Unitary and Irreducible Human Beings Martha Rogers's theory synthesized from theories of the sciences to incorporate the proposition that the human is an open system embedded in larger open systems; living systems are pattern and organization; and man is sentient, capable of awareness, feeling, and choosing.

Self-actualization In humanistic theories (e.g., Maslow), refers to the process of developing human potential and talents.

Self-Care Deficit Nursing Theory (SCDNT) Dorothea Orem's work, consisting of three nested theories: the theories of self-care, self-care deficit, and nursing systems. This needs-based theory seeks to provide for as many contingencies as possible in the care of the patient, ill or well.

Self-transcendence In Reed's theory, a characteristic of developmental maturity in which there is an expansion of self-boundaries and orientation toward broadened life perspectives and purposes.

Shared (or borrowed) theory Theories that arise or are derived from other disciplines but are applied in nursing situations.

Simultaneity Conceptualization in which humans and environment including the universe are in constant interaction all at the same time.

Simultaneity paradigm Parse's depiction of a group of theories based on the science of unitary and irreducible human beings and meaning that the paradoxes of living go on all at once, continuously. The human is a system embedded in the universal energy system and enters into all that is taking place, in some way, at all times.

Situation-specific theories (practice theories) Theories that are specific, narrow in scope, contain few concepts, and are easily defined. They tend to be prescriptive.

Social-Ecological Models (SEMs) Contemporary applications of the bio-psycho-social perspective to examine the patient/family experience of health or illness within the social ecological context. The SEMs have been used in various forms for several decades to examine the complex interplay among individuals, social groups, and other entities which influence health-related behaviors.

Stress, coping, and adaptation theory Lazarus and Folkman's explanation of the psychological responses that occur as a person copes with stressful situations. Successful coping results in adaptation, which is the capacity of a person to survive and flourish.

Symbolic interactionism A sociologic paradigm that synthesizes the concepts of self, mind, and society. In this viewpoint, humans adapt to and survive in their environment by sharing common symbols, both verbal and nonverbal. Within symbolic interactions, humans can imagine themselves in social roles and internalize the attitudes, values, and norms of a social group.

Synergy Model A model that describes nurses' contributions, activities, and outcomes with regard to caring for critically ill patients. The model identifies eight patient needs or characteristics and eight competencies of nurses in critical care situations. When patient characteristics and nurse competencies match and synergize, outcomes for the patient are optimal.

Teaching The intentional act of communicating information; may be defined as the facilitation of learning.

The Future of Nursing A publication from the Institute of Medicine (IOM), which has been viewed as a challenge and strategy to (1) make quality health care accessible to the diverse populations of the United States, (2) intentionally promote wellness and disease prevention, (3) improve health outcomes, and (4) provide compassionate care across the life span.

Theoretical framework A set of interrelated concepts that symbolically represents and conveys a mental image of a phenomenon.

Theory A systematic explanation of an event in which constructs and concepts are identified and relationships are proposed and predications made; a set of interpretive assumptions, principles, or propositions that help explain or guide action.

Theory-based nursing practice Application of various models, theories, and principles from nursing science and the biologic, behavioral, medical, and sociocultural disciplines to clinical nursing practice.

Theory evaluation (or theory analysis)   The process of systematically examining a theory and ascertaining how well the theory serves its purpose; results in a decision or action about the use of the theory.

Theory of Chronic Sorrow   A theory that initially described grief observed in the parents of children with mental deficiencies; expanded to include individuals who experience a variety of loss situations and to their family caregivers.

Theory of Goal Attainment and Transactional Process   Imogene King's nursing framework, which focuses on the transactions between nurse and client to attain the goals of the nurse–patient relationship.

Theory of Reasoned Action/Theory of Planned Behavior   A theory that explains the relationship among beliefs, attitudes, intentions, and behavior. According to the theory, the most important determinant of a person's behavior(s) is intention.

Theory of Self-Transcendence   Pamela Reed's explanation of the expansion of self-boundaries and orientation toward broadened life perspectives and purpose in which the individual moves beyond the immediate or constricted view of self and the world. The theory can be used by nurses to develop interventions to attend to spiritual and psychosocial expressions of self-transcendence in clients who are confronted with end-of-life issues.

Theory of Unpleasant Symptoms   A theory that seeks to improve understanding of the symptom experience in various contexts and to provide information useful for designing effective means to prevent, ameliorate, or manage unpleasant symptoms and their negative effects.

Theory–practice gap   The notion that there is a "gap" between theory and practice; a common perception among nurses because nurses in clinical practice rarely use the language of nursing theory, nursing diagnosis, or the nursing process.

Totality paradigm   The paradigm in which the person and the world are known by the sum of their parts and the workings thereof.

Transactional leader   A leader who is viewed as the traditional manager; one who is concerned with day-to-day operations.

Transformational leader   A leader who is a long-term visionary able to inspire and empower others with his or her vision.

Transitions Theory   Afaf Meleis's theory, which describes the interactions between nurses and patients, explaining how nurses are concerned with the experiences of people as they undergo transitions, whenever health and well-being are the desired outcome. The goal of nursing is to address the potential problems that individuals encounter during transitional experiences and develop preventative and therapeutic interventions to support the patient during these occasions.

Transtheoretical Model (TTM) and Stages of Change   A theory that describes how behavior change unfolds through a series of stages; each stage involves different change processes. At its core, the TTM focus on the six "Stages of Change" which are not necessarily linear; rather, change is seen as fluid or dynamic and occurs through the unfolding of the processes over a period of time.

Uncertainty in Illness Theory   Merle Mishel's theory describing how individuals process illness-related stimuli and structure meaning for those events. Adaptation is the desirable end state achieved after coping with the uncertainty. Nurses may develop interventions to influence the person's cognitive process to address the uncertainty, which should produce positive coping and adaptation.

Unitary   Concept in which all things are part of a universal energy system and in constant and changing interaction.

Utilitarianism   Philosophical perspective that is exemplified by choosing actions that maximize the pleasure and happiness and minimize the pain and suffering the choices may cause. Utilitarianism supports "the greatest good for the greatest number of people."

Variable   A phenomenon that has properties that can differ or change based on circumstances; anything that varies.

Virtue Ethics (or Virtue Theory)   Term used to describe Aristotle's views on ethics, focusing on character traits one needs in order to have good judgment, or a habit of character that predisposes one to do what is right.

Web of Causation (Chain of Causation)   A disease model used to explain chronic diseases or disability not attributable to one or two factors or causative agents; rather, they result from the interaction of multiple factors.

Worldview   The philosophical frame of reference used by a social or cultural group to describe that group's outlook on and beliefs about reality.

AUTHOR INDEX

Note: Page numbers followed by b indicate material in boxes; those followed by f indicate material in figures, and those followed by t indicate material in tables.

SUBJECT INDEX

Note: Page numbers followed by b indicate material in boxes; those followed by f indicate material in figures, and those followed by t indicate material in tables.

A

AACN. *See* American Association of Colleges of Nursing; American Association of Critical-Care Nurses
Abortion, ethics of, 363
Abstract concepts, 50–52
Abstraction level, of relational statements, 80
Abstraction level, of theories, 34–38, 37f, 73–75, 75f
  in categorization of grand theories, 118–119
  in middle range theories, 211, 224
  in theory evaluation, 97
ACA. *See* Patient Protection and Affordable Care Act
Academic Center for Evidence-Based Practice (ACE) Star Model, 261–263, 262b, 262f, 269t
Academic discipline. *See* Discipline(s)
Acceptance, of theory, 103
Accessibility, of theory, 101
Accommodation
  in conflict handling, 397
  in learning, 418
Accountability
  in patient care delivery models, 483
  in shared governance, 480–482
Accountable care organizations (ACOs), 492–493, 531
Accreditation, nursing curriculum and, 503–504
Accreditation Commission for Education in Nursing (ACEN), 504
Accuracy, of theory, 103, 105t, 106
ACEN. *See* Accreditation Commission for Education in Nursing
ACE Star Model, of evidence-based practice, 261–263, 262b, 262f, 269t
Achievement, need for, 389, 389t
Achievement–Motivation Theory, 389, 389t
Achievement-oriented leader, 384
Achievement system, 148
ACOs. *See* Accountable care organizations
Action Research, 289–290
Action stage, of change, 323, 323f
Active potential assessment model (APAM), 166
Activities for client assistance, 137–138, 138b
Actual caring moment occasion, 180t, 207
Actualizing tendency, 313
Acupuncture, prescriptive theory of, 40

Acute pain management, theories of, 211, 217, 244t
Adaptation
  in Artinian Intersystem Model, 162
  of borrowed or shared theories, 78. *See also* Borrowed theory
  in Complex Adaptive Systems, 294–295
  in Modeling and Role-Modeling, 166, 167t
  in Roy Adaptation Model, 172–177, 174t. *See also* Roy Adaptation Model
  in stress theories, 315–317, 341–342
  in systems, 276
  in Uncertainty in Illness Theory, 237
Adaptation to Chronic Pain, Theory of, 215, 244t
Adaptive equilibrium, 166
Adaptive modes, in Roy Adaptation Model, 175–176, 175f
Adaptive Spirituality, Theory of, 85–86, 176, 213, 456t
Administration and management. *See also* Management
  application of theory in, 475–500
  borrowed theory from, 78, 78t
  future issues in, 526–529, 528b
Administrative model, of shared governance, 481
Adulthood, transition to, 443t
Adult Learning Theory, 412, 423–425, 426t
  application to nursing, 425
  application to nursing education, 513–514
  assumptions of, 423–424, 424b
Adult Uncertainty in Illness Scale, 237
Adult Uncertainty in Illness Scale–Community Form, 237
Advanced practice nurses (APNs), 32
  in accountability care organizations, 493
  administrative or management role of, 376–377
  authority and responsibility of, 479
  case management by, 489
  chain of command, 477
  in community-based health care systems, 525
  disease management role of, 492
  in evidence-based practice, 405, 496
  learning theory and, 412, 412b
  management level of, 479
  theoretical knowledge and skills of, 523, 523b
  work specialization of, 477

Advances in Nursing Science, 453
Advancing Research and Clinical Practice Through Close Collaboration (ARCC) Model, 261, 263, 264b, 269t
Affective learning, 411
Affiliated-individuation, 167t
Affiliation, need for, 389, 389t
Affiliative subsystem, 148
Affordable Care Act. *See* Patient Protection and Affordable Care Act
"Against medical advice" (AMA), 367
Ageism, 282
Agency, concept of, 287–288, 288t
Agency for Healthcare Research and Quality, 255, 257
Agenda for Change (The Joint Commission), 398
Agents, in Complex Adaptive Systems, 294
Aggressive subsystem, 148
Aging, successful, theories of, 214, 236t, 446–447
Aging population, 520b
AIM. *See* Artinian Intersystem Model
Aim of instinct, 304
Alarm, as stage of stress, 315, 316t, 341, 342t
Allostasis, 340–341
Allostatic Load Theory, 343
Alzheimer disease, information processing in, 423
AMA. *See* American Medical Association
AMA ("against medical advice"), 367
American Academy of Nursing, 488
American Association of Colleges of Nursing (AACN)
  on Chaos Theory and Complexity Science, 293b
  Commission on Collegiate Nursing Education (CCNE), 504, 505
  on competencies and skills needed by generalist nurses, 521, 521b
  on concept application, 50b
  doctor of nursing practice proposed, 32
  on evidence-based practice, 255b
  on genetics, 345b
  on learning theories, 412b
  on middle range theory, 224b
  on scientific foundation of nursing, 5b
  on theoretical knowledge and skills, 523, 523b
American Association of Critical-Care Nurses (AACN), Synergy Model of, 95, 233–234. *See also* Synergy Model